SISKIYOU COUNTY LIBRARY

3 2871 00467115 8

D0702156

DATE DUE

CDC
YELLOW BOOK 2018
Health Information for
International Travel

OFFICIALLY
DISCARDED

SISKIYOU COUNTY PUBLIC LIBRARY
719 FOURTH STREET
YREKA, CALIFORNIA 96097

Wishing you safe travels
and a healthy return!

SISKIYOU COUNTY PUBLIC HEALTH

SISKIYOU COUNTY PUBLIC HEALTH

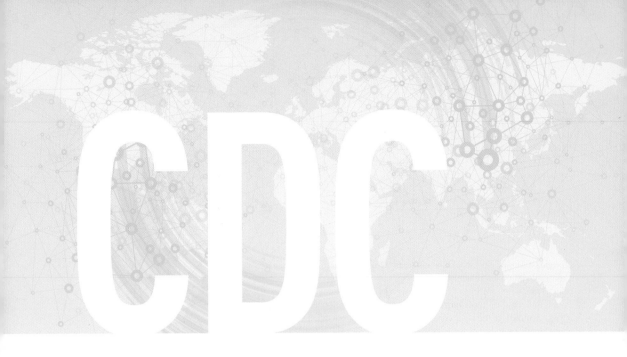

YELLOW BOOK 2018

Health Information for International Travel

Editor in Chief Gary W. Brunette, MD, MS

CHIEF MEDICAL EDITOR
Phyllis E. Kozarsky, MD

MEDICAL EDITORS
Clive M. Brown, MBBS, DTM&H
Nicole J. Cohen, MD, MS
Douglas H. Esposito, MD, MPH
Mark D. Gershman, MD
Stephen M. Ostroff, MD
Edward T. Ryan, MD
David R. Shlim, MD
Richard W. Steketee, MD, MPH
Michelle Weinberg, MD, MPH
Mary Elizabeth Wilson, MD

MANAGING EDITOR
Megan Crawley O'Sullivan, MPH

TECHNICAL EDITOR
Ronnie Henry

US DEPARTMENT OF HEALTH AND
HUMAN SERVICES

PUBLIC HEALTH SERVICE

CENTERS FOR DISEASE CONTROL AND
PREVENTION

NATIONAL CENTER FOR EMERGING AND
ZOONOTIC INFECTIOUS DISEASES

DIVISION OF GLOBAL MIGRATION AND
QUARANTINE

ATLANTA, GEORGIA

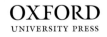

Oxford University Press is a department of the University of Oxford. It furthers
the University's objective of excellence in research, scholarship, and education
by publishing worldwide. Oxford is a registered trade mark of Oxford University
Press in the UK and certain other countries.

Published in the United States of America by Oxford University Press
198 Madison Avenue, New York, NY 10016, United States of America.

© Oxford University Press 2017

All rights reserved. No part of this publication may be reproduced, stored in
a retrieval system, or transmitted, in any form or by any means, without the
prior permission in writing of Oxford University Press, or as expressly permitted
by law, by license, or under terms agreed with the appropriate reproduction
rights organization. Inquiries concerning reproduction outside the scope of the
above should be sent to the Rights Department, Oxford University Press, at the
address above.

You must not circulate this work in any other form
and you must impose this same condition on any acquirer.

ISSN 0095–3539
ISBN 978–0–19–062861–1

9 8 7 6 5 4 3 2 1
Paperback printed by LSC Communications, United States of America

Oxford University Press is proud to pay a portion of its sales for this book to the CDC
Foundation. Chartered by Congress, the CDC Foundation began operations in 1995
as an independent, nonprofit organization fostering support for CDC through public-
private partnerships. Further information about the CDC Foundation can be found at
www.cdcfoundation.org. The CDC Foundation did not prepare any portion of this
book and is not responsible for its contents.

All CDC material in this publication is in the public domain and may be used and reprinted without special permission; however, citation of the source is appreciated.

Suggested Citation

Centers for Disease Control and Prevention. CDC Yellow Book 2018: Health Information for International Travel. New York: Oxford University Press; 2017.

Readers are invited to send comments and suggestions regarding this publication to Gary W. Brunette, Editor in Chief, Centers for Disease Control and Prevention, Division of Global Migration and Quarantine (E-03), Travelers' Health Branch (proposed), 1600 Clifton Road NE, Atlanta, GA 30333, USA.

Disclaimers

Both generic and trade names (without trademark symbols) are used in this text. In all cases, the decision to use one or the other was made based on recognition factors and was done for the convenience of the intended audience. Therefore, the use of trade names and commercial sources in this publication is for identification only and does not imply endorsement by the US Department of Health and Human Services, the Public Health Service, or CDC.

References to non-CDC Internet sites are provided as a service to readers and do not constitute or imply endorsement of these organizations or their programs by the US Department of Health and Human Services, the Public Health Service, or CDC. CDC is not responsible for the content of these sites. URL addresses were current as of the date of publication.

Notice

This material is not intended to be, and should not be considered, a substitute for medical or other professional advice. Treatment for the conditions described in this material is highly dependent on the individual circumstances. While this material is designed to offer accurate information with respect to the subject matter covered and to be current as of the time it was written, research and knowledge about medical and health issues are constantly evolving, and dose schedules for medications and vaccines are being revised continually, with new side effects recognized and accounted for regularly. Readers must, therefore, always check the product information and clinical procedures with the most up-to-date published product information and data sheets provided by the manufacturers and the most recent codes of conduct and safety regulation. Oxford University Press and the authors make no representations or warranties to readers, express or implied, as to the accuracy or completeness of this material, including without limitation that they make no representations or warranties as to the accuracy or efficacy of the drug dosages mentioned in the material. The authors and the publishers do not accept, and expressly disclaim, any responsibility for any liability, loss, or risk that may be claimed or incurred as a consequence of the use and/or application of any of the contents of this material.

The Publisher is responsible for author selection and the Publisher and the Author(s) make all editorial decisions, including decisions regarding content. The Publisher and the Author(s) are not responsible for any product information added to this publication by companies purchasing copies of it for distribution to clinicians.

For additional copies, please contact Oxford University Press. Order online at www.oup.com/us.

cont

1 Introduction   *1*

2 The Pretravel Consultation   *16*

3 Infectious Diseases Related to Travel   *139*

Select Destinations   *425*

List of Boxes, Figures, Maps, & Tables, by Topic

Zika

RESOURCES
General Resources

Insect Avoidance

Pretravel Consultation

Water Treatment

SPECIAL POPULATIONS

Cruise Ship Passengers

Health Care Workers

Immigrants and Migrants

Immunocompromised

Infants and Children

Long-Term Travelers

Medical Tourists

Military

List of Maps

DESTINATION AND REFERENCE MAPS

Editorial Staff

Editor in Chief: Gary W. Brunette

Chief Medical Editor: Phyllis E. Kozarsky

Medical Editors: Clive M. Brown, Nicole J. Cohen, Douglas H. Esposito, Mark D. Gershman, Stephen M. Ostroff, Edward T. Ryan, David R. Shlim, Richard W. Steketee, Michelle Weinberg, and Mary Elizabeth Wilson

Managing Editor: Megan Crawley O'Sullivan

Technical Editor: Ronnie Henry

Design and Production Editor: Kelly Holton

Editorial Assistant: Kelly Winter

Cartographer: R. Ryan Lash

Assistant Cartographer: C. Virginia Lee

CDC Contributors

Abanyie, Francisca

Abe, Karon

Alexander, James P.

Ansari, Armin

Appiah, Grace

Arboleda, Nelson

Arguin, Paul M.

Armstrong, Paige

Averhoff, Francisco

Baggett, Henry C.

Bair-Brake, Heather

Ballesteros, Michael F.

Barbre, Kira A.

Beavers, Suzanne

Beckman, Michele G.

Benenson, Gabrielle A.

Berro, Andre

Blaney, David D.

Bowen, Anna

Bresee, Joseph

Brogdon, William G.

Brooks, John T.

Brown, Clive M.

Brunette, Gary W.

Burdette, Erin

Burke, Heather

Cantey, Paul T.

Cardemil, Cristina V.

Chen, Tai-Ho

Chiller, Tom M.

Choi, Mary

Chosewood, Casey

Clemmons, Nakia S.

Cochi, Stephen L.

Cohen, Nicole J.

Cope, Jennifer

Czarkowski, Alan G.

Dhara, V. Ramana

Dubray, Christine

Duong, Krista Kornylo

Ederer, David J.

Erskine, Stefanie K.

Esposito, Douglas H.

Fischer, Marc

Fitzgerald, Collette

Flannery, Brendan

Fox, LeAnne M.

Francois Watkins, Louise K.

Friedman, Cindy R.

Fullerton, Katie

Gaines, Joanna

Galland, G. Gale

Galloway, Renee L.

Garrison, Laurel E.

Gastañaduy, Paul A.

Gee, Jay E.

Geissler, Aimee L.

Gerber, Susan I.

Gershman, Mark D.

Gibbins, John

Goodson, James L.

Gould, L. Hannah

Green, Michael D.

Griffin, Patricia M.

Hall, Aron J.

Hawley, William A.

Hendricks Walters, Kate

Henry, Ronnie

Herwaldt, Barbara L.

Hills, Susan L.

Hlavsa, Michele C.

Holtzman, Deborah

Hunter, Jennifer C.

Iwamoto, Martha

Jackson, Brendan

Jentes, Emily S.

Jones, Jeffrey L.

Judd, Michael C.

Kersh, Gilbert J.

Kharod, Grishma A.

Kitt, Margaret

Knust, Barbara

Kozarsky, Phyllis E.

Kroger, Andrew T.
Kutty, Preeta K.
Lebo, Emmaculate J.
Lessa, Fernanda C.
Liang, Jennifer L.
Lippold, Susan A.
LoBue, Philip
Lopez, Adriana S.
Lopman, Ben
Lyss, Sheryl
MacNeil, Jessica R.
Mahon, Barbara E.
Maloney, Susan A.
Marano, Nina
Marin, Mona
Marston, Chung K.
Martin, Diana L.
Mast, Eric E.
McCollum, Andrea M.
McCotter, Orion Z.
McFarland, Jeffrey
Mead, Paul S.
Meites, Elissa
Meyer, Sarah A.

Mintz, Eric D.
Montgomery, Susan
Montiel, Sonia H.
Morgan, Oliver W
Moro, Pedro L.
Morof, Diane F.
Mullan, Robert J.
Mutebi, John-Paul
Negron, Maria E.
Nelson, Christina A.
Nelson, Noele P.
Nguyen, Duc B.
Nicholson, William L.
Nickels, Leslie
O'Reilly, Ciara E.
Objio, Tina
Paddock, Christopher D.
Patel, Manisha
Patimeteeporn, Calvin
Perez-Padilla, Janice
Peters, Philip J.
Petersen, Brett W.
Piacentino, John
Powers, Ann M.

Rabe, Ingrid B.
Raczniak, Gregory A.
Reef, Susan E.
Regan, Joanna J.
Reyes, Nimia L.
Reynolds, Megan R.
Rollin, Pierre E.
Russell, Michelle
Schafer, Ilana J.
Schmid, D. Scott
Schneider, Eileen
Sharp, Tyler M.
Shealy, Katherine R.
Skoff, Tami H.
Sleet, David A.
Sobel, Jeremy
Sotir, Mark J.
Staples, J. Erin
Steele, Stefanie F.
Stoddard, Robyn A.
Stoney, Rhett J.
Strikas, Raymond A.
Tan, Kathrine R.
Tardivel, Kara

Teshale, Eyasu
Tiller, Rebekah
Tiwari, Tejpratap S. P.
Traxler, Rita M.
Uribe, Carolina
Van Bogaert, Donna
Villarino, Margarita E.
Walker, Allison Taylor
Wallace, Ryan M.
Wassilak, Steven G. F.
Waterman, Stephen H.
Watson, John T.
Weinberg, Michelle S.
Weinberg, Nicholas
Weston, Emily J.
Winter, Kelly
Wong, Karen K.
Workowski, Kimberly
Xiao, Lihua
Yeoman, Kristin
Yoder, Jonathan S.

External Contributors

Adler, Tina — Westat—National Center for Complementary and Integrative Health Clearinghouse, Rockville, Maryland

Ansdell, Vernon E. — University of Hawaii, Honolulu, HI

Atkinson, Gregory — Teesside University, Middlesbrough, United Kingdom

Backer, Howard D. — California Emergency Medical Services Authority, Sacramento, CA

Barbeau, Deborah Nicolls — Tulane University, New Orleans, LA

Barnett, Elizabeth D. — Boston University School of Medicine and Boston Medical Center, Boston, MA

Batterham, Alan M. — Teesside University, Middlesbrough, United Kingdom

Benenson, Michael W. — Armed Forces Research Institute of the Medical Sciences, Bangkok, Thailand (retired)

Boggild, Andrea K. — University of Toronto, Toronto, Canada

Borwein, Sarah T. — TravelSafe Medical Centre, Hong Kong, China

Carroll, I. Dale — The Pregnant Traveler, Spring Lake, MI

Changizi, Roohollah — United Family Hospital, subsidiary of United Family Healthcare, Beijing, China

Chen, Lin H. — Mount Auburn Hospital—Travel Medicine Center, Cambridge, MA, and Harvard Medical School, Boston, MA

Connor, Bradley A.	Weill Medical College of Cornell University, New York, NY
DeRomaña, Inés	University of California System, Education Abroad Program, Santa Barbara, CA
Ejike-King, Lacreisha	US Food and Drug Administration, US Department of Health and Human Services, Rockville, Maryland
Fairley, Jessica K.	Emory University School of Medicine, Atlanta, GA
Forgione, Michael	Keesler Medical Center, Keesler AFB, Mississippi
Freedman, David O.	Shoreland, Inc., Milwaukee, WI
Fukuda, Mark	Armed Forces Research Institute of Medical Sciences, Bangkok, Thailand
Gracia, J. Nadine	Office of Minority Health, US Department of Health and Human Services, Rockville, Maryland
Gushulak, Brian D.	Migration Health Consultants, Cheltenham, Canada
Hackett, Peter H.	Institute for Altitude Medicine, Telluride, CO, and Altitude Research Center, University of Colorado Denver School of Medicine, Denver, CO
Hamer, Davidson H.	Center for Global Health and Development Boston University; Department of Global Health, Boston University School of Public Health and Section of Infectious Diseases, Boston Medical Center, Boston, MA
Henderson, John	United Nations consultant, Burma
Hochberg, Natasha S.	Section of Infectious Diseases, Boston University School of Medicine, Boston, MA
Hyle, Emily P.	Massachusetts General Hospital, Boston, MA
Kain, Kevin C.	University of Toronto, Toronto, Canada
Keystone, Jay S.	University of Toronto, Toronto, Canada
Kotton, Camille Nelson	Massachusetts General Hospital and Harvard University, Boston, MA
LaRocque, Regina C.	Massachusetts General Hospital and Harvard Medical School, Boston, MA
Law, Catherine	National Center for Complementary and Integrative Health, National Institutes of Health, Bethesda, MD
Libman, Michael	McGill University, Centre for Tropical Disease, Montreal, Canada
Magill, Alan J.*	Walter Reed Army Institute of Research, Experimental Therapeutics, Silver Spring, MD
Neumann, Karl	Weill Medical College of Cornell University and New York Presbyterian Hospital/Cornell Medical Center, New York, NY
Nilles, Eric J.	Division of Health Securities and Emergencies, World Health Organization, Suva, Fiji
Nord, Daniel A.	Divers Alert Network, Durham, NC
Ostroff, Stephen M.	Food and Drug Administration, Silver Spring, MD
Parker, Salim	Dee Bee Medical Centre, Cape Town, and South African Society of Travel Medicine, Johannesburg, South Africa
Pedone, Bettina N.	Arthur Ashe Student Health & Wellness Center, University of California, Los Angeles, CA
Pogemiller, Hope	University of Minnesota Medical School, Minneapolis, MN
Prinz, Robyn K.	US Department of State Bureau of Consular Affairs, Washington D.C.
Rhodes, Gary	Center for Global Education, University of California, Los Angeles, CA
Riddle, Mark S.	Naval Medical Research Center, Silver Spring, MD
Rosselot, Gail A.	Travel Well of Westchester, Inc., Briarcliff Manor, NY
Ryan, Edward T.	Massachusetts General Hospital and Harvard University, Boston, MA
Sampson, Dana M.	Office of Minority Health, US Department of Health and Human Services, Rockville, Maryland
Shlim, David R.	Jackson Hole Travel and Tropical Medicine, Jackson Hole, WY

* Deceased

Shurtleff, David	National Center for Complementary and Integrative Health, National Institutes of Health, Bethesda, MD
Staat, Mary Allen	International Adoption Center, Cincinnati Children's Hospital Medical Center, Cincinnati, OH
Taggart, Linda R.	University of Toronto, Toronto, Canada
Takiguchi, Rodd	Department of Dermatology, Kaiser Permanente, Honolulu, Hawaii
Thompson, Andrew	University of Liverpool, Liverpool, United Kingdom
Valk, Thomas H.	VEI Inc., Marshall, VA
Van Tilburg, Christopher	Providence Hood River Memorial Hospital, Hood River, OR
Wangu, Zoon	Department of Pediatric Infectious Diseases, Boston Medical Center, Boston, MA
Wilson, Mary Elizabeth	Harvard School of Public Health, Boston, MA
Wu, Henry M.	Emory University, Department of Medicine, Atlanta, GA
Youngster, Ilan	Children's Hospital Boston and Harvard University, Boston, MA

All contributors have signed a statement indicating that they have no conflicts of interest with the subject matter or materials discussed in the document(s) that they have written or reviewed for this book and that the information that they have written or reviewed for this book is objective and free from bias.

Acknowledgments

The *CDC Yellow Book 2018: Health Information for International Travel* editorial team gratefully acknowledges all the authors and reviewers for their commitment to this new edition. We extend sincere thanks to the following people for their contributions to the production of this book:

- Elise Beltrami, Pamela Diaz and Scott Santibanez for their extensive review of the text.

- Courtney Ware, Aida Sawadogo, Laurie Dieterich and Crystal Polite for their assistance in preparing the text for publication.

Preface

To stay on the cutting edge of travel health information, this latest edition of the *CDC Yellow Book: Health Information for International Travel* has been extensively revised. The book serves as a guide to the practice of travel medicine, as well as the authoritative source of US government recommendations for immunizations and prophylaxis for foreign travel. As international travel continues to become more common in the lives of US residents, having at least a basic understanding of the medical problems that travelers face has become a necessary aspect of practicing medicine. The goal of this book is to be a comprehensive resource for clinicians to find the answers to their travel health–related questions.

Centers for Disease Control and Prevention
Anne Schuchat, MD, Acting Director
National Center for Emerging and Zoonotic Infectious Diseases
Rima Khabbaz, MD, Acting Director
Division of Global Migration and Quarantine
Martin S. Cetron, MD, Director
Gary W. Brunette, MD, MS, Chief, Travelers' Health Branch
Phyllis E. Kozarsky, MD, Expert Consultant, Travelers' Health Branch
Megan Crawley O'Sullivan, MPH, Health Communications Specialist, Travelers' Health Branch

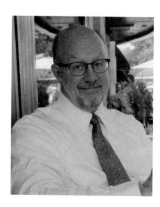

Alan J. Magill passed away on September 19, 2015, just days after work began on the *CDC Yellow Book 2018*. He was a key figure in the evolution of this publication, serving as an author and medical editor for three editions. Over the years, he provided invaluable insight and guidance as a singularly experienced and knowledgeable contributor. The editorial board of the *CDC Yellow Book* respectfully dedicate this edition to Alan.

In Memoriam: A Tribute to Alan J. Magill

Alan Magill and I were asked to become co-editors of the *Yellow Book* at the same time, during the Conference of the International Society of Travel Medicine in Vancouver, BC, in 2009. The next day we drove together from Vancouver to the ISTM Executive Board meeting in Whistler, and during that 3-hour trip, we discussed how we might revise the *Yellow Book* to make it more relevant to travel medicine practitioners. It was one of the more enjoyable conversations of my life.

Whatever Alan was involved in always seemed to go smoother, be more relevant, and even more fun. At that point in time, Alan was the president-elect of the International Society of Travel Medicine. He would subsequently serve as the president of the American Society of Tropical Medicine and Hygiene, becoming the first person to be president of both societies. During a 26-year career in the US Army Medical Corps, Alan focused mainly on malaria and leishmaniasis, but his research interests and projects spanned an extraordinary range, including diagnostics, pharmaceuticals, and vaccine development. He carried with him a nagging curiosity about the history of disease, and he often delved into original sources of research that informed our present practice in new ways. Invariably kind, enthusiastic, supportive, tireless, and insightful, Alan improved any project with which he was involved, including the *Yellow Book*.

Upon retiring from the military in 2012, Alan became the Malaria Program Director for the Gates Foundation, charged with designing a strategy that could lead to the elimination of malaria in the world. He had already played a large role in helping to shape an international strategy in this regard when he died suddenly on September 19, 2015, near his home in Seattle, leaving behind his wife and two daughters, and a devastated string of colleagues and admirers. Although tributes often end with the words, "He will be missed," in Alan's case, we are left wondering what the world has missed and what might have happened if he had been able to stay with us for many more years. He was 62 years old.

David R. Shlim, MD
Medical Editor of the *Yellow Book*
Recent Past-President of the ISTM

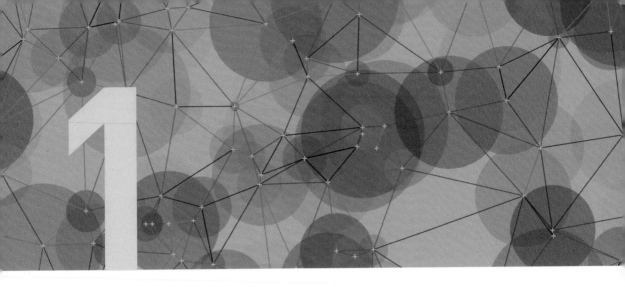

Introduction

INTRODUCTION TO TRAVEL HEALTH & THE YELLOW BOOK

Phyllis E. Kozarsky

TRAVEL HEALTH

The number of people traveling internationally has continued to grow substantially in the past decade. According to the World Tourism Organization, there were 1.2 billion worldwide international tourist arrivals in 2015, an increase of 4% from 2013; 50 million more people spent a night at an international destination than in 2014. In 2015, US residents made more than 73 million trips with at least 1 night outside the United States. The importance of protecting the health of individual travelers, as well as safeguarding the health of the communities to which they return, cannot be overstated. International travel takes on many forms, including tourism, business, study abroad, research, visiting friends and relatives, ecotourism, adventure, medical tourism, mission work, and responding to international disasters. Travelers are as unique as their itineraries, covering all age ranges and

having a variety of preexisting health concerns and conditions. The infectious disease risks that travelers face are dynamic—some travel destinations have become safer, while in other areas, new diseases have emerged and other diseases have reemerged.

The risk of becoming ill or injured during international travel depends on many factors, such as the region of the world visited, a traveler's age and health status, the length of the trip, and the diversity of planned activities. CDC provides international travel health information to address the range of health risks a traveler may face, with the aim of assisting travelers and clinicians to better understand the measures necessary to prevent illness and injury during international travel. This publication and the CDC Travelers' Health website (www.cdc.gov/travel) are 2 primary avenues of communicating CDC's travel health recommendations.

BOX 1-1. CDC contact information for clinicians

1

CDC-INFO NATIONAL CONTACT CENTER

All topics for clinicians and general public *(English and Spanish)*

- 8 AM to 8 PM Eastern, M–F: toll-free at 800-CDC-INFO (800-232-4636)
- E-mail form: www.cdc.gov/info

CDC EMERGENCY OPERATIONS CENTER

Emergency or urgent patient care assistance *(Note:This line is not intended for use by the general public.)*

- Available 24 hours per day, 7 days per week: 770-488-7100

CDC DRUG SERVICE

Distribution of special biologic agents and drugs

- Formulary:www.cdc.gov/ laboratory/drugservice/ formulary.html
- 8 AM to 4:30 PM Eastern, M–F: 404-639-3670
- After hours/weekends/ holidays: 770-488-7100
- E-mail: drugservice@cdc.gov

CHIKUNGUNYA, JAPANESE ENCEPHALITIS, TICKBORNE ENCEPHALITIS, AND YELLOW FEVER

Assistance with diagnostic testing for these diseases and for questions about antibody response to yellow fever vaccination

- Division of Vectorborne Diseases, 8 AM to 4:30 PM Mountain, M–F: 970-221-6400
- Viral Special Pathogens Branch can also assist for tickborne encephalitis, 8:30 AM to 5:30 PM Eastern, M–F: 404-639-1115

- After hours/weekends/ holidays: 770-488-7100
- State or local health departments may be able to assist: www.cdc.gov/mmwr/ international/relres.html

DENGUE

Dengue diagnostic testing assistance

- 8 AM to 5 PM Atlantic (office in Puerto Rico), M–F: 787-706-2399
- After hours/weekends/ holidays: 770-488-7100
- Clinical/laboratory guidance: www.cdc.gov/ Dengue/clinicalLab/index. html

MALARIA HOTLINE

Assistance with diagnosis or management of suspected cases of malaria

- 9 AM to 5 PM Eastern, M–F: 770-488-7788 or toll-free at 855-856-4713
- Emergency consultation after hours/weekends/ holidays: 770-488-7100, ask for a Malaria Branch clinician

PARASITIC DISEASES (OTHER THAN MALARIA)

Hotline

Assistance with evaluation and treatment of patients suspected to have a parasitic disease

- 8 AM to 4 PM Eastern, M–F: 404-718-4745
- Emergency consultation after hours/weekends/holidays: 770-488-7100, ask for an on-call clinician in Parasitic Diseases
- E-mail: parasites@cdc.gov

DPDx

Online parasitic diseases diagnostic assistance service for laboratorians, pathologists, and other health professionals

- www.cdc.gov/dpdx/contact. html

RICKETTSIAL DISEASES

Diagnostic and treatment assistance

- 8 AM to 4:30 PM Eastern, M–F: 404-639-1075
- Emergency consultation after hours/weekends/ holidays: 770-488-7100, ask for an on-call clinician in Rickettsial Diseases

VIRAL HEMORRHAGIC FEVERS

Diagnosis

Consultation for diagnosis and reporting suspected cases in or requiring evacuation to the United States

- 8:30 AM to 5:30 PM Eastern, M–F: 404-639-1115
- Emergency consultation after hours/weekends/ holidays: 770-488-7100

Treatment

Requests for ribavirin through the Food and Drug Administration (FDA) from Valeant Pharmaceuticals

- Providers should request through FDA at 301-736-3400
- Simultaneously notify Valeant at 800-548-5100, ext. 5 (domestic) or 949-461-6971 (international)

HISTORY AND ROLES OF THE YELLOW BOOK

CDC Health Information for International Travel ("The Yellow Book") has been a trusted resource since 1967. Originally, it was a small pamphlet published to satisfy the International Sanitary Regulations' requirements and the International Health Regulations (IHR), adopted by the World Health Organization (WHO) in 1951 and 1969, respectively; the IHR were completely revised in 2005. The purpose of the IHR is to ensure maximum security against the international spread of diseases, with minimum interference with world travel and commerce. A copy of the current IHR and supporting information can be found on the WHO website (www.who.int/csr/ihr/en).

In addition to reporting public health events of international concern, the United States must also inform the public about health requirements for entering other countries, such as the necessity of being vaccinated against yellow fever. The Yellow Book and the CDC Travelers' Health website aim to communicate these requirements under the IHR (2005). Although this publication includes the most current available information at the time of printing, requirements can change. The CDC Travelers' Health website (www.cdc.gov/travel) may be checked for regularly updated information to ensure that requirements for international travel are known and met.

The Yellow Book is written primarily for clinicians, including physicians, nurses, and pharmacists. Others, such as people in the travel industry, multinational corporations, missionary and volunteer organizations, and individual travelers, can also find a wealth of information here.

This text is authored by subject-matter experts from within CDC and outside the agency. The guidelines presented in this book are evidence-based and supported by best practices. Internal text citations have not been included; however, a bibliography is included at the end of each section for those who would like to obtain more detailed information. The CDC Travelers' Health program and the CDC Foundation are pleased to partner with Oxford University Press, Inc., to publish the 2018 edition. In addition to the printed copy, a searchable, online version of the Yellow Book can be found on the CDC Travelers' Health website (www.cdc.gov/yellowbook).

CONTACT INFORMATION FOR CDC

Questions, comments, and suggestions for CDC Travelers' Health, including comments about this publication, may be made through the CDC-INFO contact center, toll-free at 800-CDC-INFO (800-232-4636) 8 AM to 8 PM Eastern Time (Monday–Friday, closed on holidays) or by visiting www.cdc.gov/info to submit your question through an online form.

Pretravel or Post-travel Clinical Questions

Since CDC is not a medical facility, clinicians needing assistance with preparing patients for international travel should consider referral to a travel clinic or a clinic listed on the International Society of Travel Medicine (ISTM) website (www.istm.org).

Clinicians with post-travel health questions regarding their patients may consider referral to a clinic listed on the ISTM website, the American Society of Tropical Medicine and Hygiene website (www.astmh.org), or a medical university with specialists in infectious diseases.

Because of the complexity of some travel-related diseases, Box 1-1 lists contact information for providers needing clinical assistance.

BIBLIOGRAPHY

1. United Nations World Tourism Organization. UNWTO World Tourism Barometer, Vol. 14 (March). Madrid: United Nations World Tourism Organization; 2016 [cited 2016 Mar. 2]; Available from: http://www.e-unwto.org/toc/wtobarometereng/14/2.

2. US Department of Commerce, Office of Travel and Tourism Industries. 2015 Monthly US Outbound Air Travel to International Regions. Washington, DC: US Department of Commerce; 2016 [cited 2016 Mar. 21]; Available from: http://travel.trade.gov/tinews/archive/tinews2016/20160321.asp.

3. World Health Organization. International Health Regulations (2005). Geneva: World Health Organization; 2008 [cited 2016 Apr. 11]; 2nd: Available from: http://www.who.int/ihr/publications/9789241596664/en/.

PLANNING FOR HEALTHY TRAVEL: CDC TRAVELERS' HEALTH WEBSITE AND MOBILE APPLICATIONS

Ronnie Henry

TRAVELERS' HEALTH WEBSITE

The CDC Travelers' Health website (www.cdc.gov/travel) offers destination-specific vaccine and travel health recommendations, travel notices, help with finding a travel medicine provider, and other resources for travelers and clinicians. The home page (Figure 1-1) includes separate portals for travelers and clinicians. Users can also select special populations (such as "traveling with children" or

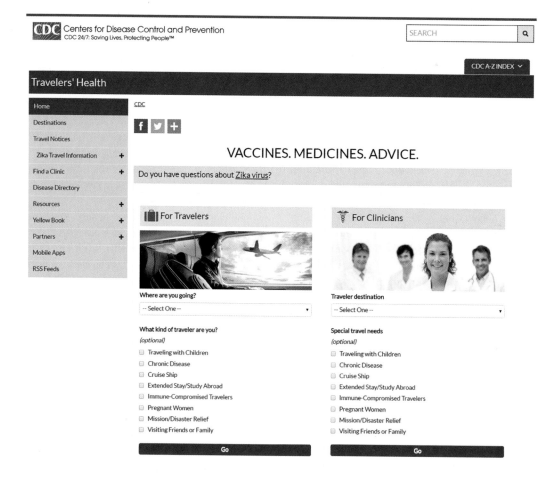

FIGURE 1-1. CDC Travelers' Health website homepage

"immune-compromised travelers") to receive customized health recommendations.

Destination Pages

The most popular feature of the Travelers' Health website are the "destination pages," each with a clinician and traveler view. Destination pages provide health recommendations for a particular destination and include the following information:

- Vaccine and medicine recommendations
- Patient counseling information (called "Stay Healthy and Safe" on the destination pages and includes information on preventing foodborne and vectorborne disease and avoiding injuries)
- Healthy travel packing list
- Travel health notices
- Post-travel health information

Information Centers

Resources for clinicians (wwwnc.cdc.gov/travel/page/clinician-information-center) includes clinical updates on travel medicine–related topics and continuing education courses on travel medicine.

Resources for travelers (http://wwwnc.cdc.gov/travel/page/resources-for-travelers) provides printable fact sheets that cover over 40 travel health topics written in plain language for the international traveler. Topics include travel health insurance, jet lag, motion sickness, cruise ship travel, and travel to high altitudes.

Resources for the travel industry (wwwnc.cdc.gov/travel/page/travel-industry-information-center) contains guidelines for the air travel and cruise ship industries. It includes information on reporting illnesses and deaths among travelers, managing ill crew members, and other guidance.

Disease Directory

The disease directory (wwwnc.cdc.gov/travel/diseases) is a list of diseases that may be related to travel. It provides a resource on rare as well as common infections, the risk to travelers, and what travelers can do to prevent them.

Travel Notices

CDC posts travel health notices about disease outbreaks and international events (such as natural disasters or mass gatherings) that may affect the health of travelers. The notices include information about what the situation or health risk is, who is affected, how travelers can protect their health, and links for more information. Travel health notices and information about travel notice categories can be found at wwwnc.cdc.gov/travel/notices.

MOBILE APPLICATIONS

CDC has developed 2 mobile applications for travelers, *Can I Eat This?* and *TravWell*, in addition to the mobile version of the Yellow Book. All are available for iOS and Android devices and can be accessed from wwwnc.cdc.gov/travel/page/apps-about.

Can I Eat This?

CDC's *Can I Eat This?* application helps international travelers avoid travelers' diarrhea by guiding their food and drink choices. Travelers select the country they are in and answer a few simple questions about what they are eating or drinking, and the application will tell them whether it is likely to be safe. In addition to helping guide their on-the-spot decisions, *Can I Eat This?* also teaches travelers general principles regarding safe food and water. All recommendations are stored locally on the user's device, so no international data connection is needed to use the application when traveling.

TravWell

CDC's *TravWell* is a companion application to the Travelers' Health destination pages. It allows users to build an itinerary and receive destination-specific vaccine and medicine recommendations. For each itinerary, it also generates a customizable, destination-specific to-do list and packing list. *TravWell* also prompts users to set reminders for healthy behaviors, such as taking malaria prophylaxis or getting booster doses of vaccines. It also provides users with a place to store electronic copies of health-related travel documents, such as prescriptions or vaccination records.

TRAVEL EPIDEMIOLOGY

Allison Taylor Walker, Regina C. LaRocque, Mark J. Sotir

1

Travelers are an epidemiologically important population because of their mobility, their potential for exposure to diseases outside their home country, and the possibility that they may carry nonendemic diseases between countries. International tourist arrivals were 1.2 billion in 2015 and are projected to increase to almost 2 billion by 2030, so the public health impact of travel will likely only increase. The destinations of travelers are also changing. Increased travel to destinations in Asia (arrivals up 5% from 2014 to 2015) and the Middle East (arrivals up 3% from 2014 to 2015) and anticipated increases in travel to Africa will place more travelers at risk for a variety of travel-related conditions, including malaria, dengue, measles, and other tropical or vaccine-preventable infections.

The risk of travel-related illness varies depending on destination and traveler characteristics. Existing information regarding the actual risk for travelers (often expressed as number of events per 100,000 travelers) is limited for several reasons. It is difficult to obtain an accurate numerator (number of cases of disease among travelers) and denominator (number of travelers overall or travelers to a specific destination). Many travelers who become infected will have returned to their home countries by the time they develop symptoms so will not be included in the visited country's surveillance data. Similarly, diseases with short incubation periods or brief durations may have resolved by the time a traveler returns home and thus may not be counted in surveillance data of the traveler's country of origin. If the illness is mild, the traveler may never seek health care, or diagnostic tests may not be performed to accurately diagnose the cause. Travelers often visit multiple locations, and it may be difficult to determine the location in which the exposure occurred.

Frequently quoted studies on the incidence of infection in travelers are based on extrapolations of limited data collected in limited samples of travelers. Often, these studies were conducted >20 years ago and might be of limited relevance to current travelers. Furthermore, these studies use a variety of methodologic designs, each with its own set of strengths and weaknesses, making the findings difficult to compare or combine. They have also, for the most part, only examined a few key diseases or conditions and have combined all travelers regardless of destination or purpose of travel. Many have been single-clinic or single-destination studies that lead to conclusions that do not apply to groups of travelers with different local, national, or cultural backgrounds.

A number of factors are relevant to epidemiologic data on travel-related diseases and adverse health events. First, the characteristics of the disease itself must be considered, including mode of transmission, incubation period, signs and symptoms, duration of illness, and diagnostic testing. Second, the presence, frequency, seasonality, and geographic distribution of the disease need to be assessed; these might change over time because of outbreaks, emergence or reemergence in new areas or populations, successful public health interventions, or other factors. Third, travelers represent a unique subset of people, and their exposures, behaviors, and disease susceptibility might differ dramatically from those of the local population at a tourist destination.

Along with demographic characteristics, additional travel-specific factors that should be considered include trip length, destinations (both current and previous), specific travel itineraries, use of preventive measures, and purpose of travel. Fourth, travelers themselves are a heterogeneous group, and different subgroups of travelers might have different risks because of activities, behaviors, and other factors during travel. For example, travelers who are visiting friends and relatives (VFR travelers) have consistently demonstrated higher proportions of serious febrile illness, particularly malaria, when compared with other types of travelers.

During the past 2 decades, the most relevant data on travel-related disease occurrence have come from surveillance of travelers themselves. Data on disease incidence in local populations may identify the most important diseases to monitor within a country, but relevance of such data to travelers—who have different risk behaviors, eating habits, accommodations, knowledge of preventive measures, and activities—is usually limited. Surveillance data that are either focused on travelers or on illnesses that affect travelers are more useful in describing travel-related disease patterns and risks.

Data collected by the Global TravEpiNet (GTEN) network of pretravel visits in health clinics across the United States provide a snapshot into the types of travelers seeking pretravel health care and their travel practices. Health care providers need to understand the epidemiologic features of the traveling population to guide their pretravel recommendations and post-travel evaluations. In examining GTEN data collected from 2009 through 2011, 13,235 travelers ranged in age from 1 month to 94 years (median 35 years). The median duration of travel that prompted the pretravel evaluation was 14 days, although 22% of travelers were taking trips of >28 days, and 3% of the travelers were taking trips of >6 months. A total of 75% were traveling to malaria-endemic countries, and 38% were visiting yellow fever–endemic countries. Immunocompromising conditions, such as HIV infection and AIDS, organ transplantation, or receipt of immunocompromising medications, were present in 3% of GTEN travelers.

Post-travel illness surveillance data are collected by the GeoSentinel Global Surveillance Network, a worldwide data collection and communication network composed of International Society of Travel Medicine (ISTM) member travel and tropical medicine clinics. Analyses of these data are used to describe the relationships between travel and travel-related illness in specific subpopulations of travelers. A 2013 summary of GeoSentinel data found that diarrheal, febrile/systemic, and respiratory illnesses are the most common diagnoses reported. Another study found that >20% of travelers visiting malarious areas reported inconsistent or no use of

malaria prophylaxis. Post-travel data from the GeoSentinel network of 53 clinics around the world collected from 2007 through 2011 indicate that Asia (33%) and sub-Saharan Africa (27%) were the most common regions where travel-related illnesses were acquired. Malaria, dengue, enteric fever, spotted-fever group rickettsioses, chikungunya, and nonspecific viral syndromes were the most frequent contributors to the acute systemic febrile illness category. Falciparum malaria was most commonly acquired in West Africa, while enteric fever was most often contracted on the Indian subcontinent; leptospirosis, scrub typhus, and murine typhus were principally acquired in Southeast Asia. Common skin and soft tissue infections, mosquito bites (often infected), and allergic dermatitis were the most common skin conditions affecting travelers. Among the more exotic diagnoses, the most important were hookworm-related cutaneous larva migrans, leishmaniasis, myiasis, and tungiasis. The relative frequency of many diseases varied by travel destination and reason for travel, and VFR travelers had a disproportionately high prevalence of serious febrile illness (malaria) and low rates of seeking advice before travel (18%). Only 40% of all ill GeoSentinel travelers reported pretravel medical visits.

Investigations of travel-related outbreaks can also provide data on epidemiologic patterns of travel-related illness. Outbreaks in travelers to the Caribbean are a reminder of travel-associated risk of illness. Incidence of chikungunya was evaluated among 102 participants returning from the Dominican Republic in 2014. Forty-two (41%) had evidence of recent chikungunya infection, and of those, 37 (90%) reported rash or joint pain. Outbreaks in travelers are sentinels to warn the international community of prevalent or unrecognized illnesses in destination countries. An outbreak investigation of sarcocystosis in travelers returning from Tioman Island, Malaysia, in 2011–2012 led to continued monitoring for additional cases and identified asymptomatic infection and late presentation. Diseases identified through medical tourism, a booming yet unregulated industry, can also highlight local transmission of health care–associated infections. *Mycobacterium abscessus* infections in postsurgical wounds of medical tourists returning from the Dominican Republic and Venezuela have been reported.

Familiarity with the epidemiology and prevalence of these and other infections, coupled with demographic information on travelers and their particular travel details, can help clinicians provide optimal health-related information and advice to their travelers. Clinical networks and surveillance systems provide epidemiologic data on new and prevalent global infectious disease threats. These data contribute to the evidence base in this growing field and allow for informed preparation before travel, as well as clinical awareness of travel epidemiology.

BIBLIOGRAPHY

1. Adachi K, Coleman MS, Khan N, Jentes ES, Arguin P, Rao SR, et al. Economics of malaria prevention in US travelers to West Africa. Clin Infect Dis. 2014 Jan;58(1):11–21.

2. CDC. Malaria surveillance—United States, 2011. MMWR Surveill Summ. 2013 Nov 1;62(5):1–17.

3. Esposito DH, Stich A, Epelboin L, Malvy D, Han PV, Bottieau E, et al. Acute muscular sarcocystosis: an international investigation among ill travelers returning from Tioman Island, Malaysia, 2011–2012. Clin Infect Dis. 2014 Nov 15;59(10):1401–10.

4. Harvey K, Esposito DH, Han P, Kozarsky P, Freedman DO, Plier DA, et al. Surveillance for travel-related disease—GeoSentinel Surveillance System, United States, 1997–2011. MMWR Surveill Summ. 2013 Jul. 19;62:1–23.

5. LaRocque RC, Rao SR, Lee J, Ansdell V, Yates JA, Schwartz BS, et al. Global TravEpiNet: a national consortium of clinics providing care to international travelers—analysis of demographic characteristics, travel destinations, and pre-travel healthcare of high-risk US international travelers, 2009–2011. Clin Infect Dis. 2012 Feb. 15;54(4):455–62.

6. Leder K, Torresi J, Libman MD, Cramer JP, Castelli F, Schlagenhauf P, et al. GeoSentinel surveillance of illness in returned travelers, 2007–2011. Ann Intern Med. 2013 Mar. 19;158(6):456–68.

7. Millman AJ, Esposito DH, Biggs HM, Decenteceo M, Klevos A, Hunsperger E, et al. Chikungunya and dengue virus infections among United States community service volunteers returning from the Dominican Republic. Am J Trop Med Hyg. 2014 Mar. 14;64(6):1336–41.

8. Sharp TM, Pillai P, Hunsperger E, Santiago GA, Anderson T, Vap T, et al. A cluster of dengue cases in American missionaries returning from Haiti. Am J Trop Med Hyg. 2010 Jan.;86(1):6–22.

9. Sotir M, Freedman D. Basic epidemiology of infectious diseases, including surveillance and reporting. In: Zuckerman J, Leggat P, Brunette G, editors. Essential Travel Medicine. Chichester (UK): John Wiley & Sons; 2015.

10. United Nations World Tourism Organization. UNWTO Tourism Highlights, 2016 ed. [Internet]. Madrid: World Tourism Organization; 2016 [cited 2016 Mar. 26]. Available from: http://media.unwto.org/press-release/2016-01-18/international-tourist-arrivals-4-reach-record-12-billion-2015.

WHY GUIDELINES DIFFER

David R. Shlim, Alan J. Magill*

INTRODUCTION

Numerous international, national, and professional organizations publish guidelines and recommendations that assist travel health providers in giving the best possible advice to prospective travelers. The CDC Yellow Book is one example of published recommendations. However, it is quickly apparent to both clinicians and patients that guidelines and recommendations differ, sometimes dramatically. Conflicting messages from authoritative sources may confuse patients and clinicians and undermine the credibility of the source. It can be unsettling for patients to receive travel medicine advice, vaccines, and an antimalarial drug prescription from a provider, only to find that the recommendations conflict with what they have obtained from other sources or even heard from other advisors. The skillful travel health provider will be able to help the traveler run this gauntlet of conflicting advice by knowing more about why guidelines differ.

HOW ARE GUIDELINES CREATED?

Most guidelines of interest to travel health providers

and travelers focus on recommendations for immunizations, prophylactic medications, and self-treatment regimens (such as those for travelers' diarrhea). Guidelines come from many sources. A regulatory agency in each country must review and approve an application from the sponsor of a product in order for the product to be commercially distributed. Regulatory authorities review data from prelicensure clinical trials and also assess the manufacturing process. International organizations such as the World Health Organization (WHO) promote their own sets of guidelines. At national levels, agencies such as CDC make recommendations for the use of approved vaccines and medications for travelers. In addition, professional organizations may create consensus clinical practice guidelines based on published medical literature and expert opinion. Travel medicine–specific subscription services use experts to organize and present travel medicine recommendations for clinicians. However, these services can use information and sources that may not be

fully validated by national and international authorities. Finally, vast quantities of unregulated opinions are published on the Internet. People new to travel medicine may not be aware of the decision-making process or the source information that results in formal recommendations from these organizations.

Regulatory Authorities

Countries typically have a national regulatory authority which acts as the government body that approves vaccines and drugs. In the United States, this is the Food and Drug Administration (FDA). For the vaccines and medications commonly prescribed in a pretravel consultation, providers are expected to use the products in accordance with the product label as approved by the FDA. The product label is a valuable source of information that is accurate at the time it is published. Manufacturers submit a detailed application that undergoes rigorous, multidisciplinary review. The approved product label reflects the information

* Deceased.

provided by the manufacturer in response to the requirements specified by a large body of regulatory law developed over many years. Since each country has different laws and requirements, approved products and their product labels may differ from country to country. This difference is then reflected in the national guidelines that relate to that product.

International Organizations

Travelers' health information is provided by WHO's publication *International travel and health* (the "Green Book") and also in the WHO International Health Regulations 2005. The Green Book is currently out of print; however, WHO updates factual or evidence-based essential information on the International travel and health website (www.who.int/ith). Countries with less-developed or nonexistent regulatory agencies often default to the WHO guidelines, while more-developed countries with resources devoted to travelers' health may be aware of the WHO recommendations but may not be able to reconcile WHO recommendations with their own country's recommendations in every situation.

US National Organizations

CDC provides recommendations for travel health and publishes those recommendations in this book. Subject-matter experts at CDC review information in their area of expertise and formulate recommendations. For vaccines, the Advisory Committee on Immunization Practices (ACIP) develops written recommendations for the administration of vaccines, including travelers' vaccines, to children and adults in the civilian population. Recommendations include age for vaccine administration, number of doses and dosing interval, and precautions and contraindications. ACIP, which is the only entity appointed by the federal government to make such recommendations, consists of 15 experts in fields associated with immunization who have been selected to provide advice and guidance to the Department of Health and Human Services and CDC on the control of vaccine-preventable diseases (Box 2-1).

Professional Organizations

Professional organizations often develop, write, and publish practice guidelines using committees of experts from their membership. These practice guidelines typically follow an evidence-based medicine approach that links recommendations to the strength and quality of the evidence as assessed by the committee members. The Infectious Diseases Society of America has published a travel medicine practice guideline that many find useful.

Peer-Reviewed Medical Literature and Open Sources

As experience with a vaccine or a drug is acquired over the years, these results are often published in the peer-reviewed medical literature. In addition, people who use these products gain experience over time and develop their own opinions ("experience-based medicine"). The data that would be most useful in deciding how to use a vaccine or medication may not be available in published reports, so expert opinion attempts to interpret available information or provide background perspective.

The use of medications to treat or prevent disease is up to the discretion of the prescribing health practitioner. An example is whether to provide travelers with empiric treatment for travelers' diarrhea, and if so, what medication to recommend and what course to prescribe. The travel medicine practitioner needs to review the available literature to keep up with changing antibiotic resistance and the epidemiology of diarrhea in various destinations.

WHY DO GUIDELINES DIFFER?

Guidelines in different countries and organizations may differ in substantial ways. Some of the reasons why guidelines differ include availability of products in different countries, a different cultural perception of risk, lack of evidence (or differing interpretations of the same evidence), and sometimes just honest differences in opinion among experts. Occasionally, public opinion may influence recommendations (for example, the widespread adverse publicity about mefloquine that was reported in the media).

Availability of Products

Travel health providers can only use the products that are available to them. Availability is determined by the regulatory approval status of the product and, to a lesser extent, the marketing and distribution plan of the manufacturer. Among the various vaccines and antimalarial drugs commercially available worldwide, the process for regulatory approvals varies greatly. For example, registering a new vaccine or antimalarial drug in the United States is a costly and rigorous process. If the market is insufficient to justify the expense of registration, then a commercial company may not seek registration in a particular country. The standards for licensure vary, and what may be sufficient for one regulatory authority may not suffice for another. For example, primaquine, an option for malaria chemoprophylaxis in the United States, is not registered or commercially available in Switzerland. Atovaquone-proguanil was available for malaria chemoprophylaxis in the United States before many other countries. On the other hand, a vaccine against tickborne encephalitis is approved for use and widely available in many countries, but is not approved by the FDA; therefore, CDC and ACIP guidelines do not include any recommendations for the use of this vaccine.

Even when the same products are available, the recommendations for their use may differ. The injectable capsular polysaccharide typhoid vaccine and the oral typhoid vaccine are examples. In the United States, a booster of the polysaccharide vaccine is recommended after 2 years, but in most European countries, a booster is recommended after 3 years. In the United States, a packet of 4 oral typhoid capsules is dispensed, whereas in Europe, 3 doses are considered adequate. The regulatory agencies may have reviewed the same data and drawn different conclusions, or they may have reviewed different data at separate times and reached different conclusions. Regulatory submissions to various agencies rarely are ready and occur at the same time; therefore, the data available for review by each agency may not be the same, for legitimate reasons.

Perception of Risk

People from varying backgrounds can view the same risk data and come to different conclusions as to the cost and benefit of preventing that risk. For example, national-level recommendations to prevent malaria while traveling to India vary widely. Germany does not recommend using standard prophylaxis for any travel to an Indian destination; standby emergency treatment (SBET or self-treatment) is the recommendation for identified risk destinations.

(continued)

The guidelines in the United Kingdom recommend only awareness and mosquito bite prevention as the default recommendation for more than half the Indian subcontinent, including large cities and popular tourist destinations in the north and south, while recommending an individual risk assessment that is based on activities and types of travel for consideration of chemoprophylaxis. For some defined higher-risk areas, the recommendation is for standard chemoprophylaxis for most travelers, with the option to consider mosquito avoidance for low-risk travelers. However, CDC recommends malaria chemoprophylaxis for any Indian destination except for some mountainous areas of northern states above 2,000 m (6,561 ft) as the default recommendation for most travelers, with consideration of individual risk and benefit. Is one of these recommendations better than the others? Not necessarily, as the recommendations may be based on the national experience with different types of travelers and the risk assessment approach of the organization formulating the national guidelines.

Lack of Evidence

In many cases, limited or no data are available to inform an evidence-based assessment. In this setting, travel health providers defer to expert opinion or an extrapolation from limited data in conjunction with expert opinion. In travel medicine, it is rare to have actual prospective numerator and denominator data on the risk of any vaccine-preventable diseases in travelers. For example, any data on the risk of hepatitis A in travelers would have to account for the immunization rate with hepatitis A vaccine. These data are rarely available, and therefore, we often rely on historical data that captured few actual cases.

CAN WE HARMONIZE GUIDELINES?

The complex nature of how we obtain, evaluate, and verify data, combined with the fundamental differences in risk perception, makes it likely that multiple, overlapping, and at times conflicting guidelines will continue to exist. However, given the international nature of travel medicine and the existence of the International Society of Travel Medicine, conflicting guidelines have

decreased in the past decade. In one example of an effort to harmonize guidelines, from 2008 through 2010, WHO convened an international group of yellow fever and travel medicine experts to review available data on yellow fever virus transmission. The product of this collaboration was a country-specific list of yellow fever vaccine recommendations based on the geographic distribution of risk (see Chapter 3, Yellow Fever & Malaria Information, by Country).

In summary, the role of the travel health provider is to become more sophisticated in his or her understanding of the various differences in guidelines, in interpreting this information, and in conveying it in an assured and comforting manner to travelers.

BIBLIOGRAPHY

1. CDC. Malaria surveillance— United States, 2011. MMWR Surveill Summ. 2013 Nov 1;62(5):1–17.

2. CDC. Advisory Committee on Immunization Practices (ACIP). Atlanta: CDC; 2014 [cited 2016 Sep. 10]; Available from: http://www.cdc.gov/vaccines/acip/.

3. Chiodini PL, Field VK, Whitty CJM, Lalloo DG. Guidelines for malaria prevention in travellers from the United

Kingdom. London: Public Health England; 2014 [cited 2016 Sep. 16]. Available from: https://www.gov.uk/government/uploads/system/uploads/attachment_data/file/337761/Guidelines_for_malaria_prevention_in_travellers_UK_PC.pdf.

4. Committee to Advise on Tropical Medicine and Travel (CATMAT). Canadian recommendations for the prevention and treatment of malaria. Ottawa: Public Health Agency of Canada; 2014 [cited 2016 June 14]. Available from: http://publications.

gc.ca/collections/collection_2014/aspc-phac/HP40-102-2014-eng.pdf.

5. German Society for Tropical Medicine and International Health Association (DTG). [Recommendations for malaria prevention]. 2015 [cited 2016 June 14]; Available from: http://www.dtg.org/malaria.html.

6. Hill DR, Ericsson CD, Pearson RD, Keystone JS, Freedman DO, Kozarsky PE, et al. The practice of travel medicine: guidelines by the Infectious Diseases Society of

America. Clin Infect Dis. 2006 Dec. 15;43(12):1499–539.

7. World Health Organization. International Health Regulations (2005). Geneva: World Health Organization; 2008 [cited 2016 June 14]; Available from: http://www.who.int/ihr/9789241596664/en/index.html.

8. World Health Organization. International Travel and Health. Geneva: World Health Organization; 2012 (with 2016 updates) [cited 2016 June 14]; Available from: http://www.who.int/ith/en/.

Perspectives sections are written as editorial discussions aiming to add depth and clinical perspective to the official recommendations contained in the book. The views and opinions expressed in this section are those of the authors and do not necessarily represent the official position of CDC.

AIR TRAVEL TRENDS

Andre D. Berro

The increased complexity and extent of the global aviation network can accelerate the spread of communicable diseases of public health concern. Recently, air travel has been a factor in the spread of Ebola, Middle East respiratory syndrome (MERS), and Zika. International airlines connect approximately 40,000 global cities and carry about 3 billion total passengers per year. Growth in air travel over time reflects a volume growth on established routes and a nodal growth where more airports and cities globally are connected. Understanding the overall trends of global air travel can inform the response to issues of public health concern and allow for targeted mitigating measures to limit the spread of communicable diseases.

About 100 million passengers flew from the United States to overseas destinations during 2015. Map 1-1 shows the spatial distribution of these passengers by destination country. Five destination countries (Mexico, Canada, United Kingdom, Japan, and China) account for 40% of all outbound international air travel from the United States. Table 1-1 below shows the volume and proportion of air travelers from the United States into each of the top 10 destination countries in 2015.

Seasonal trends in travel are discernible from year to year; overall outbound travel peaks in the summer and has its nadir in February. Seasonal trends also vary by destination. For example, although outbound travel volume to Europe peaks in June, the volume of passengers to the Caribbean, Latin America, and sub-Saharan Africa peaks during December.

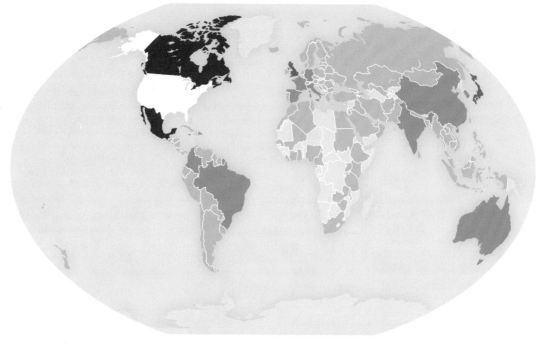

Estimated number of air passengers by destination

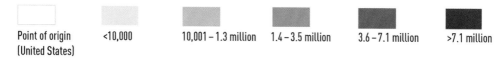

| Point of origin (United States) | <10,000 | 10,001 – 1.3 million | 1.4 – 3.5 million | 3.6 – 7.1 million | >7.1 million |

MAP 1-1. Estimated number of US air travelers received[1]

[1] Diio Market Intelligence, Fares and Market Sizes, Global (at www.diio.net).

Table 1-1. Estimated number of US air passengers departing to the top 10 destination countries, 2015

DESTINATION COUNTRY	DEPARTING PASSENGERS	PERCENTAGE OF ALL US OUTBOUND TRAVEL
Mexico	12,200,000	12.4%
Canada	12,100,000	12.3%
United Kingdom	7,100,000	7.2%
Japan	4,500,000	4.6%
China	3,500,000	3.5%
Dominican Republic	3,100,000	3.1%
Germany	2,800,000	2.8%
Brazil	2,800,000	2.8%
India	2,600,000	2.6%
Italy	2,500,000	2.5%
Other Countries	45,400,000	45.9%

During 2014, approximately 83% of the US residents who traveled overseas did so for vacation or to visit family and friends and 17% for business. US residents traveling abroad made reservations on average 68 days before departure. This period should allow travelers time to schedule a pretravel consultation to get recommended vaccinations and learn about health precautions.

PROJECTIONS

According to the International Air Transport Association (IATA), the combined global volume of inbound and outbound air travel is projected to more than double and reach 7 billion total passengers per year by 2034. China and the United States are anticipated to lead the growth volume.

The fastest-growing routes include those to Africa, Asia, and South America; travel to countries such as the Central African Republic, Ethiopia, Malawi, Rwanda, Sierra Leone, Tanzania, and Uganda, considered to be at high risk for travel-related diseases, is expected to double in volume over the next decade. This growth could lead to increased exposures to communicable diseases.

Public health planners, responders, and clinicians will need to take these projections into account when developing strategies to prevent the spread of communicable diseases of public health concern through international travel.

BIBLIOGRAPHY

1. Chen LH, Wilson ME. The role of the traveler in emerging infections and magnitude of travel. Med Clin North Am. 2008 Nov;92(6):1409–32.

2. Hui DS, Perlman S, Zumla A. Spread of MERS to South Korea and China. Lancet Respir Me. 2015 Jun 4;3(7):509–10.

3. International Air Transport Association. 100 Years of Commercial Flight | Small World, Big Future. [cited 2016 Mar. 21]; Available from: http://flying100years.com/.

4. International Air Transport Association. IATA Air Passenger Forecast Shows Dip in Long-Term Demand. The International Air Transport Association (IATA), 2015 [updated Nov. 2015; cited 2016 Apr. 5]; Available from: http://www.iata.org/pressroom/pr/Pages/2015-11-26-01.aspx.

5. International Air Transport Association. FMg DM. Global passengers volume based on ticket settlement data from ARC and IATA. 2015 [cited 2016 Apr. 05].

6. Musa EO, Adedire E, Olayinka A, Adeoye O, Adewuyi P, Waziri N, et al. Epidemiological profile of the Ebola virus disease outbreak in Nigeria July–September 2014. Pan Afr Med J. 2014;21(1):331.

7. Musso D. Zika Virus Transmission from French Polynesia to Brazil (Letter). Emerg Infect Dis. 2015 Oct;21(10).

8. US Department of Commerce International Trade Administration. Profile of U.S. Resident Travelers Visiting Overseas Destinations: 2014 Outbound. 2014 [cited 2016 Apr. 05]; Available from: http://travel.trade.gov/outreachpages/download_data_table/2014_Outbound_Profile.pdf.

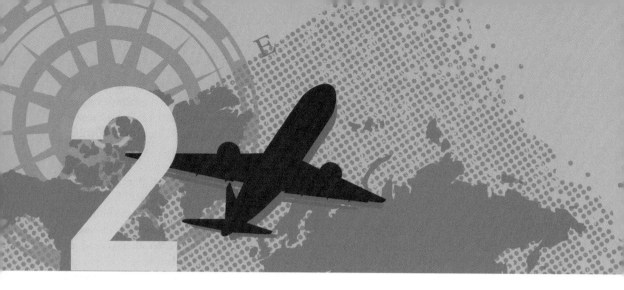

The Pretravel Consultation

THE PRETRAVEL CONSULTATION

Lin H. Chen, Natasha S. Hochberg, Alan J. Magill

The pretravel consultation offers a dedicated time to prepare travelers for the health concerns that might arise during their trips. The objectives of the pretravel consultation are:

1. To perform an individual risk assessment.

2. To educate the traveler regarding anticipated health risks and methods for prevention.

3. To provide immunizations for vaccine-preventable diseases and medications for prophylaxis, self-treatment, or both.

THE TRAVEL HEALTH SPECIALIST

The outcome of a pretravel consultation likely depends on the fund of knowledge, expertise, and communication skills of the provider, as well as the health beliefs of the traveler. Counseling by trained staff can effectively deliver many messages, such as those regarding the need for appropriate immunizations, and malaria risk and prevention. Familiarity with the traveler's destination, its culture, infrastructure, and disease patterns can assist the travel health advisor in providing more personalized advice.

Travel medicine specialists have in-depth knowledge of immunizations, risks associated with specific destinations, and the implications of traveling with underlying conditions. Therefore, a comprehensive consultation with a travel medicine expert is indicated for any traveler with a complicated health history, special risks (such as traveling at high altitudes or working in refugee camps), or exotic or complicated itineraries. Those clinicians who wish to be travel health providers are encouraged to take advantage of one of the many travel health educational opportunities available, join the International Society of Travel Medicine, attend conferences, and obtain their Certificate in Travel Health.

COMPONENTS OF A PRETRAVEL CONSULTATION

Effective pretravel consultations require attention to the health background of the traveler and incorporate the itinerary, trip duration, travel purpose, and activities, all of which determine health risks (Table 2-1). The pretravel consultation is the major opportunity to educate the traveler about health risks at the destination and how to mitigate them. The typical pretravel consultation does not include a physical examination; a separate appointment with the same or a different provider may be necessary to assess a person's fitness to travel. Because the traveler does not need to be physically present to receive pretravel education, pretravel consultations are ideally suited to be done remotely. In addition, because travel medicine clinics are not available in many communities, remote consultations can give more travelers access to the information they need.

Travel health advice should be personalized, highlighting the likely exposures and also

Table 2-1. Information necessary for a risk assessment during pretravel consultations

Health Background	
Past medical history	• Age • Sex • Underlying conditions • Allergies (especially any pertaining to vaccines, eggs, or latex) • Medications
Special conditions	• Pregnancy (including trimester) • Breastfeeding • Disability or handicap • Immunocompromising conditions or medications • Older age • Psychiatric condition • Seizure disorder • Recent surgery • Recent cardiopulmonary event • Recent cerebrovascular event • History of Guillain-Barré syndrome
Immunization history	• Routine vaccines • Travel vaccines
Prior travel experience	• Experience with malaria chemoprophylaxis • Experience with altitude • Illnesses related to prior travel
Trip Details	
Itinerary	• Countries and specific regions, including order of countries if >1 country • Rural or urban
Timing	• Trip duration • Season of travel • Time to departure

(continued)

Table 2-1. Information necessary for a risk assessment during pretravel consultations (continued)

Reason for travel	• Tourism • Business • Visiting friends and relatives • Volunteer, missionary, or aid work • Research or education • Adventure • Pilgrimage • Adoption • Seeking health care (medical tourism)
Travel style	• Independent travel or package tour • Propensity for "adventurous" eating • Traveler risk tolerance • General hygiene standards at destination • Modes of transportation • Accommodations (such as tourist or luxury hotel, guest house, hostel or budget hotel, dormitory, local home or host family, or tent)
Special activities	• Disaster relief • Medical care (providing or receiving) • High altitude • Diving • Cruise ship • Rafting or other water exposure • Cycling • Extreme sports • Spelunking • Anticipated interactions with animals

reminding the traveler of ubiquitous risks, such as injury, foodborne and waterborne infections, vectorborne disease, respiratory tract infections, and bloodborne and sexually transmitted infections. Written information is essential to supplement the discussion and highlight key advice for travelers. Balancing the cautions with an appreciation of the positive aspects of the journey leads to a more meaningful pretravel consultation. Attention to the cost of recommended interventions may be critical. Some travelers may not be able to afford all of the recommended immunizations and medications, a situation that requires prioritizing interventions. (See *Perspectives:* Prioritizing for the Resource-Limited Traveler later in this chapter.)

Assess Individual Risk

Many elements merit consideration in assessing a traveler's health risks (Table 2-1). Certain travelers may confront special risks. Recent hospitalization for serious problems may lead the advisor to recommend delaying travel. Air travel is contraindicated for certain conditions, such as <3 weeks after an uncomplicated myocardial infarction and <10 days after thoracic or abdominal surgery. The travel health provider and traveler should consult with the relevant health care providers most familiar with the underlying illnesses. Other travelers with specific risks include travelers who are visiting friends and relatives, long-term travelers, travelers with chronic illnesses, immunocompromised travelers, pregnant travelers, and travelers with small children. More comprehensive discussion on advising travelers with specific needs is available in Chapter 8. Providers should determine whether recent outbreaks or other safety notices have been posted for the traveler's destination; information is available on the CDC website and in various other resources.

In addition to recognizing the traveler's characteristics, health background, and destination-specific risks, the exposures related to special activities also merit discussion. For example, river rafting could expose a traveler to schistosomiasis or leptospirosis, and spelunking in Central America could put the traveler at risk of histoplasmosis. Flying from lowlands to high-altitude areas and trekking or climbing in mountainous regions introduces the risk of altitude illness. Therefore, the provider should inquire about plans for specific activities.

Manage Risk

Immunizations are a crucial component of pretravel consultations, and the risk assessment forms the basis of recommendations for travel vaccines. For example, providers should consider whether there is sufficient time before travel to complete a vaccine series; the purpose of travel and specific destination within a country will inform the need for particular vaccinations. At the same time, the pretravel consultation presents an opportunity to update routine vaccines (Table 2-2). Particular attention should be paid to vaccines for which immunity may have waned over time or a recent immunocompromising condition (such as after a hematopoietic stem cell transplant). Asking the question, "Do you have any plans to travel again in the next 1–2 years?" may help the traveler justify an immunization for this particular trip, such as rabies preexposure or Japanese encephalitis. Travelers should receive a record of immunizations administered and instructions to follow up as needed to complete a vaccine series.

Table 2-2. Vaccines to update or consider during pretravel consultations

VACCINE	TRAVEL-RELATED OCCURRENCES AND RECOMMENDATIONS
Routine Vaccines	
Haemophilus influenzae type b	No report of travel-related infection, although organism is ubiquitous.
Hepatitis B	Recommended for travelers visiting countries where HBsAg prevalence is ≥2%. Vaccination may be considered for all international travelers, regardless of destination, depending upon the traveler's behavioral risk and potential for exposure as determined by the provider and traveler.
Human papillomavirus (HPV)	No report of travel-acquired infection; however, sexual activity during travel may lead to HPV and other sexually transmitted infections.
Influenza	Year-round transmission may occur in tropical areas. Outbreaks have occurred on cruise ships, and 2009 influenza A (H1N1) illustrated the rapidity of spread via travel. Novel influenza viruses such as avian influenza H5N1 and H7N9 can be transmitted to travelers visiting areas with circulation of these viruses.
Measles, mumps, rubella	Infections are common in countries and communities that do not immunize children routinely, including Europe. Outbreaks have occurred in the United States as a result of infection in returning travelers.
Meningococcal	Outbreaks occur regularly in sub-Saharan Africa in the "meningitis belt" during the dry season, generally December through June, although transmission may occur at other times for those with close contact with local populations. Outbreaks have occurred with Hajj pilgrimage, and the Kingdom of Saudi Arabia requires the quadrivalent vaccine for pilgrims.

(continued)

Table 2-2. Vaccines to update or consider during pretravel consultations (continued)

VACCINE	TRAVEL-RELATED OCCURRENCES AND RECOMMENDATIONS
Pneumococcal	Organism is ubiquitous, and causal relationship to travel is difficult to establish.
Polio	Unimmunized or underimmunized travelers can become infected with either wild poliovirus or vaccine-derived poliovirus. Because the international spread of wild poliovirus in 2014 was declared a Public Health Emergency of International Concern under the International Health Regulations, temporary recommendations for polio vaccination are in place for countries with wild poliovirus circulation for their residents, long-term visitors, and international travelers.
Rotavirus	Common in developing countries, although not a common cause of travelers' diarrhea in adults. The vaccine is only recommended in young children.
Tetanus, diphtheria, pertussis	Rare cases of diphtheria have been attributed to travel. Pertussis has occurred in travelers, recently in adults whose immunity has waned.
Varicella	Infections are common in countries that do not immunize children routinely, as in most developing countries. Naturally occurring disease also occurs later in tropical countries.
Zoster	Travel (a form of stress) may trigger varicella zoster reactivation, but causal relationship is difficult to establish.
Travel Vaccines	
Cholera	Cases in travelers have occurred recently in association with travel to the Dominican Republic and Haiti.
Hepatitis A	Prevalence patterns of hepatitis A virus infection may vary among regions within a country, and missing or obsolete data present a challenge. Serologic testing may be considered in travelers from highly endemic countries since they may already be immune. Some expert travel clinicians advise people traveling outside the United States to consider hepatitis A vaccination regardless of their country of destination.
Japanese encephalitis	Rare cases have occurred, estimated at <1 case/1 million travelers to endemic countries.
Rabies	Rabies preexposure immunization simplifies postexposure immunoprophylaxis, as adequately screened immunoglobulin may be difficult to obtain in many destinations.
Tickborne encephalitis (vaccine not available in the United States)	Cases have been identified in travelers with an estimated risk of 1/10,000 person-months in travelers. Endemic areas are expanding in Europe.
Typhoid	UK surveillance found the highest risk to be travel to India (6 cases/100,000 visits), Pakistan (9 cases/100,000 visits), and Bangladesh (21 cases/100,000 visits), although risk is substantial in many destinations.
Yellow fever	Risk occurs mainly in defined areas of sub-Saharan Africa and the Amazonian regions of South America. Some countries require proof of vaccination for entry. For travelers visiting multiple countries, order of travel may make a difference in the requirements.

Abbreviation: HBsAg, hepatitis B surface antigen.

Another major focus of pretravel consultations for many destinations is the prevention of malaria. Malaria continues to cause substantial morbidity and mortality in travelers. In 2011, the number of US malaria cases reported to CDC was the highest since 1971; therefore, pretravel consultation must carefully assess travelers' risk for malaria and recommend preventive measures. For travelers going to malaria-endemic countries, it is imperative to discuss malaria transmission, ways to reduce risk, and recommendations for chemoprophylaxis.

Travelers with underlying health conditions require attention to their health issues as they relate to the destination and activities. For example, a traveler with a history of cardiac disease should carry medical reports, including a recent electrocardiogram. Asthma may flare in a traveler visiting a polluted city or from physical exertion during a hike; travelers should be encouraged to discuss with their primary care provider how to plan for treatment and bring necessary medication in case of asthma exacerbation. Travelers should be counseled on how they can find reputable medical facilities at their destination, such as using the ISTM website (www.istm.org) or the American Society of Tropical Medicine and Hygiene website (www.astmh.org) to find suitable clinics. Any allergies or serious medical conditions should be identified on a bracelet or a card to expedite medical care in emergency situations.

The pretravel consultation also provides another setting to remind travelers of basic health practices during travel, including frequent handwashing, wearing seatbelts, and using car seats for infants and children. Topics to be explored are numerous and could be organized into a checklist, placing priority on the most serious and frequently encountered issues (Table 2-3). General issues such as

Table 2-3. Major topics for discussion during pretravel consultations

Immunizations	• Review routine immunizations and those travel immunizations indicated for the specific itinerary and based on the traveler's medical history. • Discuss utility of titers when records are unavailable or unreliable, particularly for measles, mumps, rubella, and hepatitis A. • Screen for chronic hepatitis B for people born in countries with HBsAg prevalence ≥2% (see Map 3-4). • Discuss indications for, effectiveness of, and adverse reactions to immunizations.
Malaria chemoprophylaxis	• Determine if there is a risk of malaria. • Discuss personal protective measures. • Discuss risks and benefits of chemoprophylaxis and recommended choices of chemoprophylaxis for the itinerary.
Other vectorborne diseases	• Define risk of disease in specific itinerary and insect precautions needed.
Respiratory illnesses	• Discuss areas of particular concern (such as avian influenza in Asia or MERS in the Arabian Peninsula). • Consider influenza treatment for high-risk travelers.
Travelers' diarrhea	• Recommend strategies to decrease risk of diarrhea. • Discuss antibiotics for self-treatment, adjunct medications such as loperamide, and staying hydrated.
Altitude illness	• Determine if the itinerary puts the traveler at risk of altitude illness. • Discuss preventive measures such as gradual ascent, adequate hydration, and medications to prevent and treat.

(continued)

Table 2-3. Major topics for discussion during pretravel consultations (continued)

Other environmental hazards	• Caution travelers to avoid contact with animals to reduce the potential for bites and scratches that can transmit rabies. • Advise travelers to avoid walking barefoot to avoid certain parasitic infections. • Advise travelers to avoid wading or swimming in freshwater where there is risk for schistosomiasis or leptospirosis. • Remind travelers to apply sunscreen to skin exposed to the sun.
Personal safety	• Discuss precautions travelers can take to minimize risks specific to the trip, such as traffic accidents, alcohol excess, personal assault, robbery, or drowning. • Provide information on travel health and medical evacuation insurance. • Advise travelers to look for security bulletins related to their destination and consider areas to avoid.
Sexual health and bloodborne pathogens	• Caution the traveler to avoid activities that can lead to sexually transmitted infections, unwanted pregnancy, or bloodborne infections. • Remind travelers to use condoms if they do have sex. • Inform travelers who will provide health care overseas what to do in case of needlestick or bloodborne pathogen exposure.
Disease-specific counseling	• Remind travelers to hand carry medications and supplies. • Advise travelers to prepare for exacerbations or complications from underlying disease.

Abbreviations: HBsAg, hepatitis B surface antigen; MERS, Middle East respiratory syndrome.

preventing injury and sunburn also deserve mention. Written information is essential to supplement oral advice and enable travelers to review the instructions from their clinic visits; educational material is available on the CDC Travelers Health webpage (http://www.cdc.gov/travel). Advice on self-treatable conditions may minimize the need for travelers to seek medical care while abroad and possibly lead to faster return to good health.

Self-Treatable Conditions

Despite providers' best efforts, some travelers will become ill. Obtaining reliable and timely medical care during travel can be problematic in many destinations. As a result, prescribing certain medications in advance can empower the traveler to self-diagnose and treat common health problems. With some activities in remote settings, such as trekking, the only alternative to self-treatment would be no treatment. Pretravel counseling may actually result in a more accurate self-diagnosis and treatment than relying on local medical care in some areas. In addition, the increasing awareness of substandard and counterfeit drugs in pharmacies in the developing world (as many as

50% of the drugs on the shelves) makes it more important for travelers to bring quality manufactured drugs with them from a reliable supplier in their own country (see *Perspectives: Pharmaceutical Quality & Falsified Drugs* later in this chapter).

Travel health providers need to recognize the conditions for which the traveler may be at risk and educate the traveler about the diagnosis and treatment of those particular conditions. The keys to successful self-treatment strategies are providing a simple disease or condition definition, providing a treatment, and educating the traveler about the expected outcome of treatment. Using travelers' diarrhea as an example, a practitioner could provide the following advice:

● "Travelers' diarrhea" is the sudden onset of abnormally loose, frequent stools.

● Most cases will resolve within 2–5 days, and symptoms can be managed with loperamide or bismuth subsalicylate.

● For diarrhea severe enough to interrupt travel plans, an antibiotic can be prescribed that travelers can carry with them (see Travelers' Diarrhea section in this chapter).

- The traveler should feel better within 6–24 hours.

- If symptoms persist for 24–36 hours despite self-treatment, it may be necessary to seek medical attention.

To minimize the potential negative effects of a self-treatment strategy, the recommendations should follow a few key points:

- Drugs recommended must be safe, well tolerated, and effective for use as self-treatment.

- A drug's toxicity or potential for harm, if used incorrectly or in an overdose situation, should be minimal.

- Simple and clear directions are critical. Consider providing handouts describing how to use the drugs. Keeping the directions simple will increase the effectiveness of the strategy.

The following are some of the most common situations in which people would find self-treatment useful. The extent of self-treatment recommendations offered to the traveler should reflect the remoteness and difficulty of travel and the availability of reliable medical care at the particular destination. The recommended self-treatment options for each disease are provided in the designated section of the Yellow Book or discussed below.

- Travelers' diarrhea (see section in this chapter)

- Altitude illness (see section in this chapter)

- Jet lag (see section in this chapter)

- Motion sickness (see section in this chapter)

- Respiratory infections (see section in this chapter)

- Skin conditions: skin reactions due to allergic or irritant triggers usually respond to topical steroids; discomfort from superficial fungal infections respond to antifungal creams. See Chapter 5, Skin and Soft Tissue Infections in Returned Travelers.

- Urinary tract infections: common among many women; carrying an antibiotic for empiric treatment may be valuable.

- Vaginal yeast infections: self-treatment course of patient's preferred antifungal medication can be prescribed for women who are prone to infections, sexually active, or who may be receiving antibiotics for other reasons (including doxycycline for malaria chemoprophylaxis).

- Occupational exposure to HIV (see Chapter 8, Health Care Workers)

- Malaria self-treatment (see Chapter 3, Malaria)

In sum, travelers should be encouraged to carry a travel health kit with prescription and nonprescription medications. Providers should review medication lists for possible drug interactions. More detailed information for providers and travelers is given in Chapter 2, Travel Health Kits; supplementary travel health kit information for travelers with specific needs is given in Chapter 8.

BIBLIOGRAPHY

1. Freedman DO, Chen LH, Kozarsky P. Medical considerations before travel. N Engl J Med. 2016 July 21;375:247–60.

2. Hatz CFR, Chen LH. Pre-travel consultation. In: Keystone JS, Freedman DO, Kozarsky PE, Connor BA, Nothdurft HD, editors. Travel Medicine. 3rd ed. Philadelphia: Saunders Elsevier; 2013. pp. 31–6.

3. Hill DR, Ericsson CD, Pearson RD, Keystone JS, Freedman DO, Kozarsky PE, et al. The practice of travel medicine: guidelines by the Infectious Diseases Society of America. Clin Infect Dis. 2006 Dec 15;43(12):1499–539.

4. International Society of Travel Medicine. Body of knowledge for the practice of travel medicine—2012. Atlanta: International Society of Travel Medicine; 2012 [cited 2016 Oct. 1]; Available from: http://www.istm.org/bodyofknowledge.

5. LaRocque RC, Rao SR, Lee J, Ansdell V, Yates JA, Schwartz BS, et al. Global TravEpiNet: a national consortium of clinics providing care to international travelers—analysis of demographic characteristics, travel destinations, and pretravel healthcare of high-risk US international travelers, 2009–2011. Clin Infect Dis. 2012 Feb 15;54(4):455–62.

6. Leder K, Chen LH, Wilson ME. Aggregate travel vs. single trip assessment: arguments for cumulative risk analysis. Vaccine. 2012 Mar 28;30(15):2600–4.

7. Leder K, Torresi J, Libman MD, Cramer JP, Castelli F, Schlagenhauf P, et al. GeoSentinel surveillance of illness in returned travelers, 2007–2011. Ann Intern Med. 2013 Mar 19;158(6):456–68.

8. Schwartz BS, Larocque RC, Ryan ET. In the clinic: travel medicine. Ann Intern Med. 2012 Jun 5;156(11):ITC6:1–16.

9. Steffen R, Behrens RH, Hill RD, Greenaway C, Leder K. Vaccine-preventable travel health risks: what is the evidence—what are the gaps? J Travel Med. 2015;22(1):1–12.

10. Steffen R, Hill DR, DuPont HL. Traveler's Diarrhea: a clinical review. JAMA. 2015 Jan 6, 2015;313(1):71–80.

2

TRAVELERS' PERCEPTION OF RISK

David R. Shlim

Travel medicine is based on the concept of the reduction of risk. In the context of travel medicine, "risk" refers to the possibility of harm during the course of a planned trip. Some risks may be avoidable, and others may not. Vaccine-preventable diseases may be mostly avoidable, depending on the risk of the disease and the protective efficacy of the vaccine. Non-disease risks, such as motor vehicle accidents or drowning, account for a much higher percentage of deaths among travelers than infectious diseases.

For many years, travel medicine practitioners have felt that if they knew the statistics for a given risk, they could objectively advise travelers about that risk. However, it has become clear that the perception and tolerance of risk are subjective factors that must be considered when addressing risks of travel. Travel health providers may know statistics for a given risk, but whether the risk is considered high or low depends on the perception of the traveler or the travel medicine provider. For example, the risk of dying while trekking in Nepal is 15

deaths per 100,000 trekkers, but there is no objective way to determine whether this risk is high or low. When the manuscript that reported this risk of dying while trekking was peer-reviewed, one reviewer wrote, "You need to emphasize that these data show how dangerous trekking actually is." The other reviewer wrote, "You should make a point of stating that these data show how safe trekking is."

The subjective sense of risk is based on one's perception of risk ("15 per 100,000 means it's dangerous") and one's tolerance for risk ("it may be 15 per 100,000, but it's worth it"). This subjective sense of risk suffuses the field of travel medicine, but it is rarely discussed. Some travelers canceled travel plans to Asia because of their fear of H5N1 avian influenza, even though the actual risk to travelers was virtually zero. Other travelers plan to ascend Mount Everest, even though the risk of dying during an Everest climb is 1 in 40.

Regardless of the perception and tolerance of risk, the hazards associated with travel cannot be eliminated,

just as the risks of staying home are not zero. Even the act of trying to prevent a risk—such as yellow fever—can lead to a fatal reaction to the vaccine in rare cases. Therefore, the goal in travel and in travel medicine should be skillfully managing risk, rather than trying to eliminate risk. The pretravel consultation is an opportunity to discuss risks and develop plans that minimize these risks. Each traveler will have individual concepts about the risks and benefits of vaccines, prophylaxis, and behavior modification.

Travelers should also consider the psychological and emotional aspects of foreign travel. Culture shock can occur on either end of a journey: on arrival when one encounters an entirely strange new world, and on return when one's own world may temporarily appear unfamiliar. Travelers with underlying psychiatric conditions should be cautious when heading out to a stressful new environment, particularly if they are traveling alone.

Travel medicine providers should promote the understanding of the concept of

(continued)

TRAVELERS' PERCEPTION OF RISK (CONTINUED)

commitment, the idea that certain parts of a journey cannot easily be reversed. A person trekking into a remote area may need to accept that rescue, if available at all, may be delayed for days. A person who has a myocardial infarction in a country with no advanced cardiac services may have a difficult time getting to definitive medical care. If the traveler has already contemplated these concerns and accepted them, it will be easier to deal with them if they come to pass.

Travel medicine practitioners should explore their own perception and tolerance of risk, so that they can help travelers find their individual comfort level when making decisions about destinations, activities, and prophylactic measures.

Perspectives sections are written as editorial discussions aiming to add depth and clinical perspective to the official recommendations contained in the book. The views and opinions expressed in this section are those of the author and do not necessarily represent the official position of CDC.

PRIORITIZING CARE FOR THE RESOURCE-LIMITED TRAVELER

Zoon Wangu, Elizabeth D. Barnett

Travelers seen in pretravel clinic consultations often have financial constraints. Prioritizing immunizations and prophylactic medications should be part of an individualized assessment based on the travel itinerary, efficacy and safety of vaccines and medications, and associated costs. Travelers must often pay out of pocket for pretravel care, as many health insurance plans do not cover travel immunizations or prophylaxis. As an example, the estimated cost of a US pretravel consultation for a backpacker planning a 4-week trip to West Africa may be as high as $1,400 for the initial consultation and vaccinations, excluding malaria chemoprophylaxis. Travelers with limited budgets may be at higher risk for travel-associated infections, as they often visit remote areas, stay in lower-grade accommodations, and are more likely to eat local street food. Therefore, the cost of disease (such as malaria) may, in many cases, outweigh costs of vaccination and prophylaxis. The financial benefits of obtaining travel

health insurance and evacuation insurance before travel must also be considered (see Travel Insurance, Travel Health Insurance, & Medical Evacuation Insurance later in this chapter). Clinicians need to understand travelers' financial constraints in order to provide realistic recommendations. The variety of insurance plans, number of travelers without adequate insurance coverage, and number of student and budget travelers challenges even the most savvy travel medicine clinicians. This section provides guidance for busy practitioners in prioritizing vaccine and prophylaxis choices.

VACCINES
Required Vaccines

Only 2 vaccines are required categorically for some travelers: meningococcal vaccine for pilgrims traveling to Mecca during the Hajj and yellow fever vaccine for travelers to certain countries in Africa and South America (see Chapter 3, Yellow Fever & Malaria Information, by Country). If either of these vaccines is required for an itinerary, prioritize it since

the traveler may be denied entry to the country without proof of vaccination. Note that travelers who may be staying in a yellow fever–endemic country only briefly (such as during an airport layover) may still need evidence of vaccination to enter other countries on their itinerary. In a few specific circumstances, travelers to countries that are exporting polio may be asked to show proof of polio vaccination before they are allowed to leave those countries if they have spent >4 weeks in the country (see Chapter 3, Poliomyelitis).

Routine Vaccines

All travelers should be up-to-date with routine vaccines before international travel, regardless of destination. The benefits of vaccines extend beyond the travel period, and in many cases lifelong immunity is achieved. Routine vaccines are generally associated with lower costs, since they are mass-produced as part of the scheduled national childhood and adult vaccination programs, and many health insurance plans will

(continued)

reimburse the patient for the cost of vaccine administration. If cost of routine vaccines is a limitation, a traveler can explore opportunities for obtaining them in a health department or primary care setting, where cost may be lower than in a travel clinic. Prioritize the routine vaccines that protect against diseases for which the traveler is most likely to be at general risk. At this time, top priorities for most destinations would include vaccines against influenza, measles, and hepatitis A and B.

Some travelers may be immune to the disease for which immunization is being considered. Testing for antibody concentrations may be covered by insurance when vaccines are not. Testing for immunity to diseases such as measles, varicella, and hepatitis A and B can help determine whether vaccination is needed.

Recommended Vaccines

Consider time until departure, risk of disease at the destination, effectiveness and safety of vaccine, and likelihood of repeat travel. For example, parenteral typhoid vaccine may be less cost-effective for certain travelers (especially when departures are imminent and trip duration is short) because of the relatively low efficacy, short duration of protection, and time needed for onset of protection (≥2 weeks). On the other hand, oral typhoid vaccine has a longer duration of protection, and time to protection is shorter, approximately 1 week.

When considering rabies vaccine for resource-limited travelers, consider the risk of animal exposure, access to local health care, and availability of rabies immune globulin and rabies vaccine at the traveler's destination. Travelers who decline pre-exposure immunization should have a plan of action if an exposure occurs. In up to 37% of locations worldwide, rabies vaccine or immune globulin are available only sometimes or never.

Review the itinerary in detail to determine the need for Japanese encephalitis vaccine. Some travelers may be able to obtain vaccine at lower cost outside the United States. Those who decline vaccine should have a clear understanding of when and how to use insect repellents and other measures to prevent mosquito bites.

MALARIA CHEMOPROPHYLAXIS

Every pretravel consultation should include detailed advice about preventing mosquito bites (see Protection against Mosquitoes, Ticks, & Other Arthropods later in this chapter). Malaria chemoprophylaxis, if needed, should be offered based on the risk profile of the traveler, taking into account possible financial burden. The risk of acquiring malaria varies widely, depending on destination, accommodations, and activities during travel. Malaria risk is decreasing in many countries, and up-to-date sources of risk areas in the destination country should be used to advise travelers. Costs associated with the different regimens vary widely. For example, based on current prices in the United States, a prophylactic treatment course for a 3-week trip to a malaria-endemic destination would cost $120–$250 for doxycycline, $50–$100 for chloroquine, $95–$120 for mefloquine, and $200–$225 for atovaquone-proguanil (depending on health insurance and other factors). Atovaquone-proguanil cost may be equivalent to that of mefloquine for short trips, but mefloquine (or chloroquine, in the few regions where malaria remains susceptible) will be more cost-effective for trips lasting ≥2 weeks. Travelers who raise the question of purchasing antimalarial drugs at their destination must be advised about the risk of inappropriate, substandard, and counterfeit medications and discouraged from this practice (see *Perspectives:* Pharmaceutical Quality & Falsified Drugs later in this chapter).

PREVENTIVE BEHAVIORS

Educate about alternative ways to reduce risk, especially when immunization is not possible. For example, advise travelers to avoid animal bites, use insect precautions, and observe food and water precautions to the best of their ability.

Budget travelers and those who cannot afford travel vaccines will continue to challenge travel medicine practitioners. All travelers can benefit from multiple strategies to safeguard their health during travel, in addition to vaccination and prophylaxis. These strategies include following safety (especially road traffic safety) and security guidelines, observing sun protection, avoiding food hazards, and following safe sex practices. Following insect precautions is essential to prevent dengue and chikungunya viruses and has become especially pertinent with the emergence of Zika virus in Latin America. Travelers can be reassured that the actions they take to avoid these preventable hazards may, in the long run, protect against travel-associated risks that are more prevalent than are certain vaccine-preventable diseases.

BIBLIOGRAPHY

1. Adachi K, Coleman MS, Khan N, Jentes ES, Arguin P, Rao SR, et al. Economics of malaria prevention in US travelers to West Africa. Clin Infect Dis. 2014 Jan;58(1):11–21.

2. Jentes ES, Blanton JD, Johnson KJ, Petersen BW, Lamias MJ, Robertson K, et al. The global availability of rabies immune globulin and rabies vaccine in clinics providing indirect care to travelers. J Travel Med. 2014 Jan-Feb;21(1):62–6.

3. Johnson DF, Leder K, Torresi J. Hepatitis B and C infection in international travelers. J Travel Med. 2013 May-Jun;20(3):194–202.

4. Mangtani P, Roberts JA. Economic evaluations of travelers' vaccinations. In: Zuckerman JN, Jong EC, editors. Travelers' Vaccines. 2nd ed. Shelton (CT): People's Medical Publishing House; 2010. pp. 553–67.

5. Steffen R, Connor BA. Vaccines in travel health: from risk assessment to priorities. J Travel Med. 2005 Jan-Feb;12(1):26–35.

6. Wu D, Guo CY. Epidemiology and prevention of hepatitis A in travelers. J Travel Med. 2013 Nov-Dec;20(6):394–9.

Perspectives sections are written as editorial discussions aiming to add depth and clinical perspective to the official recommendations contained in the book. The views and opinions expressed in this section are those of the authors and do not necessarily represent the official position of CDC.

THE NEED FOR A COST ANALYSIS TO JUSTIFY THE TRAVEL MEDICINE CONSULT

Emily P. Hyle, Edward T. Ryan

CLINICAL BENEFITS OF THE PRETRAVEL MEDICAL ENCOUNTER

The pretravel medical encounter usually consists of 3 components—vaccination, prophylaxis, and education—each of which is intended to reduce the risk of illness during travel. Vaccination and prophylaxis prevent disease among travelers. Fewer data exist on the effect of pretravel education and advice. For example, educating travelers on ways to limit exposure to foodborne and waterborne diseases has not been shown to have a demonstrable effect on the risk of travelers' diarrhea.

The pretravel encounter has more clinical benefit when the risks of acquiring a travel-related illness are greater. Such risks are influenced by regional destination, itinerary, travel duration, and season, but few data quantify the risk to travelers. Our best data for estimating disease risk at a destination often reflect disease prevalence among the local population and may not correlate with the risk to travelers. Vaccine efficacy data are also too often extrapolated from studies unrelated to travel. Travel-related risks fluctuate and are affected by evolving destination infrastructure and economy, advancements in disease-control programs, and the emergence of infections into new zones. The risk of travel-related illness is also traveler-specific. Some travelers participate in more high-risk behavior, and some travelers (such as those who are immunocompromised) may be more predisposed to infection or complications.

Benefits of a pretravel encounter may also extend beyond the immediate duration of travel, and immunity resulting from vaccination can overlap multiple itineraries. Travelers are known to spread extremely contagious infections (such as measles), highly morbid diseases (such as Middle East respiratory syndrome or Ebola), and highly drug-resistant pathogens (such as NDM-1–expressing bacteria or multidrug-resistant *Mycobacterium tuberculosis*). Reducing importations of communicable diseases by returning travelers can have far-reaching public health implications by diminishing outbreaks.

ECONOMICS OF THE PRETRAVEL ENCOUNTER

The pretravel encounter incurs direct costs, including clinic visit fees (as a component of a primary care visit or dedicated specialist visit), vaccines, and prescribed drugs, as well as indirect costs associated with travel to clinic and missed work. When considering costs and other components of resource use, it is essential to consider the perspective of who pays and who benefits: the traveler, the health care payer, or society.

Economic benefits include when the pretravel encounter prevents a travel-related illness; therefore, costs of the travel-related illness prevented should be considered as cost savings. A frequently overlooked economic aspect linked to the pretravel medical encounter is its potential to reduce the incidence of many travel-related illnesses that have public health implications. The introduction of measles or hepatitis A into a community by a returning traveler prompts expensive public health and infection-control responses. Such costs are largely borne by the public health sector and therefore do not usually appear in the financial calculus of the individual traveler or the insurance carrier.

MATHEMATICAL MODELING FOR TRAVEL MEDICINE

Mathematical modeling allows for a comprehensive investigation of the value of the pretravel medical encounter. By incorporating best estimates of benefits and costs for pretravel encounters, travel exposures, and travel-related illness, a model can project possible outcomes and costs for different travelers, exposures, risks of infection, and effectiveness of pretravel interventions singly or in combination.

A comprehensive model of the pretravel encounter would examine the range of possible illnesses posed by an itinerary, including those that present long after return (such as tuberculosis or HIV) or that lead to chronic sequelae (such as neurologic damage from cerebral malaria, Japanese encephalitis, or Zika infection). Such a model would incorporate the effect of any pretravel intervention on mitigating the risk of infection while traveling as well as possible side effects of the intervention. Models should incorporate the costs of public health–related resources and expenditures relating to the importation of pathogens,

not only to trace and limit ongoing disease transmission but also to mitigate the risk of establishing environmental or animal reservoirs in home communities. Such a model could then be used to examine the effect of a pretravel encounter on different populations of travelers. Because only some travelers seek pretravel evaluation, a model could examine the effect when different percentages of the traveling population obtain pretravel evaluation.

A modeling approach can also be used to perform sensitivity analyses, in which a range of values for a specific input parameter is examined in terms of the impact on the outcome of interest. Sensitivity analyses can evaluate thresholds, or the specific value at which a parameter results in a meaningful change in clinical outcomes or costs. Uncertain data estimates or assumptions are assessed by using a model in a similar fashion, investigating at what values such estimates will result in clinically meaningful changes. Results from a pretravel model could highlight where further data would be high-yield and worth investing research dollars.

A logical way forward is to begin by focusing initial analyses around a number of core areas. Studies have been published that investigate a specific component of the pretravel encounter, including malaria prophylaxis, hepatitis

A vaccination, typhoid vaccination, and travelers' diarrhea strategies. Unfortunately, many of these analyses were performed decades ago. A reasonable approach would therefore be to develop modeling approaches for major groups of travel-related illnesses, using available current data regarding the pretravel encounter from the GlobalTravEpiNet (GTEN) consortium (see Chapter 1, Travel Epidemiology) and other large consortiums. The goals of such analyses could include defining core metrics for pretravel encounters, improving the value of pretravel encounters, and examining where improvements in pretravel medicine would result in maximally improved patient outcomes and cost-effectiveness. These separate models could then be incorporated into a single integrated analysis that would address a comprehensive pretravel encounter. Such an approach will not be easy, but it is necessary.

BIBLIOGRAPHY

1. Adachi K, Coleman MS, Khan N, Jentes ES, Arguin P, Rao SR, et al. Economics of malaria prevention in US travelers to West Africa. Clin Infect Dis. 2014 Jan;58(1):11–21.

2. Behrens RH, Roberts JA. Economic appraisal of prophylactic measures against malaria, hepatitis A, and typhoid in travellers. BMJ Clinical Research Ed. 1994 Oct 8;309(6959):918–22.

(continued)

THE NEED FOR A COST ANALYSIS TO JUSTIFY THE TRAVEL MEDICINE CONSULT (CONTINUED)

3. Ortega-Sanchez IR, Vijayaraghavan M, Barskey AE, Wallace GS. The economic burden of sixteen measles outbreaks on United States public health departments in 2011. Vaccine. 2014;32(11):1311–7.

4. Papadimitropoulos V, Vergidis PI, Bliziotis I, Falagas ME. Vaccination against typhoid fever in travellers: a

cost-effectiveness approach. Clin Microbiol Infect. 2004 Aug;10(8):681–3.

5. Reves RR, Johnson PC, Ericsson CD, DuPont HL. A cost-effectiveness comparison of the use of antimicrobial agents for treatment or prophylaxis of travelers' diarrhea. Arch Intern Med. 1988;148(11):2421–7.

6. Siegel JE, Weinstein MC, Russell LB, Gold MR. Recommendations for reporting cost-effectiveness analyses. JAMA. 1996;276(16): 1339–41.

7. Van Doorslaer E, Tormans G, Van Damme P. Cost-effectiveness analysis of vaccination against hepatitis A in travellers. J Med Virol. 1994;44(4):463–9.

Perspectives sections are written as editorial discussions aiming to add depth and clinical perspective to the official recommendations contained in the book. The views and opinions expressed in this section are those of the authors and do not necessarily represent the official position of CDC.

GENERAL RECOMMENDATIONS FOR VACCINATION & IMMUNOPROPHYLAXIS

Andrew T. Kroger, Raymond A. Strikas

Recommendations for the use of vaccines and other biologic products (such as immune globulin [IG] products) in the United States are developed by the Advisory Committee on Immunization Practices (ACIP) and are harmonized with ACIP liaison organizations including the American Academy of Pediatrics, the American Academy of Family Physicians, the American College of Physicians, the American College of Obstetricians and Gynecologists, and others. Recommendations voted on by the ACIP are reviewed by the CDC director and, if adopted, become official recommendations of the Department of Health and Human Services/CDC upon publication in CDC's *Morbidity and Mortality Weekly Report* (MMWR). ACIP recommendations are based on scientific evidence of benefits (disease immunity) and risks (vaccine adverse reactions) and, where few or no data are available, on expert opinion. Recommendations include information on general

immunization issues and the use of specific vaccines. Box 2-1 provides more information about ACIP. This section is based primarily on the ACIP General Recommendations on Immunization.

Evaluation of people before travel should include a review and provision of routine vaccines recommended based on age and other individual characteristics. Additionally, some routine vaccines are recommended at earlier ages for international travelers. For example, MMR (measles-mumps-rubella) vaccine is recommended for infants aged 6–11 months who travel abroad to protect them from measles. Recommendations for specific vaccines related to travel will depend on itinerary, duration of travel, and host factors. Vaccinations against diphtheria, tetanus, pertussis, measles, mumps, rubella, varicella, poliomyelitis, hepatitis A, hepatitis B, *Haemophilus influenzae* type b (Hib), rotavirus, human papillomavirus (HPV), and pneumococcal and meningococcal

2

BOX 2-1. The Advisory Committee on Immunization Practices (ACIP)

In 1964, the Department of Health, Education, and Welfare chartered the Advisory Committee on Immunization Practices (ACIP) to provide guidance to CDC for making immunization policy. Guidance includes scheduling of vaccine doses, specific risk groups for whom vaccination is recommended, and vaccine contraindications and precautions.

ACIP is composed of 15 voting members selected by the Secretary of Health and Human Services. The ACIP chair, a consumer representative, and 13 members are balanced among various sectors, including academic immunology, medicine, and public health. In addition to the 15 voting members, the committee includes 8 ex officio members representing federal agencies and 35 nonvoting representatives of liaison organizations with broad responsibilities for vaccine development, administration of vaccines to various segments of the population,

and operation of immunization programs. ACIP is subdivided into 4 permanent workgroups that address child/adolescent immunization schedules, adult immunization schedules, influenza vaccine, and general immunization issues. In addition to the 4 permanent workgroups, additional workgroups focus on particular vaccines. Input into the development of immunization schedules is shared with professional organizations, including the American Academy of Pediatrics, American College of Physicians, American Academy of Family Physicians, American College of Obstetricians and Gynecologists, and American College of Nurse-Midwives.

ACIP workgroups are led by a member of ACIP who works in close collaboration with a CDC workgroup lead staff member. Members of the vaccine pharmaceutical industry may not serve as workgroup members. The workgroup develops consensus

on various policy points, then the CDC workgroup lead writes specific content for presentation to the ACIP at large. When it is difficult to achieve consensus, options with plans are developed and presented to the ACIP at large for a vote.

ACIP holds 3 public meetings a year during which the various workgroups present content that has been developed and is ready for discussion or voting. Sometimes ACIP members are involved in academic vaccine research supported by the pharmaceutical industry. These members must state these conflicts and must recuse themselves from votes regarding vaccines manufactured by companies from which they receive support. The result of various discussions and votes is an ACIP document published in CDC's *Morbidity and Mortality Weekly Report* (www.cdc.gov/mmwr), representing the official policy of the Department of Health and Human Services.

invasive disease are routinely administered in the United States, usually in childhood or adolescence. Influenza vaccine is routinely recommended for all people aged ≥6 months, each year. A dose of herpes zoster (shingles) vaccine is recommended for adults aged ≥60 years. If a person does not have a history of adequate protection against these diseases, immunizations appropriate to age and previous immunization status should be obtained, whether or not international travel is planned. A visit to a clinician for travel-related immunizations should be seen as an opportunity to bring an incompletely vaccinated person up-to-date on his or her routine vaccinations.

Both the child and adolescent vaccination schedules, and an adult vaccination schedule, are published annually. Clinicians should obtain the

most current schedules from the CDC Vaccines and Immunization website (www.cdc.gov/vaccines/schedules). The text and many tables of this publication present recommendations for the use, number of doses, dose intervals, adverse reactions, precautions, and contraindications for vaccines and toxoids that may be indicated for travelers. Recommendations for travelers are not always the same as routine recommendations. For instance, most adults born after 1956 are recommended to receive 1 dose of MMR vaccine; however, international travelers of this age are recommended to receive 2 doses. For specific vaccines and toxoids, additional details on background, adverse reactions, precautions, and contraindications, refer to the respective ACIP recommendations (www.cdc.gov/vaccines/acip/index.html).

SPACING OF IMMUNOBIOLOGICS

Simultaneous Administration

With some exceptions (such as PCV13 and PPSV23, as well as PCV13 and MenACWY-D [Menactra]), all commonly used vaccines can safely and effectively be given simultaneously (on the same day) at separate sites without impairing antibody responses or increasing rates of adverse reactions. This knowledge is particularly helpful for international travelers, for whom exposure to several infectious diseases might be imminent. Simultaneous administration of all indicated vaccines is encouraged for people who are the recommended age to receive these vaccines and for whom no contraindications exist. If not administered on the same day, an inactivated vaccine may be given at any time before or after a different inactivated vaccine or a live-virus vaccine.

The immune response to an injected or intranasal live-virus vaccine (such as MMR, varicella, yellow fever, or live attenuated influenza vaccines) might be impaired if administered within 28 days of another live-virus vaccine (within 30 days for yellow fever vaccine). Whenever possible, injected live-virus vaccines administered on different days should be given ≥28 days apart (≥30 days for yellow fever vaccine). If 2 injected or intranasal live-virus vaccines are not administered on the same day but <28 days apart (<30 days for yellow fever vaccine), the second vaccine should be repeated in ≥28 days (≥30 days for yellow fever vaccine).

Measles and other live-virus vaccines may interfere with the response to tuberculin skin testing and the interferon-γ release assay. Tuberculin testing, if otherwise indicated, can be done either on the day that live-virus vaccines are administered or 4–6 weeks later. Tuberculin skin testing is not a prerequisite for administration of any vaccine. Oral typhoid vaccine, a live attenuated bacterial vaccine, has not been associated with suppressing the response to tuberculosis testing.

Missed Doses and Boosters

All vaccines require a primary dose or series to ensure immunity, and some require periodic repeat, or booster, doses to maintain immunity. Occasionally, the demand for a vaccine may exceed its supply, and providers may have difficulty obtaining vaccines. Information on vaccine shortages and recommendations can be found on the CDC Vaccines and Immunization website at www.cdc.gov/vaccines/hcp/clinical-resources/shortages.html.

In some cases, a scheduled dose of vaccine may not be given on time. If this occurs, the dose should be given at the next visit. However, travelers may forget to return to complete a series or for a booster at the specified time. Available data indicate that intervals between doses longer than those routinely recommended do not affect seroconversion rate or titer when the schedule is completed. Consequently, it is not necessary to restart the series or add doses of any vaccine because of an extended interval between doses. There are some exceptions to this rule. Some experts recommend repeating the series of oral typhoid vaccine if the 4-dose series is extended to more than 3 weeks. If an extended interval passes between doses of the preexposure rabies vaccine series, immune status should be assessed by serologic testing 7–14 days after the final dose in the series.

Antibody-Containing Blood Products

Antibody-containing blood products from the United States, such as immune globulin (IG) products, do not interfere with the immune response to yellow fever vaccine and are not believed to interfere with the response to live typhoid, live attenuated influenza, rotavirus, or zoster vaccines. When MMR and varicella vaccines are given shortly before, simultaneously with, or after an antibody-containing blood product, response to the vaccine can be diminished. The duration of inhibition of MMR and varicella vaccines is related to the dose of IG in the product. MMR and varicella vaccines either should be administered ≥2 weeks before receipt of a blood product or should be delayed 3–11 months after receipt of the blood product, depending on the dose and type of blood product (Table 2-4).

IG administration may become necessary for another indication after MMR or varicella vaccines have been given. In such a situation, the IG may interfere with the immune response to the MMR or varicella vaccines. Vaccine virus replication and stimulation of immunity usually occur 2–3 weeks

Table 2-4. Recommended intervals between administration of antibody-containing products and measles-containing vaccine or varicella-containing vaccine[1]

INDICATION	DOSE AND ROUTE	RECOMMENDED INTERVAL BEFORE MEASLES OR VARICELLA VACCINATION
Blood transfusion		
Red blood cells (RBCs), washed	10 mL/kg (negligible IgG/kg) IV	None
RBCs, adenine-saline added	10 mL/kg (10 mg IgG/kg) IV	3 months
Packed RBCs (hematocrit 65%)[2]	10 mL/kg (60 mg IgG/kg) IV	6 months
Whole blood (hematocrit 35%–50%)[2]	10 mL/kg (80–100 mg IgG/kg) IV	6 months
Plasma/platelet products	10 mL/kg (160 mg IgG/kg) IV	7 months
Botulism immune globulin, intravenous	1.5 mL/kg (75 mg IgG/kg) IV	6 months
Cytomegalovirus prophylaxis (CMV IGIV)	150 mg/kg IV (maximum)	6 months
Hepatitis A (IG), duration of international travel		
≤3-month stay	0.02 mL/kg (3.3 mg IgG/kg) IM	3 months
≥3-month stay	0.06 mL/kg (10 mg IgG/kg) IM	3 months
Hepatitis B prophylaxis (HBIG)	0.06 mL/kg (10 mg IgG/kg) IM	3 months
Intravenous immune globulin (IVIG)		
Replacement therapy	300–400 mg/kg IV	8 months
Immune thrombocytopenic purpura (ITP)	400 mg/kg IV	8 months
	800 mg/kg IV or 1 g/kg IV	10 months[3]
Postexposure measles prophylaxis (includes immunocompromised people)	400 mg/kg IV	8 months
Postexposure varicella prophylaxis[4]	400 mg/kg IV	8 months
Kawasaki disease	2 gm/kg IV	11 months
Measles prophylaxis (IG)		
Immunocompetent contact	0.5 mL/kg (80 mg IgG/kg) IM	6 months
Monoclonal antibody to respiratory syncytial virus (RSV) F protein (Synagis [MedImmune])[5]	15 mg/kg IM	None
Rabies prophylaxis (HRIG)	20 IU/kg (22 mg IgG/kg) IM	4 months

(continued)

Table 2-4. Recommended intervals between administration of antibody-containing products and measles-containing vaccine or varicella-containing vaccine (continued)

INDICATION	DOSE AND ROUTE	RECOMMENDED INTERVAL BEFORE MEASLES OR VARICELLA VACCINATION
Tetanus (TIG)	250 units (10 mg IgG/kg) IM	3 months
Varicella zoster immune globulin[4]	125 units/10 kg (60–200 mg IgG/kg) IM (maximum 625 units)	5 months

Abbreviations: IG, immune globulin; IM, intramuscular; IV, intravenous.

[1] Adapted from Table 5, CDC. General recommendations on immunization: recommendations of the Advisory Committee on Immunization Practices (ACIP). MMWR Recomm Rep. 2011 Jan 28;60(RR-2):1–61. Updated with information from CDC. Prevention of measles, rubella, congenital rubella syndrome, and mumps, 2013: summary recommendations of the Advisory Committee on Immunization Practices (ACIP). MMWR Recomm Rep. 2013 Jun 14; 62(RR-04):1–34. This table is not intended for determining the correct indications and dosage for the use of IG preparations. Unvaccinated people may not be fully protected against measles during the entire recommended interval, and additional doses of IG or measles vaccine may be indicated after measles exposure. Concentrations of measles antibody in an IG preparation can vary by manufacturer's lot. For example, more than a 4-fold variation in the amount of measles antibody titers has been demonstrated in different IG preparations. Rates of antibody clearance after receipt of an IG preparation can also vary. Recommended intervals are extrapolated from an estimated half-life of 30 days for passively acquired antibody and an observed interference with the immune response to measles vaccine for 5 months after a dose of 80 mg IgG/kg. Does not include zoster vaccine. Zoster vaccine may be given with antibody-containing products.

[2] Assumes a serum IgG concentration of 16 mg/mL.

[3] Recommendation adapted from Neunert C, Lim W, Crowther M, Cohen A, Solberg L, Crowther MA. The American Society of Hematology 2011 evidence-based practice guideline for immune thrombocytopenia. Blood. 2011;117(16):4190–207

[4] If varicella zoster immune globulin is not available, IVIG can be used. The recommendation for use of IVIG is based on best judgment of experts and is supported by reports comparing varicella IgG titers measured in both IVIG and varicella zoster immune globulin preparations and patients given IVIG and varicella zoster immune globulin. Although licensed IVIG preparations contain antivaricella antibodies, the titer of any specific lot of IVIG is uncertain, because IVIG is not tested routinely for antivaricella antibodies. No clinical data demonstrating effectiveness of IVIG for postexposure prophylaxis of varicella are available. The recommended IVIG dose for postexposure prophylaxis of varicella is 1 dose of 400 mg/kg, intravenously (see http://redbook.solutions.aap.org/chapter.aspx?sectionid=88187270&bookid=1484).

[5] Contains only antibody to respiratory syncytial virus.

after vaccination. If the interval between administration of one of these vaccines and the subsequent administration of an IG preparation is ≥14 days, the vaccine need not be readministered. If the interval is <14 days, the vaccine should be readministered after the interval shown in Table 2-4, unless serologic testing indicates that antibodies have been produced. Such testing should be performed after the interval shown in Table 2-4, to avoid detecting antibodies from the IG preparation.

If administration of IG becomes necessary, MMR or varicella vaccines can be administered simultaneously with IG, with the recognition that vaccine-induced immunity can be compromised. The vaccine should be administered at a body site different from that chosen for the IG injection. Vaccination should be repeated after the interval noted in Table 2-4, unless serologic testing indicates antibodies have been produced.

When IG is given with the first dose of hepatitis A vaccine, the proportion of recipients who develop a protective level of antibody is not affected, but antibody concentrations are lower. Because the final concentrations of antibody are many times higher than those considered protective, this reduced immunogenicity is not expected to be clinically relevant. However, the effect of reduced antibody concentrations on long-term protection is unknown.

IG preparations interact minimally with other inactivated vaccines and toxoids. Other inactivated vaccines may be given simultaneously, or at any time interval before or after an antibody-containing blood product is used. However, such vaccines should be administered at different sites from the IG.

VACCINATION OF PEOPLE WITH ACUTE ILLNESSES

Every opportunity should be taken to provide needed vaccinations. The decision to delay vaccination because of a current or recent acute illness depends on the severity of the symptoms and their cause. Although a moderate or severe acute illness is sufficient reason to postpone vaccination, minor illnesses (such as diarrhea, mild upper respiratory infection with or without low-grade fever, or other low-grade febrile illness) are not contraindications to vaccination.

People with moderate or severe acute illness, with or without fever, should be vaccinated as soon as the condition improves. This precaution is to avoid superimposing adverse effects from the vaccine on underlying illness, or mistakenly attributing a manifestation of underlying illness to the vaccine. Antimicrobial therapy is not a contraindication to vaccination, with several exceptions:

- Antibacterial agents may interfere with the response to oral typhoid vaccine.

- Antiviral agents active against herpesviruses (such as acyclovir) may interfere with the response to varicella-containing vaccines.

- Antiviral agents active against influenza virus (such as zanamivir and oseltamivir) may interfere with the response to live attenuated influenza vaccine.

- Antibiotics may interfere with the response to the new oral cholera vaccine.

A physical examination or temperature measurement is not a prerequisite for vaccinating a person who appears to be in good health. Asking if a person is ill, postponing a vaccination for someone with moderate or severe acute illness, and vaccinating someone who does not have contraindications are appropriate procedures for clinic immunizations.

ALTERED IMMUNOCOMPETENCE

Altered immunocompetence is a general term that is often used interchangeably with the terms immunosuppression, immunodeficiency, and a weakened immune system. It can be caused either by a disease (leukemia, HIV infection) or by drugs or other therapies (cancer chemotherapy, radiation therapy, prolonged high-dose corticosteroids). It can also include conditions such as asplenia and chronic renal disease.

Determination of altered immunocompetence is important because the incidence or severity of some vaccine-preventable diseases is higher in people with altered immunocompetence. Therefore, certain vaccines (such as meningococcal B vaccine, pneumococcal polysaccharide vaccines) are recommended specifically for people with altered immunocompetence. Inactivated vaccines may be safely administered to a person with altered immunocompetence, although response to such vaccines may be suboptimal. These vaccines may need to be repeated after immune function has improved. If immunocompetence does not improve, the usual doses and schedules for inactivated vaccines are recommended. Again, the effectiveness of such vaccinations might be suboptimal.

People with altered immunocompetence may be at increased risk for an adverse reaction after administration of live attenuated vaccines because of reduced ability to mount an effective immune response. Live vaccines should generally be deferred until immune function has improved. If immune function does not improve, live vaccines are contraindicated. This is particularly important when planning to give yellow fever vaccine (see Chapter 3, Yellow Fever). For HIV-infected people with mild or moderate immunosuppression, MMR vaccine is recommended and varicella vaccine can be considered. For an in-depth discussion, see Chapter 8, Immunocompromised Travelers.

VACCINATION SCHEDULING FOR LAST-MINUTE TRAVELERS

As noted, for people anticipating imminent travel, most vaccine products can be given during the same visit. Unless the vaccines given are booster doses of those typically given during childhood, vaccines may require a month or more to induce a sufficient immune response, depending on the vaccine and the number of doses in the series. Some vaccines require more than 1 dose for best protection. Recommended spacing should be maintained between doses (Table 2-5). Doses given at less than minimum intervals may induce

Table 2-5. Recommended and minimum ages and intervals between vaccine doses[1,2]

VACCINE AND DOSE NUMBER	RECOMMENDED AGE FOR THIS DOSE	MINIMUM AGE FOR THIS DOSE	MINIMUM INTERVAL TO NEXT DOSE[3]
Diphtheria and tetanus toxoids and acellular pertussis vaccine, pediatric (6 weeks through 6 years) (DTaP)-1[4]	2 months	6 weeks	4 weeks
DTaP-2	4 months	10 weeks	4 weeks
DTaP-3	6 months	14 weeks	6 months[5]
DTaP-4	15–18 months	12 months	6 months[5]
DTaP-5	4–6 years	4 years	NA
Haemophilus influenzae type b (Hib)-1[6]	2 months	6 weeks	4 weeks
Hib-2	4 months	10 weeks	4 weeks
Hib-3[7]	6 months	14 weeks	8 weeks
Hib-4	12–15 months	12 months	NA
Hepatitis A (HepA)-1	12–23 months	12 months	6 months[5]
HepA-2	≥18 months	18 months	NA
Hepatitis B (HepB)-1[4]	Birth	Birth	4 weeks
HepB-2	1–2 months	4 weeks	8 weeks
HepB-3[8]	6–18 months	24 weeks	NA
Herpes zoster[9]	≥60 years	60 years	NA
Human papillomavirus (HPV)-1[10]	11–12 years	9 years	4 weeks
HPV-2	2 months after dose 1	9 years and 4 weeks	12 weeks
HPV-3[11]	6 months after dose 1	9 years and 24 weeks	NA
Inactivated poliovirus (IPV)-1[4]	2 months	6 weeks	4 weeks
IPV-2	4 months	10 weeks	4 weeks
IPV-3	6–18 months	14 weeks	6 months[5]

(continued)

Table 2-5. Recommended and minimum ages and intervals between vaccine doses (continued)

VACCINE AND DOSE NUMBER	RECOMMENDED AGE FOR THIS DOSE	MINIMUM AGE FOR THIS DOSE	MINIMUM INTERVAL TO NEXT DOSE[3]
IPV-4[12]	4–6 years	4 years	NA
Influenza, inactivated[13]	≥6 months	6 months[14]	4 weeks
Influenza, live attenuated[13]	2–49 years	2 years	4 weeks
Japanese encephalitis, Vero cell (Ixiaro)-1[15]	≥2 months	≥2 months	28 days
Ixiaro-2	28 days after dose 1	≥2 months and 28 days	NA
Measles, mumps, and rubella (MMR)-1[16]	12–15 months	12 months[17]	4 weeks
MMR-2[16]	4–6 years	13 months	NA
Meningococcal conjugate (MenACWY-1)[18]	11–12 years	2 months (Menveo) or 9 months (Menactra)	8 weeks[19]
MenACWY-2	16 years	4 months (Menveo) or 11 months (Menactra)	3–5 years if at increased risk of disease[19]
Meningococcal polysaccharide (MPSV4)-1[18]	NA	2 years	5 years
MPSV4-2	NA	7 years	NA
Pneumococcal conjugate (PCV)-1[6]	2 months	6 weeks	4 weeks
PCV-2	4 months	10 weeks	4 weeks
PCV-3	6 months	14 weeks	8 weeks
PCV-4	12–15 months	12 months	NA
Pneumococcal polysaccharide (PPSV)-1	NA	2 years	5 years
PPSV-2[20]	NA	7 years	NA
Rabies-1 (preexposure)	See footnote 21	See footnote 21	7 days
Rabies-2	7 days after dose 1	7 days after dose 1	14 days
Rabies-3	21 days after dose 1	21 days after dose 1	NA
Rotavirus (RV)-1[22]	2 months	6 weeks	4 weeks

(continued)

Table 2-5. Recommended and minimum ages and intervals between vaccine doses (continued)

VACCINE AND DOSE NUMBER	RECOMMENDED AGE FOR THIS DOSE	MINIMUM AGE FOR THIS DOSE	MINIMUM INTERVAL TO NEXT DOSE[3]
RV-2[22]	4 months	10 weeks	4 weeks
RV-3[22]	6 months	14 weeks	NA
Tetanus and reduced diphtheria toxoids (Td)	11–12 years	7 years	5 years
Tetanus toxoid, reduced diphtheria toxoid, and reduced acellular pertussis vaccine (Tdap)[23]	≥11 years	7 years	NA
Typhoid, inactivated (ViCPS)	≥2 years	≥2 years	NA
Typhoid, live attenuated (Ty21a)	≥6 years	≥6 years	See footnote 24
Varicella (Var)-1[16]	12–15 months	12 months	12 weeks[25]
Varicella (Var)-2	4–6 years	15 months	NA
Yellow fever	≥9 months[26]	≥9 months[26]	10 years

[1] Adapted from Table 1, CDC. General recommendations on immunization: recommendations of the Advisory Committee on Immunization Practices (ACIP). MMWR Recomm Rep. 2011 Jan 28;60(RR-2):1–61.

[2] Combination vaccines are available. Use of licensed combination vaccines is generally preferred over separate injections of their equivalent component vaccines (CDC. Combination vaccines for childhood immunization. MMWR Recomm Rep. 1999 May 14;48[RR-5]:1–14.). When administering combination vaccines, the minimum age for administration is the oldest age for any of the individual components (exception: the minimum age for the first dose of MenHibrix is 6 weeks); the minimum interval between doses is equal to the largest interval of any of the individual components.

[3] See www.cdc.gov/vaccines/schedules for recommended revaccination (booster) schedules.

[4] Combination vaccines containing the HepB component are available (DTaP-HepB-IPV, HepA-HepB). DTaP-HepB-IPV should not be administered to infants aged <6 weeks because of the other components (DTaP, IPV). HepA-HepB is not licensed in the United States for children aged <18 years.

[5] Calendar months.

[6] For Hib and PCV, children receiving the first dose of vaccine at ≥7 months of age require fewer doses to complete the series (see the current childhood and adolescent immunization schedule at www.cdc.gov/vaccines).

[7] If PRP-OMP (Pedvax-Hib, Merck Vaccine Division) was administered at 2 and 4 months of age, a dose at 6 months of age is not indicated. The final dose has a minimum age of 12 months.

[8] HepB-3 should be administered ≥8 weeks after Hep B-2 and ≥16 weeks after Hep B-1; it should not be administered before age 24 weeks.

[9] Herpes zoster (shingles) vaccine is recommended as a single dose for people aged ≥60 years.

[10] Bivalent HPV vaccine is approved for girls/women aged 10–26 years. It is recommended to prevent cervical and other anogenital cancers and precursors for girls/women aged 11–26 years. Quadrivalent HPV and 9vHPV vaccines are approved for boys/men and girls/women aged 9–26 years. They are recommended to prevent cervical and other anogenital cancers, precursors, and genital warts for girls/women aged 11–26 years. They are recommended for boys/men aged 11–21 years and high-risk boys or men (men who have sex with men, HIV-positive men, or immunocompromised men) aged 22–26 years. They may be given to girls aged 9–10 years to prevent the same diseases, and to boys/men aged 9–10 years and 22–26 years to prevent genital warts.

[11] The third dose of HPV should be administered ≥12 weeks after the second and ≥24 weeks after the first. Dose 3 need not be repeated if administered ≥16 weeks after dose 1, as long as a minimum interval of 4 weeks is maintained between dose 1 and dose 2 and as long as a minimum interval of 12 weeks is maintained between dose 2 and dose 3.

[12] For people receiving an all-IPV or all-OPV series, if the third dose is given after the fourth birthday, a fourth dose is not needed. For IPV, the next-to-last and the last dose must be spaced by 6 months.

[13] Two doses of influenza vaccine are recommended for children aged <9 years who are receiving the vaccine for the first time, and for certain incompletely vaccinated children (see reference 2).

[14] The minimum age for inactivated influenza vaccine varies by vaccine manufacturer. See package insert for vaccine-specific minimum ages.

[15] Ixiaro is approved by the Food and Drug Administration for people aged ≥2 months.

[16] Combination MMR-varicella (MMRV) can be used for children aged 12 months through 12 years

[17] If an infant 6–11 months of age is traveling internationally, a dose of MMR is recommended but does **not** count toward the 2-dose recommended series. The next dose should be administered at 12–15 months of age and a minimum of 4 weeks from the international travel dose.

(continued)

Table 2-5. Recommended and minimum ages and intervals between vaccine doses (continued)

[18] **Infants aged 2–18 months.** Routine vaccination with HibMenCY – TT (MenHibrix) or Menveo (4-dose primary series) is recommended for infants aged 2–18 months who are at increased risk for meningococcal disease. The first dose of either vaccine may be administered as early as age 6 weeks. The fourth dose may be administered as late as age 18 months. Infants and children who received Hib-MenCY-TT and are traveling to areas with high endemic rates of meningococcal disease such as the African "meningitis belt" are not protected against serogroups A and W-135 and should receive a quadrivalent meningococcal vaccination before travel.

 People aged 9 months through 55 years. People aged 9 months through 55 years at increased risk for meningococcal disease should receive Menveo or Menactra. Infants aged 9–23 months are recommended to receive a 2-dose primary series with a dosing interval of 12 weeks.

 People aged ≥56 years. Menomune is the only licensed meningococcal vaccine for adults aged ≥56 years and is immunogenic in older adults. For adults who have received a conjugate meningococcal vaccine previously, limited data demonstrate a higher antibody response after a subsequent dose of a conjugate vaccine compared with a subsequent dose of Menomune. For meningococcal vaccine-naïve people aged ≥56 years who anticipate requiring a single dose of meningococcal vaccine (such as travelers and people at risk as a result of a community outbreak), Menomune is preferred. For people now aged ≥56 years who were vaccinated previously with a meningococcal conjugate vaccine and are recommended for revaccination or for whom multiple doses are anticipated (such as people with asplenia and microbiologists), a conjugate vaccine is preferred.

[19] Revaccination with meningococcal vaccine is recommended for people previously vaccinated who remain at high risk for meningococcal disease. MenACWY is preferred for revaccinating people aged 2–55 years (CDC. Prevention and control of meningococcal disease. Recommendations of the Advisory Committee on Immunization Practices [ACIP]. MMWR Recomm Rep. 2013 Mar 22;62[RR-2]:1–28.).

[20] A second dose of PPSV is recommended for people aged ≥65 years who received a first dose at an age <65 years and at a 5-year minimum interval. A second dose is also recommended for people aged <65 years at highest risk for serious pneumococcal infection and those who are likely to have a rapid decline in pneumococcal antibody concentration (CDC. Updated recommendations for prevention of invasive pneumococcal disease among adults using the 23-valent pneumococcal polysaccharide vaccine [PPSV23]. MMWR Recomm Rep. 2010;59[34]:1102–6.).

[21] There is no minimum age for preexposure immunization for rabies (CDC. Human rabies prevention—United States, 2008: recommendations of the Advisory Committee on Immunization Practices. MMWR Recomm Rep. 2008 May 23;57[RR-3]:1–28.).

[22] The first dose of RV must be administered by 14 weeks and 6 days of age. The vaccine series should not be started at ≥15 weeks of age. The final dose in the series should be administered by age 8 months, 0 days. If Rotarix rotavirus vaccine is administered at 2 and 4 months of age, a dose at 6 months of age is not indicated.

[23] Only 1 dose of Tdap is recommended. Subsequent doses should be given as Td. Children aged 7–10 years who are not fully vaccinated against pertussis and for whom no contraindication to pertussis vaccine exists should receive a single dose of Tdap. If additional doses of tetanus and diphtheria toxoid-containing vaccines are needed, then children aged 7–10 years should be vaccinated according to catch-up guidance, with Tdap preferred as the first dose. Tdap vaccine, when indicated, should be administered regardless of the interval since the last dose of Td vaccine. For management of a tetanus-prone wound, the minimum interval after a previous dose of any tetanus-containing vaccine is 5 years. A dose of Tdap is recommended for pregnant women, preferably at 27–36 weeks' gestation, regardless of history of previous Tdap vaccination.

[24] Oral typhoid vaccine is recommended to be administered 1 hour before a meal with a cold or lukewarm drink (temperature not to exceed body temperature—98.6°F [37°C]) on alternate days, for a total of 4 doses.

[25] The minimum interval from Var-1 to Var-2 for people beginning the series at ≥13 years of age is 4 weeks.

[26] Yellow fever vaccine may be administered to children aged <9 months in certain situations (CDC. Yellow fever vaccine: recommendations of the Advisory Committee on Immunization Practices [ACIP]. MMWR Recomm Rep. 2010 Jul 30;59[RR-7]:1–27.).

lower antibody response than if given according to the recommended schedule. Intervals between doses longer than those routinely recommended do not decrease the immune response when the schedule is completed. Consequently, it is not necessary to restart the series or add doses of any vaccine because of an extended interval between doses, with the exceptions mentioned previously (oral typhoid vaccine and rabies vaccine). If a traveler needs yellow fever vaccination to meet a country requirement under the International Health Regulations, the yellow fever vaccine is not considered valid until 10 days after administration.

Administration of a vaccine earlier than the recommended minimum age or at an interval shorter than the recommended minimum is discouraged. Table 2-5 lists the minimum age and minimum interval between doses for vaccines routinely recommended in the United States.

Because some travelers visit their health care providers at the last minute before departure, studies have been performed to determine whether accelerated scheduling is adequate. This concern is primarily the case for hepatitis B vaccine or the combined hepatitis A and B vaccine. An accelerated schedule for combined hepatitis A and B vaccine has been approved by the Food and Drug Administration (FDA). It is unclear what level of protection any given traveler will have if he or she does not complete a full series of multi-dose vaccination.

ALLERGY TO VACCINE COMPONENTS

Vaccine components can cause allergic reactions in some recipients. These reactions can be local or systemic and can include anaphylaxis or anaphylactic-like responses. The vaccine components responsible can include the vaccine antigen, animal proteins, antibiotics, preservatives (such as thimerosal), or stabilizers (such as gelatin). The most common animal protein allergen is egg protein in vaccines prepared by using embryonated chicken eggs (influenza and yellow fever vaccines). People with a history of egg allergy who have experienced only hives after exposure to egg should receive influenza vaccine. Any licensed influenza vaccine that is otherwise appropriate for the recipient's age and health status may be used.

People who report having had reactions to egg involving symptoms other than hives, such as angioedema, respiratory distress, lightheadedness, or recurrent emesis, or who required epinephrine or another emergency medical intervention, may similarly receive any licensed influenza vaccine that is otherwise appropriate for the recipient's age and health status. If a person has a severe egg sensitivity or has a positive skin test to yellow fever vaccine but the vaccination is recommended because of their travel destination-specific risk, desensitization can be performed under direct supervision of a physician experienced in the management of anaphylaxis. In such circumstances, both yellow fever and influenza vaccines should be administered in an inpatient or outpatient medical setting. Vaccine administration should be supervised by a health care provider who is able to recognize and manage severe allergic reactions. A previous severe allergic reaction to any vaccine, regardless of the component suspected of being responsible for the reaction, is a contraindication to future receipt of the vaccine.

Some vaccines contain a preservative or trace amounts of antibiotics to which people might be allergic. Providers administering the vaccines should carefully review the prescribing information before deciding if the rare person with such an allergy should receive the vaccine. No recommended vaccine contains penicillin or penicillin derivatives. Some vaccines (MMR vaccine, inactivated polio vaccine [IPV], hepatitis A vaccine, some hepatitis B vaccines, some influenza vaccines, rabies vaccine, varicella vaccine, and smallpox vaccine) contain trace amounts of neomycin or other antibiotics; the amount is less than would normally be used for the skin test to determine hypersensitivity. However, people who have experienced anaphylactic reactions to this antibiotic generally should not receive these vaccines. Most often, neomycin allergy is a contact dermatitis—a manifestation of a delayed-type (cell-mediated) immune response rather than anaphylaxis. A history of delayed-type reactions to neomycin is not a contraindication to receiving these vaccines.

Thimerosal, an organic mercurial compound in use since the 1930s, has been added to certain immunobiologic products as a preservative. Thimerosal is present at preservative concentrations in multidose vials of some brands of vaccine. Receiving thimerosal-containing vaccines has been postulated to lead to induction of allergy. However, there is limited scientific evidence for this assertion. Allergy to thimerosal usually consists of local delayed-type hypersensitivity reactions. Thimerosal elicits positive delayed-type hypersensitivity patch tests in 1%–18% of people tested, but these tests have limited or no clinical relevance. Most people do not experience reactions to thimerosal administered as a component of vaccines, even when patch or intradermal tests for thimerosal indicate hypersensitivity. A localized or delayed-type hypersensitivity reaction to thimerosal is not a contraindication to receipt of a vaccine that contains thimerosal.

Since mid-2001, vaccines routinely recommended for infants have been manufactured without thimerosal as a preservative. Additional information about thimerosal and the thimerosal content of vaccines is available on the FDA website (www.fda.gov/cber/vaccine/thimerosal.htm).

REPORTING ADVERSE EVENTS AFTER IMMUNIZATION

Modern vaccines are extremely safe and effective. Benefits and risks are associated with the use of all immunobiologics—no vaccine is completely effective or completely safe for all recipients. Adverse events after immunization have been reported with all vaccines, ranging from frequent, minor, local reactions to extremely rare, severe, systemic illness, such as that associated with yellow fever vaccine. Adverse events following specific vaccines and toxoids are discussed in detail in each ACIP statement. In the United States, clinicians are required by law to report selected adverse events occurring after vaccination with any vaccine in the recommended childhood series. In addition, CDC strongly recommends that all vaccine adverse events be reported to the Vaccine Adverse Event Reporting System (VAERS), even if a causal relation to vaccination is not certain. VAERS reporting forms and information are available electronically at www.vaers.hhs.gov, or they may be requested by telephone: 800-822-7967 (toll-free). Clinicians are encouraged to report electronically at https://vaers.hhs.gov/esub/step1.

INJECTION ROUTE AND INJECTION SITE

Injectable vaccines are administered by intramuscular, intradermal, and subcutaneous routes.

The method of administration of injectable vaccines depends in part on the presence of an adjuvant in some vaccines. The term *adjuvant* refers to a vaccine component distinct from the antigen, which enhances the immune response to the antigen. Vaccines containing an adjuvant (DTaP, DT, HPV, Td, Tdap, pneumococcal conjugate, Hib, hepatitis A, hepatitis B) should be injected into a muscle mass, because administration subcutaneously or intradermally can cause local irritation, induration, skin discoloration, inflammation, and granuloma formation. Detailed discussion and recommendations about vaccination of people with bleeding disorders or receiving anticoagulant therapy are available in the ACIP general recommendations on immunization.

Routes of administration are recommended by the manufacturer for each immunobiologic. Deviation from the recommended route of administration may reduce vaccine efficacy or increase local adverse reactions. Detailed recommendations on the route and site for all vaccines have been published in ACIP recommendations; a compiled list of these publications is available on the CDC website at www.cdc.gov/vaccines/hcp/acip-recs (also see Table B-1 in Appendix B).

BIBLIOGRAPHY

1. CDC. General recommendations on immunization: recommendations of the Advisory Committee on Immunization Practices (ACIP). MMWR Recomm Rep. 2011 Jan 28;60(2):1–64.

2. CDC. Updated recommendations for use of tetanus toxoid, reduced diphtheria toxoid, and acellular pertussis (Tdap) vaccine in adults aged 65 years and older—Advisory Committee on Immunization Practices (ACIP), 2012. MMWR Morb Mortal Wkly Rep. 2012 Jun 29;61(25):468–70.

3. Cohn AC, MacNeil JR, Clark TA, Ortega-Sanchez IR, Briere EZ, Meissner HC, et al. Prevention and control of meningococcal disease: recommendations of the Advisory Committee on Immunization Practices (ACIP). MMWR Recomm Rep. 2013 Mar 22;62(2):1–28.

4. Grohskopf LA, Sokolow LZ, Olsen SJ, Bresee JS, Broder KR, Karron RA, et al. Prevention and control of seasonal influenza with vaccines: recommendations of the Advisory Committee on Immunization Practices—United States, 2013–2014. MMWR Recomm Rep. 2015 Aug 7;64(30):818–25.

5. Kobayashi M, Bennett NM, Gierke R, Almendares O, Moore MR, Whitney CG, et al. Intervals between PCV13 and PPSV23 vaccines: recommendations of the Advisory Committee on Immunization Practices (ACIP). MMWR Morb Mortal Wkly Rep. 2015 Sep 4;64(64):944–7.

6. Kretsinger K, Broder KR, Cortese MM, Joyce MP, Ortega-Sanchez I, Lee GM, et al. Preventing tetanus, diphtheria, and pertussis among adults: use of tetanus toxoid, reduced diphtheria toxoid and acellular pertussis vaccine recommendations of the Advisory Committee on Immunization Practices (ACIP) and recommendation of ACIP, supported by the Healthcare Infection Control Practices Advisory Committee (HICPAC), for use of Tdap among health-care personnel. MMWR Recomm Rep. 2006 Dec 15;55(RR-17):1–37.

7. McLean HQ, Fiebelkorn AP, Temte JL, Wallace GS, CDC. Prevention of measles, rubella, congenital rubella syndrome, and mumps, 2013: summary recommendations of the Advisory Committee on Immunization Practices (ACIP). MMWR Recomm Rep. 2013 Jun 14;62(RR-04):1–34.

8. Nuorti JP, Whitney CG, CDC. Prevention of pneumococcal disease among infants and children—use of 13-valent pneumococcal conjugate vaccine and 23-valent

pneumococcal polysaccharide vaccine: recommendations of the Advisory Committee on Immunization Practices (ACIP). MMWR Recomm Rep. 2010 Dec 10;59(RR-11):1–18.

9. Shimabukuro TT, Nguyen M, Martin D, DeStefano F. Safety monitoring in the Vaccine Adverse Event Reporting System (VAERS). Vaccine. 2015 Aug 26;33(36):4398–405.

10. Staples JE, Gershman M, Fischer M, CDC. Yellow fever vaccine: recommendations of the Advisory Committee on Immunization Practices (ACIP). MMWR Recomm Rep. 2010 Jul 30;59(RR-7):1–27.

2

INTERACTIONS AMONG TRAVEL VACCINES & DRUGS

Ilan Youngster, Elizabeth D. Barnett

Vaccines and medications are prescribed frequently in pretravel consultations, and potential interactions between vaccines and medications, including those already taken by the traveler, must be considered. The importance of this topic is highlighted by a study identifying potential drug–drug interactions with travel-related medications in 45% of travelers using chronic medications. Although a comprehensive list of interactions is beyond the scope of this section, some of the more serious interactions of commonly used travel-related vaccines and medications are discussed here.

INTERACTIONS BETWEEN VACCINES

In general, concomitant administration of multiple vaccines, including live attenuated immunizations, is safe and effective. Administering a live-virus vaccine within 4 weeks after administration of another live-virus vaccine can decrease immunogenicity to the second administered vaccine. This observation has given rise to the recommendation that live-virus vaccines should be administered the same day or ≥4 weeks apart. If the 4-week span is not achievable, the second vaccine may be administered sooner to afford some protection, but it should be readministered ≥4 weeks later if the traveler is at continued risk. A study examining concurrent administration of the yellow fever vaccine with the measles-mumps-rubella (MMR) vaccine in 12-month-old children showed slightly reduced immunogenicity

to yellow fever and mumps components, compared with responses following separate vaccination with MMR and yellow fever vaccines 30 days apart. (See "Simultaneous Administration" in Yellow Fever section, Chapter 3.) A single study suggested that in adults, concomitant administration of the 13-valent pneumococcal conjugate vaccine with the trivalent inactivated influenza vaccine results in lower immunogenicity to the PCV13 components. However, the clinical significance of this observation is uncertain, as responses still met FDA criteria of noninferiority. In infants given PCV13 and inactivated influenza vaccine concomitantly, the risk of fever and febrile seizure is slightly increased. However, this risk must be weighed against the need for both vaccines before travel and the time available to separate them.

INTERACTIONS BETWEEN TRAVEL VACCINES AND DRUGS

Live Attenuated Oral Typhoid and Cholera Vaccines

Live attenuated vaccines should generally be avoided in immunocompromised travelers, including those who are taking immunomodulators, calcineurin inhibitors, cytotoxic agents, antimetabolites, and high-dose steroids (see Table 8-1).

Antimicrobial agents may be active against the vaccine strain in the oral typhoid and cholera vaccines and may prevent an adequate immune response to the vaccine. Therefore, oral typhoid or cholera vaccine should not be given to people taking antibacterial agents. Vaccination with oral typhoid vaccine should be delayed for >72 hours after the administration of any such agent. Parenteral typhoid vaccine may be a more appropriate choice for these people. Live attenuated oral cholera vaccine should not be given to people who have received oral or parenteral antibiotics within 14 days prior to vaccination. There is no parenteral cholera vaccine currently available, and no killed oral cholera vaccines are licensed in the United States.

Chloroquine and atovaquone-proguanil at doses used for malaria chemoprophylaxis may be given concurrently with the oral typhoid vaccine. Data from an older formulation of the CVD 103-HgR oral cholera vaccine suggest that the immune response to the vaccine may be diminished when it is given concomitantly with chloroquine. Live attenuated oral cholera vaccine should be given at least 10 days before beginning antimalarial prophylaxis with chloroquine, although a study in children using the oral cholera vaccine suggested no decrease in immunogenicity when given with atovaquone-proguanil.

Rabies Vaccine

Concomitant use of chloroquine may reduce the antibody response to intradermal rabies vaccine administered for preexposure vaccination. The intramuscular route should be used for people taking chloroquine concurrently. (Currently, intradermal administration of rabies vaccine is not approved in the United States.)

INTERACTIONS BETWEEN ANTIMALARIALS AND SELECTED OTHER DRUGS

This section describes some of the more commonly encountered drug interactions. Any time a new medication is prescribed, clinicians should check for any interactions and inform the traveler of the potential risk.

Mefloquine

Mefloquine may interact with several categories of drugs, including other antimalarial drugs, drugs that alter cardiac conduction, and anticonvulsants. Mefloquine is associated with increased toxicities of the antimalarial drug lumefantrine (available in the United States in fixed combination to treat people with uncomplicated *Plasmodium falciparum* malaria), potentially causing fatal prolongation of the QTc interval. Lumefantrine should therefore be avoided or used with caution in patients taking mefloquine prophylaxis. Although no conclusive data are available with regard to coadministration of mefloquine and other drugs that may affect cardiac conduction, mefloquine should be used with caution or avoided in patients taking antiarrhythmic or β-blocking agents, calcium-channel blockers, antihistamines, H_1-blocking agents, tricyclic antidepressants, selective serotonin reuptake inhibitors (SSRIs), or phenothiazines. Mefloquine may also lower plasma levels of a number of anticonvulsants, such as valproic acid, carbamazepine, phenobarbital, and phenytoin; concurrent use of mefloquine with these agents should be avoided. In general, mefloquine should be avoided in travelers with a history of seizures, mood disorders or psychiatric disease. Mefloquine can also lead to increased levels of calcineurin inhibitors and mTOR inhibitors (tacrolimus, cyclosporine A, and sirolimus). Potent CYP3A4 inhibitors such as macrolides (azithromycin, clarithromycin, erythromycin), azole antifungals (ketoconazole, voriconazole, posaconazole and itraconazole), SSRIs (fluoxetine, sertraline, fluvoxamine), (antiretroviral protease inhibitors (ritonavir, lopinavir, darunavir, atazanavir, saquinavir), and cobicistat (available in a combination with elvitegravir) may increase the levels of mefloquine, increasing the risk for QT prolongation. CYP3A4 inducers such as efavirenz, nevirapine, etravirine, rifampin, rifabutin, St John's wort and glucocorticoids may reduce plasma concentrations of mefloquine, and concurrent use should be avoided. Concurrent use of mefloquine with the direct-acting protease inhibitors boceprevir and telaprevir used to treat hepatitis C should also be avoided. The newer direct-acting protease inhibitors (grazoprevir, paritaprevir, simeprevir) are believed to be associated with fewer drug–drug interactions, but as safety data are lacking, alternatives to mefloquine could be considered pending additional data.

Chloroquine

Chloroquine may increase risk of prolonged QTc interval when given with other QT-prolonging agents (such as sotalol, amiodarone, and lume-fantrine), and the combination should be avoided. The antiretroviral rilpivirine has also been shown to prolong QTc, and coadministration should be avoided. Chloroquine inhibits CYP2D6; when given concomitantly with substrates of this enzyme (such as metoprolol, propranolol, fluoxetine, paroxetine, flecainide), increased monitoring for side effects may be warranted. Chloroquine absorption may be reduced by antacids or kaolin; ≥4 hours should elapse between doses of these medications. Concomitant use of cimetidine and chloroquine should be avoided, as cimetidine can inhibit the metabolism of chloroquine and may increase drug levels. CYP3A4 inhibitors such as ritonavir, ketoconazole, and erythromycin may also increase chloroquine levels, and concomitant use should be avoided. Chloroquine inhibits bioavailability of ampicillin, and 2 hours should elapse between doses. Chloroquine is also reported to decrease the bioavailability of ciprofloxacin and methotrexate. Chloroquine may increase digoxin levels; increased digoxin monitoring is warranted. Use of chloroquine could possibly also lead to increased levels of calcineurin inhibitors and should be used with caution.

Atovaquone-Proguanil

Tetracycline, rifampin, and rifabutin may reduce plasma concentrations of atovaquone and should not be used concurrently with atovaquone-proguanil. Metoclopramide may reduce bioavailability of atovaquone; unless no other antiemetics are available, this antiemetic should not be used to treat the vomiting that may accompany use of atovaquone at treatment doses. Atovaquone-proguanil should not be used with other medications that contain proguanil. Patients on warfarin may need to reduce their anticoagulant dose or monitor their prothrombin time more closely while taking atovaquone-proguanil, although coadministration of these drugs is not contraindicated. The use of novel oral anticoagulants (dabigatran, rivaroxaban and apixaban) is not expected to cause significant interactions, and their use has been suggested as an alternative in patients in need of anticoagulation. Atovaquone-proguanil may interact with the antiretroviral protease inhibitors ritonavir, darunavir, atazanavir, indinavir, and lopinavir, in addition to the nonnucleoside

reverse transcriptase inhibitors nevirapine, etravirine, and efavirenz, resulting in decreased levels of atovaquone-proguanil. Despite the potential for interactions, atovaquone-proguanil is well tolerated in most patients receiving these antivirals and is the preferred antimalarial for short-term travel. Cimetidine and fluvoxamine interfere with the metabolism of proguanil and should therefore be avoided.

Doxycycline

Phenytoin, carbamazepine, and barbiturates may decrease the half-life of doxycycline. Patients on anticoagulants may need to reduce their anticoagulant dose while taking doxycycline because of its ability to depress plasma prothrombin activity. Absorption of tetracyclines may be impaired by bismuth subsalicylate, preparations containing iron, and antacids containing calcium, magnesium, or aluminum; these preparations should not be taken within 3 hours of taking doxycycline. Doxycycline may interfere with the bactericidal activity of penicillin, so these drugs, in general, should not be taken together. Doxycycline has no known interaction with antiretroviral agents, but concurrent use may lead to increased levels of calcineurin inhibitors and mTOR inhibitors (sirolimus).

INTERACTIONS WITH DRUGS FOR TREATMENT OF TRAVELERS' DIARRHEA

Azithromycin

Close monitoring for side effects of azithromycin is recommended when azithromycin is used with nelfinavir. Increased anticoagulant effects have been noted when azithromycin is used with warfarin; monitoring prothrombin time is recommended for people taking these drugs concomitantly. Additive QTc prolongation may occur when azithromycin is used with the antimalarial artemether, and concomitant therapy should be avoided. Drug interactions have been reported with macrolides and antiretroviral protease inhibitors, as well as efavirenz and nevirapine, and can increase risk of QTc prolongation, though a short treatment course is not contraindicated for those without an underlying cardiac abnormality. Concurrent use with macrolides may lead to increased levels of calcineurin inhibitors.

Fluoroquinolones

Increase in the international normalized ratio has been reported when levofloxacin and warfarin are used concurrently. Concurrent administration of ciprofloxacin and antacids that contain magnesium or aluminum hydroxide may reduce bioavailability of ciprofloxacin. Ciprofloxacin decreases clearance of theophylline and caffeine; theophylline levels should be monitored when ciprofloxacin is used concurrently. Ciprofloxacin and other fluoroquinolones should not be used with tizanidine. Sildenafil should not be used in patients on ciprofloxacin, as concomitant use is associated with increased rates of adverse effects. Fluoroquinolones have no known interaction with antiretroviral agents, but concurrent use may increase levels of calcineurin inhibitors and fluoroquinolone levels, and use should reflect renal function.

Rifaximin

Rifaximin is not absorbed in appreciable amounts by intact bowel, and no clinically significant drug interactions have been reported to date with rifaximin.

INTERACTIONS WITH DRUGS USED FOR TRAVEL TO HIGH ALTITUDES

Acetazolamide

Acetazolamide produces alkaline urine that can increase the rate of excretion of barbiturates and salicylates and may potentiate salicylate toxicity, particularly if taking a high dose of aspirin. Decreased excretion of dextroamphetamine, anticholinergics, mecamylamine, ephedrine, mexiletine, or quinidine may also occur. Hypokalemia caused by corticosteroids may be potentiated by concurrent use of acetazolamide. Acetazolamide should not be given to patients taking the anticonvulsant topiramate, as concurrent use is associated with increased toxicity. Increased monitoring of cyclosporine, tacrolimus, and sirolimus is warranted if these drugs are given with acetazolamide. Concurrent administration of metformin and acetazolamide should be done with caution as there may be an additive risk for lactic acidosis. Acetaminophen and diclofenac sodium form complex bonds with acetazolamide in the stomach's acidic environment, impairing absorption.

These agents should not be taken within 30 minutes of acetazolamide.

Dexamethasone

Dexamethasone interacts with multiple classes of drugs. Using this drug to treat altitude illness may, however, be life-saving. Interactions may occur with dexamethasone and the following drugs and drug classes: macrolide antibiotics, anticholinesterases, anticoagulants, hypoglycemic agents, isoniazid, digitalis preparations, oral contraceptives, and phenytoin.

DRUG INTERACTIONS IN PATIENTS ON HIV MEDICATIONS

Patients with HIV can be a challenge in the pretravel consultation (See Chapter 8, Immunocompromised Travelers). A study in Europe showed that as many as 29% of HIV-positive travelers do not disclose their disease and medication status when seeking pretravel advice. Antiretroviral medications have multiple drug interactions, especially through activation or inhibition of CYP3A4 and CYP2D6. There are several reports of antimalarial treatment failure and prophylaxis failure in patients on protease inhibitors and both nucleoside and nonnucleoside reverse transcriptase inhibitors, whereas entry and integrase inhibitors are not a common cause of drug–drug interactions with commonly administered travel-related medications. A number of the potential interactions are listed above, and 2 excellent resources for HIV medication interactions can be found at www.hiv-druginteractions.org and at www.aidsinfo.nih.gov.

INTERACTIONS WITH HERBAL OR NUTRITIONAL SUPPLEMENTS

As many as 30% of travelers take herbal or nutritional supplements, and many consider them to be of no clinical relevance, and will not disclose their use unless specifically asked during the pretravel consultation. Special attention should be given to supplements that activate or inhibit CYP2D6 or CYP3A4 like ginseng, hypericum, St. John's wort and grapefruit extract. Coadministration with medications that are substrates of CYP2D6 or 3A4 should be avoided (chloroquine, mefloquine, macrolides).

BIBLIOGRAPHY

1. Frenck RW Jr, Gurtman A, Rubino J, Smith W, van Cleeff M, Jayawardene D, et al. Randomized, controlled trial of a 13-valent pneumococcal conjugate vaccine administered concomitantly with an influenza vaccine in healthy adults. Clin Vaccine Immunol. 2012 Aug;19(8):1296–303.

2. Jabeen E, Qureshi R, Shah A. Interaction of antihypertensive acetazolamide with nonsteroidal anti-inflammatory drugs. J Photochem Photobiol B. 2013 Aug 5;125:155–63.

3. Kollaritsch H, Que JU, Kunz C, Wiedermann G, Herzog C, Cryz SJ Jr. Safety and immunogenicity of live oral cholera and typhoid vaccines administered alone or in combination with antimalarial drugs, oral polio vaccine, or yellow fever vaccine. J Infect Dis. 1997 Apr;175(4):871–5.

4. Nascimento Silva JR, Camacho LA, Siqueira MM, Freire Mde S, Castro YP, Maia Mde L, et al. Mutual interference on the immune response to yellow fever vaccine and a combined vaccine against measles, mumps and rubella. Vaccine. 2011 Aug 26;29(37):6327–34.

5. Nielsen US, Jensen-Fangel S, Pedersen G, Lohse N, Pedersen C, Kronborg G, et al. Travelling with HIV: a cross sectional analysis of Danish HIV-infected patients. Travel Med Infect Dis. 2014 Jan-Feb;12(1):72–8.

6. Ridtitid W, Wongnawa M, Mahatthanatrakul W, Raungsri N, Sunbhanich M. Ketoconazole increases plasma concentrations of antimalarial mefloquine in healthy human volunteers. J Clin Pharm Ther. 2005 Jun;30(3):285–90.

7. Stienlauf S, Meltzer E, Kurnik D, Leshem E, Kopel E, Streltsin B, et al. Potential drug interactions in travelers with chronic illnesses: a large retrospective cohort study. Travel Med Infect Dis. 2014 Sep-Oct;12(5):499–504.

Self-Treatable Conditions

TRAVELERS' DIARRHEA

Bradley A. Connor

Travelers' diarrhea (TD) is the most predictable travel-related illness. Attack rates range from 30% to 70% of travelers, depending on the destination and season of travel. Traditionally, it was thought that TD could be prevented by following simple recommendations such as "boil it, cook it, peel it, or forget it," but studies have found that people who follow these rules may still become ill. Poor hygiene practice in local restaurants is likely the largest contributor to the risk for TD.

TD is a clinical syndrome that can result from a variety of intestinal pathogens. Bacterial pathogens are the predominant risk, thought to account for up to 80%–90% of TD. Intestinal viruses usually account for at least 5%–8% of illnesses, although improved diagnostics may increase recognition of norovirus infections in the future. Infections with protozoal pathogens are slower to manifest symptoms and collectively account for approximately 10% of diagnoses in longer-term travelers. What is commonly known as "food poisoning" involves the ingestion of preformed toxins in food. In this syndrome, vomiting and diarrhea may both be present, but symptoms usually resolve spontaneously within 12 hours.

INFECTIOUS AGENTS

Bacteria are the most common cause of TD. Overall, the most common pathogen is enterotoxigenic *Escherichia coli*, followed by *Campylobacter jejuni*, *Shigella* spp., and *Salmonella* spp. Enteroaggregative and other *E. coli* pathotypes are also commonly found in cases of TD. There is increasing discussion of *Aeromonas* spp., *Plesiomonas* spp., and newly recognized pathogens (*Acrobacter*, *Larobacter*, enterotoxigenic *Bacteroides fragilis*) as potential causes of TD as well. Viral diarrhea can be caused by a number of pathogens, including norovirus, rotavirus, and astrovirus.

Giardia is the main protozoal pathogen found in TD. *Entamoeba histolytica* is a relatively uncommon cause of TD, and *Cryptosporidium* is also relatively uncommon. The risk for *Cyclospora* is highly geographic and seasonal: the most well-known risks are in Nepal, Peru, Haiti, and Guatemala. *Dientamoeba fragilis* is a flagellate occasionally associated with diarrhea in travelers. Most of the individual pathogens are discussed in their own sections in Chapter 3, and persistent diarrhea in returned travelers is discussed in Chapter 5.

OCCURRENCE

The most important determinant of the causative organism and risk for TD is travel destination. The world is generally divided into 3 grades of risk: low, intermediate, and high.

- Low-risk countries include the United States, Canada, Australia, New Zealand, Japan, and countries in Northern and Western Europe.

- Intermediate-risk countries include those in Eastern Europe, South Africa, and some Caribbean islands.

- High-risk areas include most of Asia, the Middle East, Africa, Mexico, and Central and South America.

RISK FOR TRAVELERS

TD occurs equally in male and female travelers and is more common in young adult travelers than in older travelers. In short-term travelers, bouts of TD do not appear to protect against future attacks, and >1 episode of TD may occur during a single trip. A cohort of expatriates residing in Kathmandu, Nepal, experienced an average of 3.2 episodes of TD per person in their first year. In more temperate regions, there may be seasonal variations in diarrhea risk. In south Asia, for example, much higher TD attack rates are reported during the hot months preceding the monsoon.

In environments in warmer climates where large numbers of people do not have access to plumbing or latrines, the amount of stool contamination in the environment will be higher and more accessible to flies. Inadequate electrical capacity may lead to frequent blackouts or poorly functioning refrigeration, which can result in unsafe food storage and an increased risk for disease. Lack of safe water may lead to contaminated foods and drinks prepared with such water; inadequate water supply may lead to shortcuts in cleaning hands, surfaces, utensils, and foods such as fruits and vegetables. In addition, handwashing may not be a social norm and could be an extra expense; thus there may be no handwashing stations in food preparation areas. In destinations in which effective food handling courses have been provided, the risk for TD has been demonstrated to decrease. However, even in developed countries, pathogens such as *Shigella sonnei* have caused TD linked to handling and preparation of food in restaurants.

CLINICAL PRESENTATION

Bacterial and viral TD presents with the sudden onset of bothersome symptoms that can range from mild cramps and urgent loose stools to severe abdominal pain, fever, vomiting, and bloody diarrhea, although with norovirus vomiting may be more prominent. Protozoal diarrhea, such as that caused by *Giardia intestinalis* or *E. histolytica*, generally has a more gradual onset of low-grade symptoms, with 2–5 loose stools per day. The incubation period between exposure and clinical presentation can be a clue to the etiology:

- Bacterial toxins generally cause symptoms within a few hours.

- Bacterial and viral pathogens have an incubation period of 6–72 hours.

- Protozoal pathogens generally have an incubation period of 1–2 weeks and rarely present in the first few days of travel. An exception can be *Cyclospora cayetanensis*, which can present quickly in areas of high risk.

Untreated bacterial diarrhea usually lasts 3–7 days. Viral diarrhea generally lasts 2–3 days. Protozoal diarrhea can persist for weeks to months without treatment. An acute bout of gastroenteritis can lead to persistent gastrointestinal symptoms, even in the absence of continued infection (see Chapter 5, Persistent Travelers' Diarrhea). This presentation is commonly referred to as postinfectious irritable bowel syndrome. Other postinfectious sequelae may include reactive arthritis and Guillain-Barré syndrome.

PREVENTION

For travelers to high-risk areas, several approaches may be recommended that can reduce, but never completely eliminate, the risk for TD. These include instructions regarding food and beverage selection, using agents other than antimicrobial drugs for prophylaxis, using prophylactic antibiotics, and carefully washing hands with soap where available. Carrying small containers of alcohol-based hand sanitizers (containing ≥60% alcohol) may make it easier for travelers to clean their hands before eating when handwashing is not possible. No vaccines are available for most pathogens that cause TD, but travelers should refer to the Cholera, Hepatitis A, and Typhoid & Paratyphoid Fever sections in Chapter 3 regarding vaccines that can prevent other foodborne or waterborne infections to which travelers are susceptible.

Food and Beverage Selection

Care in selecting food and beverages can minimize the risk for acquiring TD. See the Food & Water Precautions section later in this chapter for CDC's detailed food and beverage recommendations. Although food and water precautions continue to be recommended, travelers may not always be able to adhere to the advice. Furthermore, many of the factors that ensure food safety, such as restaurant hygiene, are out of the traveler's control.

Nonantimicrobial Drugs for Prophylaxis

The primary agent studied for prevention of TD, other than antimicrobial drugs, is bismuth subsalicylate (BSS), which is the active ingredient in adult formulations of Pepto-Bismol and Kaopectate. Studies from Mexico have shown that this agent (taken daily as either 2 oz of liquid or 2 chewable tablets 4 times per day) reduces the incidence of TD by approximately 50%. BSS commonly causes blackening of the tongue and stool and may cause nausea, constipation, and rarely tinnitus. BSS should be avoided by travelers with aspirin allergy, renal insufficiency, and gout, and by those taking anticoagulants, probenecid, or methotrexate. In travelers taking aspirin or salicylates for other reasons, the use of BSS may result in salicylate toxicity. BSS is not generally recommended for children aged <12 years; however, some clinicians use it off-label with caution to avoid administering BSS to children with viral infections, such as varicella or influenza, because of the risk for Reye syndrome. BSS is not recommended for children aged <3 years or pregnant women. Studies have not established the safety of BSS use for periods >3 weeks. Because of the number of tablets required and the inconvenient dosing, BSS is not commonly used as prophylaxis for TD.

The use of probiotics, such as *Lactobacillus* GG and *Saccharomyces boulardii*, has been studied in the prevention of TD in small numbers of people. Results are inconclusive, partially because standardized preparations of these bacteria are not reliably available. Studies are ongoing with prebiotics to prevent TD, but data are insufficient to recommend their use. There have been anecdotal reports of beneficial outcomes after using bovine colostrum as a daily prophylaxis agent for TD. However, commercially sold preparations of bovine colostrum are marketed as dietary supplements that are not Food and Drug Administration (FDA) approved for medical indications. Because no data from rigorous clinical trials demonstrate efficacy, there is insufficient information to recommend the use of bovine colostrum to prevent TD.

Although not available in the United States, a cholera vaccine (Dukoral) that provides partial protection against enterotoxigenic *E. coli* is available in some other countries. Several clinical trials of new vaccines against TD pathogens are in progress.

Prophylactic Antibiotics

Although prophylactic antibiotics can prevent some TD, the emergence of antimicrobial resistance has made the decision of how and when to use antibiotic prophylaxis for TD difficult. Controlled studies have shown that diarrhea attack rates are reduced by 90% or more by the use of antibiotics. The prophylactic antibiotic of choice has changed over the past few decades as resistance patterns have evolved. Fluoroquinolones have been the most effective antibiotics for the prophylaxis and treatment of bacterial TD pathogens, but increasing resistance to these agents among *Campylobacter* and *Shigella* species globally limits their potential use. Alternative considerations include azithromycin and rifaximin, a nonabsorbable broad-spectrum antibiotic.

At this time, prophylactic antibiotics should not be recommended for most travelers. Prophylactic antibiotics afford no protection against nonbacterial pathogens and can remove normally protective microflora from the bowel, increasing the risk of infection with resistant bacterial pathogens. Travelers may become colonized with extended-spectrum β-lactamase (ESBL)–producing bacteria, and this risk is increased by exposure to antibiotics while abroad. Additionally, the use of antibiotics may be associated with allergic or adverse reactions, and prophylactic antibiotics limit the therapeutic options if TD occurs; a traveler relying on prophylactic antibiotics will need to carry an alternative antibiotic to use if severe diarrhea develops despite prophylaxis. The risks associated with the use of prophylactic antibiotics should be weighed against the benefit of using prompt, early self-treatment with antibiotics when moderate to severe TD occurs, shortening the duration of illness to 6–24 hours in most cases. Prophylactic antibiotics may be considered for short-term travelers who are high-risk hosts (such as those who are immunosuppressed) or who are taking critical trips (such as engaging in a sporting event) without the opportunity for time off in the event of sickness.

TREATMENT

Oral Rehydration Therapy

Fluids and electrolytes are lost during TD, and replenishment is important, especially in young children or adults with chronic medical illness. In adult travelers who are otherwise healthy, severe dehydration resulting from TD is unusual unless vomiting is prolonged. Nonetheless, replacement of fluid losses remains an adjunct to other therapy

and helps the traveler feel better more quickly. Travelers should remember to use only beverages that are sealed, treated with chlorine, boiled, or are otherwise known to be purified. For severe fluid loss, replacement is best accomplished with oral rehydration solution (ORS) prepared from packaged oral rehydration salts, such as those provided by the World Health Organization. ORS is widely available at stores and pharmacies in most developing countries. ORS is prepared by adding 1 packet to the indicated volume of boiled or treated water—generally 1 liter. Travelers may find most ORS formulations to be relatively unpalatable due to their saltiness. In mild cases, rehydration can be maintained with any palatable liquid (including sports drinks), although overly sweet drinks, such as sodas, can cause osmotic diarrhea if consumed in quantity.

Antimotility Agents

Antimotility agents provide symptomatic relief and are useful therapy in TD. Synthetic opiates, such as loperamide and diphenoxylate, can reduce frequency of bowel movements and therefore enable travelers to ride on an airplane or bus. Loperamide appears to have antisecretory properties as well. The safety of loperamide when used along with an antibiotic has been well established, even in cases of invasive pathogens; however, acquisition of ESBL-producing pathogens may be more common when loperamide and antibiotics are coadministered. Antimotility agents alone are not recommended for patients with bloody diarrhea or those who have diarrhea and fever. Loperamide can be used in children, and liquid formulations are available. In practice, however, these drugs are rarely given to small children (aged <6 years).

Antibiotics

Antibiotics are effective in reducing the duration of diarrhea by about a day in cases caused by bacterial pathogens that are susceptible to the particular antibiotic prescribed. However, there are concerns about adverse consequences of using antibiotics to treat TD. Travelers who take antibiotics may acquire resistant organisms such as ESBL-producing organisms, resulting in potential harm to travelers—particularly those who are immunosuppressed or women who may be prone to urinary tract infections—and the possibility of introducing these resistant bacteria into the community. In addition, there is concern about the effects of antibiotic use on travelers' microbiota and the potential for adverse consequences such as *Clostridium difficile* infection as a result. These concerns have to be weighed against the consequences of TD and the role of antibiotics in shortening the acute illness and possibly preventing postinfectious sequelae (see Chapter 5, Persistent Travelers' Diarrhea).

The effectiveness of a particular antimicrobial drug depends on the etiologic agent and its antibiotic sensitivity. As empiric therapy or to treat a specific bacterial pathogen, first-line antibiotics have traditionally been the fluoroquinolones, such as ciprofloxacin or levofloxacin. Increasing microbial resistance to the fluoroquinolones, especially among *Campylobacter* isolates, may limit their usefulness in many destinations, particularly South and Southeast Asia, where both *Campylobacter* infection and fluoroquinolone resistance is prevalent. Increasing fluoroquinolone resistance has been reported from other destinations and in other bacterial pathogens, including in *Shigella* and *Salmonella*. In addition, the use of fluoroquinolones has been associated with tendinopathies and the development of *C. difficile* infection. FDA warns that the potentially serious side effects of fluoroquinolones may outweigh their benefit in treating uncomplicated respiratory and urinary tract infections; however, because of the short duration of therapy for TD, these side effects are not believed to be a significant risk.

A potential alternative to fluoroquinolones is azithromycin, although enteropathogens with decreased azithromycin susceptibility have been documented in several countries. Rifaximin has been approved to treat TD caused by noninvasive strains of *E. coli*. However, since it is often difficult for travelers to distinguish between invasive and noninvasive diarrhea, and since they would have to carry a backup drug in the event of invasive diarrhea, the overall usefulness of rifaximin as empiric self-treatment remains to be determined.

Single-dose regimens are equivalent to multidose regimens and may be more convenient for the traveler. Single-dose therapy with a fluoroquinolone is well established, both by clinical trials and clinical experience. The best regimen for azithromycin treatment may also be a single dose of 1,000 mg, but side effects (mainly nausea) may limit the acceptability of this large dose. Giving azithromycin as 2 divided doses on the same day may limit this adverse event.

Because of the competing concerns of effective treatment of TD episodes and a desire to avoid the potential negative consequences of antibiotic use, consensus guidelines have been developed by the International Society of Travel Medicine to address this (Box 2-2 and Table 2-6). See the next section in this chapter for more information on the risks and benefits of antiobiotic use for TD.

Treatment of TD Caused by Protozoa

The most common parasitic cause of TD is *Giardia intestinalis*, and treatment options include metronidazole, tinidazole, and nitazoxanide (see Chapter 3, Giardiasis). Although cryptosporidiosis is usually a self-limited illness in immunocompetent people, nitazoxanide can be considered as a treatment option. Cyclosporiasis is treated with trimethoprim-sulfamethoxazole. Treatment of amebiasis is with metronidazole or tinidazole, followed by treatment with a luminal agent such as iodoquinol or paromomycin.

Treatment for Children

Children who accompany their parents on trips to high-risk destinations can contract TD as well, with elevated risk if they are visiting friends and family. Causative organisms include bacteria responsible for TD in adults as well as viruses including norovirus and rotavirus. The main treatment for TD in children is ORS. Infants and younger children with TD are at higher risk for dehydration, which is best prevented by the early initiation of oral rehydration. Empiric antibiotic therapy should be considered if there is bloody or severe watery diarrhea or evidence of systemic infection. In older children and teenagers, treatment recommendations for TD follow those for adults, with possible adjustments in the dose of medication. Among younger children, macrolides such as azithromycin are considered first-line antibiotic therapy, although some experts now use short-course fluoroquinolone therapy (despite its not being FDA-approved

Table 2-6. Travelers' diarrhea treatment recommendations

Therapy of mild travelers' diarrhea

- Antibiotic treatment is not recommended in patients with mild travelers' diarrhea.
- Loperamide or BSS may be considered in the treatment of mild travelers' diarrhea.

Therapy of moderate travelers' diarrhea

- Antibiotics may be used to treat cases of moderate travelers' diarrhea.
- Fluoroquinolones may be used to treat moderate travelers' diarrhea.
- Azithromycin may be used to treat moderate travelers' diarrhea.
- Rifaximin may be used to treat moderate travelers' diarrhea.
- Loperamide may be used as adjunctive therapy for moderate to severe travelers' diarrhea.
- Loperamide may be considered for use as monotherapy in moderate travelers' diarrhea.

Therapy of severe travelers' diarrhea

- Antibiotics should be used to treat severe travelers' diarrhea.
- Azithromycin is preferred to treat severe travelers' diarrhea.
- Fluoroquinolones may be used to treat severe, nondysenteric travelers' diarrhea.
- Rifaximin may be used to treat severe, nondysenteric travelers' diarrhea.
- Single-dose antibiotic regimens may be used to treat travelers' diarrhea.

BOX 2-2. Travelers' diarrhea definitions

Mild (acute): diarrhea that is tolerable, is not distressing, and does not interfere with planned activities.	**Moderate (acute)**: diarrhea that is distressing or interferes with planned activities.	**Severe (acute)**: diarrhea that is incapacitating or completely prevents planned activities; all dysentery is considered severe.

for this indication in children) for travelers aged <18 years. Rifaximin is approved for use in children aged ≥12 years.

Breastfed infants should continue to nurse on demand, and bottle-fed infants can continue to drink formula. Older infants and children should be encouraged to eat and may consume a regular diet. Children in diapers are at risk for developing diaper rash on their buttocks in response to the liquid stool. Barrier creams, such as zinc oxide or petrolatum, could be applied at the onset of diarrhea to help prevent and treat rash. Hydrocortisone cream is the best treatment for an established rash. More information about diarrhea and dehydration is discussed in Chapter 7, Traveling Safely with Infants & Children.

BIBLIOGRAPHY

1. Black RE. Epidemiology of travelers' diarrhea and relative importance of various pathogens. Rev Infect Dis. 1990 Jan-Feb;12 Suppl 1:S73–9.

2. Drakoularakou A, Tzortzis G, Rastall RA, Gibson GR. A double-blind, placebo-controlled, randomized human study assessing the capacity of a novel galacto-oligosaccharide mixture in reducing travellers' diarrhoea. Eur J Clin Nutr. 2010 Feb;64(2):146–52.

3. DuPont HL, Ericsson CD, Farthing MJ, Gorbach S, Pickering LK, Rombo L, et al. Expert review of the evidence base for prevention of travelers' diarrhea. J Travel Med. 2009 May-Jun;16(3):149–60.

4. Farthing M, Salam MA, Lindberg G, Dite P, Khalif I, Salazar-Lindo E, et al. Acute diarrhea in adults and children: a global perspective. J Clin Gastroenterol. 2013 Jan;47(1):12–20.

5. Kantele A, Lääveri T, Mero S, Vilkman K, Pakkanen S, Ollgren J, et al. Antimicrobials increase travelers' risk of colonization by extended-spectrum betalactamase-producing Enterobacteriaceae. Clin Infect Dis. 2015 Mar 15;60(6):837–46.

6. Kendall ME, Crim S, Fullerton K, Han PV, Cronquist AB, Shiferaw B, et al. Travel-associated enteric infections diagnosed after return to the United States, Foodborne Diseases Active Surveillance Network (FoodNet), 2004–2009. Clin Infect Dis. 2012 Jun;54 Suppl 5:S480–7.

7. Raja MK, Ghosh AR. Laribacter hongkongensis: an emerging pathogen of infectious diarrhea. Folia Microbiol (Praha) 2014 Jul;59(4):341–7.

8. Riddle MS, DuPont HL, Connor BA. ACG clinical guideline: diagnosis, treatment, and prevention of acute diarrheal infections in adults. Am J Gastroenterol 2016 May;111(5):602–22.

9. Shlim DR. Looking for evidence that personal hygiene precautions prevent travelers' diarrhea. Clin Infect Dis. 2005 Dec 1;41(Suppl 8):S531–5.

10. Steffen R, Hill DR, DuPont HL. Traveler's diarrhea: a clinical review. JAMA. 2015 Jan 6;313(1):71–80.

ANTIBIOTICS IN TRAVELERS' DIARRHEA—BALANCING THE RISKS & BENEFITS

Mark S. Riddle, Bradley A. Connor

2

For the last 30 years, randomized controlled trials have consistently and clearly demonstrated that antibiotics slightly but significantly shorten the duration of illness and alleviate the disability associated with travelers' diarrhea (TD). Treatment with an effective antibiotic shortens the average duration of a TD episode by about a day, and if the traveler combines an antibiotic with an antimotility agent such as loperamide, the duration is shortened even further. Emerging data on the potential long-term health consequences of TD, such as irritable bowel syndrome, dyspepsia, and chronic constipation, might suggest a benefit of early antibiotic therapy given the association between more severe and longer disease and risk of postinfectious consequences.

Although these clinical results are impressive, antibiotics, like any drug, are not without consequences. Each of the antibiotics commonly used to treat TD have side effects, but these are generally mild and self-limiting, and

the benefits appear to outweigh the risks. More recently, there has been concern that antibiotics used by travelers might result in significant changes in the host microbiome as well as the acquisition of multidrug-resistant bacteria. Multiple observational studies have found that people who travel (in particular to regions of Asia), develop TD, and take antibiotics are at incrementally increasing risk for colonization with extended-spectrum β-lactamase–producing Enterobacteriaceae (ESBL-PE). The effect of colonization on the average traveler appears limited; carriage is most often transient but does persist in a small percentage of those who are colonized. However, international travel by a household member is associated with ESBL colonization among US children, which suggests that there may be larger public health consequences from acquiring ESBL-PE during travel.

The challenge that we face as providers and travelers is how to balance the risk of colonization and the global

spread of resistance with the health benefits of antibiotic treatment of TD. Although the role of travelers in the translocation of infectious disease and resistance cannot be ignored, the ecology of ESBL-PE infections is complex and includes environmental, diet, immigration, and local nosocomial transmission dynamics. ESBL-PE infections are an emerging health threat, and addressing this complex problem will require multiple strategies.

How, then, to prepare a traveler with a prescription for empiric self-treatment before a trip? There needs to be a conversation with the traveler about the multi-level (individual, community, global) risks of travel, travelers' diarrhea, preventing TD through hand hygiene and careful selection of foods and beverages, and antibiotic treatment. Reserving antibiotics for moderate to severe TD should be emphasized strongly, and using antimotility agents alone may be suggested for mild TD. Elderly travelers or those with recurrent urinary tract

(continued)

ANTIBIOTICS IN TRAVELERS' DIARRHEA—BALANCING THE RISKS & BENEFITS (CONTINUED)

infections may be at higher risk of health consequences as a result of ESBL-PE colonization. At a minimum these travelers should be made aware of this risk, and should be counseled to convey their travel exposure history to their treating providers if they become ill after travel. Though further studies are needed (and many are underway), a rational approach is advised to decrease exposure by using single-dose regimens and selecting an antibiotic agent that minimizes microbiome disruption and risk of colonization. Additionally, as travel and untreated TD increase the risk of ESBL-PE

colonization, nonantibiotic chemoprophylactic strategies, such as the use of bismuth subsalicylate, may decrease both the acute and post-travel risk concerns. Strengthening the resilience of the host microbiota to prevent infection and unwanted colonization, as with the use of prebiotics or probiotics, are promising potential strategies but need further investigation.

Finally, we must be cognizant of the fact that we expect the traveler to be the diagnostician, practitioner, and patient when it comes to managing TD. For even the most astute traveler, making such learned decisions can

be challenged by the anxiety-provoking onset of that first abdominal cramp in sometimes austere and inconvenient settings. Providing prospective travelers with clear written guidance about TD prevention and step-by-step instructions about how and when to use medications for TD is crucial (see previous section, Travelers' Diarrhea).

BIBLIOGRAPHY

1. Islam S, Selvarangan R, Chohan R, Chappell JD, McHenry R, Dighe A, et al. Antibiotic-resistant Enterobacteriaceae colonization in healthy children in the United States. Open Forum Infect Dis. 2015;2(Suppl 1):73.

Perspectives sections are written as editorial discussions aiming to add depth and clinical perspective to the official recommendations contained in the book. The views and opinions expressed in this section are those of the authors and do not necessarily represent the official position of CDC.

ALTITUDE ILLNESS

Peter H. Hackett, David R. Shlim

The high-altitude environment exposes travelers to cold, low humidity, increased ultraviolet radiation, and decreased air pressure, all of which can cause problems. The biggest concern, however, is hypoxia. At 10,000 ft (3,000 m), for example, the inspired PO_2 is only 69% of sea-level value. The magnitude of hypoxic stress depends on altitude, rate of ascent, and duration of exposure. Sleeping at high altitude produces

the most hypoxemia; day trips to high altitude with return to low altitude are much less stressful on the body. Typical high-altitude destinations include Cusco (11,000 ft; 3,300 m), La Paz (12,000 ft; 3,640 m), Lhasa (12,100 ft; 3,650 m), Everest Base Camp (17,700 ft; 5,400 m), and Kilimanjaro (19,341 ft; 5,895 m).

The human body adjusts very well to moderate hypoxia, but requires time to do so (Box 2-3).

2

BOX 2-3. Tips for acclimatization

- Ascend gradually, if possible. Avoid going directly from low altitude to more than 9,000 ft (2,750 m) sleeping altitude in 1 day. Once above 9,000 ft (2,750 m), move sleeping altitude no higher than 1,600 ft (500 m) per day, and plan an extra day for acclimatization every 3,300 ft (1,000 m).
- Consider using acetazolamide to speed acclimatization, if abrupt ascent is unavoidable.
- Avoid alcohol for the first 48 hours.
- Participate in only mild exercise for the first 48 hours.
- Having a high-altitude exposure at more than 9,000 ft (2,750 m) for 2 nights or more, within 30 days before the trip, is useful.

The process of acute acclimatization to high altitude takes 3–5 days; therefore, acclimatizing for a few days at 8,000–9,000 ft (2,500–2,750 m) before proceeding to a higher altitude is ideal. Acclimatization prevents altitude illness, improves sleep, and increases comfort and well-being, although exercise performance will always be reduced compared with low altitude. Increase in ventilation is the most important factor in acute acclimatization; therefore, respiratory depressants must be avoided. Increased red-cell production does not play a role in acute acclimatization.

RISK FOR TRAVELERS

Inadequate acclimatization may lead to altitude illness in any traveler going to 8,000 ft (2,500 m) or higher, and sometimes even at lower altitude. Susceptibility and resistance to altitude illness are genetic traits, and no simple screening tests are available to predict risk. Risk is not affected by training or physical fitness. Children are equally susceptible as adults; people aged >50 years have slightly lower risk. How a traveler has responded to high altitude previously is the most reliable guide for future trips if the altitude and rate of ascent are similar, but this is not infallible. Given certain baseline susceptibility, risk is largely influenced by the altitude, rate of ascent, and exertion (see Table 2-7). Creating an itinerary that will avoid any occurrence of altitude illness is difficult because of variations in individual susceptibility, as well as in starting points and terrain. The goal for the traveler may not be to avoid all symptoms of altitude illness but to have no more than mild illness.

Some common destinations such as the ones mentioned above require rapid ascent by airplane to >3,400 meters and thus place travelers in the high-risk category (see Table 2-7). Chemoprophylaxis may be necessary for these travelers, in addition to 2–4 days of acclimatization before going higher. In some cases, such as Cuzco and La Paz, the traveler can descend to altitudes much lower than the airport to sleep.

CLINICAL PRESENTATION

Altitude illness is divided into 3 syndromes: acute mountain sickness (AMS), high-altitude cerebral edema (HACE), and high-altitude pulmonary edema (HAPE).

Acute Mountain Sickness

AMS is the most common form of altitude illness, affecting, for example, 25% of all visitors sleeping above 8,000 ft (2,500 m) in Colorado. Symptoms are similar to those of an alcohol hangover: headache is the cardinal symptom, sometimes accompanied by fatigue, loss of appetite, nausea, and occasionally vomiting. Headache onset is usually 2–12 hours after arrival at a higher altitude and often during or after the first night. Preverbal children may develop loss of appetite, irritability, and pallor. AMS generally resolves with 12–48 hours of acclimatization.

High-Altitude Cerebral Edema

HACE is a severe progression of AMS and is rare; it is most often associated with HAPE. In addition to AMS symptoms, lethargy becomes profound, with drowsiness, confusion, and ataxia on tandem gait test, similar to alcohol intoxication. A person with

Table 2-7. Risk categories for acute mountain sickness

RISK CATEGORY	DESCRIPTION	PROPHYLAXIS RECOMMENDATIONS
Low	• People with no prior history of altitude illness and ascending to less than 9,000 ft (2,750 m) • People taking ≥2 days to arrive at 8,200–9,800 ft (2,500–3,000 m), with subsequent increases in sleeping elevation less than 1,600 ft (500 m) per day, and an extra day for acclimatization every 3,300 ft (1,000 m)	Acetazolamide prophylaxis generally not indicated.
Moderate	• People with prior history of AMS and ascending to 8,200–9,200 ft (2,500–2,800 m) or higher in 1 day • No history of AMS and ascending to more than 9,200 ft (2,800 m) in 1 day • All people ascending more than 1,600 ft (500 m) per day (increase in sleeping elevation) at altitudes above 9,900 ft (3,000 m), but with an extra day for acclimatization every 3,300 ft (1,000 m)	Acetazolamide prophylaxis would be beneficial and should be considered.
High	• History of AMS and ascending to more than 9,200 ft (2,800 m) in 1 day • All people with a prior history of HAPE or HACE • All people ascending to more than 11,400 ft (3,500 m) in 1 day • All people ascending more than 1,600 ft (500 m) per day (increase in sleeping elevation) above 9,800 ft (3,000 m), without extra days for acclimatization • Very rapid ascents (such as less than 7-day ascents of Mount Kilimanjaro)	Acetazolamide prophylaxis strongly recommended.

Abbreviations: AMS, acute mountain sickness; HACE, high-altitude cerebral edema; HAPE, high-altitude pulmonary edema.

HACE requires immediate descent; death can ensue within 24 hours of developing ataxia, if the person fails to descend.

High-Altitude Pulmonary Edema

HAPE can occur by itself or in conjunction with AMS and HACE; incidence is 1 per 10,000 skiers in Colorado and up to 1 per 100 climbers at more than 14,000 ft (4,270 m). Initial symptoms are increased breathlessness with exertion, and eventually increased breathlessness at rest, associated with weakness and cough. Oxygen or descent is life-saving. HAPE can be more rapidly fatal than HACE.

Preexisting Medical Problems

Travelers with medical conditions, such as heart failure, myocardial ischemia (angina), sickle cell disease, any form of pulmonary insufficiency or preexisting hypoxemia, or obstructive sleep apnea (OSA) should consult a physician familiar with high-altitude medical issues before undertaking high-altitude travel (see Table 2-8). The risk for new ischemic heart disease in previously healthy travelers does not appear to be increased at high altitudes. Patients with asthma, hypertension, atrial arrhythmia, and seizure disorders that are well controlled at low altitude generally do well at high altitude. All patients with OSA should receive acetazolamide; those with mild to moderate OSA may do well without their CPAP machines, while those with severe OSA should avoid altitude travel unless given supplemental oxygen in addition to their CPAP. People with diabetes can travel safely to high altitudes, but they must be accustomed to exercise and carefully monitor their blood glucose. Diabetic ketoacidosis may be triggered by altitude illness and may be more difficult to treat in those on acetazolamide. Not all glucose meters read accurately at high altitudes.

Most people do not have visual problems at high altitudes. However, at very high altitudes

Table 2-8. Ascent risk associated with various underlying medical conditions

LIKELY NO EXTRA RISK	CAUTION REQUIRED	ASCENT CONTRAINDICATED
Children and adolescents	Infants <6 weeks old	Sickle cell anemia
Elderly people	Compensated heart failure	Severe–very severe chronic obstructive
Sedentary people	Morbid obesity	pulmonary disease
Mild obesity	Cystic fibrosis (FEV$_1$ 30%–50%	Pulmonary hypertension with
Well-controlled asthma	predicted)	pulmonary artery systolic pressure
Diabetes mellitus	Poorly controlled arrhythmia	>60 mm Hg
Coronary artery disease	Poorly controlled asthma	Unstable angina
following revascularization	Poorly controlled hypertension	Decompensated heart failure
Mild chronic obstructive	Moderate chronic obstructive	High-risk pregnancy
pulmonary disease	pulmonary disease	Cystic fibrosis (FEV$_1$ <30% predicted)
Low-risk pregnancy	Severe obstructive sleep apnea	Recent myocardial infarction or stroke
Mild–moderate obstructive	Stable angina	(<90 days)
sleep apnea	Nonrevascularized coronary	Untreated cerebral vascular aneurysms
Controlled hypertension	artery disease	or arteriovenous malformations
Controlled seizure disorder	Sickle cell trait	Cerebral space-occupying lesions
Psychiatric disorders	Poorly controlled seizure disorder	
Neoplastic diseases	Cirrhosis	
	Mild pulmonary hypertension	
	Radial keratotomy surgery	

Abbreviations: FEV$_1$, forced expiratory volume in 1 s.

some people who have had radial keratotomy may develop acute farsightedness and be unable to care for themselves. LASIK and other newer procedures may produce only minor visual disturbances at high altitudes.

There are no studies or case reports of harm to a fetus if the mother travels briefly to high altitudes during pregnancy. However, it may be prudent to recommend that pregnant women do not stay at sleeping altitudes higher than 10,000 ft (3,048 m). In addition, the pregnancy should be verified as low risk and the mother in good health. The dangers of having a pregnancy complication in remote, mountainous terrain should also be discussed.

DIAGNOSIS AND TREATMENT

Acute Mountain Sickness/High-Altitude Cerebral Edema

The differential diagnosis of AMS/HACE includes dehydration, exhaustion, hypoglycemia, hypothermia, or hyponatremia. Focal neurologic symptoms, or seizures, are rare in HACE and should lead to suspicion of an intracranial lesion or seizure disorder. Patients with AMS can

descend ≥300 m, and symptoms will rapidly abate. Alternatively, supplemental oxygen at 2 L per minute will relieve headache quickly and resolve AMS over hours, but it is rarely available. People with AMS can also safely remain at their current altitude and treat symptoms with nonopiate analgesics and antiemetics, such as ondansetron. They may also take acetazolamide, which speeds acclimatization and effectively treats AMS, but is better for prophylaxis than treatment. Dexamethasone is more effective than acetazolamide at rapidly relieving the symptoms of moderate to severe AMS. If symptoms are getting worse while the traveler is resting at the same altitude, or in spite of medication, he or she must descend.

HACE is an extension of AMS characterized by neurologic findings, particularly ataxia, confusion, or altered mental status. HACE may also occur in the presence of HAPE. People developing HACE in populated areas with access to medical care can be treated at altitude with supplemental oxygen and dexamethasone. In remote areas, descent should be initiated in any person suspected of having HACE. If descent is not feasible because of logistical issues, supplemental oxygen or a portable hyperbaric chamber in addition to dexamethasone can be lifesaving.

High-Altitude Pulmonary Edema

Although the progression of decreased exercise tolerance, increased breathlessness, and breathlessness at rest is almost always recognizable as HAPE, the differential diagnosis includes pneumonia, bronchospasm, myocardial infarction, or pulmonary embolism. Descent in this situation is urgent and mandatory, and should be accomplished with as little exertion as is feasible for the patient. If descent is not immediately possible, supplemental oxygen or a portable hyperbaric chamber is critical. Patients with mild HAPE who have access to oxygen (at a hospital or high-altitude medical clinic, for example) may not need to descend to lower elevation and can be treated with oxygen at the current elevation. In the field setting, where resources are limited and there is a lower margin for error, nifedipine can be used as an adjunct to descent, oxygen, or portable hyperbaric therapy. A phosphodiesterase inhibitor may be used if nifedipine is not available, but concurrent use of multiple pulmonary vasodilators is not recommended.

Medications

In addition to the discussion below, recommendations for the usage and dosing of medications to prevent and treat altitude illness are outlined in Table 2-9.

Table 2-9. Recommended medication doses to prevent and treat altitude illness

MEDICATION	INDICATION	ROUTE	DOSE
Acetazolamide	AMS, HACE prevention	Oral	125 mg twice a day; 250 mg twice a day if >100 kg Pediatrics: 2.5 mg/kg every 12 h
	AMS treatment[1]	Oral	250 mg twice a day Pediatrics: 2.5 mg/kg every 12 h
Dexamethasone	AMS, HACE prevention	Oral	2 mg every 6 h or 4 mg every 12 h Pediatrics: should not be used for prophylaxis
	AMS, HACE treatment	Oral, IV, IM	AMS: 4 mg every 6 h HACE: 8 mg once, then 4 mg every 6 h Pediatrics: 0.15 mg/kg/dose every 6 h up to 4 mg
Nifedipine	HAPE prevention	Oral	30 mg SR version every 12 h, or 20 mg SR version every 8 h
	HAPE treatment	Oral	30 mg SR version every 12 h, or 20 mg SR version every 8 h
Tadalafil	HAPE prevention	Oral	10 mg twice a day
Sildenafil	HAPE prevention	Oral	50 mg every 8 h
Salmeterol	HAPE prevention[2]	Inhaled	125 μg twice a day

Abbreviations: AMS, acute mountain sickness; HACE, high-altitude cerebral edema; HAPE, high-altitude pulmonary edema; IM, intramuscular; IV, intravenous; SR, sustained release.
[1] Acetazolamide can also be used at this dose as an *adjunct* to dexamethasone in HACE treatment, but dexamethasone remains the primary treatment for that disorder.
[2] Should not be used as monotherapy and should only be used in conjunction with oral medications.

ACETAZOLAMIDE

Acetazolamide prevents AMS when taken before ascent and can speed recovery if taken after symptoms have developed. The drug works by acidifying the blood, which causes an increase in respiration and arterial oxygenation and thus aids acclimatization. An effective dose that minimizes the common side effects of increased urination and paresthesias of the fingers and toes is 125 mg every 12 hours, beginning the day before ascent and continuing the first 2 days at altitude, or longer if ascent continues. Allergic reactions to acetazolamide are uncommon. As a nonantimicrobial sulfonamide, it does not cross-react with antimicrobial sulfonamides. However, it is best avoided by people with history of anaphylaxis to any sulfa. People with history of severe penicillin allergy have occasionally had allergic reactions to acetazolamide. The pediatric dose is 5 mg/kg/day in divided doses, up to 125 mg twice a day.

DEXAMETHASONE

Dexamethasone is effective for preventing and treating AMS and HACE and prevents HAPE as well. Unlike acetazolamide, if the drug is discontinued at altitude before acclimatization, mild rebound can occur. Acetazolamide is preferable to prevent AMS while ascending, with dexamethasone reserved for treatment, as an adjunct to descent. The adult dose is 4 mg every 6 hours. An increasing trend is to use dexamethasone for "summit day" on high peaks such as Kilimanjaro and Aconcagua, in order to prevent abrupt altitude illness.

NIFEDIPINE

Nifedipine prevents HAPE and ameliorates it as well. For prevention, it is generally reserved for people who are particularly susceptible to the condition. The adult dose for prevention or treatment is 30 mg of extended release every 12 hours, or 20 mg every 8 hours.

OTHER MEDICATIONS

Phosphodiesterase-5 inhibitors can also selectively lower pulmonary artery pressure, with less effect on systemic blood pressure. Tadalafil, 10 mg twice a day, during ascent can prevent HAPE and is being studied for treatment. When taken before ascent, gingko biloba, 100–120 mg twice a day, was shown to reduce AMS in adults in some trials, but it was not effective in others, probably due to variation in ingredients. Ibuprofen 600 mg every 8 hours was recently found to help prevent AMS, although it was not as effective as acetazolamide. However, it is over-the-counter, inexpensive, and well-tolerated.

PREVENTION OF SEVERE ALTITUDE ILLNESS OR DEATH

The main point of instructing travelers about altitude illness is not to eliminate the possibility of mild illness but to prevent death or evacuation. Since the onset of symptoms and the clinical course are sufficiently slow and predictable, there is no reason for anyone to die from altitude illness, unless trapped by weather or geography in a situation in which descent is impossible. Three rules can prevent death or serious consequences from altitude illness:

- Know the early symptoms of altitude illness, and be willing to acknowledge when they are present.

- Never ascend to sleep at a higher altitude when experiencing symptoms of altitude illness, no matter how minor they seem.

- Descend if the symptoms become worse while resting at the same altitude.

For trekking groups and expeditions going into remote high-altitude areas, where descent to a lower altitude could be problematic, a pressurization bag (such as the Gamow bag) can be beneficial. A foot pump produces an increased pressure of 2 lb/in^2, mimicking a descent of 5,000–6,000 ft (1,500–1,800 m) depending on the starting altitude. The total packed weight of bag and pump is about 14 lb (6.5 kg).

BIBLIOGRAPHY

1. Bartsch P, Swenson ER. Acute high-altitude illnesses. N Engl J Med. 2013 Oct 24;369(17):1666–7.

2. Hackett P. High altitude and common medical conditions. In: Hornbein TF, Schoene RB, editors. High Altitude: an Exploration of Human Adaptation. New York: Marcel Dekker; 2001. p. 839–85.

3. Hackett PH, Roach RC. High altitude cerebral edema. High Alt Med Biol. 2004 Summer;5(2):136–46.

4. Hackett PH, Roach RC. High-altitude medicine and physiology. In: Auerbach PS, editor. Wilderness Medicine. 6th ed. Philadelphia: Mosby Elsevier; 2012. p. 2–32.

5. Johnson TS, Rock PB, Fulco CS, Trad LA, Spark RF, Maher JT. Prevention of acute mountain sickness by dexamethasone. N Engl J Med. 1984 Mar 15;310(11):683–6.

6. Luks AM, McIntosh SE, Grissom CK, Auerbach PS, Rodway GW, Schoene RB, et al. Wilderness Medical Society consensus guidelines for the prevention and treatment of acute altitude illness. Wilderness Environ Med. 2010 Jun;21(2):146–55.

7. Luks AM, Swenson ER. Medication and dosage considerations in the prophylaxis and treatment of high-altitude illness. Chest. 2008 Mar;133(3):744–55.

8. Maggiorini M, Brunner-La Rocca HP, Peth S, Fischler M, Bohm T, Bernheim A, et al. Both tadalafil and dexamethasone may reduce the incidence of high-altitude pulmonary edema: a randomized trial. Ann Intern Med. 2006 Oct 3;145(7):497–506.

9. Pollard AJ, Murdoch DR. The High Altitude Medicine Handbook. 3rd ed. Abingdon, UK: Radcliffe Medical Press; 2003.

10. Pollard AJ, Niermeyer S, Barry P, Bartsch P, Berghold F, Bishop RA, et al. Children at high altitude: an international consensus statement by an ad hoc committee of the International Society for Mountain Medicine, March 12, 2001. High Alt Med Biol. 2001 Fall;2(3):389–403.

JET LAG

Gregory Atkinson, Ronnie Henry, Alan M. Batterham, Andrew Thompson

RISK FOR TRAVELERS

Jet lag results from a mismatch between a person's circadian (24-hour) rhythms and the time of day in the new time zone. When establishing risk, clinicians should first determine how many time zones the traveler will cross and what the discrepancy will be between time of day at home and at the destination. During the first few days after a flight to a new time zone, a person's circadian rhythms are still "anchored" to time of day at home. Rhythms then adjust gradually to the new time zone. A useful web-based tool for world time zone travel information can be found at: www.timeanddate.com/worldclock/converter.html. If ≤3 time zones are being crossed, the risk of significant jet lag is likely to be negligible.

Many people traveling over >3 time zones for a vacation accept the risk of jet lag as a transient and mild inconvenience, while other people who are traveling on business or to compete in athletic events desire clear advice on prophylactic measures and treatments. If ≤2 days are spent in the new time zone, some people may prefer to anchor their sleep–wake schedule to time of day at home as much as is practical. Thereby, the total "burden" of jet lag resulting from the short round trip is minimized.

CLINICAL PRESENTATION

Jet-lagged travelers typically experience the following symptoms after a flight across >3 time zones:

- Poor sleep, including difficulty initiating sleep at the usual time of night (after eastward flights), early awakening (after westward flights), and fractionated sleep (after flights in either direction)

- Poor performance in physical and mental tasks during the new daytime

- Negative feelings such as fatigue, headache, irritability, anxiety, inability to concentrate, and depression

- Gastrointestinal disturbances and decreased interest in, and enjoyment of, meals

These symptoms are difficult to distinguish from the general fatigue resulting from international travel itself, as well as from other travel factors such as the hypoxia in the aircraft cabin.

TREATMENT

Since light and social contacts influence the timing of internal circadian rhythms, a traveler who is staying in the time zone for >2 days should try to follow the local people's sleep–wake habits as much as possible and as quickly as possible. This approach can be supplemented with the following information on specific treatments.

Light

Exposure to bright light can advance or delay human circadian rhythms depending on when it is received relative to a person's body clock time. Consequently, schedules have been formulated for proposed "good" and "bad" times for exposure to light after arrival in a new time zone (www.caa.co.uk/Passengers/Before-you-fly/Am-I-fit-to-fly/Health-information-for-passengers/Jet-lag/). After flights that cross a large number of time zones, the proposed best circadian time for exposure to light immediately after the flight may actually be when it is still dark in the new time zone, which raises the question of whether exposure to supplementary light from a "light box" is helpful. Unfortunately, to date, only 1 small randomized controlled trial on supplementary bright light for reducing jet lag has been conducted. No clinically relevant effects of supplementary light on jet lag symptoms were detected after a flight across 5 time zones going west.

Diet and Physical Activity

Dietary interventions do not reduce jet lag symptoms. Because gastrointestinal disturbance is a common symptom, smaller meals before and during the flight might be better tolerated than larger meals. Caffeine and physical activity may be used strategically at the destination to ameliorate any daytime sleepiness, but little evidence indicates that these interventions reduce overall feelings of jet lag. Any purported treatments that are underpinned by homeopathy, aromatherapy, and acupressure have no scientific basis.

Hypnotic Medications

Prescription medications like temazepam, zolpidem, or zopiclone may reduce sleep loss during and after travel but do not necessarily help resynchronize circadian rhythms or improve overall jet lag symptoms. The lowest effective dose of a short- to medium-acting compound should be prescribed for the initial few days, bearing in mind the adverse effects of these drugs. Taking hypnotics during a flight should be considered with caution because the resulting immobility could increase the risk of deep vein thrombosis. Alcohol should not be used by travelers as a sleep aid because it disrupts sleep and can provoke obstructive sleep apnea.

Melatonin and Melatonin-Receptor Analogs

Melatonin is secreted at night by the pineal gland and is probably the most well-known treatment for jet lag. Melatonin delays circadian rhythms when taken during the rising phase of body temperature (usually the morning) and advances rhythms when ingested during the falling phase of body temperature (usually the evening). These effects are opposite to those of bright light. The instructions on most melatonin products advise travelers to take it before nocturnal sleep in the new time zone, irrespective of number of time zones crossed or direction of travel. Studies published in the mid-1980s indicated a substantial benefit of melatonin (just before sleep) for reducing overall feelings of jet lag after flights. However, subsequent larger studies did not replicate the earlier findings. Melatonin is considered a dietary supplement in the United States and is not regulated by the Food and Drug Administration. Therefore, the advertised concentration of melatonin has not been confirmed for most melatonin products on the market, and the presence of contaminants in the product cannot be ruled out.

Ramelteon, a melatonin-receptor agonist, is an FDA-approved treatment for insomnia. A dose of 1 mg taken just before bedtime can decrease sleep onset latency after eastward travel across 5 time zones. Higher doses do not seem to lead to further improvements, and the effects of the medication on other symptoms of jet lag and the timing of circadian rhythms are not as clear.

Combination Treatments

Multiple therapies to decrease jet lag symptoms may be combined into treatment packages. Although marginal gains from multiple treatments may aggregate, evidence from robust randomized controlled trials is lacking for most of these treatment packages. One treatment package offering tailored advice via a mobile application was piloted recently to be used over several months of frequent flying. Participants reported reduced

fatigue compared with the comparator group and improved aspects of health-related behavior such as physical activity, snacking, and sleep quality but not other measures of sleep (latency, duration, use of sleep-related medication).

In conclusion, there is still no "cure" for jet lag. Counseling should focus on the factors that are known, from laboratory simulations, to alter circadian timing. Nevertheless, more randomized controlled trials of treatments prescribed before, during, or after transmeridian flights are needed before the clinician can provide robust, evidence-based advice.

BIBLIOGRAPHY

1. Atkinson G, Batterham AM, Dowdall N, Thompson A, Van Drongelen A. From animal cage to aircraft cabin: an overview of evidence translation in jet lag research. Eur J Appl Physiol. 2014 Dec;114(12):2459–68.

2. Herxheimer A. Jet lag. BMJ Clin Evid. 2014 Apr 29.

3. Herxheimer A, Petrie KJ. Melatonin for the prevention and treatment of jet lag. Cochrane Database of Systematic Reviews 2002, Issue 2. Art. No.: CD001520.

4. Sack RL. Clinical practice. Jet lag. N Engl J Med. 2010 Feb 4;362(5):440–7.

5. Samuels CH. Jet lag and travel fatigue: a comprehensive management plan for sport medicine physicians and high-performance support teams Clin J Sport Med. 2012 May;22(3):268–73.

6. Thompson A, Batterham AM, Jones H, Gregson W, Scott D, Atkinson G. The practicality and effectiveness of supplementary bright light for reducing jet-lag in elite female athletes. Int J Sports Med. 2013 Jul;34(7):582–9.

7. Van Drongelen A, Boot CR, Hlobil H, Twisk JW, Smid T, Van der Beek AJ. Evaluation of an mHealth intervention aiming to improve health-related behavior and sleep and reduce fatigue among airline pilots. Scand J Work Environ Health. 2014 Nov;40(6):557–68.

8. Waterhouse J, Reilly T, Atkinson G. Jet-lag. Lancet. 1997 Nov 29;350(9091):1611–6.

9. Waterhouse J, Reilly T, Atkinson G, Edwards B. Jet lag: trends and coping strategies. Lancet. 2007 Mar 31;369(9567):1117–29.

MOTION SICKNESS

Stefanie K. Erskine

RISK FOR TRAVELERS

Motion sickness is the term attributed to physiologic responses to motion by sea, car, train, air, and virtual reality immersion. Given sufficient stimulus all people with functional vestibular systems can develop motion sickness. However, people vary in their susceptibility. Risk factors include the following:

- Age—children aged 2–12 years are especially susceptible, but infants and toddlers are generally immune. Adults older than

50 years are less susceptible to motion sickness.

- Sex—women are more likely to have motion sickness, especially when pregnant, menstruating, or on hormones.

- Race/ethnicity—Asians may be more susceptible to motion sickness than Europeans.

- Migraines—people who get migraine headaches are more prone to motion sickness, especially during a migraine.

- Medication—some prescriptions can worsen the nausea of motion sickness.

CLINICAL PRESENTATION

Travelers suffering from motion sickness commonly exhibit some or all of the following symptoms:

- Nausea
- Vomiting/retching
- Sweating
- Cold sweats
- Excessive salivation
- Apathy
- Hyperventilation
- Increased sensitivity to odors
- Loss of appetite
- Headache
- Drowsiness
- Warm sensation
- General discomfort

PREVENTION

Nonpharmacologic interventions to prevent or treat motion sickness include the following:

- Being aware of and avoiding situations that tend to trigger symptoms.

- Optimizing position to reduce motion or motion perception—for example, driving a vehicle instead of riding in it, sitting in the front seat of a car or bus, sitting over the wing of an aircraft, holding the head firmly against the back of the seat, and choosing a window seat on flights and trains.

- Reducing sensory input—lying prone, shutting eyes, sleeping, or looking at the horizon.

- Maintaining hydration by drinking water, eating small meals frequently, and limiting alcoholic and caffeinated beverages.

- Avoiding smoking—even short-term cessation reduces susceptibility to motion sickness.

- Adding distractions—controlling breathing, listening to music, or using aromatherapy scents such as mint or lavender. Flavored lozenges may also help.

- Using acupressure or magnets is advocated by some to prevent or treat nausea, although scientific data on efficacy of these interventions for preventing motion sickness are lacking.

- Gradually exposing oneself to continuous or repeated motion sickness triggers. Most people, in time, notice a reduction in motion sickness symptoms.

TREATMENT

Nonpharmacologic treatments for preventing and treating motion sickness can be effective with few adverse side effects (see Prevention above). However, these measures can be time-consuming and unpleasant for travelers. Many patients will prefer medication.

Before deciding which medications to prescribe, consider factors such as individual susceptibility and type, magnitude, and duration of potential stimuli. Medications to treat motion sickness are most effective when taken before exposure.

A primary side effect of most efficacious medications used for motion sickness is drowsiness, along with other drug-specific side effects. Some medications may interfere with or delay acclimation to the offending movement. Because gastric stasis can occur with motion sickness, parenteral delivery may be advantageous.

Antihistamines are the most frequently used and widely available medications for motion sickness; non-sedating ones appear to be less effective. Antihistamines commonly used for motion sickness include cinnarizine (not currently available in the United States), cyclizine, dimenhydrinate, meclizine, and promethazine (oral and suppository). Other common medications used to treat motion sickness are anticholinergics such as scopolamine (hyoscine, oral, intranasal, and transdermal), antidopaminergic drugs (such as prochlorperazine), metoclopramide, sympathomimetics, and benzodiazepines. Clinical trials have not shown that ondansetron, a drug commonly used as an antiemetic in cancer patients, is effective in the prevention of nausea associated with motion sickness.

When recommending any of these medications to travelers, providers should make sure that patients understand the risks and benefits, possible undesirable side effects, and potential drug interactions. Travelers may consider trying the medication before travel to see what effect it has on them.

Medications in Children

For children aged 2–12 years, dimenhydrinate (Dramamine), 1–1.5 mg/kg per dose, or diphenhydramine (Benadryl), 0.5–1 mg/kg per dose up to 25 mg, can be given 1 hour before travel and every 6 hours during the trip. Because some children have paradoxical agitation with these medicines, a test dose should be given at home before departure.

Antihistamines are not approved by the Food and Drug Administration to treat motion sickness in children. Caregivers should be reminded to always ask a physician, pharmacist, or other clinician if they have any questions about how to use or dose antihistamines in children before they administer the medication. Oversedation of young children with antihistamines can be life-threatening.

Scopolamine can cause dangerous adverse effects in children and should not be used; prochlorperazine and metoclopramide should be used with caution in children.

Medications in Pregnancy

Drugs with the most safety data regarding the treatment of the nausea of pregnancy are the logical first choice. Alphabetical scoring of the safety of medications in pregnancy may not be helpful, and clinicians should review the actual safety data or call the patient's obstetric provider for suggestions. Web-based information may be found at the websites www.Motherisk.org and www.Reprotox.org.

BIBLIOGRAPHY

1. Golding JF, Gresty MA. Pathophysiology and treatment of motion sickness. Curr Opin Neurol. 2015 Feb;28(1):83–8.

2. Murdin L, Golding J, Bronstein A. Managing motion sickness. BMJ. 2011 Dec 2;343:d7430.

3. Priesol AJ. Motion sickness. Deschler DG, editor. Waltham MA: UpToDate; 2012.

4. Schmäl F. Neuronal mechanisms and the treatment of motion sickness. Pharmacology. 2013 May;91(3-4):229–41.

5. Shupak A, Gordon CR. Motion sickness: advances in pathogenesis, prediction, prevention, and treatment. Aviat Space Environ Med. 2006 Dec;77(12):1213–23.

6. Zhang L, Wang J, Qi R, Pan L, Li M, Cai Y. Motion sickness: current knowledge and recent advance. CNS Neurosci Ther. 2016 Jan;22(1):15–24.

RESPIRATORY INFECTIONS

Regina C. LaRocque, Edward T. Ryan

Respiratory infection is a leading cause of seeking medical care in returning travelers. Respiratory infections occur in up to 20% of all travelers, which is almost as common as travelers' diarrhea. Upper respiratory infection is more common than lower respiratory infection. In general, the types of respiratory infections that affect travelers are similar to those in nontravelers, and exotic causes are rare. Clinicians must inquire about history of travel when evaluating a patient for respiratory infections.

INFECTIOUS AGENT

Viral pathogens are the most common cause of respiratory infection in travelers; causative agents include rhinoviruses, respiratory syncytial virus, influenza virus, parainfluenza virus, human metapneumovirus, measles, mumps, adenovirus, and coronaviruses. Clinicians also need to consider novel viral causes of respiratory infection in travelers, including Middle East respiratory syndrome (MERS) coronavirus and highly pathogenic avian influenza viruses. Respiratory infection due to viral pathogens may predispose to bacterial sinusitis, bronchitis, or pneumonia. Bacterial pathogens are less common but can include *Streptococcus pneumoniae, Mycoplasma pneumoniae, Haemophilus influenzae,* and *Chlamydophila pneumoniae. Coxiella burnetii* and *Legionella pneumophila* can also cause outbreaks and sporadic cases of respiratory illness.

RISK FOR TRAVELERS

Reported outbreaks are usually associated with common exposure in hotels and cruise ships or among tour groups. A few pathogens have been associated with outbreaks in travelers, including influenza virus, *L. pneumophila,* and *Histoplasma capsulatum.* The peak influenza season in the temperate Northern Hemisphere is December through February. In the temperate Southern Hemisphere, the peak influenza season is June through August. Travelers to tropical zones are at risk all year. Exposure to an infected person from another hemisphere, such as on a cruise ship or package tour, can lead to an outbreak of influenza at any time or place.

Air-pressure changes during ascent and descent of aircraft can facilitate the development of sinusitis and otitis media. Direct airborne transmission aboard commercial aircraft is unusual because recirculated air passes through a series of filters, and cabin air generally circulates in limited areas within the aircraft. Despite this, influenza, tuberculosis, measles, and other diseases have resulted from transmission in aircraft. Transmission may occur via several pathways, including direct physical contact, fomites, direct droplet spread, and suspended small particles. Intermingling of large numbers of people in locations such as airports, cruise ships, and hotels can also facilitate transmission of respiratory pathogens.

The air quality at many travel destinations may be poor, and exposure to sulfur dioxide, nitrogen dioxide, carbon monoxide, ozone, and particulate matter is associated with a number of health risks, including respiratory tract inflammation, exacerbations of asthma and chronic obstructive pulmonary disease (COPD), impaired lung function, bronchitis, and pneumonia. Certain travelers have a higher risk for respiratory tract infection, including children, the elderly, and people with comorbid pulmonary conditions such as asthma and COPD.

The risk for tuberculosis among most travelers is low (see Chapter 3, Tuberculosis).

DIAGNOSIS

Identifying a specific etiologic agent, especially in the absence of pneumonia or serious disease, is not always clinically necessary. If indicated, the following methods of diagnosis can be used:

- Molecular methods are available to detect a number of respiratory viruses, including influenza virus, parainfluenza virus, adenovirus, human metapneumovirus, and respiratory syncytial virus, and for certain nonviral pathogens.

- Rapid tests are also available to detect some pathogens such as respiratory syncytial virus, influenza virus, *L. pneumophila,* and group A *Streptococcus.*

- Microbiologic culturing of sputum and blood, although insensitive, can help identify a causative respiratory pathogen.

- Special consideration should be given to diagnosing patients with suspected MERS (www.cdc.gov/coronavirus/mers/interim-guidance.html) or highly pathogenic avian influenza (www.cdc.gov/flu/avianflu/severe-potential.htm)

CLINICAL PRESENTATION

Most respiratory tract infections, especially those of the upper respiratory tract, are mild and not incapacitating. Upper respiratory tract infections often cause rhinorrhea or pharyngitis. Lower respiratory tract infections, particularly pneumonia, can be more severe. Lower respiratory tract infections are more likely than upper respiratory tract infections to cause fever, dyspnea, or chest pain. Cough is often present in either upper or lower tract infections. People with influenza commonly have acute onset of fever, myalgia, headache, and cough. At present, MERS should be considered in travelers who develop fever and pneumonia within 14 days after traveling from countries in or near the Arabian Peninsula. Certain other patients with illness following contact with a confirmed or suspected MERS case, or with health care facilities with MERS transmission, should also be evaluated.

Practitioners should be aware that regions associated with MERS may expand or change (www.cdc.gov/coronavirus/mers). H5N1 and H7N9 should be considered in patients with new-onset severe acute respiratory illness requiring hospitalization when no alternative etiology has been identified and if the patient has recently (within 10 days) been to a country with recently confirmed human or animal cases of H5N1 (www.cdc.gov/flu/avianflu/h5n1/case-definitions.htm) or H7N9 (www.cdc.gov/flu/avianflu/h7n9/case-definitions.htm) or has had close contact with an ill person who has traveled to these areas in the last 10 days. It should also be noted that highly pathogenic avian influenza A H5 virus has now been reported in wild birds and domestic poultry in the United States. Pulmonary embolism should be considered in the differential diagnosis of travelers who present with dyspnea, cough, or pleurisy and fever, especially those who have recently been on long car or plane rides.

TREATMENT

Affected travelers are usually managed similarly to nontravelers, although travelers with progressive or severe illness should be evaluated for illnesses specific to their travel destinations and exposure history. Most respiratory infections are due to viruses, are mild, and do not require specific treatment or antibiotics. Self-treatment with antibiotics during travel can be considered for higher-risk travelers who develop symptoms of lower respiratory tract infections, such as those who have chronic bronchitis and who have been instructed by their providers to take an antibiotic for exacerbations. A respiratory-spectrum fluoroquinolone such as levofloxacin or a macrolide such as azithromycin may be prescribed to the traveler for this purpose before travel.

The rate of influenza among travelers is not known. The difficulty in self-diagnosing influenza makes it problematic to decide whether to prescribe travelers a neuraminidase inhibitor for self-treatment. This practice should probably be limited to travelers with a specific underlying condition that may predispose them to severe influenza.

Specific situations that may require medical intervention include the following:

- Pharyngitis without rhinorrhea, cough, or other symptoms that may indicate infection with group A *Streptococcus*.

- Sudden onset of cough, chest pain, and fever that may indicate pneumonia (or pulmonary embolism), resulting in a situation where the traveler may be sick enough to seek medical care right away.

- Travelers with underlying medical conditions, such as asthma, pulmonary disease, or heart disease, who may need to seek medical care earlier than otherwise healthy travelers.

PREVENTION

Vaccines are available to prevent a number of respiratory diseases, including influenza, *S. pneumoniae* infection, *H. influenzae* type B infection (in young children), pertussis, diphtheria, varicella, and measles. Unless contraindicated, travelers should be vaccinated against influenza and be up-to-date on other routine immunizations. Preventing respiratory illness while traveling may not be possible, but common-sense preventive measures include the following:

- Minimizing close contact with people who are coughing and sneezing.

- Frequent handwashing, either with soap and water or alcohol-based hand sanitizers (containing ≥60% alcohol) when soap and water are not available.

- Using a vasoconstricting nasal spray immediately before air travel, if the traveler has a pre-existing eustachian tube dysfunction, may help lessen the likelihood of otitis or barotrauma.

Appropriate infection control measures should be used while managing any patient with a respiratory infection (www.cdc.gov/flu/professionals/infectioncontrol).

BIBLIOGRAPHY

1. Benkouiten S, Charrel R, Belhouchat K, Drali T, Nougairede A, Salez N, et al. Respiratory viruses and bacteria among pilgrims during the 2013 Hajj. Emerg Infect Dis. 2014 Nov.;20(11):1821–7.

2. Camps M, Vilella A, Marcos MA, Letang E, Munoz J, Salvado E, et al. Incidence of respiratory viruses among travelers with a febrile syndrome returning from tropical and subtropical areas. J Med Virol. 2008 Apr;80(4):711–5.

3. Foxwell AR, Roberts L, Lokuge K, Kelly PM. Transmission of influenza on international flights, May 2009. Emerg Infect Dis. 2011 Jul;17(7):1188–94.

4. Freedman DO, Weld LH, Kozarsky PE, Fisk T, Robins R, von Sonnenburg F, et al. Spectrum of disease and relation to place of exposure among ill returned travelers. N Engl J Med. 2006 Jan 12;354(2):119–30.

5. German M, Olsha R, Kristjanson E, Marchand-Austin A, Peci A, Winter AL, et al. Acute respiratory infections in travelers returning from MERS-CoV-affected areas. Emerg Infect Dis. 2015 Sep.;21(9):1654–6.

6. Jennings L, Priest PC, Psutka RA, Duncan AR, Anderson T, Mahagamasekera P, et al. Respiratory viruses in airline travellers with influenza symptoms: Results of an airport screening study. J Clin Virol. 2015 Jun;67:8–13.

7. Leder K, Sundararajan V, Weld L, Pandey P, Brown G, Torresi J. Respiratory tract infections in travelers: a review of the GeoSentinel surveillance network. Clin Infect Dis. 2003 Feb 15;36(4):399–406.

8. Leder K, Torresi J, Libman MD, Cramer JP, Castelli F, Schlagenhauf P, et al. GeoSentinel surveillance of illness in returned travelers, 2007–2011. Ann Intern Med. 2013 Mar 19;158(6):456–68.

9. Luna LK, Panning M, Grywna K, Pfefferle S, Drosten C. Spectrum of viruses and atypical bacteria in intercontinental air travelers with symptoms of acute respiratory infection. J Infect Dis. 2007 Mar 1;195(5):675–9.

10. Mangili A, Gendreau MA. Transmission of infectious diseases during commercial air travel. Lancet. 2005 Mar 1218;365(9463):989–96.

Counseling & Advice for Travelers

FOOD & WATER PRECAUTIONS

Patricia M. Griffin, Michele C. Hlavsa, Jonathan S. Yoder

Contaminated food and water often pose a risk for travelers. Many of the infectious diseases associated with contaminated food and water are caused by pathogens transmitted via the fecal–oral route. Swallowing, inhaling aerosols of, or coming in contact with contaminated water, including natural freshwater, marine water, or the water in inadequately treated swimming pools, water playgrounds (splash parks or splash pads), or hot tubs and spas can transmit pathogens that can cause diarrhea, vomiting, or infection of the ears, eyes, skin, or the respiratory or nervous system.

FOOD

Travelers should be advised to select food with care. Raw food is especially likely to be contaminated. Raw or undercooked meat, fish, and shellfish can carry various intestinal and systemic pathogens. (Some fish harvested from tropical waters can transmit toxins that survive cooking; see Food Poisoning from Marine Toxins section in this chapter.) In areas where hygiene and sanitation are inadequate or unknown, travelers should avoid consuming salads, uncooked vegetables, unpasteurized fruit juices, unpasteurized milk, or cheese made from unpasteurized milk. Raw fruits that are eaten unpeeled (such as strawberries) should be avoided, and fruits that are eaten peeled (such as bananas and mangoes) should be peeled by the person who eats them. Produce should be washed under safe running water or soaked in water that has been purified, and then rinsed with safe water just before eating (see Water Disinfection for Travelers section in this chapter). It is safest to eat only food that is fully cooked and served hot. Always refrigerate perishable cooked food within 2 hours (1 hour at temperatures >90°F [32°C]). Cooked food that has been stored should be thoroughly reheated before serving. Eggs should be thoroughly cooked, whether they are served alone or used in sauces. Consumption of food and beverages obtained from street vendors has been associated with an increased risk of illness.

Travelers should wash their hands with soap and water before preparing food, before eating, after using the bathroom or changing diapers, before and after caring for someone who is ill, and after contact with animals or their environments. If soap and water are not available, use an alcohol-based hand sanitizer (with ≥60% alcohol) and wash hands with soap and water as soon as they become available. Hand sanitizer is not very effective against *Cryptosporidium* or norovirus and does not work well when hands are visibly dirty or greasy.

The safest way to feed an infant aged <6 months is to breastfeed exclusively. If the infant is fed formula prepared from commercial powder, the powder should be reconstituted with hot water at a temperature of ≥158°F (≥70°C). This precaution will kill most pathogens with which the infant formula may have been contaminated during manufacturing or through handling after opening. To ensure that the water is hot enough, travelers should prepare formula within 30 minutes after boiling the water (see the Water Disinfection for Travelers section later in this chapter). The prepared formula should be cooled to a safe temperature for feeding (for example, by placing the bottle upright in a bath of safe water and safe ice [see below], keeping the bath water below the nipple ring) and used within 2 hours of preparation. Bottles and nipples should be washed and then sterilized (in boiling water or in an electric sterilizer). Travelers may wish to pack enough formula for their trip because manufacturing standards vary widely around the world.

Travelers should be advised not to bring perishable seafood from high-risk areas back to the United States. For example, cholera has occurred in people who ate crab that had been brought into the United States from Latin America by travelers. Moreover, travelers should not assume that food and water aboard commercial aircraft are safe; they may be obtained in the country of departure, where hygiene and sanitation may be inadequate.

WATER
Drinking Water and Other Beverages

In many parts of the world, particularly where water treatment, sanitation, and hygiene are inadequate, tap water may contain disease-causing agents, including viruses, bacteria, and parasites, or chemical contaminants such as lead. As a result, tap water in some places may be unsafe for drinking, preparing food and beverages, making ice, cooking, and brushing teeth. Infants, young children, pregnant women, the elderly, and people whose immune systems are compromised (for example, because of HIV, chemotherapy, or transplant medications) may be especially susceptible to illness.

Travelers should avoid drinking or putting into their mouths tap water unless they are reasonably certain it is safe. Many people choose to disinfect or filter their water when traveling to destinations where safe tap water may not be available. Tap water is not sterile and should not be used for sinus or nasal irrigation or rinsing, including use in neti pots and for ritual ablution (see Chapter 4, Saudi Arabia: Hajj/Umrah Pilgrimage), unless it is disinfected. Tap water should never be used to clean or rinse contact lenses. Water contaminated with toxins or chemicals will not be made safe by boiling or disinfection.

In areas where tap water may be unsafe, only commercially bottled water from an unopened, factory-sealed container or water that has been adequately disinfected should be used for drinking, preparing food and beverages, making ice, cooking, and brushing teeth. (See Water Disinfection for Travelers later in this chapter for proper disinfection techniques.)

Beverages made with boiled water and served steaming hot (such as tea and coffee) are generally safe to drink. When served in unopened, factory-sealed cans or bottles, carbonated beverages, commercially prepared fruit drinks, water, alcoholic beverages, and pasteurized drinks generally can be considered safe. Because water on the outside of cans and bottles may be contaminated, they should be wiped clean and dried before opening or drinking directly from the container.

Beverages that may not be safe for consumption include fountain drinks or other drinks made with tap water and iced drinks. Because ice might be made from contaminated water, travelers in areas with unsafe tap water should request that beverages be served without ice.

Recreational Water

Pathogens that cause gastrointestinal, respiratory, skin, ear, eye, and neurologic illnesses can be transmitted by contaminated recreational water in inadequately treated pools, water playgrounds (splash pads or spray parks), or hot tubs and spas or in freshwater or marine water. Recreational water contaminated by human feces from swimmers, sewage, animal waste, or wastewater runoff can appear clear but still contain disease-causing infectious or chemical agents. Ingesting even small amounts of such water can cause illness. To protect other people, children and adults with diarrhea should not enter recreational water. Infectious pathogens, such as *Cryptosporidium*, can survive for days even in well-maintained pools, water playgrounds, and hot tubs and spas.

Maintaining proper pH and free chlorine or bromine concentration is necessary to prevent transmission of most infectious pathogens in water in pools, water playgrounds, and hot tubs and spas. If travelers would like to test recreational water prior to use, CDC recommends pH 7.2–7.8 and a free available chlorine concentration of at least 3 ppm in hot tubs and spas and at least 1 ppm in pools and water playgrounds (or a free available bromine concentration of at least 4 ppm in hot tubs and spas and at least 3 ppm in pools and water playgrounds). Test strips may be purchased at most superstores, hardware stores, and pool supply stores. *Pseudomonas*, which can cause "hot tub rash" or "swimmer's ear," and *Legionella* (see Chapter 3, Legionellosis) can multiply in hot tubs and spas in which chlorine or bromine

concentrations are not adequately maintained. Travelers at increased risk for legionellosis, such as the elderly and those with immunocompromising conditions, may choose to avoid entering or walking near higher-risk areas such as hot tubs and spas (see Chapter 3, Legionellosis). Travelers should avoid pools, water playgrounds, and hot tubs or spas where bather limits are not enforced or where the water is cloudy. Additional guidance can be found at www.cdc.gov/healthywater/swimming.

To protect their health in oceans, lakes, and rivers, travelers should try not to swim or wade (1) near storm drains; (2) in water that may be contaminated with sewage, human or animal feces, or wastewater runoff; (3) in lakes or rivers after heavy rainfall; 4) in freshwater streams, canals, and lakes in schistosomiasis-endemic areas of the Caribbean, South America, Africa, and Asia (see Chapter 3, Schistosomiasis); (5) in water that might be contaminated with urine from animals infected with *Leptospira* (see Chapter 3, Leptospirosis); or (6) in warm seawater when they have wounds. A traveler with an open wound should stay out of the water if the wound is not covered with a water-occlusive bandage. To help prevent a rare but fatal infection caused by *Naegleria fowleri* (www.cdc.gov/parasites/naegleria), a parasite found in warm freshwater around the world, travelers should prevent water from entering the nose by holding the nose shut or wearing a nose clip when swimming, diving, or participating in similar activities in warm freshwater (including lakes, rivers, ponds, hot springs, or locations with water warmed by discharge from power plants and industrial complexes), and avoid digging in or stirring up sediment, especially in warm water. This infection has also been linked to use of contaminated tap water for sinus and nasal irrigation.

BIBLIOGRAPHY

1. Cartwright RY, Colbourne JS. Cryptosporidiosis and hotel swimming pools—a multifaceted challenge. Water SciTechnol: Water Supply. 2002 Jan 2(3):47–54.

2. CDC. Drinking water: camping, hiking, travel. Atlanta: CDC; 2012 [cited 2016 Apr. 15]; Available from: www.cdc.gov/healthywater/drinking/travel/index.html

3. CDC. *Naegleria fowleri*—Primary amebic meningoencephalitis (PAM). Atlanta, GA: CDC; 2012 [updated Sep. 24, 2015; cited 2016 Apr. 15]; Available from: www.cdc.gov/parasites/naegleria/index.html.

4. CDC. Legionellosis resource site. Atlanta: CDC; 2013 [cited 2016 Apr. 15]; Available from: www.cdc.gov/legionella/index.html.

5. CDC. Notes from the field: primary amebic meningo-encephalitis associated with ritual nasal rinsing—St. Thomas, US Virgin Islands, 2012. MMWR Morb Mortal Wkly Rep. 2013 Nov 15;62(45):903.

6. CDC. Otitis externa: Swimmer's ear. Atlanta: CDC; 2016 [updated May 4, 2016; cited 2016 Apr. 15]; Available from: www.cdc.gov/healthywater/swimming/swimmers/rwi/ear-infections.html.

7. CDC. Pseudomonas dermatitis/folliculitis: Hot tub rash. Atlanta: CDC; 2016 [updated May 4, 2016; cited 2016 Apr. 15]; Available from: www.cdc.gov/healthywater/swimming/swimmers/rwi/rashes.html.

8. Eberhart-Phillips J, Besser RE, Tormey MP, Koo D, Feikin D, Araneta MR, et al. An outbreak of cholera from food served on an international aircraft. Epidemiol Infect. 1996 Feb;116(1):9–13.

9. Finelli L, Swerdlow D, Mertz K, Ragazzoni H, Spitalny K. Outbreak of cholera associated with crab brought from an area with epidemic disease. J Infect Dis. 1992 Dec;166(6):1433–5.

10. Yoder JS, Straif-Bourgeois S, Roy SL, Moore TA, Visvesvara GS, Ratard RC, et al. Primary amebic meningoencephalitis deaths associated with sinus irrigation using contaminated tap water. Clin Infect Dis. 2012 Nov;55(9):e79–85.

WATER DISINFECTION FOR TRAVELERS

Howard D. Backer

RISK FOR TRAVELERS

Waterborne disease is a risk for international travelers who visit countries that have poor hygiene and inadequate sanitation, and for wilderness visitors who rely on surface water in any country, including the United States. The list of potential waterborne pathogens is extensive and includes bacteria, viruses, protozoa, and parasitic helminths. Most of the organisms that can cause travelers' diarrhea can be waterborne. Where treated tap water is available, most travelers' intestinal infections are probably transmitted by food, but aging or inadequate water treatment infrastructure may not effectively disinfect water or maintain water quality during distribution. Where untreated surface or well water is used and there is no sanitation infrastructure, the risk of waterborne infection is high. Microorganisms with small infectious doses (such as *Giardia, Cryptosporidium, Shigella, Escherichia coli* O157:H7, and norovirus) can even cause illness through recreational water exposure, via inadvertent water ingestion.

Bottled water has become the convenient solution for most travelers, but in some places it may not be superior to tap water. Moreover, the plastic bottles create an ecological problem, since most developing countries do not recycle plastic bottles. All international travelers, especially long-term travelers or expatriates, should become familiar with and use simple methods to ensure safe drinking water. Several methods are scalable and some can be improvised from local resources, allowing adaptation to disaster relief and refugee situations. Table 2-10 compares benefits and limitations of different methods.

FIELD TECHNIQUES FOR WATER TREATMENT

Heat

Common intestinal pathogens are readily inactivated by heat. Microorganisms are killed in a shorter time at higher temperatures, whereas temperatures as low as 140°F (60°C) are effective with a longer contact time. Pasteurization uses this principle to kill foodborne enteric pathogens and spoilage-causing organisms at temperatures between 140°F (60°C) and 158°F (70°C), well below the boiling point of water (212°F [100°C]).

Although boiling is not necessary to kill common intestinal pathogens, it is the only easily recognizable end point that does not require a thermometer. All organisms except bacterial

Table 2-10. Comparison of water disinfection techniques

TECHNIQUE	ADVANTAGES	DISADVANTAGES
Heat	• Does not impart additional taste or color • Single step that inactivates all enteric pathogens • Efficacy is not compromised by contaminants or particles in the water as for halogenation and filtration	• Does not improve taste, smell, or appearance of source water • Fuel sources may be scarce, expensive, or unavailable • Does not prevent recontamination during storage
Filtration	• Simple to operate • Requires no holding time for treatment • Large choice of commercial product designs • Adds no unpleasant taste and often improves taste and appearance of water • Can be combined with halogens to remove or kill all pathogenic waterborne microbes	• Adds bulk and weight to baggage • Many filters do not reliably remove viruses • Channeling of water or high pressure can force microorganisms through the filter • More expensive than chemical treatment • Eventually clogs from suspended particulate matter and may require some field maintenance or repair • Does not prevent recontamination during storage
Halogens (chlorine, iodine)	• Inexpensive and widely available in liquid or tablet form • Taste can be removed by simple techniques • Flexible dosing • Equally easy to treat large and small volumes • Will preserve microbiologic quality of stored water	• Impart taste and odor to water • Flexible dosing requires understanding of principles • Iodine is physiologically active, with potential adverse effects • Not readily effective against *Cryptosporidium* oocysts • Efficacy decreases with low water temperature and decreasing water clarity • Corrosive and stains clothing
Chlorine dioxide	• Low doses have no taste or color • Simple to use and available in liquid or tablet form • More potent than equivalent doses of chlorine • Effective against all waterborne pathogens	• Volatile and sensitive to sunlight: do not expose tablets to air, and use generated solutions rapidly • No persistent residual concentration, so does not prevent recontamination during storage
Ultraviolet (UV)	• Imparts no taste • Portable devices now available • Effective against all waterborne pathogens • Extra doses of UV can be used for added assurance and with no side effects • Solar UV exposure (SODIS) also provides substantial benefit	• Requires clear water • Does not improve taste or appearance of water • Relatively expensive (except solar) • Requires batteries or power source • Cannot know if devices are delivering required UV doses • No persistent residual concentration, so does not prevent recontamination during storage

spores, which are rarely waterborne enteric pathogens, are killed in seconds at boiling temperature. In addition, the time required to heat the water from 60°C to boiling works toward heat disinfection. Any water that is brought to a boil should be adequately disinfected; however, if fuel supplies are adequate, travelers may wish to boil for 1 minute to allow for a margin of safety. Although the boiling point decreases with altitude, at common terrestrial travel elevations it is still above temperatures required to inactivate enteric pathogens.

If no other means of water treatment is available, a potential alternative to boiling is to use tap water that is too hot to touch, which is probably at a temperature between 131°F (55°C) and 140°F (60°C). This temperature may be adequate to kill pathogens if the water has been kept hot in the tank for some time. Travelers with access to electricity can bring a small electric heating coil or a lightweight beverage warmer to boil water.

Filtration and Clarification

Portable hand-pump or gravity-drip filters with various designs and types of filter media are commercially available to international travelers. Filter pore size is the primary determinant of a filter's effectiveness, but microorganisms also adhere to filter media by electrochemical reactions. Microfilters with "absolute" pore sizes of 0.1– 0.4 µm are usually effective to remove cysts and bacteria but may not adequately remove viruses, which are a major concern in water with high levels of fecal contamination (Table 2-11). Filters that claim Environmental Protection Agency (EPA) designation of water "purifier" undergo company-sponsored testing that has demonstrated removal of 10^6 bacteria, 10^4 (9,999 of 10,000) viruses, and 10^3 *Cryptosporidium* oocysts or *Giardia* cysts. (EPA does not independently test the validity of these claims.)

Progressively finer levels of filtration known as ultrafiltration, nanofiltration, and reverse osmosis can remove particles of 0.01, 0.001, and 0.0001 µm, respectively. All of these filters can remove viruses. Nanofiltration will remove organic molecules, while reverse osmosis will remove monovalent salts, thus achieving desalination. One new portable filter design incorporates hollow fiber technology, which is a cluster of tiny tubules with variable pore sizes that can achieve nanofiltration and remove virus-size particles. These are now available in various designs at reasonable prices, including hand-pump, gravity drip, and drink through. All are effective, although drink-through is least practical due to the negative pressure required for flow. The high price and slow output of small hand-pump reverse-osmosis units prohibit use by land-based travelers; however, they are survival aids for ocean voyagers, and larger powered devices are used for military and refugee situations. Microfilters that commonly use ceramic, synthetic fiber, compressed carbon, or large-pore hollow-fiber filter elements are sufficient to remove bacteria and protozoan cysts in water with low levels of contamination (wilderness water with little human and animal activity), but hollow-fiber filters with ultrafiltration or nanofiltration should be used for water with high levels of human and animal activity in the watershed. A 2-step process of halogen (see below) and microfiltration can also assure virus removal.

Table 2-11. Microorganism size and susceptibility to filtration

ORGANISM	AVERAGE SIZE (µM)	MAXIMUM RECOMMENDED FILTER RATING (µM ABSOLUTE)
Viruses	0.03	Not specified (optimally 0.01, ultrafiltration)
Enteric bacteria (such as *Escherichia coli*)	0.5 × 3.0–8.0	0.2–0.4 (microfiltration)
Cryptosporidium oocyst	4–6	1 (microfiltration)
Giardia cyst	6.0–10.0 × 8.0–15.0	3.0–5.0 (microfiltration)
Nematode eggs	30 × 60	Not specified; any microfilter
Schistosome larvae	50 × 100	Not specified; any microfilter

Filters made from ceramic clay or simple sand and gravel (slow sand or biosand) filters are successfully used for households in developing countries. Gravel and sand filters can be improvised in remote or austere situations when no other means of disinfection is available.

Coagulation-flocculation (CF) removes suspended particles that cause a cloudy appearance and bad taste and do not settle by gravity; this process removes many but not all microorganisms. CF is easily applied in the field. Alum—an aluminum salt that is widely used in food, cosmetic, and medical applications— or one of several other natural substances is added to the water and stirred. The clumped particulates that form are allowed to settle, then poured through a coffee filter or fine cloth to remove the sediment. Tablets or packets of powder that combine flocculent and hypochlorite disinfection are available (products include Chlor-floc and PUR Purifier of Water [Proctor and Gamble—for humanitarian use, not sold commercially]). CF removes most microorganisms but should not be used as the sole means of disinfection. It also improves the effectiveness of filtration by causing microorganisms, including viruses, to clump with larger particles, facilitating their removal.

Granular-activated carbon (GAC) purifies water by adsorbing organic and inorganic chemicals and most heavy metals, thereby improving odor, taste, and safety. GAC is a common component of household and field filters. It may trap but does not kill organisms. In field water treatment, GAC is best used after chemical disinfection to remove disinfection byproducts as well as the taste of iodine and chlorine (see Halogens below).

Chemical Disinfection

HALOGENS

The most common chemical water disinfectants are halogens, mainly chlorine and iodine, although bromine has similar qualities. Sodium hypochlorite, the active ingredient in common household bleach, is the primary disinfectant promoted by CDC and the World Health Organization Safe Water System at a 1.5% concentration for household use in the developing world. Other chlorine-containing compounds such as calcium hypochlorite and sodium dichloroisocyanurate, available in granular or tablet formulation, are also effective for water treatment. An advantage of halogens is flexible dosing that allows use by individual travelers, small or large groups, or communities.

Given adequate concentrations and length of exposure (contact time), chlorine and iodine have similar activity and are effective against bacteria and viruses (www.cdc.gov/safewater/effectiveness-on-pathogens.html). *Giardia* cysts are more resistant to halogens; however, field-level concentrations are effective with longer contact times. For this reason, dosing and concentrations of halogen products are targeted to the cysts. Some common waterborne parasites, such as *Cryptosporidium*, are poorly inactivated by halogen disinfection at practical concentrations, even with extended contact times.

Chemical disinfection may be supplemented with filtration to remove resistant oocysts from drinking water. Cloudy water contains substances that will neutralize disinfectant, so it will require higher concentrations or contact times or, preferably, clarification through settling, CF, or filtration before disinfectant is added.

Both chlorine and iodine are available in liquid and tablet form. Because iodine has physiologic activity, WHO recommends limiting iodine water disinfection to a few weeks. Iodine use is not recommended for people with unstable thyroid disease or known iodine allergy. In addition, pregnant women should not use iodine to disinfect water over the long term because of the potential effect on the fetal thyroid. Pregnant travelers who have other options should use an alternative means such as heat, chlorine, or filtration.

Some prefer the taste of iodine to chlorine, but neither is appealing in doses often recommended for field use. The taste of halogens in water can be improved by:

- Reducing concentration and increasing contact time;

- Or, following contact time,

  > Running water through a filter containing activated carbon or

> Adding a 25mg tablet of vitamin C, a tiny pinch of powdered ascorbic acid, or a small amount of hydrogen peroxide.

IODINE RESINS

Iodine resins transfer iodine to microorganisms that come into contact with the resin but leave little iodine dissolved in the water. The resins have been incorporated into various filter designs available for field use. Most contain a 1-μm cyst filter, which should effectively remove protozoan cysts. Few models are sold in the United States because of inconsistent test results.

SALT (SODIUM CHLORIDE) ELECTROLYSIS

Passing a current through a simple brine salt solution generates oxidants, including hypochlorite, which can be used to disinfect microbes. This technique has been engineered into a pocket-sized, battery-powered product, which is commercially available.

CHLORINE DIOXIDE

Chlorine dioxide (ClO_2) can kill most waterborne pathogens, including *Cryptosporidium* oocysts, at practical doses and contact times. Tablets and liquid formulations are available to generate chlorine dioxide in the field for small-quantity water treatment. Although extensive data show the efficacy of chlorine dioxide in municipal and industrial systems, fewer data are available to show the efficacy of small-quantity treatment comparable to other halogens—mainly concentrations achieved and contact time required.

Ultraviolet (UV) Light

UV light kills bacteria, viruses, and *Cryptosporidium* oocysts in water. The effect depends on UV dose and exposure time. Portable battery-operated units that deliver a metered, timed dose of UV are an effective way to disinfect small quantities of clear water in the field. Larger units with higher output are available where a power source is available. These units have limited effectiveness in water with high levels of suspended solids and turbidity, because suspended particles can shield microorganisms from UV rays.

Solar Irradiation and Heating

UV irradiation by sunlight in the UVA range can substantially improve the microbiologic quality of water and may be used in austere emergency situations. Recent work has confirmed the efficacy and optimal procedures of the solar disinfection (SODIS) technique. Solar disinfection is not effective on turbid water. If the headlines in a newspaper cannot be read through the bottle of water, then the water must be clarified before solar irradiation is used. Under cloudy weather conditions, water must be placed in the sun for 2 consecutive days.

Silver and Other Products

Silver ion has bactericidal effects in low doses, and some attractive features include lack of color, taste, and odor, and the ability of a thin coating on the container to maintain a steady, low concentration in water. Silver is widely used by European travelers as a primary drinking water disinfectant. In the United States, silver is approved only for maintaining microbiologic quality of stored water because its concentration can be strongly affected by adsorption onto the surface of the container, and there has been limited testing on viruses and cysts. Silver is available alone or in combination with chlorine in tablet formulation.

Several other common products, including hydrogen peroxide, citrus juice, and potassium permanganate have antibacterial effects in water and are marketed in commercial products for travelers. None have sufficient data to recommend them for primary water disinfection at low doses in the field.

THE PREFERRED TECHNIQUE

Tables 2-10 and 2-12 summarize advantages and disadvantages of field water disinfection techniques and their bacteriological efficacy. It is advisable to test a method before travel.

Table 2-12. Summary of field water disinfection techniques

	BACTERIA	VIRUSES	*GIARDIA*/AMEBAS	CRYPTOSPORIDIA	NEMATODES/CERCARIAE
Heat	+	+	+	+	+
Filtration	+	+/–[1]	+	+	+
Halogens	+	+	+[2]	–	+/–[3]
Chlorine dioxide	+	+	+	+	+

[1] Most filters make no claims for viruses. Hollow-fiber filters with ultrafiltration pore size and reverse osmosis are effective.
[2] Require higher concentrations and contact time than for bacteria or viruses.
[3] Eggs are not very susceptible to halogens, but risk of waterborne transmission is very low.

BIBLIOGRAPHY

1. Backer H. Field water disinfection. In: Auerbach PS, editor. Wilderness Medicine. 6th ed. Philadelphia: Mosby Elsevier; 2012. pp. 1324–59.

2. Backer H, Hollowell J. Use of iodine for water disinfection: iodine toxicity and maximum recommended dose. Environ Health Perspect. 2000 Aug;108(8):679–84.

3. Bielefeldt AR. Appropriate and sustainable water disinfection methods for developing communities. In: Buchaman K, editor. Water Disinfection. New York City: Nova Science 2011. pp. 41–75.

4. CDC. Safe water systems for the developing world: a handbook for implementing household-based water treatment and safe storage projects. Atlanta: CDC, 2000 [cited 2016 Sep 19]. Available from: http://www.cdc.gov/safewater/pdf/sws-for-the-developing-world-manual.pdf.

5. Clasen T, Roberts I, Rabie T, Schmidt W, Cairncross S. Interventions to improve water quality for preventing diarrhoea. Cochrane Database Syst Rev. 2006;(3):CD004794.

6. Sobsey MD, Stauber CE, Casanova LM, Brown JM, Elliott MA. Point of use household drinking water filtration: a practical, effective solution for providing sustained access to safe drinking water in the developing world. Environ Sci Technol. 2008 Jun 15;42(12):4261–7.

7. Swiss Federal Institute of Aquatic Science and Technology. SODIS method. Dübendorf, Switzerland: Swiss Federal Institute of Aquatic Science and Technology; 2012 [cited 2016 Sep. 21]; Available from: www.sodis.ch/methode/index_EN.

8. World Health Organization. Boil water. Technical Brief. WHO; 2015 [cited 2016 Mar. 13]; Available from: http://apps.who.int/iris/bitstream/10665/155821/1/WHO_FWC_WSH_15.02_eng.pdf?ua=1.

9. World Health Organization. Guidelines for drinking-water quality. WHO; 2011 [cited 2016 Mar. 13]; Available from: http://apps.who.int/iris/bitstream/10665/44584/1/9789241548151_eng.pdf.

FOOD POISONING FROM MARINE TOXINS

Vernon E. Ansdell

Seafood poisoning from marine toxins is an underrecognized hazard for travelers, particularly in the tropics and subtropics. Furthermore, the risk is increasing as a result of factors such as climate change, coral reef damage, and spread of toxic algal blooms.

CIGUATERA FISH POISONING

Ciguatera fish poisoning occurs after eating reef fish contaminated with toxins such as ciguatoxin or maitotoxin. These potent toxins originate from *Gambierdiscus toxicus*, a small marine organism (dinoflagellate) that grows on and around coral reefs. Dinoflagellates are ingested by herbivorous fish. The toxins produced by *G. toxicus* are then modified and concentrated as they pass up the marine food chain to carnivorous fish and finally to humans. Ciguatoxins are concentrated in fish liver, intestines, roe, and heads.

G. toxicus may proliferate on dead coral reefs more effectively than other dinoflagellates. The risk of ciguatera is likely to increase as more coral reefs deteriorate because of climate change, ocean acidification, construction, and nutrient runoff.

Risk for Travelers

Ciguatera poisoning is underrecognized and underreported; up to 50,000 cases occur globally every year. The incidence in travelers to highly endemic areas has been estimated as high as 3 per 100. Ciguatera is widespread in tropical and subtropical waters, usually between the latitudes of 35°N and 35°S; it is particularly common in the Pacific and Indian Oceans and the Caribbean Sea. The incidence and geographic distribution of ciguatera poisoning are increasing. Newly recognized areas of risk include the Canary Islands, the eastern Mediterranean, and the western Gulf of Mexico. Medical practitioners must be aware that cases of ciguatera fish poisoning acquired by travelers in endemic areas may present in nonendemic (temperate) areas. In addition, cases of ciguatera fish poisoning are seen with increasing frequency in nonendemic areas as a result of the increasing global trade in seafood products.

Fish that are most likely to cause ciguatera poisoning are large carnivorous reef fish, such as barracuda, grouper, moray eel, amberjack, sea bass, or sturgeon. Omnivorous and herbivorous fish such as parrot fish, surgeonfish, and red snapper can also be a risk.

Clinical Presentation

Ciguatera poisoning may cause gastrointestinal, cardiovascular, neurologic, and neuropsychiatric illness. The first symptoms usually develop within 3–6 hours after eating contaminated fish but may be delayed for up to 30 hours. Symptoms include:

- Gastrointestinal: diarrhea, nausea, vomiting, and abdominal pain.

- Cardiovascular: bradycardia, heart block, hypotension.

- Neurologic: paresthesias, weakness, pain in the teeth or a sensation that the teeth are loose, burning or metallic taste in the mouth, generalized itching, sweating, and blurred vision. Cold allodynia (abnormal sensation when touching cold water or objects) has been reported as characteristic, but there can be acute sensitivity to both hot and cold. Neurologic symptoms usually last a few days to several weeks but may persist for months or even years.

- Neuropsychiatric: fatigue, general malaise, insomnia.

The overall death rate from ciguatera poisoning is <0.1% but varies according to the toxin dose and availability of medical care to deal with complications. The diagnosis of ciguatera poisoning is based on the characteristic signs and symptoms and a history of eating species of fish that are known to carry ciguatera toxin. Fish testing can be done by the Food and Drug Administration (FDA) in their laboratory at Dauphin Island. There is no readily available test for ciguatera toxins in human clinical specimens.

Prevention

Travelers can take the following precautions to prevent ciguatera fish poisoning:

- Avoid or limit consumption of reef fish.

- Never eat high-risk fish such as barracuda or moray eel.

- Avoid the parts of the fish that concentrate ciguatera toxin: liver, intestines, roe, and head.

Remember that ciguatera toxins do not affect the texture, taste, or smell of fish, and they are not destroyed by gastric acid, cooking, smoking, freezing, canning, salting, or pickling.

Treatment

There is no specific antidote for ciguatoxin or maitotoxin poisonings. Symptomatic treatment may include gabapentin or pregabalin (neuropathic symptoms), amitriptyline (chronic paresthesias, depression, and pruritus), fluoxetine (chronic fatigue), and nifedipine or acetaminophen (headaches). Intravenous mannitol has been reported in uncontrolled studies to reduce the severity and duration of neurologic symptoms, particularly if given within 48 hours of the appearance of symptoms. It should only be given to hemodynamically stable, well-hydrated patients.

After recovering from ciguatera poisoning, patients may want to avoid any fish, nuts, alcohol, or caffeine for at least 6 months as they may cause a relapse in symptoms.

SCOMBROID

Scombroid, one of the most common fish poisonings, occurs worldwide in both temperate and tropical waters. The illness occurs after eating improperly refrigerated or preserved fish containing high levels of histamine, and often resembles a moderate to severe allergic reaction.

Fish typically associated with scombroid have naturally high levels of histidine in the flesh and include tuna, mackerel, mahi mahi (dolphin fish), sardine, anchovy, herring, bluefish, amberjack, and marlin. Histidine is converted to histamine by bacterial overgrowth in fish that has been improperly stored after capture. Histamine and other scombrotoxins are resistant to cooking, smoking, canning, or freezing.

Clinical Presentation

Symptoms of scombroid poisoning resemble an acute allergic reaction and usually appear 10–60 minutes after eating contaminated fish. They include flushing of the face and upper body (resembling sunburn), severe headache, palpitations, itching, blurred vision, abdominal cramps, and diarrhea. Untreated, symptoms usually resolve within 12 hours but may last up to 48 hours. Rarely, there may be respiratory compromise, malignant arrhythmias, and hypotension requiring hospitalization. There are no long-term sequelae. Diagnosis is usually clinical. A clustering of cases helps exclude the possibility of true fish allergy.

Prevention

Fish contaminated with histamine may have a peppery, sharp, salty, taste or "bubbly" feel but will usually look, smell, and taste normal. The key to prevention is to make sure that the fish is properly iced or refrigerated at temperatures <38°F (<3.3°C), or immediately frozen after it is caught. Cooking, smoking, canning, or freezing will not destroy histamine in contaminated fish.

Treatment

Scombroid poisoning usually responds well to antihistamines (H_1-receptor blockers, although H_2-receptor blockers may also be of benefit).

SHELLFISH POISONING

Several forms of poisoning may occur after ingesting toxin-containing shellfish, such as filter-feeding bivalve mollusks (such as mussels, oysters, clams, scallops, and cockles), gastropod mollusks (such as abalone, whelks, and moon snails), or crustaceans (such as Dungeness crabs, shrimp, and lobsters). The toxins originate in small marine organisms (dinoflagellates or diatoms) that are ingested and are concentrated by shellfish.

Risk for Travelers

Contaminated (toxic) shellfish may be found in temperate and tropical waters, typically during or after phytoplankton blooms, also called harmful algal blooms (HABs). One example of a HAB is the Florida red tide caused by *Karenia brevis*.

Clinical Presentation

Poisoning results in gastrointestinal and neurologic illness of varying severity. Symptoms typically appear 30–60 minutes after ingesting toxic shellfish but can be delayed for several hours. Diagnosis is usually one of exclusion and is typically made clinically in patients who have recently eaten shellfish.

PARALYTIC SHELLFISH POISONING

Paralytic shellfish poisoning (PSP) is the most common and most severe form of shellfish poisoning. PSP is caused by eating shellfish contaminated with saxitoxins. These potent neurotoxins are produced by various dinoflagellates. A wide range of shellfish may cause PSP, but most cases occur after eating mussels or clams.

PSP occurs worldwide but is most common in temperate waters, especially off the Pacific and Atlantic Coasts of North America, including Alaska. Cases have also been reported from countries such as the Philippines, China, Chile, Scotland, Ireland, New Zealand, and Australia.

Symptoms usually appear 30–60 minutes after eating toxic shellfish and include numbness and tingling of the face, lips, tongue, arms, and legs. There may be headache, nausea, vomiting, and diarrhea. Severe cases are associated with ingestion of large doses of toxin and clinical features such as ataxia, dysphagia, mental status changes, flaccid paralysis, and respiratory failure. The case-fatality ratio is dependent on the availability of modern medical care, including mechanical ventilation. The death rate may be particularly high in children.

NEUROTOXIC SHELLFISH POISONING

Neurotoxic shellfish poisoning (NSP) is caused by eating shellfish contaminated with brevetoxins produced by the dinoflagellate *K. brevis*. NSP has been reported from the southeastern coast of the United States, the Gulf of Mexico, the Caribbean, and New Zealand.

NSP usually presents 30 minutes to 3 hours after eating toxic shellfish. Most cases present with gastroenteritis accompanied by minor neurologic symptoms resembling mild ciguatera poisoning or mild paralytic shellfish poisoning. A syndrome known as aerosolized red tide respiratory irritation (ARTRI) occurs when aerosolized brevetoxins are inhaled in sea spray. This has been reported in association with a red tide (*K. brevis* bloom) in Florida. It can induce bronchoconstriction and may cause acute, temporary respiratory discomfort in healthy people. People with asthma may experience more severe and prolonged respiratory effects.

DIARRHEIC SHELLFISH POISONING

Diarrheic shellfish poisoning (DSP) is caused by eating shellfish contaminated with toxins such as okadaic acid. It occurs worldwide, and outbreaks have been reported from China, Japan, Scandinavia, France, Belgium, Spain, Chile, Uruguay, Ireland, the United States, and Canada.

Most cases result from eating toxic bivalve mollusks such as mussels and scallops. Symptoms usually occur within 2 hours of eating contaminated shellfish and include chills, diarrhea, nausea, vomiting, and abdominal pain. Symptoms usually resolve within 2–3 days. No deaths have been reported.

AMNESIC SHELLFISH POISONING

Amnesic shellfish poisoning (ASP) is a rare form of shellfish poisoning caused by eating shellfish contaminated with domoic acid, produced by the diatom *Pseudonitzchia* spp. ASP has been reported from Canada, Scotland, Ireland, France, Belgium, Spain, Portugal, New Zealand, Australia, and Chile. Toxic mussels, scallops, razor clams, and crustaceans were responsible in those outbreaks.

In most cases, gastrointestinal symptoms such as diarrhea, vomiting, and abdominal pain develop within 24 hours of eating toxic shellfish, followed by headache, memory loss, and cognitive impairment. In severe cases there may be hypotension, arrhythmias, ophthalmoplegia, coma, and death. Survivors may have severe anterograde, short-term memory deficits.

Prevention

Shellfish poisoning can be prevented by avoiding potentially contaminated shellfish. This is particularly important in areas during or shortly after algal blooms, which may be locally referred to as "red tides" or "brown tides." Travelers to developing countries should avoid eating all shellfish, because they also carry a high risk of viral and bacterial infections. Marine shellfish toxins cannot be destroyed by cooking or freezing.

Treatment

Treatment is symptomatic and supportive. Severe cases of paralytic shellfish poisoning may require mechanical ventilation.

BIBLIOGRAPHY

1. Ansdell V. Food-borne illness. In: Keystone JS, Freedman DO, Kozarsky PE, Connor BA, Nothduft HD, editors. Travel Medicine. 3rd ed. Philadelphia: Saunders Elsevier; 2013. pp. 425–32.

2. Chan TY. Ciguatera fish poisoning in East Asia and Southeast Asia. Marine Drugs. 2015 Jun 2;13(6):3466–78.

3. Chan TY. Characteristic features and contributory factors in fatal ciguatera fish poisoning—implications for prevention and public education. Am J Trop Med Hyg. 2016 Apr;94(4):704–9.

4. Dickey RW, Plakas SM. Ciguatera: a public health perspective. Toxicon. 2010 Aug 15;56(2):123–36.

5. Hungerford JM. Scombroid poisoning: a review. Toxicon. 2010 Aug 15;56(2):231–43.

6. Isbister GK, Kiernan MC. Neurotoxic marine poisoning. Lancet Neurol. 2005 Apr;4(4):219–28.

7. Palafox NA, Buenoconsejo-Lum LE. Ciguatera fish poisoning: review of clinical manifestations. J Toxicol Toxin Rev. 2001 May;20(2):141–60.

8. Schnorf H, Taurarii M, Cundy T. Ciguatera fish poisoning: a double-blind randomized trial of mannitol therapy. Neurology. 2002 Mar 26;58(6):873–80.

9. Sobel J, Painter J. Illnesses caused by marine toxins. Clin Infect Dis. 2005 Nov 1;41(9):1290–6.

10. Stewart I, Lewis RJ, Eaglesham GK, Graham GC, Poole S, Craig SB. Emerging tropical diseases in Australia. Part 2. Ciguatera fish poisoning. Ann Trop Med Parasitol. 2010 Oct;104(7):557–71.

2

PROTECTION AGAINST MOSQUITOES, TICKS, & OTHER ARTHROPODS

John-Paul Mutebi, William A. Hawley, William G. Brogdon

Vaccines or prophylactic drugs are available to protect against some vectorborne diseases such as yellow fever, Japanese encephalitis, and malaria; however, travel health practitioners should advise travelers to use repellents and other general protective measures against biting arthropods. The effectiveness of malaria prophylaxis is variable, depending on patterns of drug resistance, bioavailability, and compliance with medication, and no similar preventive measures exist for other mosquitoborne diseases such as dengue, chikungunya, Zika, and West Nile encephalitis, or tickborne diseases such as Lyme borreliosis, tickborne encephalitis, and relapsing fever.

The Environmental Protection Agency (EPA) regulates repellent products in the United States. CDC recommends that consumers use repellent products that have been registered by EPA. EPA registration indicates the materials have been reviewed and approved for both efficacy and human safety when applied according to the instructions on the label.

GENERAL PROTECTIVE MEASURES

Avoid outbreaks. To the extent possible, travelers should avoid known foci of epidemic disease transmission. The CDC Travelers' Health website provides updates on regional disease transmission patterns and outbreaks (www.cdc.gov/travel).

Be aware of peak exposure times and places. Exposure to arthropod bites may be reduced if travelers modify their patterns or locations of activity. Although mosquitoes may bite at any time of day, peak biting activity for vectors of some diseases (such as dengue, Zika, and chikungunya) is during daylight hours. Vectors of other diseases (such as malaria) are most active in twilight periods (dawn and dusk) or in the evening after dark. Avoiding the outdoors or taking preventive actions (such as using repellent) during peak biting hours may reduce risk. Place also matters; ticks and chiggers are often found in grasses, woodlands, or other vegetated areas. Local health officials or guides may be able to point out areas with increased arthropod activity.

Wear appropriate clothing. Travelers can minimize areas of exposed skin by wearing long-sleeved shirts, long pants, boots, and hats. Tucking in shirts, tucking pants into socks, and wearing closed shoes instead of sandals may reduce risk. Repellents or insecticides, such as permethrin, can be applied to clothing and gear for added protection. (Additional information on clothing is below.)

Check for ticks. Travelers should inspect themselves and their clothing for ticks during outdoor activity and at the end of the day. Prompt removal of attached ticks can prevent some infections. Showering within 2 hours of being in a tick-infested area reduces the risk of some tickborne diseases.

Bed nets. When accommodations are not adequately screened or air conditioned, bed nets are essential in providing protection and reducing discomfort caused by biting insects. If bed nets do not reach the floor, they should be tucked under mattresses. Bed nets are most effective when they are treated with a pyrethroid insecticide. Pretreated, long-lasting bed nets can be purchased before traveling, or nets can be treated after purchase. Effective, treated nets may also be available in destination countries. Nets treated with a pyrethroid insecticide will be effective for several months if they are not washed. Long-lasting pretreated nets may be effective for much longer.

Insecticides and spatial repellents. More spatial repellent products are becoming commercially available. These products, containing active ingredients such as metofluthrin and allethrin, augment aerosol insecticide sprays, vaporizing mats, and mosquito coils that have been available for some time. Such products can help to clear rooms or areas of mosquitoes (spray aerosols) or repel mosquitoes from a circumscribed area (coils, spatial repellents). Although many of these products appear to have repellent or insecticidal activity under particular conditions, they have not yet been adequately evaluated in peer-reviewed studies for their efficacy in preventing vectorborne disease. Travelers should supplement the use of these products with repellent on skin or clothing and using bed nets in areas where vectorborne diseases are a risk or biting arthropods are noted. Since some products available internationally may contain pesticides that are not registered in the United States, it may be preferable for travelers to bring their own. Insecticides and repellent products should always be used with caution, avoiding direct inhalation of spray or smoke.

Optimum protection can be provided by applying the repellents described in the following sections to clothing and to exposed skin (Box 2-4).

BOX 2-4. **Maximizing protection from mosquitoes and ticks**

To optimize protection against mosquitoes and ticks and reduce the risk of diseases they transmit:

- Wear a long-sleeved shirt, long pants, and socks.
- Treat clothing with permethrin or purchase pretreated clothing.
  - > Permethrin-treated clothing will retain repellent activity through multiple washes.
  - > Repellents used on skin can also be applied to clothing but provide shorter duration of protection (same duration as on skin) and must be reapplied after laundering.
- Apply lotion, liquid, or spray repellent to exposed skin.
- For Mosquitoes
  - > Ensure adequate protection during times of day when mosquitoes are most active.
  - > Dengue, yellow fever, Zika, and chikungunya vector mosquitoes bite mainly from dawn to dusk.
  - > Malaria, West Nile, and Japanese encephalitis vector mosquitoes bite mainly from dusk to dawn.
  - > Use common sense. Reapply repellents as protection wanes and mosquitoes start to bite.
- For Ticks
  - > Check yourself daily (your entire body) and remove attached ticks promptly.

REPELLENTS FOR USE ON SKIN AND CLOTHING

CDC has evaluated information published in peer-reviewed scientific literature and data available from EPA to identify several types of EPA-registered products that provide repellent activity sufficient to help people reduce the bites of disease-carrying mosquitoes. Products containing the following active ingredients typically provide reasonably long-lasting protection:

- **DEET** (chemical name: *N,N*-diethyl-*m*-toluamide or *N,N*-diethyl-3-methyl-benzamide). Products containing DEET include, but are not limited to, Off!, Cutter, Sawyer, and Ultrathon.

- **Picaridin** (KBR 3023 [Bayrepel] and icaridin outside the US; chemical name: 2-(2-hydroxyethyl)-1-piperidinecarboxylic acid 1-methylpropyl ester). Products containing picaridin include, but are not limited to, Cutter Advanced, Skin So Soft Bug Guard Plus, and Autan (outside the US).

- **Oil of lemon eucalyptus (OLE) or PMD** (chemical name: para-menthane-3,8-diol), the synthesized version of OLE. Products containing OLE and PMD include, but are not limited to, Repel and Off! Botanicals. This recommendation refers to EPA-registered products containing the active ingredient OLE (or PMD). "Pure" oil of lemon eucalyptus (essential oil not formulated as a repellent) is not recommended; it has not undergone similar, validated testing for safety and efficacy and is not registered with EPA as an insect repellent.

- **IR3535** (chemical name: 3-[*N*-butyl-*N*-acetyl]-aminopropionic acid, ethyl ester). Products containing IR3535 include, but are not limited to, Skin So Soft Bug Guard Plus Expedition and SkinSmart.

- **2-undecanone** (chemical name: methyl nonyl ketone). The product BioUD contains 2-undecanone.

EPA characterizes the active ingredients DEET and picaridin as "conventional repellents" and OLE, PMD, IR3535, and 2-undecanone as "biopesticide repellents," which are either derived from or are synthetic versions of natural materials.

Repellent Efficacy

Published data indicate that repellent efficacy and duration of protection vary considerably among products and among mosquito and tick species. Product efficacy and duration of protection are also markedly affected by ambient temperature, level of activity, amount of perspiration, exposure to water, abrasive removal, and other factors. In general, higher concentrations of active ingredient provide longer duration of protection, regardless of the active ingredient. Products with <10% active ingredient may offer only limited protection, often 1–2 hours. Products that offer sustained-release or controlled-release (microencapsulated) formulations, even with lower active ingredient concentrations, may provide longer protection times. Studies suggest that concentrations of DEET above approximately 50% do not offer a marked increase in protection time against mosquitoes; DEET efficacy tends to plateau at a concentration of approximately 50%. CDC recommends using products with ≥20% DEET on exposed skin to reduce biting by ticks that may spread disease.

Recommendations are based on peer-reviewed journal articles and scientific studies and data submitted to regulatory agencies. People may experience some variation in protection from different products. Regardless of what product is used, if travelers start to get insect bites they should reapply the repellent according to the label instructions, try a different product, or, if possible, leave the area with biting insects.

Ideally, repellents should be purchased before traveling and can be found online or in hardware stores, drug stores, and supermarkets. A wide variety of repellents can be found in camping, sporting goods, and military surplus stores. When purchasing repellents overseas, look for the active ingredients specified above on the product labels; some names of products available internationally have been specified in the list above.

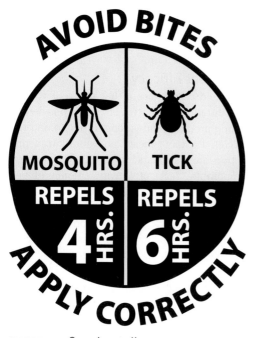

FIGURE 2-1. Sample repellency awareness graphic for skin-applied insect repellents[1]

[1] Image from: www.epa.gov/insect-repellents/repellency-awareness-graphic

Repellency Awareness Graphic

The Environmental Protection Agency (EPA) allows companies to apply for permission to include a new repellency awareness graphic on the labels of insect repellents that are applied to the skin (Figure 2-1). The graphic helps consumers easily identify the time a repellent is effective against mosquitoes and ticks. EPA reviews products that apply to use the graphic to ensure that their data meet current testing protocols and standard evaluation practices. Use of this graphic by manufacturers is voluntary. For more information, visit www.epa.gov/insect-repellents/repellency-awareness-graphic

Repellents and Sunscreen

Repellents that are applied according to label instructions may be used with sunscreen with no reduction in repellent activity; however, limited data show a one-third decrease in the sun protection factor (SPF) of sunscreens when DEET-containing insect repellents are used after a sunscreen is applied. Products that combine sunscreen and repellent are not recommended, because sunscreen may need to be reapplied more often and in larger amounts than needed for the repellent component to provide protection from biting insects. In general, the recommendation is to use separate products, applying sunscreen first and then applying the repellent. Due to the decrease in SPF when using a DEET-containing insect repellent after applying sunscreen, travelers may need to reapply the sunscreen more frequently.

Repellents and Insecticides for Use on Clothing

Clothing, hats, shoes, bed nets, jackets, and camping gear can be treated with permethrin for added protection. Products such as Permanone and Sawyer, Permethrin, Repel, and Ultrathon Permethrin Clothing Treatment are registered with EPA specifically for use by consumers to treat clothing and gear. Alternatively, clothing pretreated with permethrin is commercially available, marketed to consumers in the United States as Insect Shield, BugsAway, or Insect Blocker.

Permethrin is a highly effective insecticide, acaricide and repellent. Permethrin-treated clothing repels and kills ticks, chiggers, mosquitoes, and other biting and nuisance arthropods. Clothing and other items must be treated 24–48 hours in advance of travel to allow them to dry. As with all pesticides, follow the label instructions when using permethrin clothing treatments.

Permethrin-treated materials retain repellency or insecticidal activity after repeated laundering but should be retreated, as described on the product label, to provide continued protection. Clothing that is treated before purchase is labeled for efficacy through 70 launderings. Clothing treated with the other repellent products described above (such as DEET) provides protection from biting arthropods but will not last through washing and will require more frequent reapplications.

Precautions when Using Insect Repellents

Travelers should take the following precautions:

- Apply repellents only to exposed skin or clothing, as directed on the product label. Do not apply repellents under clothing.

- Never use repellents over cuts, wounds, or irritated skin.

- When using sprays, do not spray directly on face—spray on hands first and then apply to face. Do not apply repellents to eyes or mouth, and apply sparingly around ears.

- Wash hands after application to avoid accidental exposure to eyes or ingestion.

- Children should not handle repellents. Instead, adults should apply repellents to their own hands first, and then gently spread on the child's exposed skin. Avoid applying directly to children's hands. After returning indoors, wash your child's treated skin and clothing with soap and water or give the child a bath.

- Use just enough repellent to cover exposed skin or clothing. Heavy application and saturation are generally unnecessary for effectiveness. If biting insects do not respond to a thin film of repellent, apply a bit more.

- After returning indoors, wash repellent-treated skin with soap and water or bathe. Wash treated clothing before wearing it again. This precaution may vary with different repellents—check the product label.

If a traveler experiences a rash or other reaction, such as itching or swelling, from an insect repellent, the repellent should be washed off with mild soap and water and its use discontinued. If a severe reaction has occurred, a local poison-control center should be called for further guidance, if feasible. Travelers seeking health care because of the repellent should take the repellent to the doctor's office and show the doctor. Permethrin should *never* be applied to skin but only to clothing, bed nets, or other fabrics as directed on the product label.

Children and Pregnant Women

Most repellents can be used on children aged >2 months. Protect infants aged <2 months from mosquitoes by using an infant carrier draped with mosquito netting with an elastic edge for a tight fit. Products containing OLE specify that they should not be used on children aged <3 years. Other than the safety tips listed above, EPA does not recommend any additional precautions for using registered repellents on children or on pregnant or lactating women.

Useful Links

- Insect Repellents: Use and Effectiveness (EPA): http://cfpub.epa.gov/oppref/insect/

- Using Insect Repellents Safely (EPA): www.epa.gov/insect-repellents/using-insect-repellents-safely-and-effectively

- FAQ: Insect Repellent Use and Safety (CDC): www.cdc.gov/westnile/faq/repellent.html

- Choosing and Using Insect Repellents (National Pesticide Information Center): http://npic.orst.edu/ingred/ptype/repel.html

BED BUGS

There has been a recent resurgence in bed bug infestations worldwide, particularly in developed countries. Although bed bugs do not transmit diseases, their bites may be a nuisance. Travelers can take measures to avoid bed bug bites and avoid transporting them in luggage and clothing (Box 2-5).

BOX 2-5. Bed bugs and international travel

A recent resurgence in bed bug infestations worldwide, particularly in developed countries, is thought to be related to the increase in international travel, pest control strategy changes in travel lodgings, and insecticide resistance. Bed bug infestations have been increasingly reported in hotels, theaters, and any locations where people congregate, even in the workplace, dormitories, and schools. Bed bugs may be transported in luggage and on clothing. Transport of personal belongings in contaminated transport vehicles is another means of spread of these insects.

Bed bugs are small, flat insects that are reddish-brown in color, wingless, and range from 1 to 7 mm in length. Although bed bugs have not been shown to transmit disease, their bites can produce strong allergic reactions and considerable emotional stress.

PROTECTIVE MEASURES AGAINST BED BUGS

Travelers should be encouraged to take the following precautions to avoid or reduce their exposure to bed bugs:

- Inspect the premises of hotels or other sleeping locations for bed bugs on mattresses, box springs, bedding, and furniture, particularly built-in furniture with the bed, desk, and closets as a continuous structural unit. Travelers who observe evidence of bed bug activity—whether it be the bugs themselves or physical signs such as blood-spotting on linens—should seek alternative lodging.

- Keep suitcases closed when they are not in use and try to keep them off the floor.
- Remove clothing and personal items (such as toiletry bags and shaving kits) from the suitcase only when they are in use.
- Carefully inspect clothing and personal items before returning them to the suitcase.
- Keep in mind that bed bug eggs and nymphs are very small and can be easily overlooked.

Prevention is by far the most effective and inexpensive way to protect oneself from these pests. The costs of ridding a personal residence of these insects are considerable, and efforts at control are often not immediately successful even when conducted by professionals.

BIBLIOGRAPHY

1. Barnard DR, Xue RD. Laboratory evaluation of mosquito repellents against *Aedes albopictus*, *Culex nigripalpus*, and *Ochlerotatus triseriatus* (Diptera: Culicidae). J Med Entomol. 2004 Jul;41(4):726–30.

2. Fradin MS, Day JF. Comparative efficacy of insect repellents against mosquito bites. N Engl J Med. 2002 Jul 4;347(1):13–8.

3. Goodyer LI, Croft AM, Frances SP, Hill N, Moore SJ, Onyango SP, et al. Expert review of the evidence base for arthropod bite avoidance. J Travel Med. 2010 May-Jun;17(3):182–92.

4. Lupi E, Hatz C, Schlagenhauf P. The efficacy of repellents against *Aedes*, *Anopheles*, *Culex* and *Ixodes* spp.—a literature review. Travel Med Infect Dis. 2013 Nov-Dec;11(6):374–411.

5. Montemarano AD, Gupta RK, Burge JR, Klein K. Insect repellents and the efficacy of sunscreens. Lancet. 1997 Jun 7;349(9066):1670–1.

6. Murphy ME, Montemarano AD, Debboun M, Gupta R. The effect of sunscreen on the efficacy of insect repellent: a clinical trial. J Am Acad Dermatol. 2000 Aug;43(2 Pt 1):219–22.

7. Pages F, Dautel H, Duvallet G, Kahl O, de Gentile L, Boulanger N. Tick repellents for human use: prevention of tick bites and tick-borne diseases. Vector Borne Zoonotic Dis. 2014 Feb;14(2):85–93.

SUN EXPOSURE

Vernon E. Ansdell, Rodd Takiguchi

Increased exposure to ultraviolet (UV) radiation occurs near the equator, during summer months, at high elevation, and between 10 AM and 4 PM. Reflection from the snow, sand, and water increases exposure, a particularly important consideration for snow skiing, beach activities, swimming, and sailing. In addition, several common medications may cause photosensitivity reactions:

- Acetazolamide

- Amiodarone

- Antibiotics (fluoroquinolones, sulfonamides, and tetracyclines)

- Diuretics (furosemide, hydrochlorothiazide)

- Nonsteroidal anti-inflammatory drugs (celecoxib, ibuprofen, ketoprofen, naproxen, piroxicam)

- Sulfonylureas (glipizide, glyburide)

Medical conditions such as connective tissue diseases, polymorphous light eruption, rosacea, and vitiligo can increase sun sensitivity. Alcohol consumption can lead to behavioral changes that increase the risk of sunburn.

Both UVA rays (320–400 nm) and UVB rays (290–320 nm) are carcinogenic. UVA rays are present throughout the day and can pass through window glass. UVA rays cause premature aging of the skin and are primarily responsible for drug-related phototoxicity and photoallergic reactions. UVB rays are most intense from 10 AM to 4 PM, are blocked by window glass, and are most responsible for sunburn.

Serious burns are painful, and the skin may be red, tender, swollen, and blistered. These sunburns may be accompanied by fever, headache, itching, and malaise. Cumulative overexposure to the sun leads to premature aging of the skin, including wrinkling and age spots, as well as an increased risk for skin cancer, including basal cell carcinoma, squamous cell carcinoma, and melanoma. Repeated exposure to sunlight in the eyes can also result in ocular pterygium formation, cataracts, and macular degeneration.

PREVENTION

Avoid Overexposure to the Sun

Sun exposure is the most preventable risk factor for skin cancer, including melanoma. Staying indoors or seeking shade between 10 AM and 4 PM is very important in limiting exposure to UV rays, particularly UVB rays. The intensity of UV rays varies seasonally, peaking at the solstice, and gets stronger at the equator and at high altitudes. Be aware that sunburn and sun damage can occur even on cloudy days. Sunburn can occur in a fair-skinned person after as little as 10–15 minutes of unprotected sun exposure. Tanning beds and sun lamps are also carcinogenic and should be avoided.

Protective Clothing

Wide-brimmed hats, long sleeves, and long pants protect against UV rays. Tightly woven clothing and darker fabrics provide additional protection. High-UPF (ultraviolet protection factor >30) clothing is recommended for travelers at increased risk of sunburn or with a history of skin cancer. This type of clothing contains colorless compounds, fluorescent brighteners, or treated resins that absorb UV rays. Sunglasses that provide 100% protection against both UVA and UVB radiation are strongly recommended.

Sunscreens

Sun protection factor (SPF) defines the extra protection against UVB rays that a person receives by using a sunscreen. Although higher-SPF sunscreens provide more protection than lower-SPF sunscreens, SPF is not linear. An SPF 30 sunscreen does not offer twice the protection of SPF 15. Sunscreens with at least an SPF of 15 and that offer protection from both UVA and UVB rays (labeled "broad-spectrum SPF") are recommended for best protection.

Physical sunscreens contain titanium dioxide or zinc oxide, inorganic molecules that are confined to the stratum corneum and reflect and scatter both visible and UV light. They are effective, broad-spectrum sunscreens that protect against both UVA and UVB radiation. With the advent of nanotechnology, these products no longer cause an opaque white film on the skin and have become cosmetically acceptable for widespread use. They are recommended for people who burn easily or who take medications that may cause photosensitivity reactions.

Chemical sunscreens absorb rather than reflect UV radiation. A combination of chemical agents is recommended to provide broad-spectrum protection against UVA and UVB rays. The Food and Drug Administration (FDA) recommends using sunscreen with 15 SPF or higher regularly and as directed.

Travelers should consider the following key points regarding physical and chemical sunscreens:

- Choose a broad-spectrum sunscreen with ≥15 SPF to ensure adequate UVA and UVB protection.

- For UVA protection, look for the following active ingredients: zinc oxide, titanium dioxide, avobenzone, ecamsule, oxybenzone, dioxybenzone, or sulisobenzone.

- Select a waterproof or water-resistant product. Waterproof sunscreens confer approximately 80 minutes of protection in the water, and water-resistant products offer 40 minutes of protection.

- Apply to dry skin 15 minutes to one-half hour before exposure to the sun.

- At least 1 oz (2 tablespoons or enough to fill a shot glass) of sunscreen is needed to cover the exposed areas of the body. Most people only apply 25%–50% of the recommended amount of sunscreen, which decreases the achieved SPF.

- Apply to all exposed areas, including the ears, scalp, back of the neck, tops of the feet, and backs of the hands.

- Use a lip balm or lipstick with broad-spectrum SPF ≥15.

- Reapply every 2 hours and after sweating, swimming, or towel-drying (even on cloudy days).

- The FDA requires that all sunscreens retain their original strength for at least 3 years. Always check the expiration date and discard all expired product.

- Sunscreens should be applied to the skin before insect repellents. (Note: DEET-containing insect repellents may decrease the SPF of sunscreens by one-third. Sunscreens may increase absorption of DEET through the skin.)

- Avoid products that contain both sunscreens and insect repellents, because sunscreen may need to be reapplied more often and in larger amounts than the repellent.

TREATMENT

Travelers with sunburn should maintain hydration and stay in a cool, shaded, or indoor environment. Topical and oral nonsteroidal anti-inflammatory drugs decrease skin redness if used before or soon after sun exposure and may relieve symptoms such as headache, fever, and local pain. Pain is usually most intense 6–48 hours after sun exposure, and skin usually peels 4–7 days later. Topical steroids are of limited benefit, and systemic steroids appear to be ineffective in alleviating pain. Cool compresses, colloidal oatmeal baths, moisturizing creams, and topical aloe vera gel may relieve symptoms. Oral diphenhydramine may relieve itching. If blisters occur, they should be left intact to promote faster healing. Open erosions should be coated with petroleum jelly and covered with sterile gauze to decrease the risk of infection. If infection occurs, oral antibiotics may be necessary. In severe cases of sunburn, dehydration and hypovolemia may occur, presenting with severely inflamed or reddened skin, disorientation, dizziness or fainting, nausea, chills, high fever, and headache. Hospitalization for intravenous rehydration and narcotic analgesics for pain relief may be required in these extreme cases.

BIBLIOGRAPHY

1. Gu X, Wang T, Collins DM, Kasichayanula S, Burczynski FJ. In vitro evaluation of concurrent use of commercially available insect repellent and sunscreen preparations. Br J Dermatol. 2005 Jun;152(6):1263–7.

2. Han A, Maibach HI. Management of acute sunburn. Am J Clin Dermatol. 2004;5(1):39–47.

3. Henry WL, Steven QW. The Skin Cancer Foundation's Guide to Sunscreens New York: Skin Cancer Foundation; 2012 [cited 2016 Sep. 22]; Available from: www.skincancer.org/prevention/sun-protection/sunscreen/the-skin-cancer-foundations-guide-to-sunscreens.

4. Krakowski AC, Kaplan LA. Exposure to radiation from the sun. In: Auerbach PS, editor. Wilderness Medicine. 6th ed. Philadelphia: Mosby Elsevier; 2012. pp. 294–313.

5. McLean DI, Gallagher R. Sunscreens. Use and misuse. Dermatol Clin. 1998 Apr;16(2):219–26.

6. Wang SQ, Stanfield JW, Osterwalder U. In vitro assessments of UVA protection by popular sunscreens available in the United States. J Am Acad Dermatol. 2008 Dec;59(6):934–42.

7. Wang SQ, Tooley IR. Photoprotection in the era of nanotechnology. Semin Cutan Med Surg. 2011 Dec;30(4):210–3.

PROBLEMS WITH HEAT & COLD

Howard D. Backer, David R. Shlim

International travelers encounter environments that may include extremes of climate to which the traveler is not accustomed. Exposure to heat and cold can result in serious injury or death. Travelers should investigate climate extremes that they will face during their journey and prepare with proper clothing, knowledge, and equipment.

PROBLEMS ASSOCIATED WITH A HOT CLIMATE

Risk for Travelers

Many of the most popular travel destinations are tropical or desert areas. Travelers who sit on the beach or by the pool and do only short walking tours incur minimal risk of heat illness. Those who do strenuous hiking, biking, or work in the heat are at risk, especially travelers coming from cool or temperate climates who are not in good physical condition and are not acclimatized to the heat.

Clinical Presentations

PHYSIOLOGY OF HEAT INJURIES

Tolerance to heat depends largely on physiologic factors, unlike cold environments where adaptive behaviors are more important. The major means of heat dissipation are radiation while at rest and evaporation of sweat during exercise, both of which become minimal with air temperatures above 95°F (35°C) and high humidity.

The major organs involved in temperature regulation are the skin, where sweating and heat exchange take place, and the cardiovascular system, which must increase blood flow to shunt heat from the core to the surface, while meeting the metabolic demands of exercise. Cardiovascular status and conditioning are the major physiologic variables affecting the response to heat stress at all ages. Many chronic illnesses limit tolerance to heat and predispose to heat illness, including cardiovascular disease, extensive skin disorders or scarring that limits sweating, diabetes, and renal disease.

In addition to environmental conditions and intensity of exercise, dehydration is the most important predisposing factor in heat illness. Dehydration also reduces exercise performance, decreases time to exhaustion, and increases internal heat load. Temperature and heart rate increase in direct proportion to the level of dehydration.

Sweat is a hypotonic fluid containing sodium and chloride. Sweat rates commonly reach 1 L per hour and may even exceed this level, which results in substantial fluid and sodium loss.

MINOR HEAT DISORDERS

Heat cramps are painful muscle contractions following exercise. They begin an hour or more after stopping exercise and most often involve heavily used muscles in the calves, thighs, and abdomen. Rest and passive stretching of the muscle, supplemented by commercial rehydration solutions or water and salt, will rapidly relieve symptoms. Water with a salty snack is sufficient. An oral salt solution can be made by adding one-fourth to one-half teaspoon of table salt (or two 1-g salt tablets) to 1 L of water. To improve taste, add a few teaspoons of sugar and/or orange juice or lemon juice.

Heat syncope is sudden fainting that occurs in unacclimatized people while standing in the heat or after 15–20 minutes of exercise. Consciousness rapidly returns to normal when the patient is supine. Rest, relief from heat, and oral fluids are sufficient treatment.

Heat edema is mild swelling of the hands and feet (more frequent in women) during the first few days of heat exposure. It resolves spontaneously and should not be treated with diuretics, which may delay heat acclimatization and cause dehydration.

Prickly heat (miliaria or heat rash) manifests as small, red, raised itchy bumps on the skin caused by obstruction of the sweat ducts. It resolves spontaneously, aided by avoiding continued sweating and relief from heat. It is best prevented by wearing light, loose clothing and avoiding heavy, continuous sweating.

MAJOR HEAT DISORDERS

HEAT EXHAUSTION

Most people who experience acute collapse or other symptoms associated with exercise in the heat are suffering from heat exhaustion—the inability to continue exertion in the heat. The presumed cause of heat exhaustion is loss of fluid and electrolytes, but there are no objective markers to define the syndrome, which is a spectrum ranging from minor complaints to a vague boundary shared with heat stroke. Transient mental changes, such as irritability, confusion, or irrational behavior may be present in heat exhaustion, but major neurologic signs such as seizures or coma indicate heat stroke or hyponatremia. Body temperature may be normal or mildly to moderately elevated.

Most cases can be treated with supine rest in the shade or other cool place and oral water or fluids containing glucose and salt; subsequently, spontaneous cooling occurs, and patients recover within hours. An oral solution for treating heat exhaustion can be made by adding one-fourth to one-half teaspoon of table salt (or two 1-g salt tablets) to 1 L of water plus 4–6 teaspoons of sugar. To further improve taste, add one-quarter cup of orange juice or 2 teaspoons of lemon juice. Commercial sports-electrolyte drinks are also effective. Plain water plus salty snacks may be more palatable and equally effective. Subacute heat exhaustion may develop over several days and is often misdiagnosed as "summer flu" because of findings of weakness, fatigue, headache, dizziness, anorexia, nausea, vomiting, and diarrhea. Treatment is as described for acute heat exhaustion.

EXERCISE-ASSOCIATED HYPONATREMIA

Hyponatremia (low sodium [salt] levels in the blood) occurs in both endurance athletes and recreational hikers, likely due to replacement of fluids with excessive amounts of water. The kidneys fail to correct the excess water because of the influence of inappropriate amounts of antidiuretic hormone that act on the kidney to cause retention of water and loss of sodium. Loss of sodium through sweat also contributes to hyponatremia.

In the field setting, altered mental status with normal body temperature and a history of large volumes of water intake suggest hyponatremia. The vague and nonspecific symptoms are the same as those described for hyponatremia in other settings, including anorexia, nausea, emesis, headache, muscle weakness, lethargy, confusion, and seizures. Symptoms of heat exhaustion and early hyponatremia are similar. Hyponatremia can be distinguished from other heat illnesses by persistent alteration of mental status without elevated temperature, delay in onset of major neurologic symptoms (confusion, seizures, or coma), or deterioration up to 24 hours after cessation of exercise and removal from heat. In organized events, measurement of serum sodium should be used to diagnose hyponatremia and guide treatment. Gaining weight or failure to lose weight increases risk of symptomatic hyponatremia.

The recommendation to force fluid intake during prolonged exercise and the attitude that "you can't drink too much" are major contributors to exercise-associated hyponatremia. Prevention includes drinking only enough to relieve thirst. During prolonged exercise (>12 hours) or heat exposure, supplemental sodium should be taken. Most sports-electrolyte drinks do not contain sufficient amounts of sodium to prevent hyponatremia; on the other hand, salt tablets often cause nausea and vomiting. For hikers, food is the most efficient vehicle for salt replacement. Trail snacks should include not just sweets, but salty foods such as trail mix, crackers, and pretzels.

If hyponatremia is suspected along with neurologic symptoms in the absence of hyperthermia or other diagnoses, restrict fluid. In conscious patients who can tolerate oral intake, salty snacks may be given with sips of water or a solution of concentrated broth (2–4 bouillon cubes in 1/2 cup of water). Obtunded patients may require hypertonic saline.

HEAT STROKE

Heat stroke is an extreme medical emergency requiring aggressive cooling measures and hospitalization for support. Heat stroke is the only form of heat illness in which the mechanisms for thermal homeostasis have failed, and the body does not spontaneously restore the temperature to normal. As a result of uncontrolled fever and circulatory collapse, organ damage can occur in the brain, liver, kidneys, and heart. Damage is related to duration as well as peak elevation of body temperature. The onset of heat stroke may be acute (exertional heat stroke), which can affect healthy people who are exercising in the heat, or gradual (nonexertional heat stroke, also referred to as classic or epidemic), which occurs from passive heat exposure in those with chronic illness.

Early symptoms are similar to those of heat exhaustion, with confusion or change in personality, loss of coordination, dizziness, headache, and nausea that progress to more severe symptoms. A presumptive diagnosis of heat stroke is made in the field when people have elevation of body temperature (hyperpyrexia) and marked alteration of mental status, including delirium, convulsions, and coma. Body temperatures in excess of 106°F (41°C) can occur in heat stroke; even without a thermometer, people will feel hot to the touch. If a thermometer is available, a rectal temperature is the safest and most reliable way to check the temperature of someone who may have heat stroke; an axillary temperature may give a reasonable estimation.

In the field, immediately institute cooling measures by these methods:

- Maintain the airway if victim is unconscious.

- Move to the shade or a cool place out of the sun.

- Use evaporative cooling: remove excess clothing to maximize skin exposure, spray tepid water on the skin, and maintain air movement over the body by fanning. Alternatively, place cool or cold wet towels over the body and fan to promote evaporation.

- Apply ice or cold packs to the neck, axillas, groin, and as much of the body as possible. Vigorously massage the skin to limit constriction of blood vessels and prevent shivering, which will increase body temperature.

- Immerse the person in cool or cold water, such as a nearby pool or natural body of water or bath—an ice bath cools fastest. Always attend and hold the person while in the water.

- Encourage rehydration for those able to take oral fluids.

Heat stroke victims usually have significant dehydration, so intravenous or oral fluid replacement is indicated. Heat stroke is life threatening, and many complications may occur in the first 24–48 hours, including liver or kidney damage and abnormal bleeding. Most victims require hospital intensive care management. If evacuation to a hospital will be delayed, monitor closely for several hours for temperature swings.

Prevention of Heat Disorders

HEAT ACCLIMATIZATION

Heat acclimatization is a process of physiologic adaptation to a hot environment that occurs in both residents and visitors. The result of acclimatization is increased sweating with less salt content, and decreased energy expenditure with lower rise in body temperature for a given workload. Only partial adaptation occurs by passive exposure to heat. Full acclimatization, especially cardiovascular response, requires 1–2 hours of exercise in the heat each day. Most acclimatization changes occur within 10 days, provided a suitable amount of daily exercise. After this time, only increased physical fitness will result in further exercise tolerance. Decay of acclimatization occurs within days to weeks if there is no heat exposure.

PHYSICAL CONDITIONING AND ACCLIMATIZATION

Higher levels of physical fitness improve exercise tolerance and capacity in heat, but not as much as acclimatization. If possible, travelers should acclimatize before leaving by exercising ≥1 hour daily in the heat. If this is not possible before departing, limit exercise intensity and duration during the first week of travel in a hot climate. It is a good idea to conform to the local practice in most hot regions and avoid strenuous activity during the hottest part of the day.

CLOTHING

Clothing should be lightweight, loose, and light-colored to allow maximum air circulation for evaporation yet give protection from the sun. A wide-brimmed hat markedly reduces radiant heat exposure.

FLUID AND ELECTROLYTE REPLACEMENT

During exertion, fluid intake improves performance and decreases the likelihood of illness. Reliance on thirst alone is not sufficient to prevent mild dehydration, but forcing a person who is not thirsty to drink water creates the potential danger of hyponatremia. During mild to moderate exertion, electrolyte replacement offers no advantage over plain water. However, for those exercising many hours in heat, salt replacement is recommended. Eating salty snacks or lightly salting mealtime food or fluids is the most efficient way to replace salt losses. Salt tablets, when swallowed whole, may cause gastrointestinal irritation and vomiting but may be better tolerated if 2 tablets are dissolved in 1 L of water. Urine volume and color are a reasonable means to monitor fluid needs.

PROBLEMS ASSOCIATED WITH A COLD CLIMATE

Risk for Travelers

Travelers do not have to be in an arctic or high-altitude environment to encounter problems with the cold. Humidity, rain, and wind can produce hypothermia even with temperatures around 50°F (10°C). Even in a temperate climate, a traveler in a small boat that overturns in cold water can rapidly become hypothermic. However, reports of severe hypothermia in international travelers are rare. Many high-altitude destinations are not wilderness areas, and villages offer an escape from extreme weather. In Nepal, trekkers almost never experience hypothermia except in the rare instance in which they get lost in a storm.

Clinical Presentations

HYPOTHERMIA

Hypothermia can be defined as having a core body temperature below 95°F (35°C). When people are faced with an environment in which they cannot keep warm, they first feel chilled, then begin to shiver, and eventually stop shivering as their metabolic reserves are exhausted. Body temperature continues to decrease, depending on the ambient temperatures. As the core temperature falls, neurologic functioning decreases until almost all hypothermic people with a core temperature of 86°F (30°C) or lower are comatose. The record low core body temperature in an adult who survived is 56°F (13°C). Travelers headed to a cold climate should ask questions and research clothing and equipment. Modern clothing, gloves, and particularly footwear have greatly decreased the chances of suffering cold injury in extreme climates. Cold injuries occur more often after accidents, such as avalanches or unexpected nights outside, than during normal recreational activities.

Travelers engaging in recreational activities or working around cold water face a different sort of risk. Immersion hypothermia can render a person unable to swim or keep floating in <15 minutes. In these cases, a personal flotation device is critical, as is knowledge about self-rescue and righting a capsized boat.

The other medical conditions associated with cold affect mainly the skin and the extremities. These can be divided into nonfreezing cold injuries and freezing injuries (frostbite).

NONFREEZING COLD INJURY

Nonfreezing cold injuries include trench foot (immersion foot), pernio (chilblains), and cold urticaria. Trench foot is caused by prolonged immersion of the feet in cold water (32°F–59°F; 0°C–15°C). The damage is mainly to nerves and blood vessels, and the result is pain that is aggravated by heat and a dependent position of the limb. Severe cases can take months to resolve. Unlike the treatment for frostbite, immersion foot should not be rapidly rewarmed, which can make the damage much worse.

Pernio are localized, inflammatory lesions that occur mainly on the hands and with exposure to only moderately cold weather. The bluish-red lesions are thought to be caused by prolonged, cold-induced vasoconstriction. As with trench foot, rapid rewarming should be avoided, as it makes the pain worse. Nifedipine may be an effective treatment.

Cold urticaria involves the formation of localized or general wheals and itching. It is not the absolute temperature that induces this form of urticaria but the rate of change of temperature in the skin.

FREEZING COLD INJURY

Frostbite is the term that is used to describe tissue damage from direct freezing of the skin. Modern equipment and clothing have decreased the risk of frostbite resulting from adventure tourism, and frostbite occurs mainly during an accident, severe unexpected weather, or as a result of poor planning.

Once frostbite has occurred, little can be done to reverse the changes. Therefore, taking great care to prevent frostbite is crucial. Frostbite is usually graded like burns. First-degree frostbite involves reddening of the skin without deeper damage. The prognosis for complete healing is virtually 100%. Second-degree frostbite involves blister formation. Blisters filled with clear fluid have a better prognosis than blood-tinged blisters. Third-degree frostbite represents full-thickness injury to the skin and possibly the underlying tissues. No blister forms, the skin darkens over time and may turn black. If the tissue is completely devascularized, amputation will be necessary.

Frostbitten skin is numb and appears whitish or waxy. The generally accepted method for treating a frozen digit or limb is through rapid rewarming in water heated to 104°F–108°F (40°C–42°C). The frozen area should be completely immersed in the warm water. A thermometer is needed to ensure the water is kept at the correct temperature. Rewarming can be associated with severe pain, so analgesics can be given if needed. Once the area is rewarmed, it must be safeguarded against freezing again. It is better to keep digits frozen a little longer and rapidly rewarm them, than to allow them to thaw out slowly or to thaw and refreeze. A cycle of freeze-thaw-refreeze is devastating to tissue and can lead to amputation.

Once the area has rewarmed, it can be examined. If blisters are present, note whether they extend to the end of the digit. Proximal blisters usually mean that the tissue distal to the blister has suffered full-thickness damage. For treatment, avoid further mechanical trauma to the area and prevent infection. In the field, wash the area thoroughly with a disinfectant such as povidone-iodine, put dressings between the toes or fingers to prevent maceration, use fluffs (expanded gauze sponges) for padding, and cover with a roller gauze bandage. These dressings can safely be left on for up to 3 days at a time. By leaving the dressings on longer, the traveler can preserve what may be limited supplies of bandages. Prophylactic antibiotics are not needed in most situations.

In the rare situation in which a foreign traveler suffers frostbite and can be evacuated to an advanced medical setting within 24–72 hours, there may be a role for thrombolytics, such as prostacyclin and recombinant tissue plasminogen activator. If you are managing frostbite in the first 72 hours, you should consult someone with expertise in frostbite as soon as possible. The risks and benefits of using these drugs should be carefully considered in each patient. Beyond 72 hours after thawing, these interventions are probably not beneficial.

Once the patient has reached a definitive medical setting, there should be no rush to do surgery. The usual time from injury to surgery is 4–5 weeks. Technetium (Tc)-99 scintigraphy and magnetic resonance imaging can be used to help define the extent of the damage. Once the delineation between dead tissue and viable becomes clear, surgery that preserves the remaining digits can be planned.

BIBLIOGRAPHY

1. Armstrong LE, Casa DJ, Millard-Stafford M, Moran DS, Pyne SW, Roberts WO. American College of Sports Medicine position stand. Exertional heat illness during training and competition. Med Sci Sports Exerc. 2007 Mar;39(3):556–72.

2. Bennett BL, Hew-Butler T, Hoffman MD, Roger sIR, Rosner MH, Wilderness Medical Society. Wilderness Medical Society practice guidelines for treatment of exercise-associated hyponatremia: 2014 update. Wilderness Environ Med. 2014 Dec;25(4 Suppl):S30–42.

3. Cauchy E, Cheguillaume B, Chetaille E. A controlled trial of a prostacyclin and rt-PA in the treatment of severe frostbite. N Engl J Med. 2011 Jan 13;364(2): 189–90.

4. Epstein Y, Moran DS. Extremes of temperature and hydration. In: Keystone JS FD, Kozarsky PE, Connor BA, Nothdurft HD, editor. Travel Medicine. Philadelphia: Saunders Eslevier; 2013. pp. 381–90.

5. Freer L, Imray CHE. Frostbite. In: Auerbach PS, editor. Wilderness Medicine. 6th ed. Philadelphia: Mosby Elsevier; 2012. pp. 181–201.

6. Hadad E, Rav-Acha M, Heled Y, Epstein Y, Moran DS. Heat stroke: a review of cooling methods. Sports Med. 2004;34(8):501–11.

7. Lipman GS, Eifling KP, Ellis MA, Gaudio FG, Otten EM, Grissom CK, et al. Wilderness Medical Society practice guidelines for the prevention and treatment of heat-related illness: 2014 update. Wilderness Environ Med. 2014 Dec;25(4 Suppl):S55–65.

8. O'Brien KK, Leon LR, Kenefick RW. Clinical management of heat-related illnesses. In: Auerbach PS, editor. Wilderness Medicine. 6th ed. Philadelphia: Mosby Elsevier; 2012. pp. 232–8.

9. Rogers IR, Hew-Butler T. Exercise-associated hyponatremia: overzealous fluid consumption. Wilderness Environ Med. 2009 Summer;20(2):139–43.

INJURY PREVENTION

David A. Sleet, David J. Ederer, Michael F. Ballesteros

According to the World Health Organization (WHO), injuries are among the leading causes of death and disability in the world, and they are the leading cause of preventable death in travelers. An estimated 18%–24% of deaths among travelers in foreign countries are caused by injuries, compared with only 2% of deaths caused by infectious diseases. Contributing to the injury toll while traveling are unfamiliar and perhaps risky environments, differences in language and communications, less stringent product safety and vehicle standards, unfamiliar rules and regulations, and a carefree holiday or vacation spirit leading to more risk-taking behavior.

In 2013 and 2014, an estimated 1,670 US citizens died from nonnatural causes, such as injuries and violence, while in foreign countries (excluding deaths occurring in the wars in Iraq and Afghanistan). Motor vehicle crashes—not crime or terrorism—are the number 1 killer of healthy US citizens living, working, or traveling overseas. In 2013 and 2014, 456 Americans died in road traffic crashes abroad (27% of nonnatural deaths). Another 350 were victims of homicide (21%), 286 committed suicide (17%), and 220 drowned (13%) (Figure 2-2).

If a traveler is seriously injured in a foreign country, emergency care may not be available

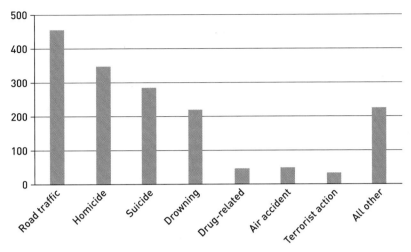

FIGURE 2-2. Leading causes of injury death for US citizens in foreign countries, 2013 & 2014[1,2]

[1] Data from US Department of State. Death of US citizens abroad by non-natural causes. Washington, DC: US Department of State; 2016 [cited 2016 Mar. 24]. Available from: http://travel.state.gov/content/travel/english/statistics/deaths.html.
[2] Excludes deaths of US citizens fighting wars in Afghanistan or Iraq, and deaths that were not reported to the nearest US Embassy or Consulate.

or acceptable by US standards. Trauma centers capable of providing optimal care for serious injuries are uncommon outside urban areas in many foreign destinations. Travelers should be aware of the increased risk of certain injuries while traveling or residing abroad, particularly in developing countries, and be prepared to take preventive steps.

ROAD TRAFFIC INJURIES

Globally, an estimated 3,300 people, including 720 children, are killed each day in road traffic crashes involving cars, buses, motorcycles, bicycles, trucks, and pedestrians. Annually, 1.24 million are killed and 20–50 million are injured in traffic crashes—a number likely to double by 2030. Although only 53% of the world's vehicles are in developing countries, more than 90% of road traffic casualties occur in these countries.

According to US Department of State data, road traffic crashes are the leading cause of injury deaths to US citizens while abroad (Figure 2-2). Motorcycle use is a risk factor for road traffic crashes; in 2013 and 2014, approximately 20% of road traffic deaths while abroad involved motorcycles. Road deaths per million trips are highest in Thailand and Vietnam, and most American

deaths were related to motorcycle use in these countries. The reported rate of motorbike injuries in Bermuda is much higher in tourists than in the local population, and the rate is highest among those aged 50–59 years. Motor vehicle rentals for tourists in Bermuda and some other small Caribbean islands are typically limited to motorbikes, possibly contributing to the higher rates of motorbike injuries. Loss of vehicular control, unfamiliar equipment, and inexperience with motorized 2-wheelers contribute to crashes and injuries, even at speeds <30 miles per hour.

Road traffic crashes are common among foreign travelers for a number of reasons: lack of familiarity with the roads, driving on the opposite side of the road, lack of seat belt use, the influence of alcohol, poorly made or maintained vehicles, travel fatigue, poor road surfaces without shoulders, unprotected curves and cliffs, and poor visibility due to lack of adequate lighting. In many developing countries, unsafe roads and vehicles and an inadequate transportation infrastructure contribute to the traffic injury problem. In many of these countries, motor vehicles often share the road with vulnerable road users such as pedestrians, bicyclists, and motorcycle users. The mix of traffic including cars, buses, taxis, rickshaws, large trucks, and even animals increases the risk for crashes and injuries.

Strategies to reduce the risk of traffic injury are shown in Table 2-13. The Association for International Road Travel (www.asirt.org) and Make Roads Safe (www.makeroadssafe.org) have useful safety information for international travelers, including road safety checklists and

Table 2-13. Recommended strategies to reduce injuries while abroad

MECHANISM OR TYPE OF INJURY	PREVENTION STRATEGIES
Road Traffic Crashes	
Lack of seat belts and child safety seats	Always use safety belts and child safety seats. Rent vehicles with seat belts; when possible, ride in taxis with seat belts and sit in the rear seat; bring child safety seats and booster seats from home for children to ride properly restrained.
Driving hazards	When possible, avoid driving at night in developing countries; always pay close attention to the correct side of the road when driving in countries that drive on the left.
Country-specific driving hazards	Check the Association for Safe International Road Travel website for driving hazards or risks by country (www.asirt.org).
Motorcycles, motorbikes, and bicycles	Always wear helmets (bring a helmet from home, if needed). When possible, avoid driving or riding on motorcycles or motorbikes, including motorcycle and motorbike taxis. Traveling overseas is a bad time to learn to drive a motorcycle or motorbike.
Alcohol-impaired driving	Alcohol increases the risk for all causes of injury. Do not drive after consuming alcohol, and avoid riding with someone who has been drinking. Penalties can be severe overseas.
Cellular telephones	Do not use a cellular telephone or text while driving. Many countries have enacted laws banning cellular telephone use while driving, and some countries have made using any kind of telephone, including hands-free, illegal while driving.
Taxis or hired drivers	Ride only in marked taxis, and try to ride in those that have safety belts accessible. Hire drivers familiar with the area.
Bus travel	Avoid riding in overcrowded, overweight, or top-heavy buses or minivans and avoid riding in mountainous terrains, at night, and with a drinking or distracted bus driver.
Pedestrian hazards	Be alert when crossing streets, especially in countries where motorists drive on the left side of the road. Walk with a companion or someone from the host country.
Other Tips	
Airplane travel	Avoid using local, unscheduled aircraft. If possible, fly on larger planes (>30 seats), in good weather, during the daylight hours, and with experienced pilots. Children <2 years should sit in a child safety seat, not on a parent's lap. Whenever possible, parents should travel with a safety seat for use before, during, and after a plane ride.
Drowning	Avoid swimming alone or in unfamiliar waters. Wear life jackets while boating or during water recreation activities.
Burns	In hotels, stay below the 6th floor to maximize the likelihood of being rescued in a fire. Bring your own smoke alarm.

country-specific driving risks. The Department of State has safety information useful to international travelers, including road safety and security alerts, international driving permits, and travel insurance (www.travel.state.gov).

WATER AND AQUATIC INJURIES

In 2013 and 2014, drowning accounted for 13% of all deaths of US citizens abroad. Although risk factors have not been clearly defined, these deaths are most likely related to unfamiliarity with local water currents and conditions, inability to swim, and the absence of lifeguards on duty. Rip currents can be especially dangerous, as are sea animals such as urchins, jellyfish, coral, and sea lice. Alcohol also contributes to drowning and boating mishaps.

Drowning is often the leading cause of injury death to US citizens visiting countries where water recreation is a major activity, such as Fiji, the Bahamas, Jamaica, and Costa Rica. Young men are particularly at risk of head and spinal cord injuries from diving into shallow water, and alcohol is a factor in some cases.

Boating can be a hazard, especially if boaters are unfamiliar with the boat, do not know proper boating etiquette or rules for watercraft navigation, or are new to the water environment in a foreign country. In 2013 and 2014, maritime accidents resulted in 16 deaths to healthy Americans abroad. Many boating fatalities result from inexperience or failure to wear lifejackets.

Scuba diving is a frequent pursuit of travelers in coastal destinations. The death rate among all divers worldwide is thought to be 15–20 deaths per 100,000 divers per year. Travelers should either be experienced divers or dive with a reliable dive shop and instructors. See the Scuba Diving section later in this chapter for a more detailed discussion about diving risks and preventive measures.

OTHER UNINTENTIONAL INJURIES

In 2013 and 2014, other unintentional injuries such as aviation incidents, drug-related incidents, natural disasters, and deaths classified as "other unintentional injuries" (including fires and falls) accounted for 19% of deaths to healthy US citizens abroad. Fires can be a substantial risk in developing countries where building codes do not exist or are not enforced, there are no smoke alarms, there is no access to emergency services, and the fire department's focus is on putting out fires rather than on fire prevention or victim rescue.

In 2013 and 2014, an estimated 50 US citizens abroad were killed in aircraft crashes. Travel by local, lightweight aircraft in many countries can be risky. Travel on unscheduled flights, in small aircraft, at night, in inclement weather, and with inexperienced pilots carries the highest risk.

Before flying with children, parents and caregivers should check to make sure that their child restraint system is approved for use on an aircraft. This approval should be printed on the system's information label or on the device itself. The Federal Aviation Administration (FAA) recommends that a child weighing <20 pounds use a rear-facing child restraint system. A forward-facing child safety seat should be used for children weighing 20–40 pounds. FAA has also approved a harness-type device for children weighing 22–44 pounds.

TRAVEL TIPS

Health care providers, vendors of travel services, and travelers themselves should consider the following:

- Travelers may wish to purchase special travel health and medical evacuation insurance if their destinations include countries where there may not be access to good medical care (see the Travel Insurance, Travel Health Insurance, & Medical Evacuation Insurance section later in this chapter).

- Adventure activities, such as mountain climbing, skydiving, whitewater rafting, dune-buggying, kayaking, skiing, and snowboarding are popular with travelers. The lack of rapid emergency trauma response, inadequate trauma care in remote locations, and sudden, unexpected weather changes that compromise safety and hamper rescue efforts can delay care and reduce survivability.

- Travelers should avoid using local, unscheduled, small aircraft and refrain if possible from flying in bad weather and at night. If available, choose larger aircraft (>30 seats), as they are more likely to have undergone more strict and regular safety inspections. Larger aircraft also provide more protection in the event of a crash. For country-specific airline crash events, see www.airsafe.com.

- When traveling by air with young children, consider bringing a child safety seat approved for use on an aircraft, helmets if considering riding bicycles or motorbikes, and life preservers if travelers will be in the water.

- To prevent fire-related injuries, travelers should select accommodations no higher than the sixth floor (fire ladders generally cannot reach higher than the sixth floor). Hotels should be checked for smoke alarms and preferably sprinkler systems. Travelers may want to bring their

own smoke alarm. Two escape routes from buildings should always be identified. Crawling low under smoke and covering one's mouth with a wet cloth are helpful in escaping a fire. Families should agree on a meeting place outside the building in case a fire erupts.

- Improperly vented heating devices may cause poisoning from carbon monoxide. Carbon monoxide (CO) at the back of boats near the engine can be especially dangerous. Travelers may want to carry a personal CO detector that can sound an alert in the presence of this lethal gas.

- Travelers should consider learning basic first aid and CPR before travel overseas with another person. Travelers should bring a travel health kit, which should be customized to the anticipated itinerary and activities.

BIBLIOGRAPHY

1. Balaban V, Sleet DA. Pediatric travel injuries: risk, prevention, and management. In: Kamat DM, Fischer PR, editors. American Academy of Pediatrics Textbook of Global Child Health. 2nd ed. Elk Grove Village, IL: American Academy of Pediatrics; 2015.

2. Ederer D, Parker E, Sleet DA. Motorcycle helmets as a vaccine: CDC and Asia Injury Prevention Foundation Partner in Cambodia and Uganda. CDC's Division of Global Health Protection; 2014 [cited 2016 Sep. 29]; Spring 2014, Issue 14. Available from: www.cdc.gov/globalhealth/healthprotection/fieldupdates/pdf/dghp-field-updates-2014-spring.pdf.

3. Guse CE, Cortes LM, Hargarten SW, Hennes HM. Fatal injuries of US citizens abroad. J Travel Med. 2007 Sep-Oct;14(5):279–87.

4. Lawson CJ, Dykewicz CA, Molinari NA, Lipman H, Alvarado-Ramy F. Deaths in international travelers arriving in the United States, July 1, 2005 to June 30, 2008. J Travel Med. 2012 Mar-Apr;19(2):96–103.

5. Li G, Pressley JC, Qiang Y, Grabowski JG, Baker SP, Rebok GW. Geographic region, weather, pilot age, and air carrier crashes: a case-control study. Aviat Space Environ Med. 2009 Apr;80(4):386–90.

6. Lozano R, Naghavi M, Foreman K, Lim S, Shibuya K. Global and regional mortality from 235 causes of death for 20 age groups in 1990 and 2010: a systematic analysis for the Global Burden of Disease Study 2010. Lancet. 2012 Dec 15;380(9859):2095–128.

7. Sherry MK, Mossallam M, Mulligan M, Hyder AA, Bishai D. Rates of intentionally caused and road crash deaths of US citizens abroad. Inj Prev. 2015 Apr;21(e1):e10–4.

8. US Department of Commerce. 2015 US travel and tourism statistics. Washington, DC: US Department of Commerce; 2016 [cited 2016 Sep. 29]; Available from: http://travel.trade.gov/outreachpages/outbound.general_information.outbound_overview.asp.

9. US Department of State. Tips for traveling abroad. Washington, DC: US Department of State; 2012 [cited 2016 Sep. 22]; Available from: https://travel.state.gov/content/passports/en/go/checklist.html.

10. World Health Organization. WHO global status report on road safety 2015. Geneva: World Health Organization; 2015 [cited 2016 Sep. 22] Available from http://www.who.int/violence_injury_prevention/road_safety_status/2015/en/.

SAFETY & SECURITY

Robyn K. Prinz, Ronnie Henry

Violence is a leading worldwide public health problem and a growing concern of US citizens traveling, working, or residing abroad. International terrorism and crime are risks anywhere in the world, but international travelers operating in an unfamiliar environment face particular hurdles. Travelers may not have access to networks of friends or family to assist them. Local government responses to problems may be different from what US residents expect, or an effective local government may not exist to respond at all. Language barriers, unexpected costs, or different cultural mores can also complicate what happens in an emergency. The best way for US residents going overseas to manage their risk is to prepare before they travel. Travelers should research conditions at their destination to learn what risks they are likely to face and have a plan to mitigate those risks while they are abroad.

RESEARCH AND PREPARATION

Travelers need information to make good decisions about risks while traveling and to make plans to deal with those risks. The Department of State's Bureau of Consular Affairs publishes comprehensive information on safety and security concerns for every independent nation, along with basic advice for safe travel anywhere, at http://travel.state.gov. More information can also be found at individual embassy and consulate websites, all of which can be found at www.usembassy.gov. The Department of State also publishes travel alerts and travel warnings that focus on emergent or chronic safety issues in countries around the world. They encourage all US citizens to avoid travel to areas with major threats to safety and security. Travelers should take these warnings seriously as they cover areas where security threats and instability severely limit the help the US government can offer to its citizens in those areas.

Travelers should enroll with the Department of State's Smart Traveler Enrollment Program (STEP) before leaving on their trip. This will allow them to receive updated information about safety and security conditions and messages about emergent threats while they are abroad. The governments of the United Kingdom, Canada, and Australia also have excellent websites with safety and security information for travelers.

CRIME

One of the most common threats to the safety of US citizens abroad comes from criminal activity. Travelers to foreign countries are viewed by many criminals as wealthy, naïve targets, who are inexperienced, unfamiliar with the culture, and inept at seeking assistance if victimized. Traveling in high-poverty areas or regions of civil unrest, using alcohol or drugs, and traveling in unfamiliar environments at night increase the likelihood that a traveler will be the victim of crime.

Travelers should take the time to research crime trends and patterns at their destination through the Overseas Security Advisory Council at www.osac.gov. Strategies for avoiding becoming the victim of a crime overseas are, for the most part, the same common-sense habits that people should follow everywhere, but the following actions should be stressed with international travelers:

- Limit travel at night, travel with a companion, and vary routine travel habits.

- Do not wear expensive clothing or accessories.

- Avoid accommodations on the ground floor or immediately next to the stairs, and lock all doors and windows.

- Take only recommended and safe modes of local transportation.

- If confronted in a robbery, give up all valuables and do not resist attackers. Resistance can escalate to violence and result in injury or death.

Victims of a crime overseas should contact the nearest US embassy, consulate, or consular agency.

The Department of State can help replace a stolen passport, contact family and friends, obtain appropriate medical care, explain the local criminal justice process, and connect victims of crime with available resources. However, they do not have the legal authority to conduct a criminal investigation and prosecution.

TERRORISM

International terrorism is also a threat to US citizens abroad. The Department of State maintains a worldwide caution addressing this threat on its consular affairs website. Terrorist groups continue to plan attacks against Western interests in multiple regions, including Europe, Asia, Africa, and the Middle East. These attacks may employ a wide variety of tactics, including suicide operations, assassinations, kidnappings, hijackings, and bombings. Possible targets include high-profile sporting events, public transportation systems, residential areas, business offices, hotels, clubs, restaurants, places of worship, schools, shopping malls, and other tourist destinations where US citizens gather in large numbers.

Although terrorism is a worldwide threat and can be a major cause of concern to travelers, it should be seen in context. In 2014, 24 private US citizens were killed in terrorist attacks overseas, 8 were injured, and 3 were kidnapped. Although threats of this type cannot be totally eliminated, travelers can lower the chance they will be a victim through knowledge and planning:

- Look out for unattended packages or bags in public places and other crowded areas.

- Be cautious of unexpected packages.

- When packing, choose clothing that does not identify one as a tourist (such as T-shirts emblazoned with the US flag or logos of the traveler's local sports team).

- Try to blend in with the locals.

These strategies incorporate the same defensive alertness and good judgment that people should use to keep safe from crime at home or abroad. Awareness is key—taking precautions to be aware of surroundings and adopting protective measures.

OTHER ISSUES

Just as important as learning about safety and security conditions at a traveler's destination country is to learn about legal differences that may cause problems for US citizens. Many countries have weapons laws that are much stricter than those in the United States, such that a single loose bullet in a suitcase can lead to arrest and possible jail time. Some countries prohibit certain religious activities or the possession of religious literature. Prescription medications that are commonly used in the United States may be illegal in another country. Some countries do not have the same free speech protections as those in the United States, and statements made in public or online can lead to arrest or detention. These and other legal differences can be researched online at the Department of State website.

Since travelers may become the victim of a crime, regardless of the precautions they take, they should have plans for what they will do in an emergency. Travelers should make photocopies of their travel documents and leave a copy with a friend or relative at home along with a detailed itinerary and contact information if possible. They should also have the contact information for the nearest US embassy or consulate where they are traveling. Many medical insurance programs, including Medicare and Medicaid, will not pay for medical treatment overseas. Travelers should ensure they have adequate medical coverage before going overseas. If their current insurance does not cover their trip abroad, they should consider additional insurance that can pay for their medical expenses abroad or help return them to the United States if that becomes necessary. For more information, see Travel Insurance, Travel Health Insurance, & Medical Evacuation Insurance in this chapter.

USEFUL WEBSITES
Department of State Consular Affairs

- Know Before You Go: http://travel.state.gov/content/passports/english/go.html

- Alerts and Warnings: http://travel.state.gov/content/passports/en/alertswarnings.html

- Country Information: http://travel.state.gov/content/passports/english/country.html

- US Citizen Deaths Overseas: http://travel.state.gov/content/travel/english/statistics/deaths.html

Federal Bureau of Investigation, Crime Statistics: https://ucr.fbi.gov

Overseas Security Advisory Council: www.osac.gov

ANIMAL-ASSOCIATED HAZARDS

Heather Bair-Brake, Ryan M. Wallace, G. Gale Galland, Nina Marano

HUMAN INTERACTION WITH ANIMALS: A RISK FACTOR FOR INJURY AND ILLNESS

Animals, even those in close association with humans, such as dogs, can attack if they feel threatened, are protecting their young or territory, or are injured or ill. Travelers should be aware that attacks by domestic animals are far more common than attacks by wildlife, and secondary infections of wounds may result in serious illness or death. This section will cover the most common routes of transmission of illness and injury from animals and insects. However, most animals can transmit infection by more than one route. This section provides examples of high-priority diseases and injuries from animals and refers the reader to other sections for more detailed descriptions of the specific diseases.

BITES AND SCRATCHES

Bites from certain mammals frequently encountered during foreign travel, such as monkeys, dogs, bats, and rodents, can present a risk for serious infection. These animals' saliva can be so heavily contaminated with pathogens that a bite may not even be necessary to cause infection if saliva enters a preexisting cut or scratch or mucous membrane.

Prevention

Before departure, travelers should have a current tetanus vaccination or documentation of a booster vaccination in the previous 5–10 years (see Chapter 3, Tetanus). Travel health providers should assess a traveler's need for preexposure rabies immunization (see Chapter 3, Rabies). While traveling, people should never try to pet, handle, or feed unfamiliar animals (whether domestic or wild, even in captive settings such as game ranches or petting zoos), particularly in areas where rabies is endemic. Young children should be watched closely around unfamiliar animals as they are more likely to be bitten and to sustain more severe injuries from animal bites.

Management

To prevent infection, all bite and scratch wounds should be promptly cleaned with soap and water, and the wound should be promptly debrided by a health care professional if necrotic tissue, dirt, or other foreign materials are present. Often, a course of antibiotics is appropriate after dog or cat bites or scratches as these can lead to local or systemic infections. Wound care is especially important for exposures where rabies or tetanus is a concern. Travelers who might have been exposed to rabies should contact a health care provider as soon as possible for advice about rabies postexposure prophylaxis (PEP). Travelers who received their most recent tetanus toxoid–containing vaccine >5 years previously, or who have not received ≥3 doses of tetanus toxoid–containing vaccines, may require a dose of tetanus toxoid–containing vaccine (Tdap, Td, or DTaP).

DOGS AND CATS

Although travelers may assume that most dogs and cats are pets and therefore safe to interact with, more rabies cases in humans occur because of bites from free-roaming dogs and cats than from any other animals in the world. Rabies infections in dogs and cats may be difficult to detect, particularly early in the onset of clinical signs. Rabies also cannot be definitively diagnosed in a live animal. Travelers who are bitten or scratched by dogs or cats should promptly clean the wound and seek medical care. To further mitigate the risk of exposure to rabies, unfamiliar dogs should be avoided, and travelers should avoid the temptation to adopt a stray dog from abroad.

BATS

Like any other wild animal, bats, whether sick or healthy, may bite if handled. Any suspected or documented bite or scratch from a bat anywhere in the world should be considered a rabies risk, and the traveler should be evaluated for rabies PEP. It is not possible to tell if a bat has rabies without laboratory confirmation; however, any bat that is active by day, is found where bats are not usually seen (for example, indoors or outdoors in areas near humans), or is unable to fly is far more likely to be rabid. People may not know when they have been bitten by a bat, as most bats have tiny teeth, and not all wounds are apparent. Furthermore, because bat bites rarely cause much trauma, people may trivialize the bite and not seek care. Travelers should seek medical advice even in the absence of an obvious bite wound if they wake up to find a bat in the room or see a bat in the room of an unattended child or other person who could not reliably report a bite.

MONKEYS

After a monkey bite or scratch, travelers should be advised to thoroughly clean the wound and seek medical care immediately to be evaluated for possible rabies and herpes B PEP. Macaque bites can transmit herpes B virus, a virus related to the herpes simplex viruses (see Chapter 3, B virus). Additional information and photos of macaques can be found at the website for the National B Virus Resource Center at the Georgia State University Viral Immunology Center (www2.gsu.edu/~wwwvir).

RODENTS

Wild rodents are unlikely to have rabies; however, rodent bites and scratches can transmit rat-bite fever, *Salmonella*, lymphocytic choriomeningitis virus, and monkeypox. Each rodent bite or scratch needs to be evaluated on a case-by-case basis to determine the need for treatment.

STINGS AND ENVENOMATIONS

Snakes

Poisonous snakes are hazards in many locations, although deaths from snakebites are uncommon. Snakebites usually occur in areas where dense human populations coexist with dense snake populations, such as Southeast Asia, sub-Saharan Africa, and tropical areas in the Americas.

PREVENTION

Common sense is the best precaution. Most snakebites result from startling, handling, or harassing snakes. Therefore, all snakes should be left alone. Travelers should be aware of their surroundings, especially at night and during warm weather when snakes tend to be more active. For extra precaution, when practical, travelers should wear heavy, ankle-high or higher boots and long pants when walking outdoors in areas possibly inhabited by venomous snakes.

MANAGEMENT

Travelers should be advised to seek immediate medical attention any time a bite wound breaks the skin or when snake venom is ejected into their eyes or other mucous membranes. Immobilization of the affected limb and application of a pressure bandage that does not restrict blood flow are recommended first aid measures while the victim is moved as quickly as possible to a medical facility. Incision of the bite site and tourniquets that restrict blood flow to the affected limb are not recommended. Specific therapy for snakebites is controversial and should be left to the judgment of local emergency medical personnel. Specific antivenoms are available for some snakes in some areas, so trying to ascertain the species of snake that bit the victim may be critical.

Insects and Other Arthropods

Bites and stings from spiders and scorpions can be painful and can result in illness and death, particularly among infants and children. Other insects and arthropods, such as mosquitoes and ticks, can transmit infections. See the Protection against Mosquitoes, Ticks, & Other Arthropods section earlier in this chapter.

Marine Animals

Most marine animals are generally harmless unless threatened. Most injuries are the result of chance encounters or defensive maneuvers. Resulting wounds have many common characteristics: bacterial contamination, foreign bodies, and occasionally venom. Venomous injuries from marine fish and invertebrates are increasing with the popularity of surfing, scuba diving, and snorkeling. Most species responsible for human injuries, including stingrays, jellyfish, stonefish, sea urchins, and scorpionfish, live in tropical coastal waters.

PREVENTION

Travelers should be advised to maintain vigilance while engaging in recreational water activities. Prevention is the best defense:

- Avoid contact. This may be difficult in conditions of poor visibility, rough water, currents, and confined areas.

- Do not attempt to feed, handle, tease, or annoy marine animals.

- Wear protective clothing, such as protective footwear.

- Try to find out which animals may be encountered at the destination and learn about their characteristics and habitats before engaging in recreational water activities.

MANAGEMENT

In case of injury, identifying the species involved can help determine the best course of treatment. Signs and symptoms may not appear for hours after contact, or the animal may not have been seen or recognized at the time of injury. In such cases, treatment is based on the injury. Symptoms of venomous injuries can range from mild swelling and redness at the site to more severe symptoms, such as difficulty breathing or swallowing, chest pain, or intense pain at the site of the sting, for which immediate medical treatment should be sought. Management will vary according to the severity of symptoms and can include medications, such as diphenhydramine, steroids, pain medication, and antibiotics.

OTHER HAZARDS

Travelers should be aware that animals do not have to be sick or appear sick to be a risk to humans. Some animals such as poultry, reptiles, and goats carry human pathogens as normal gut flora. Other animals, such as rodents, bats, and nonhuman primates, can be subclinical carriers of pathogens.

Bats

Viral infections such as rabies and viral hemorrhagic fevers can be transmitted from bats to people. Histoplasmosis is a fungal infection that may be associated with bat droppings. Exposure to bats can occur during adventure activities such as caving or spelunking and can include mucosal or cutaneous exposure to bat saliva or droppings, in addition to bites and scratches. A recent example of an indirect exposure is an imported case of Marburg fever in a tourist who had visited a "python cave" inhabited by bats in western Uganda. This case illustrates the risk of acquiring diseases from indirect contact with cave-dwelling bats. This same cave was the source of a fatal case of Marburg hemorrhagic fever in a Dutch tourist in 2008.

Bats should never be handled. If a traveler touches a bat or if infectious material (such as saliva) from a bat gets into the eyes, nose, mouth, or a wound, the traveler should wash the affected area thoroughly and seek medical advice immediately. Travelers should be discouraged from going into caves or mines that have bat infestations. If travelers will be entering densely populated bat habitats, they should wear protective equipment and clothing (face shield, respirator, gloves). Dirty clothing should be removed and washed as soon as possible after leaving the cave. If travelers, particularly adventure travelers, know they will entering high-density bat habitats or plan on having direct contact with bats or other rabies reservoir species, preexposure rabies vaccination should be considered.

Rodents

Rodents carry a variety of viral, bacterial, and parasitic agents that may pose a threat to human health. Human exposure can occur directly by a bite or scratch or indirectly by exposure to surfaces or water contaminated with urine or feces. Rodents can also be reservoirs for vectorborne infections carried by fleas, ticks, and mites.

Wild rodents should never be handled. Travelers should avoid places that have evidence of rodent infestation and should avoid contact with rodent feces. Travelers should not eat or drink anything that is suspected to be contaminated by rodent feces or urine.

Travelers who were exposed to rodents or who have a history of flea or tick bites or mite infestation may develop febrile illness shortly after exposure and should be evaluated by a clinician. Depending on the history and symptoms, diseases such as plague, leptospirosis, hantavirus, rickettsial infections, Lyme disease, lymphocytic choriomeningitis, Lassa fever, tickborne encephalitis, poxvirus, tularemia, and bartonellosis (see Chapter 3) should be included in the list of possible diagnoses.

Birds

Both ill and asymptomatic birds have been associated with cases of highly pathogenic avian influenza in humans. When traveling in an area where outbreaks of avian influenza have been reported, travelers should avoid contact with live poultry (such as chickens, ducks, geese, pigeons, turkeys, and quail) or any wild birds and should avoid settings where avian influenza A (H5N1 or H7N9)–infected poultry may be present, such as commercial or backyard poultry farms and live poultry markets. Other pathogens from birds may infect humans through infected feces or by aerosol. These cause diseases such as histoplasmosis (see Chapter 3, Histoplasmosis), salmonellosis (see Chapter 3, Salmonellosis [Nontyphoidal]), psittacosis, and avian mycobacteriosis.

Travelers should not eat uncooked or undercooked poultry or poultry products, including dishes that contain uncooked eggs or poultry blood. Travelers should wash their hands if they come in contact with bird feces.

BIBLIOGRAPHY

1. Callahan M. Bites, stings and envenoming injuries. In: Keystone JS, Freedman DO, Kozarsky PE, Connor BA, Nothdurft HD, editors. Travel Medicine. 3rd ed. Philadelphia: Saunders Elsevier; 2013. pp. 413–24.

2. Cohen JI, Davenport DS, Stewart JA, Deitchman S, Hilliard JK, Chapman LE. Recommendations for prevention of and therapy for exposure to B virus (cercopithecine herpesvirus 1). Clin Infect Dis. 2002 Nov 15;35(10):1191–203.

3. Diaz JH. The global epidemiology, syndromic classification, management, and prevention of spider bites. Am J Trop Med Hyg. 2004 Aug;71(2):239–50.

4. Gibbons RV. Cryptogenic rabies, bats, and the question of aerosol transmission. Ann Emerg Med. 2002 May;39(5):528–36.

5. Gold BS, Dart RC, Barish RA. Bites of venomous snakes. N Engl J Med. 2002 Aug 1;347(5):347–56.

6. Lankau EW, Cohen NJ, Jentes ES, Adams LE, Bell TR, Blanton JD, et al. Prevention and control of rabies in an age of global travel: a review of travel- and trade-associated rabies events—United States, 1986–2012. Zoonoses Public Health. 2014 Aug;61(5):305–16.

7. Meerburg BG, Singleton GR, Kijlstra A. Rodent-borne diseases and their risks for public health. Crit Rev Microbiol. 2009;35(3):221–70.

8. Pan American Health Organization. Rabies. In: Acha PN, Szyfres B, editors. Zoonoses and Communicable Diseases Common to Man and Animals. 3rd ed. Washington, DC: Pan American Health Organization; 2003. pp. 246–76.

9. Smith KE, Dunn JR, Castrodale L, Daly R, Wohrle R, Journal of the American Veterinary Medical Association. Compendium of measures to prevent disease associated with animals in public settings, 2013. J Am Vet Med Assoc. 2013 Nov 1;243(9):1270–88.

10. World Health Organization. WHO Expert Consultation on rabies. World Health Organ Tech Rep Ser. 2005;931:1–88.

ENVIRONMENTAL HAZARDS

Armin Ansari, Suzanne Beavers

AIR

Air pollution has decreased in many parts of the world, but it is worsening in certain industrializing countries. Polluted air can be difficult or impossible to avoid, but the risk to healthy short-term travelers is most likely low. People with preexisting heart and lung disease, children, and older adults are at higher risk.

Travelers should be familiar with the air quality at their destination. The AirNow website (http://airnow.gov/) provides information about the effects of particulate matter and ozone, as well as links to international air quality sites. Historical data on outdoor air pollution in urban areas are available from the World Health Organization at http://gamapserver.who.int/gho/interactive_charts/phe/oap_exposure/atlas.html.

Travelers should also limit exposure to indoor air pollution and carbon monoxide. Possible sources of indoor air pollutants include cooking or combustion sources (such as kerosene, coal, wood, or animal dung). Major sources of indoor carbon monoxide include gas ranges and ovens, unvented gas or kerosene space heaters, and coal- or wood-burning stoves. Another important source of indoor air pollution is secondhand smoke produced from smoking tobacco.

Travelers to countries where air pollution may be a problem should consider the following:

- For people with preexisting conditions such as asthma, chronic obstructive pulmonary disease, and heart disease, limit strenuous or prolonged outdoor activity, particularly in cities.

- For long-term travelers and expatriates, consider investing in an indoor air filtration system.

- Avoid indoor areas with high levels of indoor air pollutants such as tobacco smoke. For additional information on tobacco laws and smoke-free places in 201 countries, visit www.tobaccocontrollaws.org/legislation.

- As much as possible, look for lodging with working smoke and carbon monoxide detectors.

Travelers to areas where air pollution is reported to be high might inquire about the advisability of wearing face masks. CDC has no recommendations regarding the use of face masks for travelers. One small study in Beijing showed that wearing a valved dust respirator appeared to mitigate the effects of air pollution on blood pressure and heart rate. However, it should be noted that the respirators used in the study had better filtration than the surgical masks commonly worn in some countries. The decision to wear a mask should be left to the traveler's discretion.

MOLD CONTAMINATION

Extensive water damage after hurricanes or floods can lead to mold contamination in buildings. Travelers may visit flooded areas overseas as part of emergency, medical, or humanitarian missions. Mold is a more serious health hazard for people who are immunocompromised or have respiratory problems. To prevent exposure that could result in adverse health effects from disturbed mold, people should adhere to the following recommendations:

- Avoid areas where mold contamination is obvious.

- If the traveler will be working in a moldy environment (such as on a medical or humanitarian mission), use personal protective equipment (PPE), such as gloves, goggles, and a fit-tested N95 respirator or higher. These travelers should take sufficient PPE with them, as these may be scarce in the countries visited.

- Keep hands, skin, and eyes clean and free from mold-contaminated dust.

- Review the CDC guidance, Mold Prevention Strategies and Possible Health Effects in the Aftermath of Hurricanes and Major Floods (www.cdc.gov/mmwr/preview/mmwrhtml/rr5508a1.htm), which provides recommendations for dealing with mold in these settings.

RADIATION

Natural background radiation levels can vary substantially from region to region, but these variations are not a health concern. Travelers should be aware of regions known to have been contaminated with radioactive materials, such as the areas surrounding the Chernobyl nuclear power plant in Ukraine and the Fukushima Daiichi nuclear power plant in Japan.

The Chernobyl plant is located 100 km (62 miles) northwest of Kiev. The 1986 accident contaminated regions in 3 republics—Ukraine, Belarus, and Russia—but the highest radioactive ground contamination is within 30 km (19 miles) of Chernobyl.

The Fukushima Daiichi plant is located 240 km (150 miles) north of Tokyo. After the accident in 2011, the area within a 20-km (32-mile) radius of the plant was evacuated, and Japanese authorities also advised evacuation from locations farther away to the northwest of the plant. As Japanese authorities continue to clean the affected areas and monitor the situation, access requirements and travel advisories change. The Department of State recommends against all unnecessary travel to areas designated by the Japanese government. For up-to-date information or any travel advisories, see the Department of State's information for Japan (http://travel.state.gov/content/passports/english/country/japan.html).

In most countries, areas of known radioactive contamination are fenced or marked with signs. Any traveler seeking long-term (more than a few months) residence near a known or suspected contaminated area should consult with staff of the nearest US embassy and inquire about any advisories regarding drinking water quality or purchase of meat, fruit, and vegetables from local farmers. Radiation emergencies are rare events. In case of such an emergency, however, travelers should follow instructions provided by local authorities. If such information is not forthcoming, US travelers should seek advice from the nearest US embassy or consulate.

Natural disasters (such as floods) may also displace industrial or clinical radioactive sources. In all circumstances, travelers should exercise caution when they encounter unknown objects or equipment, especially if they bear the basic radiation tri-foil symbol or other radiation signs (see www.remm.nlm.gov/radsign.htm for examples). Travelers who encounter a questionable object should not touch or move the object and should notify local authorities.

BIBLIOGRAPHY

1. Ansari A. Radiation threats and your safety: a guide to preparation and response for professionals and community. Boca Raton (FL): Chapman & Hall/CRC; 2009.

2. Brandt M, Brown C, Burkhart J, Burton N, Cox-Ganser J, Damon S, et al. Mold prevention strategies and possible health effects in the aftermath of hurricanes and major floods. MMWR Recomm Rep. 2006 Jun 9;55(RR-8):1–27.

3. Brook RD, Rajagopalan S, Pope CAr, Brook JR, Bhatnagar A, Diez-Roux AV, et al. Particulate matter air pollution and cardiovascular disease: An update to the scientific statement from the American Heart Association. Circulation. 2010 Jun 1;121(21):2331–78.

4. Eisenbud M, Gesell TF. Environmental Radioactivity: from Natural, Industrial, and Military Sources. 4th ed. San Diego Academic Press; 1997.

5. Guarnieri M, Balmes JR. Outdoor air pollution and asthma. Lancet. 2014;383(9928):1581–92.

6. Langrish JP, Mills NL, Chan JK, Leseman DL, Aitken RJ, Fokkens PH, et al. Beneficial cardiovascular effects of reducing exposure to particulate air pollution with a simple facemask. Part Fibre Toxicol. 2009;6:8.

7. Nuclear Emergency Response Headquarters, Government of Japan. Report of Japanese Government to IAEA Ministerial Conference on Nuclear Safety: the accident at TEPCO's Fukushima nuclear power stations. 2011 [cited 2016 Sep. 19]. Available from: http://japan.kantei.go.jp/kan/topics/201106/iaea_houkokusho_e.html

8. Scientific Committee on the Effects of Atomic Radiation. Annex J: exposure and effects of the

Chernobyl accident. In: Sources and Effects of Ionizing Radiation. New York: United Nations; 2000. pp. 451–556.

9. Shofer S, Chen TM, Gokhale J, Kuschner WG. Outdoor air pollution: counseling and exposure risk reduction. Am J Med Sci. 2007 Apr;333(4):257–60.

10. US Department of Health and Human Services. The health consequences of involuntary exposure to tobacco smoke: a report of the Surgeon General. Atlanta, GA: U.S. Department of Health and Human Services, Centers for Disease Control and Prevention, Coordinating Center for Health Promotion, National Center for Chronic Disease Prevention and Health Promotion, Office on Smoking and Health; 2006 [cited 2016 Sep. 22]; Available from: www.ncbi.nlm.nih.gov/books/NBK44324/.

SCUBA DIVING

Daniel A. Nord, Gregory A. Raczniak

Published estimates report anywhere from one-half to 4 million people who participate in recreational diving in the United States, and many travel to tropical areas of the world to dive. Divers can face a variety of medical challenges, but because dive injuries are generally rare, few clinicians are trained in their diagnosis and treatment. Therefore, the recreational diver must be able to assess potential risks before diving, recognize the signs of injury, and find qualified dive medicine help when needed.

PREPARING FOR DIVE TRAVEL

Planning for dive-related travel should take into account any recent changes in health, including injuries or surgery, and medication use. Respiratory diseases (such as asthma or chronic obstructive pulmonary disease), disorders that affect central nervous system higher function and consciousness (such as seizures) or the peripheral nervous system (such as diabetic or autonomic neuropathy), mental health dysfunction (such as anxiety, claustrophobia, or substance abuse), cardiovascular disease that limits physical exertion, and pregnancy raise special concerns about diving fitness.

Special mention must be made regarding cardiovascular fitness. Diving should be considered a potentially strenuous activity that can make substantial demands on the cardiovascular system. People with known risk factors for coronary artery disease, including but not limited to abnormal lipid profile, elevated blood pressure, diabetes, and smoking history, who wish to either begin a dive program or continue diving should undergo a physical examination to assess their cardiovascular fitness. This may include an electrocardiogram and exercise treadmill test.

Health care workers providing travel medicine examinations for divers should also remind their patients of preventive actions they can take before a dive. Every dive should begin with identifying potential hazards (such as weather and water conditions, planned depth and bottom time, environment), assessing these hazards and the associated risk, and making decisions about acceptable risk. The diver should be able to implement controls to eliminate or reduce the risk (by using correct and well-maintained protective equipment, for example), make sure the dive is supervised, and ensure that medical care is available in the event of an emergency.

DIVING DISORDERS

Barotrauma

EAR AND SINUS

Ear barotrauma is the most common injury in divers. On descent, failure to equalize pressure changes in the middle ear space creates a pressure gradient across the eardrum. This pressure change must be controlled through proper equalization techniques to avoid bleeding or fluid accumulation in the middle ear and avoid stretching or rupture of the eardrum and the membranes covering the windows of the inner ear. Symptoms of barotrauma include the following:

- Pain

- Tinnitus (ringing in the ears)

- Vertigo (dizziness or sensation of spinning)

- Sensation of fullness

- Effusion (fluid accumulation in the ear)

- Decreased hearing

Paranasal sinuses, because of their relatively narrow connecting passageways, are especially susceptible to barotrauma, generally on descent. With small changes in pressure (depth), symptoms are usually mild and subacute but can be exacerbated by continued diving. Larger pressure changes, especially with forceful attempts at equilibration (such as the Valsalva maneuver), can be more injurious. Additional risk factors for ear and sinus barotrauma include the following:

- Use of solid earplugs

- Medications (such as decongestants)

- Ear or sinus surgery

- Nasal deformity or polyps

- Chronic nasal and sinus disease that interferes with equilibration during the large barometric pressure changes encountered while diving

A diver who may have sustained ear or sinus barotrauma should discontinue diving and seek medical attention.

PULMONARY

A scuba diver must reduce the risk of lung overpressure problems by breathing normally and ascending slowly when breathing compressed gas. Overinflation of the lungs can result if a scuba diver ascends toward the surface without exhaling, which may happen, for example, when a novice diver panics. During ascent, compressed gas trapped in the lung increases in volume until the expansion exceeds the elastic limit of lung tissue, causing damage and allowing gas bubbles to escape into 3 possible locations:

- Gas entering the pleural space can cause lung collapse or pneumothorax.

- Gas entering the space around the heart, trachea, and esophagus (the mediastinum) causes mediastinal emphysema and

frequently tracks under the skin (subcutaneous emphysema) or into the tissue around the larynx, sometimes precipitating a change in voice characteristics.

- Gas rupturing the alveolar walls can enter the pulmonary capillaries and pass via the pulmonary veins to the left side of the heart, where it is distributed according to relative blood flow, resulting in arterial gas embolism (AGE).

While mediastinal or subcutaneous emphysema may resolve spontaneously, pneumothorax generally requires specific treatment to remove the air and reinflate the lung. AGE is a medical emergency, requiring urgent intervention with hyperbaric oxygen recompression treatment.

Lung overinflation injuries from scuba diving can range from dramatic and life threatening to mild symptoms of chest pain and dyspnea. Although pulmonary barotrauma is relatively uncommon in divers, prompt medical evaluation is necessary, and evidence for this condition should always be considered in the presence of respiratory or neurologic symptoms following a dive.

Decompression Illness

Decompression illness (DCI) describes the dysbaric injuries (such as AGE) and decompression sickness (DCS). Because the 2 diseases are considered to result from separate causes, they are described here separately. However, from a clinical and practical standpoint, distinguishing between them in the field may be impossible and unnecessary, since the initial treatment is the same for both. DCI can occur even in divers who have carefully followed the standard decompression tables and the principles of safe diving. Serious permanent injury or death may result from either AGE or DCS.

ARTERIAL GAS EMBOLISM

Gas entering the arterial blood through ruptured pulmonary vessels can distribute bubbles into the body tissues, including the heart and brain, where they can disrupt circulation or damage vessel walls. The presentation of AGE ranges from minimal neurologic symptoms to dramatic symptoms that require immediate attention. Common signs and symptoms include the following:

- Numbness
- Weakness
- Tingling
- Dizziness
- Blurred vision
- Chest pain
- Personality change or difficulty thinking
- Bloody sputum
- Paralysis or seizures
- Loss of consciousness

In general, any scuba diver who surfaces unconscious or loses consciousness within 10 minutes after surfacing should be suspected to have AGE. Intervention with basic life support is indicated, including the administration of the highest fraction of oxygen, followed by rapid evacuation to a hyperbaric oxygen treatment facility.

DECOMPRESSION SICKNESS

Breathing air under pressure causes excess inert gas (usually nitrogen) to dissolve in body tissues and can saturate these tissues. The amount of gas dissolved is proportional to and increases with depth and time. As the diver ascends back to the surface, the excess dissolved gas must be cleared through respiration via the bloodstream. Depending on the amount dissolved and the rate of ascent, some gas can supersaturate tissues, where it separates from solution to form bubbles, interfering with blood flow and tissue oxygenation and causes the following signs and symptoms:

- Joint aches or pain
- Numbness or tingling
- Mottling or marbling of skin
- Coughing spasms or shortness of breath
- Itching

- Unusual fatigue
- Dizziness
- Weakness
- Personality changes
- Loss of bowel or bladder function
- Staggering, loss of coordination, or tremors
- Paralysis
- Collapse or unconsciousness

FLYING AFTER DIVING

The risk of developing decompression sickness is increased when divers are exposed to increased altitude too soon after a dive. The cabin pressure of commercial aircraft may be the equivalent of 6,000–8,000 ft (1,829–2,438 m). Thus, divers should avoid flying or an altitude exposure >2,000 ft (610 m) for:

- ≥12 hours after surfacing from a single no-decompression dive
- ≥18 hours after repetitive dives or multiple days of diving
- 24–48 hours after a dive that required decompression stops

These recommended preflight surface intervals do not eliminate risk of DCS, and longer surface intervals will further reduce this risk.

PREVENTING DIVING DISORDERS

Recreational divers should dive conservatively and well within the no-decompression limits of their dive tables or computers. Risk factors for DCI are primarily dive depth, dive time, and rate of ascent. Additional factors such as repetitive dives, strenuous exercise, dives to depths >60 ft (18 m), altitude exposure soon after a dive, and certain physiological variables also increase risk. Divers should be cautioned to stay hydrated and rested and dive within the limits of their training. Diving is a skill that requires training and certification and should be done with a companion.

TREATMENT OF DIVING DISORDERS

Definitive treatment of DCI begins with early recognition of symptoms, followed by recompression with hyperbaric oxygen. A high concentration (100%) of supplemental oxygen is recommended. Surface-level oxygen given for first aid may relieve the signs and symptoms of DCI and should be administered as soon as possible. Divers are often dehydrated, either because of incidental causes, immersion, or DCI itself, which can cause capillary leakage. Administration of isotonic glucose-free intravenous fluid is recommended in most cases. Oral rehydration fluids may also be helpful, provided they can be safely administered (for example, if the diver is conscious and can maintain his or her airway). The definitive treatment of DCI is recompression and oxygen administration in a hyperbaric chamber.

Divers Alert Network (DAN) maintains 24-hour emergency consultation and evacuation assistance at 919-684-9111 (collect calls are accepted). DAN will help with managing the injured diver,

help decide if recompression is needed, provide the location of the closest recompression facility, and help arrange patient transport. DAN can also be contacted for routine, nonemergency consultation by telephone at 919-684-2948, extension 6222, or by accessing the DAN website (www.diversalertnetwork.org).

Travelers who plan to scuba dive may want to ascertain whether recompression facilities are available at their destination before embarking on their trip.

HAZARDOUS MARINE LIFE

The oceans and waterways are filled with creatures and, although some are capable of wounding and poisoning, most marine animals are generally harmless unless threatened. Most injuries are the result of chance encounters or defensive maneuvers. Resulting wounds have many common characteristics: bacterial contamination, foreign bodies, and occasionally venom. See the Animal-Associated Hazards section earlier in this chapter for prevention and injury management recommendations.

BIBLIOGRAPHY

1. Brubakk AO, Neuman TS, Bennett PB, Elliott DH. Bennett and Elliott's Physiology and Medicine of Diving. 5th ed. London: Saunders; 2003.

2. Dear G, Pollock NW. DAN America Dive and Travel Medical Guide. 5th ed. Durham, NC: Divers Alert Network; 2009.

3. Moon RE. Treatment of decompression illness. In: Bove AA, Davis JC, editors. Bove and Davis' Diving Medicine. 4th ed. Philadelphia: WB Saunders; 2004. pp. 195–223.

4. Neuman TS, Thom SR. Physiology and medicine of hyperbaric oxygen therapy. Philadelphia, PA: Saunders; 2008.

5. Sheffield P, Vann RD. Flying after recreational diving, workshop proceedings of the Divers Alert Network 2002 May 2. Durham, NC: Divers Alert Network; 2004 [cited 2016 Sep. 22]; Available from: http://www.diversalertnetwork.org/research/projects/fad/workshop/FADWorkshopProceedings.pdf.

6. US Navy Diving Manual Revision 6 Change A. Publication Number SS521-AG-PRO-010 0910-LP-106-0957. 2011 [cited 2016 Mar, 16]; Revision 6 [Available from: http://www.alohashoredivers.com/links/DiveMan_rev6_Frontmatter_index.pdf.

MEDICAL TOURISM

Duc B. Nguyen, Joanna Gaines

Medical tourism is the term commonly used to describe people traveling outside their home country for medical treatment. Patients may pursue medical care abroad for a variety of reasons, such as decreased cost, a preference for care from providers from a similar culture, or to receive a procedure or therapy not available in their country of residence. In the United States, medical tourism generally refers to people traveling to less-developed countries for medical care. Medical tourism is a worldwide, multibillion-dollar phenomenon that is expected to grow substantially in the next 5–10 years. Studies have estimated that hundreds of thousands of medical tourists travel from the United States annually. Little reliable epidemiologic data on medical tourism exist, but ongoing case reports and outbreaks of infections serve as a reminder that medical tourism is not without risks.

Common categories of procedures that US travelers pursue during medical tourism trips include orthopedic surgery, cosmetic surgery, cardiology (cardiac surgery), oncologic care, and dentistry. Common destinations include Thailand, Mexico, Singapore, India, Malaysia, Cuba, Brazil, Argentina, and Costa Rica. The type of procedure and the destination need to be considered when reviewing the risk of travel for medical care.

Most medical tourists pay for their care at time of service, and rely on private companies or medical concierge services to identify foreign health care facilities. These companies may not require accreditation of foreign providers, track patient outcome data, or maintain formal medical record security policies. Some health insurance companies and large employers have formed alliances with overseas hospitals to control health care costs, and several major medical schools in the United States have developed joint initiatives with overseas providers, such as the Harvard Medical School Dubai Center, the Johns Hopkins Singapore International Medical Center, and the Duke-National University of Singapore.

RISKS ASSOCIATED WITH MEDICAL TOURISM

Medical tourism has been associated with complications, including infections caused by antibiotic-resistant strains of bacteria not commonly seen in the United States. Patients who are considering seeking medical care overseas should be aware of this risk. It is wise for travelers to bring home outer packaging and package inserts from medications they receive or purchase abroad. Health care providers should be vigilant for the possibility of resistant infections among patients who have traveled for medical procedures and take measures to control their spread in the United States.

Several outbreaks of infectious disease have been documented among medical tourists after their return to the United States. Recent examples include nontuberculous mycobacteria infections among patients who had cosmetic surgery in the Dominican Republic and Q fever among patients who received sheep cell injections in Germany. Patients who experience complications after receiving medical care overseas should inform their providers of their travel history and their medical history, but may lack adequate documentation of the care they received. Some may be reluctant to share such information if they have had complications.

PRETRAVEL ADVICE FOR MEDICAL TOURISTS

Patients who travel for medical reasons should consult a travel medicine specialist in the United States for advice tailored to individual health needs, preferably ≥4–6 weeks before travel. In addition to regular considerations for healthy travel related to their destination, medical tourists should consider the additional risks associated with surgery and travel, either while being treated or while recovering from treatment. Flying and surgery both increase the risk of blood clots and pulmonary emboli. Air pressure in most commercial aircraft is equivalent to the pressure at an altitude of approximately 6,000–8,000 ft (1,829–2,438 m). Patients should not travel for 10 days after chest or abdominal surgery to avoid risks associated with this change in pressure. The American Society of Plastic Surgeons advises people who have had cosmetic procedures of the face, eyelids, or nose, or who have had laser treatments, to wait 7–10 days before flying. Patients are also advised to avoid typical vacation activities such as sunbathing, drinking alcohol, swimming, and taking long tours or engaging in strenuous activities or exercise after surgery. The Aerospace Medical Association has published medical guidelines for airline travel that provide useful information on the risks of travel with certain medical conditions (www.asma.org/asma/media/asma/Travel-Publications/paxguidelines.pdf).

GUIDANCE FOR TRAVELERS SEEKING MEDICAL CARE ABROAD

Several professional organizations have developed guidance that includes questions useful for travelers when discussing medical or dental care abroad, either with the facility providing the care or with the group facilitating the trip. When considering a trip overseas for medical care, travelers should be aware of the guiding principles developed by the American Medical Association (Box 2-6). The American College of Surgeons (ACS) issued a similar statement on medical and surgical tourism with the additional recommendation that travelers obtain a complete set of medical records before returning home to ensure that details of their care are available to providers in the United States, which helps facilitate continuity of care and proper follow-up if needed. ACS also recommends that prospective medical tourists use facilities that are internationally accredited. Examples of accrediting

entities include Joint Commission International, DNV International Accreditation for Hospitals, and the International Society for Quality in Health Care, which have lists of standards that facilities need to meet to be accredited. However, using a facility that is accredited does not guarantee a lack of complications, similar to any hospital or procedure performed in the United States. Similarly, the American Dental Association provides informational documents, including "Traveler's Guide to Safe Dental Care," through the Global Dental Safety Organization for Safety and Asepsis Procedures (Box 2-7). Although this guidance was not developed for medical tourists, it provides useful information for travelers to consider when selecting a facility or planning a trip for medical or dental care. These guides indicate the types of questions that people considering travel for medical care should discuss with their regular health care provider. Additional resources exist to assist both providers and prospective medical tourists (Box 2-8).

BOX 2-6. ## Guiding principles on medical tourism[1]

The American Medical Association advocates that employers, insurance companies, and other entities that facilitate or promote medical care outside the United States adhere to the following principles:

(a) Medical care outside the United States must be voluntary.

(b) Financial incentives to travel outside the United States for medical care should not limit the diagnostic and therapeutic alternatives that are offered to patients or restrict treatment or referral options.

(c) Patients should be referred for medical care only to institutions that have been accredited by recognized international accrediting

bodies (such as the Joint Commission International or the International Society for Quality in Health Care).

(d) Before travel, local follow-up care should be coordinated and financing should be arranged to ensure continuity of care when patients return from medical care outside the United States.

(e) Coverage for travel outside the United States for medical care must include the costs of necessary follow-up care upon return to the United States.

(f) Patients should be informed of their rights and legal recourse before agreeing to travel outside the United States for medical care.

(g) Access to physician licensing and outcome data, as well as facility accreditation and outcomes data, should be arranged for patients seeking medical care outside the United States.

(h) The transfer of patient medical records to and from facilities outside the United States should be consistent with Health Insurance Portability and Accountability Action (HIPAA) guidelines.

(i) Patients choosing to travel outside the United States for medical care should be provided with information about the potential risks of combining surgical procedures with long flights and vacation activities.

[1] From American Medical Association. New AMA Guidelines on Medical Tourism. Chicago: AMA; 2008.

2

BOX 2-7. Patient checklist for obtaining safe dental care during international travel[1]

Before you leave:

- Visit your dentist for a check-up to reduce the chances you will have a dental emergency.
- See a health care provider to receive any needed vaccinations, medications, and advice related to your travel destination.

When seeking treatment for a dental emergency during your trip:

- Consult hotel staff or the American Embassy or consulate for assistance in finding a dentist.
- If possible, consider recommendations from Americans living in the area or from other trusted sources.

If the answers to any of the asterisked (*) items below are "No," you should have reservations about the office's infection control standards. If the answer to a two-star item (**) is "No," consider making a swift but gracious exit.

When making the appointment, ask the following:

- Do you use new gloves for each patient?*
- Do you use an autoclave (steam sterilizer) or dry heat oven to sterilize your instruments between patients?**
- Do you sterilize your handpieces (drills)?* (If not, do you disinfect them?)**
- Do you use new needles for each patient?**

- Is sterile (or boiled) water used for surgical procedures?** (In areas where drinking water is unsafe, the water also may cause illness if used for dental treatment.)

Upon arriving at the office, observe the following:

- Is the office clean and neat?
- Do staff wash their hands, with soap, between patients?**
- Do they wear gloves for all procedures?**
- Do they clean and disinfect or use disposable covers on surfaces touched during treatment?

[1] Excerpt from Organization for Safety and Asepsis Procedures. Traveler's guide to safe dental care. Annapolis, MD: Organization for Safety and Asepsis Procedures; 2001. Available from: http://www.osap.org/?page=TravelersGuide.

Many websites that market directly to travelers provide information on medical tourism. These sites may not include comprehensive details on the qualifications or certifications of a facility or provider. Furthermore, local standards for facility accreditation and provider certification can vary. The ACS recommends that patients considering treatment abroad seek care from providers certified in their specialties through a process that is equivalent to that established by the member boards of the American Board of Medical Specialties. ACS, American Society of Plastic Surgeons, and the International Society of Aesthetic Plastic Surgery all accredit overseas physicians. Again, however, the traveler should realize that accreditation does not ensure a good outcome, and travelers should be encouraged to do as much research as possible on a health care facility they are considering using.

TRANSPLANT TOURISM

One of the newer and more controversial forms of medical tourism is "transplant tourism," which is travel for the purpose of receiving an organ or stem cell purchased from an unrelated donor for transplant or receiving other biomaterial (cell, tissue) from nonhuman species (xenotransplantation). Xenotransplantation is regulated differently among countries; no scientific evidence supports its therapeutic benefit, and adverse events have been reported. Additionally, several studies of medical tourism identified potential problems that travelers and clinicians need to be aware of when considering transplantation overseas: the donor and the procedures lacked documentation, most patients received fewer immunosuppressive drugs than is current practice in the United States, and most patients did not receive antibiotic prophylaxis. In 2004, to protect vulnerable populations from becoming

BOX 2-8. Helpful resources on medical tourism

- Aerospace Medical Association guidelines for airline travel provide useful information on the risks of travel with certain medical conditions: www.asma.org/asma/media/asma/Travel-Publications/paxguidelines.pdf
- American Academy of Orthopaedic Surgeons Bulletin, July 2007, discusses safety issues that patients should consider: www.aaos.org/news/bulletin/jul07/cover1.asp
- American Academy of Orthopaedic Surgeons discusses liability implications of medical tourism: www.aaos.org/news/aaosnow/feb08/managing7.asp
- American College of Surgeons. Statement on medical and surgical tourism: www.facs.org/fellows_info/statements/st-65.html
- American Society for Aesthetic Plastic Surgery. Guidelines for patients seeking cosmetic procedures abroad: www.surgery.org/consumers/consumer-resources/consumer-tips/guidelines-for-patients-seeking-cosmetic-procedures-abroad
- American Society of Plastic Surgeons (ASPS). The dangers of plastic surgery tourism: www.plasticsurgery.org/articles-and-galleries/dangers-of-plastic-surgery-tourism.html
- American Society of Plastic Surgeons' Find-a-surgeon tool helps identify ASPS member surgeons in the United States and overseas: www1.plasticsurgery.org/find_a_surgeon
- European Commission. Cross-border care policy: http://ec.europa.eu/health/cross_border_care/policy/index_en.htm
- International Society for Aesthetic Plastic Surgery's Find-a-surgeon tool helps identify a surgeon: www.isaps.org/find-a-surgeon
- Joint Commission International list of its accredited facilities outside of the United States: www.jointcommissioninternational.org/JCI-Accredited-Organizations/
- Organization for Safety and Asepsis Procedures. Traveler's guide to safe dental care: www.osap.org/?page=TravelersGuide
- World Health Organization. Guiding principles on human cell, tissue and organ transplantation: www.who.int/transplantation/Guiding_PrinciplesTransplantation_WHA63.22en.pdf
- US Department of States: Your Health Abroad https://travel.state.gov/content/passports/en/go/health.html#healthy.html

victims of transplant tourism, the World Health Assembly Resolution 57.18 encouraged member countries to "take measures to protect the poorest and vulnerable groups [the donors] from 'transplant tourism' and the sale of tissues and organs." A meeting in 2008 in Istanbul addressed the issue of transplant tourism and organ trafficking, which resulted in a call for these activities to be prohibited. In view of those events, the World Health Organization revised the Guiding Principles on Human Cell, Tissue and Organ Transplantation and released those revised principles in March 2009. These guidelines emphasize that cells, tissues, and organs should only be donated freely without any form of financial incentive.

BIBLIOGRAPHY

1. Budiani-Saberi DA, Delmonico FL. Organ trafficking and transplant tourism: a commentary on the global realities. Am J Transplant. 2008 May;8(5):925–9.

2. Chen LH, Wilson ME. The globalization of healthcare: implications of medical tourism for the infectious disease clinician. Clin Infect Dis. 2013 Dec;57(12):1752–9.

3. Mathers AJ, Hazen KC, Carroll J, Yeh AJ, L. CH, Bonomo RA, et al. First clinical cases of OXA-48-producing carbapenem-resistant Klebsiella pneumoniae in the United States: the "menace" arrives in the new world. J Clin Microbiol. 2013 Feb;51(2):680–3.

4. Merion RM, Barnes AD, Lin M, Ashby VB, McBride V, Ortiz-Rios E, et al. Transplants in foreign countries among patients removed from the US transplant

waiting list. Am J Transplant. 2008 Apr;8(4 Pt 2): 988–96.

5. Organ Procurement and Transplantation Network, Scientific Registry of Transplant Recipients. United States organ transplantation annual data report, 2011. Rockville (MD): US Department of Health and Human Services; 2012 [cited 2016 Sep. 22]; Available from: http://srtr.transplant.hrsa.gov/annual_reports/2011/default.aspx.

6. Reed CM. Medical tourism. Med Clin North Am. 2008 Nov;92(6):1433–46, xi.

7. Robyn MP, Newman AP, Amato M, Walawander M, Kothe C, Nerone JD, et al. Q Fever outbreak among travelers to Germany who received live cell therapy—United States and Canada, 2014. MMWR Morb Mortal Wkly Rep 2015 Oct;64(38):1071–3.

8. Rogers BA, Aminzadeh Z, Hayashi Y, Paterson DL. Country-to-country transfer of patients and the risk of

multi-resistant bacterial infection. Clin Infect Dis. 2011 Jul 1;53(1):49–56.

9. Schnabel D, Gaines J, Nguyen DB, Esposito DH, Ridpath A, Yacisin K, et al. Notes from the field: rapidly growing nontuberculous Mycobacterium wound infections among medical tourists undergoing cosmetic surgeries in the Dominican Republic—multiple states, March 2013–February 2014. MMWR Morb Mortal Wkly Rep. 2014 Mar 7;63(9):201–2.

10. US Department of Health and Human Services. 2007 annual report of the US Organ Procurement and Transplantation Network and the Scientific Registry of Transplant Recipients: transplant data 1997–2006. Rockville, MD: US Department of Health and Human Services; 2007 [cited 2016 Sep. 22]; Available from: http://www.ustransplant.org/annual_reports/current/ar_archives.htm.

DISCUSSING COMPLEMENTARY & INTEGRATIVE HEALTH APPROACHES WITH TRAVELERS

Catherine Law, Tina Adler, David Shurtleff

Travelers often ask their health care providers about the use of complementary or integrative health approaches for travel-related illnesses and conditions. This should come as no surprise, given that many people—approximately 1 in 3 Americans—report using products or practices that have origins outside of conventional medicine to complement treatment for a variety of medical conditions or to promote general wellness. Some of these approaches for travel-related health problems are promoted widely in advertising or discussed on the Internet. However, little of this information is supported by research evidence, and some of it is misleading or false. This section focuses on what scientifically credible research says about some of the herbal remedies, dietary supplements (see Box 2-9), and other complementary health approaches frequently suggested for travel-related ailments and hazards.

TRAVEL-RELATED AILMENTS AND COMPLEMENTARY HEALTH APPROACHES

Malaria Prophylaxis and Treatment

ARTEMISIA (*ARTEMISIA ANNUA* L. OR SWEET WORMWOOD) AND QUININE

Standard treatments for malaria in most of the world depend on plant derivatives. Quinine from the cinchona tree (*Cinchona* spp.) may be used in combination with other antimalarial medications to treat malaria. There is no evidence that quinine prevents malaria. Travelers should not attempt to use quinine to self-treat or prevent malaria. An important component of the antimalarial drug artemether-lumefantrine comes from artemisinin, isolated from the qinghao plant (*Artemisia annua*). Consumer websites and news stories have claimed that using the herb artemisia alone may prevent malaria, but studies

2

BOX 2-9. About dietary supplements and unproven therapies

- The Food and Drug Administration (FDA) regulates dietary supplements, but the regulations are different and generally less strict than those for prescription or over-the-counter drugs. Learn more at https://nccih.nih.gov/health/supplements/wiseuse.htm.
- Two major safety concerns about dietary supplements are potential drug interactions and product contamination. Analyses of supplements sometimes find differences between labeled and actual ingredients. For example, an herbal supplement may not contain the correct plant species, or the amounts of the ingredients may be lower or higher than the label states.
- Consult the FDA's safety advisories to learn the latest regarding product recalls and safety alerts: www.fda.gov/Food/RecallsOutbreaksEmergencies/SafetyAlertsAdvisories/default.htm.
- Unproven therapies are discussed in this section only for educational purposes and are not recommended for use. The Centers for Disease Control and Prevention (CDC) endorses only FDA-approved therapies.

show it does not. The World Health Organization recommends against using artemisia plant material in any form (including tea) for treating or preventing malaria. The use of artemisia alone has contributed to the increase in malaria parasites resistant to artemisinin. Recommended drugs used to prevent and treat malaria are described in Chapter 3, Malaria.

VITAMIN AND MINERAL SUPPLEMENTS

Limited research suggests that when children with malaria are nutritionally deficient, supplements of vitamin A and zinc may help lower their fever and blood levels of the malaria parasite; however, there is no evidence that vitamin A or zinc prevent malaria infection. Vitamin A is fat soluble, and large or frequent doses may accumulate in the body and cause acute or chronic toxicity. High intake of vitamin A has been linked to birth defects. Taking beta-carotene, a precursor of vitamin A, has been linked to an increased risk of lung cancer and cardiovascular disease in some smokers. Zinc supplements can interact with several types of medications. Anyone taking high levels of zinc should be monitored for adverse health effects.

Zika Prophylaxis and Treatment

Consumer websites and online videos are claiming, without credible evidence, that herbs or other products, such as activated charcoal or diatomaceous earth, will protect against or treat the Zika virus. There is no evidence that any of these products can prevent or treat Zika virus infection. For more information see Chapter 3, Zika.

Travelers' Diarrhea Prevention and Treatment

PROBIOTICS

Probiotics are often suggested to help prevent travelers' diarrhea (TD). Research on their use in treating acute infectious diarrhea is generally positive. Results from studies on preventing TD are mixed but encouraging. Given current data, it must be assumed that effects of probiotics in any given study are specific to the strain or strains tested. The US Food and Drug Administration (FDA) has not approved any health claims for probiotics.

In healthy people, probiotics usually have only minor side effects, if any. For more information see "Nonantimicrobial Drugs for Prophylaxis" in the Travelers' Diarrhea section in this chapter.

GOLDENSEAL

Goldenseal is an herb that has been touted as a treatment for a variety of ailments. No high-quality research on goldenseal for TD has been conducted. Studies show that goldenseal inhibits cytochrome P450 enzymes, raising concerns that it may increase the toxicity or alter the effects of many commonly used drugs.

ACTIVATED CHARCOAL

There is no solid evidence to support claims that activated charcoal helps with TD, bloating, stomach cramps, or gas. The side effects of activated charcoal have not been well documented but were mild when it was tested on healthy people.

Warning: Children **should not** be given activated charcoal for diarrhea and dehydration. It may absorb nutrients, enzymes, and antibiotics in the intestine and mask the severity of fluid loss.

GRAPEFRUIT SEED EXTRACT

Claims that grapefruit seed extract can prevent bacterial foodborne illnesses are unfounded and not supported by research.

Altitude Illness Prevention and Treatment

There is little, if any, evidence that dietary or herbal supplements help prevent or treat altitude illness (often referred to as mountain sickness).

COCA

Coca tea has been used for altitude illness, but there is no strong evidence on whether it works or has adverse effects. It will result in a positive drug test for cocaine metabolites. For more information see Chapter 4, Peru: Cusco, Machu Picchu, & Other Regions.

GARLIC

There is no evidence supporting claims that garlic helps reduce altitude illness. Garlic supplements appear safe for most adults. Possible side effects of taking garlic include breath and body odor, heartburn, and upset stomach. Some people have allergic reactions to garlic. Short-term use of most commercially available garlic supplements poses only a limited risk for causing herb–drug interactions, including interfering with the effectiveness of the HIV drug saquinavir.

GINKGO BILOBA

Results from several small studies of ginkgo for preventing altitude illness show conflicting, but mostly negative, results. Whether these differences relate to the different preparations used in these studies cannot be determined. Products made from standardized ginkgo leaf extracts

appear to be safe when used as directed. However, ginkgo may increase the risk of bleeding in some people and interact with certain conventional medications, including anticoagulants. In addition, studies by the National Toxicology Program showed that rodents developed tumors after being given a ginkgo extract for up to 2 years.

VITAMIN E

Only one small study has investigated vitamin E, in combination with other antioxidants, for altitude illness, and the results were negative. Taking supplements of vitamin E, a fat-soluble vitamin, has been linked to an increased risk of hemorrhagic stroke. They also have the potential to interact with several types of medications, including statins, niacin, and warfarin.

Motion Sickness Prevention and Treatment

ACUPRESSURE AND MAGNETS

Using acupressure or magnets is advocated by some to prevent or treat motion sickness. However, research does not support the use of acupressure or magnets for this purpose.

GINGER

Although some studies have shown that ginger may ease pregnancy-related nausea and vomiting, there is no strong evidence that ginger helps with motion sickness. Several studies have found no evidence of harm from taking ginger during pregnancy, but it's uncertain whether ginger is always safe for pregnant women; women should always talk with their health care provider before trying any dietary supplements during pregnancy, especially if traveling overseas. In some people, ginger can have mild side effects such as abdominal discomfort. Research has not definitely shown whether ginger interacts with medications, but concerns have been raised that it might interact with anticoagulants. The effect of using ginger supplements with common over-the-counter drugs for motion sickness (such as dimenhydrinate [Dramamine]) is unknown.

PYRIDOXINE (VITAMIN B6)

While The American Congress of Obstetrics and Gynecology's 2015 Practice Bulletin Summary recommends pyridoxine alone or in combination with doxylamine as a safe and effective treatment for nausea and vomiting associated with pregnancy, there is no evidence supporting claims that pyridoxine prevents or alleviates motion sickness. Excessive use of pyridoxine supplements can affect nerve function.

HOMEOPATHIC PRODUCTS

There is no evidence supporting claims that homeopathic products prevent or alleviate motion sickness.

Jet Lag/Sleep Problems

MELATONIN

Melatonin supplements may help with sleep problems caused by jet lag. Travelers report having less jet lag on eastward and westward flights when given melatonin compared with placebo. In a 2007 clinical practice guideline, the American Academy of Sleep Medicine supported using melatonin to reduce jet lag symptoms and improve sleep after traveling across >1 time zone. A systematic literature review suggested taking 0.5–5 mg of melatonin appeared to be effective for easing jet lag.

Before recommending melatonin, consider the following:

- People with epilepsy or who take an oral anti-coagulant should **never** use melatonin without medical supervision.

- Melatonin supplements appear to be safe for most people when used short-term; less is known about their long-term safety.

- Melatonin should not be taken early in the day, as it may cause sleepiness and delay adaptation to local time.

- The amount of melatonin in products and the dosages recommended on labels can vary significantly.

Side effects from melatonin are uncommon but can include drowsiness, headache, dizziness, or nausea.

RELAXATION TECHNIQUES

Relaxation techniques, such as progressive relaxation and mindfulness-based stress reduction, may help with insomnia, but it has not been established whether they are effective for jet lag.

OTHER

There is very little evidence that aromatherapy, chamomile, or valerian help with insomnia. None have significant side effects, but chamomile can cause allergic reactions. Kava is also advertised for sleep but good research on kava for insomnia is lacking. More importantly, kava supplements have been linked to a risk of severe liver damage.

For more information see the Jet Lag section in this chapter.

Colds and Flu

ZINC

Zinc supplements taken orally may reduce the duration of a cold. Zinc, particularly in large doses, can have side effects including nausea and diarrhea. The intranasal use of zinc can cause anosmia (loss of sense of smell), which may be long-lasting or permanent. In 2009, the FDA warned consumers to stop using several intranasal zinc products that had been linked to cases of anosmia.

SALINE IRRIGATION

Nasal saline irrigation, such as with neti pots, may be useful and safe for chronic sinusitis. However, even in places where tap water is safe to drink, people should use only sterile or distilled water for nasal irrigation to avoid the risk of introducing waterborne pathogens. Nasal saline irrigation may help relieve the symptoms of acute upper respiratory tract infections, but the evidence is not definitive.

VITAMIN C

Taking vitamin C supplements regularly may slightly reduce the duration and severity of colds in some people. Vitamin C supplements appear safe, even at high doses.

PROBIOTICS

Probiotics might reduce susceptibility to colds or other upper respiratory tract infections and the length of the illnesses, but the quality of the evidence is low or very low.

OTHER

There is no strong evidence that echinacea, garlic, Chinese herbs, oil of oregano, or eucalyptus essential oil prevent or treat colds, or that the homeopathic product Oscillococcinum prevents or treats influenza or influenzalike illness.

Other Common or Travel-Related Infections

HEPATITIS C

Herbal supplements should never be used to treat hepatitis C outside of well-designed, randomized clinical trials. A randomized clinical trial found no evidence of benefit from silymarin (an extract from milk thistle seeds) in patients with chronic hepatitis C. In addition, a systematic review of 10 randomized clinical trials found no firm evidence of efficacy of any herbal supplements for hepatitis C. Two of the trials studied a single herb or herbal ingredient; the others studied different compounds made from herbs.

VAGINAL INFECTIONS AND URINARY TRACT INFECTIONS

Probiotics have been studied for treating vaginal or urinary tract infections, but there is not enough supporting evidence to suggest that they are helpful.

Insect Protection: Botanical Repellents

MOSQUITOES

Laboratory-based studies found that botanicals, including citronella products, worked for shorter periods than products containing DEET. For people wishing to use botanicals, CDC recommends Environmental Protection Agency (EPA)–registered products containing oil of lemon eucalyptus (OLE), such as the products Repel and Off! Botanicals.

There are no high-quality studies on the effectiveness or safety of neem oil for preventing mosquito bites. Neem oil is used in agricultural insecticide products and promoted on some websites for human use.

BED BUGS

Essential oils and other natural products are marketed for travelers to repel bed bugs, but there is no evidence that they are effective. Experts recommend against using any insect repellents or pesticides on clothing or luggage. Instead, travelers should be encouraged to follow steps to detect and avoid bed bugs, such as inspecting their mattress and keeping their luggage off the floor or bed. A guide for the public, *How to Find Bed Bugs*, is available at www.epa.gov/bedbugs/how-find-bed-bugs. Information is also available on CDC's website at www.cdc.gov/parasites/bedbugs. For more information see Box 2-5.

Sunscreens

Skin cancer is the most common type of cancer in the United States. Experts recommend using a broad-spectrum sunscreen, limiting your sun exposure, and wearing protective clothing to protect against sunburns and to possibly lower the risk of skin cancer. There are many "natural" sunscreen products available online, recipes for making your own, and advice on consuming dietary supplements or drinking teas to protect against sun damage. Sunscreens are promoted as containing aloe vera and green tea, among other natural ingredients, but studies have not proven that any herbal product or dietary supplement, including aloe, beta carotene, selenium, or epigallocatechin gallate (EGCG), an extract in green tea, reduce the risk of skin cancer or sun damage. For more information see Sun Exposure in this chapter.

Homeopathic Vaccines

There is no credible scientific evidence or plausible scientific rationale to support claims that certain homeopathic products (sometimes called nosodes or homeopathic immunizations) are effective substitutes for conventional immunizations. For more information see General Recommendations for Vaccination & Immunoprophylaxis in this chapter.

Untested Therapies in Other Countries

CDC does not recommend traveling to other countries for untested medical interventions or to buy medications that are not approved in the United States. For more information see Medical Tourism in this chapter.

TALKING TO TRAVELERS ABOUT COMPLEMENTARY HEALTH APPROACHES

Given the vast number of complementary or integrative interventions and the wealth of potentially misleading information about them that can be found on the Internet, discussing the use of these approaches with patients may seem daunting. However, it is important to be proactive, as surveys show that many patients are reluctant to raise the topic with their health care providers.

Federal agencies, such as the National Center for Complementary and Integrative Health (NCCIH), offer evidence-based resources (nccih.nih.gov/health/providers) to help you and your patients have a meaningful discussion about complementary approaches.

ACKNOWLEDGMENTS

The authors thank Dr. John Williamson of NCCIH for his scientific review and Ms. Karen Kaplan and Ms. Patricia Andersen of Westat for their editorial assistance.

BIBLIOGRAPHY

1. Hao Q, Lu Z, Dong BR, Huang CQ, Wu T. Probiotics for preventing acute upper respiratory tract infections. Cochrane Database Syst Rev. 2011 Sep 7(2):CD006895.

2. Hemilä H, Chalker E. Vitamin C for preventing and treating the common cold. Cochrane Database Syst Rev. 2013 Jan 31(1):CD000980.

3. Karsch-Völk M, Barrett B, Kiefer D, Bauer R, Ardjomand-Woelkart K, Linde K. Echinacea for preventing and treating the common cold. Cochrane Database of Syst Rev. 2014 (2):CD000530.

4. King D, Mitchell B, Wlilliams CP, Spurling GK. Saline nasal irrigation for acute upper respiratory tract infections. Cochrane Database Syst Rev. 2015 Apr 20(4):CD006821.

5. Lissiman E, Bhasale AL, Cohen M. Garlic for the common cold. Cochrane Database of Syst Rev. 2014 Nov 11(11):CD006206.

6. Liu J, Manheimer E, Tsutani K, Gluud C. Medicinal herbs for hepatitis C virus infection. Cochrane Database of Syst Rev. 2001 Oct 23(4):CD003183.

7. Mathie RT, Frye J, Fisher P. Homeopathic Oscillococcinum® for preventing and treating influenza and influenza-like illness. Cochrane Database of Syst Rev. 2015 (1):CD001957.

8. Schwenger EM, Tejani AM, Loewen PS. Probiotics for preventing urinary tract infections in adults and children. Cochrane Database of Syst Rev. 2015 Dec 23(12):CD008772.

9. Wang C, Lü L, Zhang A, Liu C. Repellency of selected chemicals against the bed bug (Hemiptera: Cimicidae). J Econ Entomol. 2013 Dec;106(6):2522–9.

10. World Health Organization. Global Malaria Programme. WHO position statement: effectiveness of non-pharmaceutical forms of Artemisia annua L. against malaria. WHO; 2012 [cited 2016 Sep. 22]; Available from: http://www.who.int/malaria/diagnosis_treatment/position_statement_herbal_remedy_artemisia_annua_l.pdf?ua=1.

DEEP VEIN THROMBOSIS & PULMONARY EMBOLISM

Nimia L. Reyes, Michele G. Beckman, Karon Abe

Deep vein thrombosis (DVT) is a condition in which a blood clot develops in the deep veins, most commonly in the lower extremities. A part of the clot can break off and travel to the lungs, causing a pulmonary embolism (PE), which can be life threatening. Venous thromboembolism (VTE) refers to DVT, PE, or both. VTE is often recurrent, and long-term complications, such as postthrombotic syndrome after a DVT or chronic thromboembolic pulmonary hypertension after a PE, are frequent.

People traveling for extended periods of time may be at increased risk for DVT/PE because they have prolonged limited mobility. More than 300 million people travel on long-distance flights each year. An association between VTE and air travel was first reported in the early 1950s, and since then, long-distance air travel has become more common, leading to increased concerns about travel-related VTE.

PATHOGENESIS

Virchow's classic triad for thrombus formation is venous stasis, vessel wall damage, and the hypercoagulable state. Prolonged cramped sitting during long-distance travel interferes with venous flow in the legs and causes venous stasis. Seat-edge pressure on the popliteal area may contribute to vessel wall damage as well as venous stasis. Coagulation activation may result from an interaction between cabin conditions (such as hypobaric hypoxia) and individual risk factors for VTE. Studies of the pathophysiologic mechanisms for the increased risk of VTE after long-distance travel have not produced consistent results, but venous stasis appears to play a major role; other factors specific to air travel may increase coagulation activation, particularly in travelers with preexisting risk factors for VTE.

INCIDENCE

The annual incidence of VTE in the general population has been estimated at 0.1% but is higher in subpopulations with risk factors for VTE (Box 2-10). The actual incidence of travel-related VTE is difficult to determine, since there is no national surveillance for VTE and no consensus on the definition of travel-related VTE, particularly in regard to duration of travel and period of observation after travel. Estimates of travel-related VTE incidence vary because of differences between studies in duration of travel, measured outcome, period of observation after the flight, and the populations observed.

In general, the overall incidence of travel-related VTE is low. Two studies reported that the absolute risk of VTE for flights >4 hours is 1 in 4,656 flights and 1 in 6,000 flights. People who travel on long-distance flights are generally healthier and therefore are at lower risk for VTE than the general population. Five prospective studies that assessed the incidence of DVT among travelers at low to intermediate risk for VTE after travel >8 hours yielded an overall incidence of VTE of 0.5%, while the incidence of symptomatic VTE was 0.3%.

ASSOCIATION WITH TRAVEL

Numerous studies have examined the association between travel, particularly air travel, and VTE with varying results due to differing study methods. Outcomes ranged from asymptomatic DVT to symptomatic DVT/PE and to severe or fatal PE. Asymptomatic DVT is estimated to be 5- to 20-fold more common than symptomatic events, is of uncertain clinical significance, and often resolves spontaneously. Definitions of long-distance travel ranged from flight duration >3 hours to >10 hours (most >4 hours). The period of observation after the flight ranged from hours after landing to ≥8 weeks (most 4 weeks).

Overall, these studies indicate that long-distance air travel may increase a person's risk for

---

BOX 2-10. **Venous thromboembolism (VTE) risk factors**

General risk factors for VTE include the following:

- Older age (increasing risk after age 40)
- Obesity (BMI ≥30 kg/m²)
- Estrogen use (hormonal contraceptives or hormone replacement therapy)

- Pregnancy and the postpartum period
- Thrombophilia (such as factor V Leiden mutation or antiphospholipid syndrome) or a family history of VTE
- Previous VTE
- Active cancer

- Serious medical illness (such as congestive heart failure or inflammatory bowel disease)
- Recent surgery, hospitalization, or trauma
- Limited mobility

VTE by 2- to 4-fold. However, published results from these studies vary; some studies found that long-distance travel increased the risk of VTE, and others either found no definitive evidence that it increased the risk of VTE or found that it increased the risk only if ≥1 additional risk factors were present.

A similar increase in risk is also seen with other modes of travel, such as car, bus, or train, implying that the increase in risk is caused mainly by prolonged limited mobility rather than by the cabin environment. The risk is the same for economy-class and business-class travel. The risk increases with increasing travel duration and with preexisting risk factors for VTE. The risk decreases with time after air travel and returns to baseline by 8 weeks; most air travel–related VTE occurs within the first 1–2 weeks after the flight.

RISK FACTORS

Most travel-related VTE occurs in travelers with preexisting risk factors for VTE (Box 2-10). The combination of air travel with preexisting individual risk factors may have a synergistic effect on the risk for VTE. Some studies have shown that 75%–99.5% of those who developed travel-related VTE had ≥1 preexisting risk factor; one study showed that 20% had ≥5 risk factors. For travelers without preexisting risk factors, the risk of travel-related VTE is low. However, a person may not be aware that he or she has a risk factor such as inherited thrombophilia.

For air travelers, height appears to be an additional risk factor. Risk of travel-related VTE increases with height <1.6 m (5 ft, 3 in). Airplane seats are higher than car seats and cannot be adjusted to a person's height; therefore, shorter people who travel by air may experience seat-edge pressure to the popliteal area. Risk of travel-related VTE also increases with height >1.9 m (6 ft, 3 in), possibly because taller travelers have less leg room.

CLINICAL PRESENTATION

Signs and symptoms of DVT/PE are nonspecific:

- Typical signs or symptoms of DVT in the extremities include pain or tenderness, swelling, increased warmth in the affected area, and redness or discoloration of the overlying skin.

- The most common signs or symptoms of acute PE include unexplained shortness of breath, pleuritic chest pain, cough or hemoptysis, and syncope.

DIAGNOSIS

Imaging studies are needed for diagnosis:

- Duplex ultrasonography is the standard imaging procedure for diagnosis of DVT.

- Computed tomographic pulmonary angiography is the standard imaging procedure for diagnosis of PE. Ventilation-perfusion scan is the second-line imaging procedure.

TREATMENT

Anticoagulants are the medications most commonly used to treat DVT or PE. Bleeding can be a complication of anticoagulant therapy.

The most frequently used injectable anticoagulants are unfractionated heparin, low molecular weight heparin (LMWH), and fondaparinux. Oral anticoagulants include warfarin, dabigatran, rivaroxaban, apixaban, and edoxaban.

It is critical that patients who are at increased risk be evaluated with enough time prior to departure so that travelers understand how to take the medication and the health provider can evaluate whether there are any potential adverse effects of the combination of these medications with others that the travel health provider has prescribed.

PREVENTIVE MEASURES FOR LONG-DISTANCE TRAVELERS

The American College of Chest Physicians published the 9th edition of their *Antithrombotic Therapy and Prevention of Thrombosis Evidence-Based Clinical Practice Guidelines* in February 2012. Recommendations for long-distance travelers (considered grade 2C: weak recommendation, low- or very low-quality evidence) are the following:

1. For long-distance travelers at increased risk of VTE (Box 2-10), frequent ambulation, calf muscle exercise, and sitting in an aisle seat if feasible are suggested.

2. For long-distance travelers at increased risk of VTE (Box 2-10), use of properly fitted, below-knee graduated compression stockings (GCS) providing 15–30 mm Hg of pressure at the ankle during travel is suggested. For all other long-distance travelers, use of GCS is not recommended.

3. For long-distance travelers, the use of aspirin or anticoagulants to prevent VTE is not recommended.

There is no evidence for an association between dehydration and travel-related VTE and no direct evidence that drinking plenty of nonalcoholic beverages to ensure adequate hydration or avoiding alcoholic beverages has a protective effect. Therefore, while maintaining hydration is reasonable and unlikely to cause harm, it cannot be recommended specifically to prevent travel-related VTE.

There is evidence that immobility while flying is a risk for VTE and indirect evidence that maintaining mobility may prevent VTE. In view of the role of venous stasis in the pathogenesis of travel-related VTE, it would be reasonable to recommend frequent ambulation and calf muscle exercises for long-distance travelers.

Compared with aisle seats, window seats in one study were reported to increase the general risk of VTE by 2-fold, while obese travelers had a 6-fold increase in risk. Aisle seats are reported to have a protective effect, compared with window or middle seats, probably because travelers are freer to move around.

GCS are indicated for long-distance travelers at increased risk. GCS appear to reduce asymptomatic DVT in travelers and are generally well tolerated.

Global use of anticoagulants for long-distance travel is not indicated. Pharmacologic prophylaxis for long-distance travelers at particularly high risk should be decided on an individual basis. In cases where the potential benefits of pharmacologic prophylaxis outweigh the possible adverse effects, anticoagulants rather than antiplatelet drugs (such as aspirin) are recommended.

RECOMMENDATIONS

1. General measures for long-distance travelers:
   a. Calf muscle exercises
   b. Frequent ambulation
   c. Aisle seating when feasible
2. Additional measures for long-distance travelers at increased risk of VTE:
   a. Properly fitted below-knee GCS
   b. Anticoagulant prophylaxis only in particularly high-risk cases where the potential benefits outweigh the risks

BIBLIOGRAPHY

1. Aryal KR, Al-Khaffaf H. Venous thromboembolic complications following air travel: what's the quantitative risk? A literature review. Eur J Vasc Endovasc Surg. 2006 Feb;31(2):187–99.

2. Bartholomew JR, Schaffer JL, McCormick GF. Air travel and venous thromboembolism: minimizing the risk. Cleve Clin J Med. 2011 Feb;78(2):111–20.

3. Chandra D, Parisini E, Mozaffarian D. Meta-analysis: travel and risk for venous thromboembolism. Ann Intern Med. 2009 Aug 4;151(3):180–90.

4. Eklof B, Maksimovic D, Caprini JA, Glase C. Air travel-related venous thromboembolism. Disease-a-month : DM. 2005 Feb-Mar;51(2-3):200–7.

5. Gavish I, Brenner B. Air travel and the risk of thromboembolism. Intern Emerg Med. 2011 Apr;6(2):113–6.

6. Kahn SR, Lim W, Dunn AS, Cushman M, Dentali F, Akl EA, et al. Prevention of VTE in nonsurgical patients: antithrombotic therapy and prevention of thrombosis, 9th ed: American College of Chest Physicians evidence-based clinical practice guidelines. Chest. 2012 Feb;141(2 Suppl):e195S–226S.

7. Schobersberger W, Schobersberger B, Partsch H. Travel-related thromboembolism: mechanisms and avoidance. Expert Rev Cardiovasc Ther. 2009 Dec;7(12):1559–67.

8. Schreijer AJ, Cannegieter SC, Caramella M, Meijers JC, Krediet RT, Simons RM, et al. Fluid loss does not explain coagulation activation during air travel. Thromb Haemost. 2008 Jun;99(6):1053–9.

9. Schreijer AJ, Cannegieter SC, Doggen CJ, Rosendaal FR. The effect of flight-related behaviour on the risk of venous thrombosis after air travel. Br J Haematol. 2009 Feb;144(3):425–9.

10. Watson HG, Baglin TP. Guidelines on travel-related venous thrombosis. Br J Haematol. 2011 Jan;152(1):31–4.

MENTAL HEALTH

Thomas H. Valk

2

International travel is stressful. Stressors vary to some extent with the type of travel; short-term tourist travel likely offers the least stress and frequent travel and expatriation the most. Given the stressors of travel, preexisting psychiatric disorders can recur, latent or undiagnosed problems can become apparent, and new problems can arise. In addition, short-term travelers may suffer from anxiety and aggravated depressive symptoms triggered by jet lag, fatigue, and work or family pressures. Remaining aware of these issues is important for providers when evaluating the ill patient who may have trouble distinguishing physical and psychological problems after travel.

OCCURRENCE IN TRAVELERS

Incidence data based on population surveys of travelers are nonexistent. Data from clinical populations include the following:

- Patel et al. conducted a study of urgent repatriation of British diplomats and found that 11% of medical evacuations were "nonphysical," or psychological in nature. Using the authors' data, an overall incident rate of 0.34% for psychological evacuations occurred for their population. Of these, 41% were for some form of depression.

- Another study examined psychiatric evacuations over a 5-year period in the US Foreign Service population from 1982 through 1986. Using an unpublished estimate of the population served in this study, an overall incidence rate of 0.16% for psychiatric evacuations occurred. Of these, fully 50% were for substance abuse or affective disorder. Mania and hypomanic states accounted for 2.8% of these evacuations.

- Streltzer studied psychiatric emergencies in travelers to Hawaii and estimated a rate of 0.22% for tourists and 2.25% for transient travelers (those arriving in Hawaii with no immediate plans to leave) versus a rate of 1.25% for nontravelers. In order of decreasing frequency, diagnoses in this population were schizophrenia, alcohol abuse, anxiety reactions, and depression.

- Quigley et al. studied repatriations over a 2-year period (2010–2012) comparing American-sponsored college students studying abroad with American-sponsored corporate business travelers and expatriates. They found a 23-times higher rate of repatriation because of mental health problems for the student population. In this population of repatriated students, in order of decreasing frequency, diagnoses were mood disorders, personality disorders, substance abuse, eating disorders, and schizophrenia or other psychotic disorders.

THE PRETRAVEL CONSULTATION AND MENTAL HEALTH EVALUATION

Any pretravel consultation should include a mental health screening, especially for those planning extended travel or residence in a foreign country. Since travel medicine specialists rarely have mental health credentials, a full mental health inquiry with mental status examination and a psychiatric review of symptoms would not be practicable. Rather, a brief inquiry aimed at eliciting previously diagnosed psychiatric disorders should be undertaken. To introduce this portion of the consultation and to elicit the most cooperation, the practitioner could enumerate the following facts:

- International travel is stressful for everyone and has been associated with the emergence or reemergence of mental health problems.

- The availability of culturally compatible mental health services varies widely.

- Laws regarding the use of illicit substances can be severe in some countries.

The practitioner can then ask about factors that might indicate a mental health problem:

- Any previously treated or diagnosed psychiatric disorders and the type of treatment involved (inpatient, outpatient, medications)

- Current treatment for any psychiatric disorders and their nature

- Current or past use of illicit substances

- Any diagnosis of substance use disorder, or suggestion from medical service providers, friends, or family that the traveler might be using alcohol or other substances to excess

- Any immediate family history of serious mental health problems

In general, any history of inpatient treatment, psychotic episode, violent or suicidal behavior, affective disorder (including mania, hypomania, or major depression), any treatment for substance use problems, and any current treatments would warrant further evaluation by a mental health professional, preferably one who has had some experience in problems relating to international travel. On occasion, the patient's mental status upon examination may be notably abnormal, which would also warrant a referral.

Other issues that may be encountered and should be addressed during the pretravel consultation include the following:

- Availability of culturally compatible mental health treatment in the destination country for long-term travelers or expatriates.

- Customs regulations: Traveling through customs with medications for personal use can be problematic in countries where those medications are prohibited. What substances are prohibited in any given country varies. Stimulants frequently used for attention deficit disorders, such as amphetamine or methylphenidate, may be problematic, along with narcotics. This list is not exhaustive, and travelers should check with the host country's embassy if anything is questionable. A health care provider or pharmacist in the destination country may also be able to provide guidance about medication restrictions. It

is always wise to carry medications in their original containers, along with a letter from the prescribing physician indicating that the medications have been prescribed for medical reasons. Even with these precautions, problems may still occur at customs.

- Psychotropic medication refills: Obtaining these medications while living overseas can be problematic, as availability or even legality of the medication varies from country to country. Again, a check with the country's embassy may be helpful, as would a check with a reputable in-country pharmacy or health care provider.

- Measuring drug levels: Locating laboratory facilities for the determination of lithium levels or for other mood-stabilizing medications may be challenging and should be investigated prior to travel. High ambient temperatures and increased sweating could lead to lithium toxicity, even on the same dose.

- Mefloquine: In general, patients with mental health issues should not be prescribed mefloquine for malarial chemoprophylaxis because of its potential for neuropsychiatric side effects. Please see the discussion of mefloquine in Chapter 3, Malaria.

- Alcoholics Anonymous (AA) and Narcotics Anonymous (NA) meetings: Currently sober patients with substance use disorders should consider seeking out AA and NA meetings, depending upon their length of stay and stability of their sobriety. AA and NA maintain, by country, lists of such meetings on their websites, although availability can change. Language of meetings should also be checked.

- Evacuation insurance: Travelers with mental health problems should consider travel health and medical evacuation insurance that does not exclude psychiatric evacuations for emergencies when abroad.

POST-TRAVEL MENTAL HEALTH ISSUES

Travel health practitioners may be in a unique position to inquire about traumatic experiences a traveler might have had that may lead to acute stress disorder (ASD) or posttraumatic stress disorder (PTSD). Travelers exposed to life-threatening events, such as disaster relief workers or war correspondents, may experience subclinical or outright ASD or PTSD.

If the traveler has had such experiences, clinicians should inquire about possible symptoms:

- Reexperiencing the event can include recurrent, intrusive recollections, distressing dreams of the event, and feeling as if the event is happening again.

- Avoidance symptoms can include avoiding thoughts, feelings, activities, places, or people that lead to memories of the event.

- Changes in mood or cognition associated with the event can include diminished interest in activities, inability to experience positive emotions, or an inability to remember significant details of the event.

- Arousal symptoms can include difficulty sleeping or concentrating, irritability, or an exaggerated startle response.

As symptoms of PTSD may occur months or even years after an event, education about the possibility of having such symptoms in the future is worthwhile. If there is any concern about a possible reaction to a traumatic event, referral to a psychiatrist is warranted.

BIBLIOGRAPHY

1. American Psychiatric Association. Diagnostic and Statistical Manual of Mental Disorders. 5th ed. Arlington, VA: American Psychiatric Association; 2013.

2. Benedek DM, Wynn GH. Clinical manual for management of PTSD. Arlington, VA: American Psychiatric Publishing, Inc.; 2011.

3. Feinstein A, Owen J, Blair N. A hazardous profession: war, journalists, and psychopathology. Am J Psychiatry. 2002 Sep;159(9):1570–5.

4. Liese B, Mundt KA, Dell LD, Nagy L, Demure B. Medical insurance claims associated with international business travel. Occup Environ Med. 1997 Jul;54(7):499–503.

5. Patel D, Easmon CJ, Dow C, Snashall DC, Seed PT. Medical repatriation of British diplomats resident overseas. J Travel Med. 2000 Mar-Apr;7(2):64–9.

6. Quigley RL, Copeland R. Mental health and study abroad: incidence and mitigation strategies. Oral presentation at: 13th Conference of the International Society of Travel Medicine; 2013 May 19-23; Maastricht, The Netherlands.

7. Streltzer J. Psychiatric emergencies in travelers to Hawaii. Compr Psychiatry. 1979 Sep-Oct;20(5): 463–8.

8. Valk TH. Psychiatric medical evacuations within the Foreign Service. Foreign Serv Med Bull. 1988;268: 9–11.

9. Valk TH. Psychiatric disorders of travel In: Keystone JS, Freedman DO, Kozarsky PE, Connor BA, Nothdurft HO, editors. Travel Medicine. 3rd ed. Philadelphia: Saunders Elsevier; 2013. pp. 439–48.

TRAVEL HEALTH KITS

Kelly Winter

Regardless of the destination, all international travelers should assemble and carry a travel health kit. The contents of a travel health kit should be tailored to the traveler's needs, type and length of travel, and destinations. Kits can be assembled at home or purchased at a local store, pharmacy, or online.

A travel health kit can help to ensure travelers have supplies they need to:

- Manage preexisting medical conditions and treat any exacerbations of these conditions.

- Prevent illness and injury related to traveling.

- Take care of minor health problems as they occur.

By bringing medications from home, travelers avoid having to purchase them at their destination. See *Perspectives:* Pharmaceutical Quality & Falsified Drugs later in this chapter for information about the risks associated with purchasing medications abroad. Even when the quality of medications is reliable, medications people are used to taking at home may be sold under different names or with different ingredients and dosage units in other countries, presenting additional challenges.

TRAVELING WITH MEDICATIONS

All medications should be carried in their original containers with clear labels, so the contents are easily identified. The patient's name and dosing regimen should be on each container. Although many travelers prefer placing medications into small containers or packing them in daily-dose containers, officials at ports of entry may require proper identification of medications.

Travelers should carry copies of all prescriptions, including their generic names and preferably translated into the local language of the destination. For controlled substances and injectable medications, travelers should carry a note from the prescribing clinician or from the travel clinic on letterhead stationery. Translating the letter into the local language of the destination and attaching this translation to the original document may prove helpful if the document is needed during the trip. Some countries do not permit certain medications. If there is a question about these restrictions, particularly regarding controlled substances, travelers should contact the embassy or consulate of the destination country.

A travel health kit is useful only when it is easily accessible. It should be carried with the traveler at all times (such as in a carry-on bag), although sharp objects must remain in checked luggage. Travelers should make sure that any liquid or gel-based items packed in the carry-on bags do not exceed size limits. Exceptions are made for certain medical reasons; check the Transportation Security Administration for US outbound and inbound travel (call toll-free at 866-289-9673 M–F 8 AM to 11 PM, weekends and holidays 9 AM to 8 PM, or e-mail TSA-ContactCenter@dhs.gov) and the embassy or consulate of the destination country for their restrictions.

SUPPLIES FOR PREEXISTING MEDICAL CONDITIONS

Travelers with preexisting medical conditions should carry enough medication for the duration of their trip and an extra supply, in case the trip is extended for any reason. If additional supplies or medications would be needed to manage exacerbations of existing medical conditions, these should be carried as well. The clinician managing a traveler's preexisting medical conditions should be consulted for the best plan of action (see Chapter 8, Travelers with Chronic Illnesses).

People with preexisting conditions, such as diabetes or allergies, should consider wearing an alert bracelet and making sure this information (in English and preferably translated into the local language of the destination) is on a card in their wallet and with their other travel documents.

GENERAL TRAVEL HEALTH KIT SUPPLIES

Although the following is not a comprehensive list, basic items that should be considered for a travel health kit are listed below. See Chapter 8 for additional suggestions that may be useful in planning the contents of a kit for travelers with specific needs.

Prescription Medications and Supplies

- Medications taken on a regular basis at home

- Antibiotic for self-treatment of moderate to severe diarrhea[1]

---

[1] For factors to consider when deciding whether to use an antibiotic for self-treatment of moderate to severe travelers' diarrhea, see Perspectives: Antibiotics in Travelers' Diarrhea, earlier in this chapter.

- Medication to prevent malaria, if needed

- Medication to prevent or treat altitude illness, if needed

- Prescription glasses/contact lenses (consider packing an extra pair of each in case lenses are damaged)

- Epinephrine auto-injectors[2] (such as an EpiPen 2-Pak), especially if history of severe allergic reaction or anaphylaxis; smaller-dose packages are available for children

- Diabetes testing supplies and insulin

- Needles or syringes, if needed for injectable medication. Needles and syringes can be difficult to purchase in some locations, so take more than what is needed for the length of the trip. (These items will require a letter from the prescribing clinician on letterhead stationery.)

- Medical alert bracelet or necklace

Over-the-Counter Medications

- Medications taken on a regular basis at home

- Treatment for pain or fever (one or more of the following, or an alternative):
  > Acetaminophen
  > Aspirin
  > Ibuprofen

- Treatment for stomach upset or diarrhea:
  > Antidiarrheal medication (such as lopera-mide [Imodium] or bismuth subsalicylate [Pepto-Bismol])
  > Packets of oral rehydration salts for dehydration
  > Mild laxative
  > Antacid

- Treatment for upper respiratory tract discomfort:
  > Antihistamine
  > Decongestant, alone or in combination with antihistamine
  > Cough suppressant or expectorant
  > Cough drops

- Anti–motion sickness medication

- Mild sedative or sleep aid

- Saline eye drops

- Saline nose drops or spray

Basic First Aid Items

- Disposable latex-free gloves (≥2 pairs)

- Adhesive bandages, multiple sizes

- Gauze

- Adhesive tape

- Antiseptic wound cleanser

- Cotton swabs

- Antifungal and antibacterial spray or creams

- 1% hydrocortisone cream

- Anti-itch gel or cream for insect bites and stings

- Aloe gel for sunburns

- Moleskin or molefoam for blister prevention and treatment

- Digital thermometer

- Tweezers[3]

- Scissors[3]

- Safety pins

[2] Injectable epinephrine and antihistamines should always be carried on one's person, including during air, sea, and land travel, for immediate treatment of a severe allergic reaction. Travelers with a history of severe allergic reactions should consider bringing along a short course of oral steroid medication (prescription required from doctor) and antihistamines as additional treatment of a severe allergic reaction.

[3] If traveling by air, travelers should pack these sharp items in checked baggage, since they could be confiscated by airport or airline security if packed in carry-on bags. Small bandage scissors with rounded tips may be available for purchase in certain stores or online.

- Elastic/compression bandage wrap for sprains and strains

- Triangular bandage to wrap injuries and to make an arm or shoulder sling

- For travel in remote areas, consider a commercial suture kit

- First aid quick reference card

Supplies to Prevent Illness or Injury

- Antibacterial hand wipes or an alcohol-based hand sanitizer, containing ≥60% alcohol

- Insect repellents for skin and clothing (see the Protection against Mosquitoes, Ticks, & Other Arthropods section earlier in this chapter for recommended types)

- Bed net (if needed, for protection against insect bites while sleeping)

- Sunscreen (≥15 SPF with UVA and UVB protection)

- Water purification tablets (if visiting remote areas, camping, or staying in areas where access to clean water is limited)

- Latex condoms

- Ear plugs

- Personal safety equipment (such as child safety seats and bicycle helmets)

Documents

Travelers should carry the following documents and leave a copy of these documents with a family member or close contact who will remain in the United States, in case of an emergency.

- Proof of vaccination on an International Certificate of Vaccination or Prophylaxis (ICVP) card or medical waiver (if vaccinations are required)

- Copies of all prescriptions for medications, eye glasses/contacts, and other medical supplies (including generic names and preferably translated into the local language of the destination)

- Documentation of preexisting conditions, such as diabetes or allergies (in English and preferably translated into the local language of the destination)

- Health insurance, supplemental travel health insurance, medical evacuation insurance, and travel insurance information (carry contact information for all insurance providers and copies of claim forms)

- Contact card to be carried with the traveler at all times, including street addresses, phone numbers, and e-mail addresses of the following:
  > Family member or close contact remaining in the United States
  > Health care provider(s) at home
  > Place(s) of lodging at the destination(s)
  > Hospitals or clinics (including emergency services) in your destination(s)
  > US embassy or consulate in the destination country or countries

See the Obtaining Health Care Abroad section later in this chapter for information about how to locate local health care and embassy or consulate contacts.

COMMERCIAL MEDICAL KITS

Commercial medical kits are available for a wide range of circumstances, from basic first aid to advanced emergency life support. For more adventurous travelers, a number of companies produce advanced medical kits and will even customize kits based on specific travel needs. In addition, specialty kits are available for managing diabetes, dealing with dental emergencies, and handling aquatic environments. Many pharmacy, grocery, retail, and outdoor sporting goods stores, as well as online retailers, sell their own basic first aid kits. Travelers who choose to purchase a preassembled kit should review the contents of the kit carefully to ensure that it has everything needed. Additional items may be necessary and can be added to the purchased kit.

BIBLIOGRAPHY

1. Goodyer L. Travel medical kits. In: Keystone JS, Freedman DO, Kozarsky PE, Connor BA, Nothdurft HD, editors. Travel Medicine. 3rd ed. Philadelphia: Saunders Elsevier; 2013. pp. 63–6.

2. Harper LA, Bettinger J, Dismukes R, Kozarsky PE. Evaluation of the Coca-Cola company travel health kit. J Travel Med. 2002 Sep-Oct;9(5):244–6.

3. Rose SR, Keystone JS. Chapter 2, trip preparation. In: Rose SR, Keystone JS, editors. International Travel Health Guide. 2016 online ed. Northampton: Travel Medicine, Inc; 2016.

2

PHARMACEUTICAL QUALITY & FALSIFIED DRUGS

Michael D. Green

The quality of medicines available outside the United States should not always be taken for granted. In many countries, national drug regulatory authorities lack the resources to effectively monitor drug quality and keep poor-quality pharmaceuticals off the market. These poor-quality drugs include falsified (the product's identity or source is falsely represented), counterfeit (a product bearing an unauthorized representation of a registered trademark), and substandard (a medicine not conforming to the specifications set by an accepted pharmacopeia) medications. Poor-quality medicines also include products that are not stored correctly, such that high temperature and humidity can alter the chemical composition. These drugs are an international problem contributing to illness, toxicity, drug resistance, and death. Although this problem exists on a worldwide scale, reliable global estimates of its prevalence are scarce because consensus is lacking on harmonized international definitions of poor-quality medicines

and surveillance methods. Recent survey studies of antimicrobial drug quality in Africa and Southeast Asia revealed that 9%–41% failed quality specifications. Previous reports have shown that global estimates of drug counterfeiting range from 1% of sales in developed countries to >10% in developing countries. In specific regions in Africa, Asia, and Latin America, chances of purchasing a counterfeit drug may be >30%.

Since counterfeit drugs are not made by the legitimate manufacturer and are produced under unlawful circumstances, toxic contaminants or lack of proper ingredients may cause serious harm. For example, the active pharmaceutical ingredient may be completely lacking, present in small quantities, or substituted by a less-effective compound. In addition, the wrong inactive ingredients (excipients) can contribute to poor drug dissolution and bioavailability. As a result, a patient may not respond to treatment or may have adverse reactions to unknown substituted or toxic ingredients.

Before international departure, travel health care providers should alert travelers to the dangers of counterfeit and substandard drugs and provide suggestions on how to avoid them.

HOW TO AVOID COUNTERFEIT DRUGS WHEN TRAVELING

The best way to avoid counterfeit drugs is to reduce the need to purchase medications abroad. Anticipated amounts of medications for chronic conditions (such as hypertension, sinusitis, arthritis, and hay fever), medications for gastroenteritis (such as travelers' diarrhea), and prophylactic medications for infectious diseases (such as malaria) should all be purchased before traveling. Purchasing these drugs via the Internet is not recommended, since the source of the medicines is always questionable. The traveler should also be aware that other health-related items such as medical devices, mosquito nets, and insect repellents could also be counterfeit, falsified, or substandard.

(continued)

PHARMACEUTICAL QUALITY & FALSIFIED DRUGS (CONTINUED)

Before departure, travelers should do the following:

- Obtain all medicines and other health-related items needed for the trip in advance. Prescriptions written in the United States usually cannot be filled overseas, and over-the-counter medicines may not be available in many foreign countries. Checked baggage can get lost; therefore, travelers should pack as much as possible in a carry-on bag and bring extra medicine in case of travel delays.

- Make sure medicines are in their original containers. If the drug is a prescription, the patient's name and dose regimen should be on the container.

- Bring the "patient prescription information" sheet. This sheet provides information on common generic and brand names, use, side effects, precautions, and drug interactions.

Many countries have restrictions on medicines (including over-the-counter medications) entering their borders. Check with the embassies of your destination countries for prohibited items. A listing of foreign embassies and consulates in the United States is available on the Department of State's website at www.state.gov/s/cpr/rls/dpl/32122.htm.

If travelers run out and require additional medications, they should take steps to ensure the medicines they buy are safe:

- Obtain medicines from a legitimate pharmacy. Patients should not buy from open markets, street vendors, or suspicious-looking pharmacies; they should request a receipt when making the purchase. The US embassy may be able to help find a legitimate pharmacy in the area.

- Do not buy medicines that are substantially cheaper than the typical price. Although generics are usually less expensive, many counterfeit brand names are sold at prices substantially lower than the normal price for that particular brand.

- Make sure the medicines are in their original packages or containers. If travelers receive medicines as loose tablets or capsules supplied in a plastic bag or envelope, they should ask the pharmacist to see the container from which the medicine was originally dispensed. The traveler should record the brand, batch number, and expiration date. Sometimes a wary consumer will prompt the seller into supplying quality medicine.

- Be familiar with medications. The size, shape, color, and taste of counterfeit medicines may be different from the authentic. Discoloration, splits, cracks, spots, and stickiness of the tablets or capsules are indications of a possible counterfeit. These defects may also indicate improper storage. Travelers should keep examples of authentic medications to compare if they purchase the same brand.

- Be familiar with the packaging. Different color inks, poor-quality print or packaging material, and misspelled words are clues to counterfeit drugs. Travelers should keep an example of packaging for comparison and observe the expiration date.

If the authentic packaging is not available or if you are not familiar with the brand, compare the distinguishing features of the package with that of the insert or blister pack. For example, batch/lot numbers, manufacturing date, and expiration date should match.

USEFUL WEBSITES

General Information about Counterfeit Drugs

- CDC: wwwnc.cdc. gov/travel/page/ counterfeit-medicine

- World Health Organization: www. who.int/mediacentre/ factsheets/fs275/en

- Food and Drug Administration: www.fda. gov//Drugs/DrugSafety/ ucm170314.htm

- US Pharmacopeia: www. usp.org/worldwide

Traveling and Customs Guidelines

Researching what travelers can pack and bring back into the United States, especially for travelers with disabilities and medical conditions, is helpful in preparing for travel.

- Transportation Security Administration: www.tsa. gov/traveler-information/ travelers-disabilities-and- medical-conditions

- Customs and Border Protection: www. cbp.gov/newsroom/ local-media-release/ 2015-04-22-000000/

cbp-advises-travelers- entry-regulations- pertaining

BIBLIOGRAPHY

1. Gaurvika ML, Nayyar JG, Bremen JG, Herrington JE. The global pandemic of falsified medicines: laboratory and field innovations and policy perspectives. Am J Trop Med Hyg 2012 Jun;92(6 suppl):2–7.

2. Institute of Medicine. Countering the problem of falsified and substandard drugs. Washington, DC: The National Academics Press; 2013 Feb.

3. World Health Organization. Medicines: counterfeit medicines [fact sheet no. 275]. Geneva: World Health Organization; 2012 [cited 2016 Sep. 22]; Available from: www. who.int/mediacentre/factsheets/ fs275/en/.

2

Perspectives sections are written as editorial discussions aiming to add depth and clinical perspective to the official recommendations contained in the book. The views and opinions expressed in this section are those of the author and do not necessarily represent the official position of CDC.

OBTAINING HEALTH CARE ABROAD

Carolina Uribe

The quality and availability of medical care abroad may be variable. Before departure, travelers should consider how they would access health care during their trip should a medical problem or emergency arise. Travelers may seek medical care for a variety of reasons, ranging from minor infections and care for chronic conditions to major illness or injury.

Some insurance plans cover emergency health care, but travelers should check with their carriers to confirm what coverage is offered and what requirements exist. At a minimum, travelers may need to provide copies of bills and invoices to initiate reimbursement. Emergency health coverage does not usually cover emergency evacuation or the costs of altered itineraries. Travelers may purchase specific policies to cover these expenses, understanding that such policies often do not cover expenses related to preexisting conditions. Supplemental medical insurance plans acquired before travel will often enable access to local providers in many countries through a 24-hour emergency hotline (see Travel Insurance, Travel Health Insurance, & Medical Evacuation Insurance section later in this chapter).

In addition to identifying quality health care, travelers, especially those with chronic or complicated medical issues, should know the names of their chronic conditions and allergies, their blood type, and current medications (including generic names), ideally in the local language. Travelers should also wear medical identification jewelry (such as a MedicAlert bracelet), if appropriate. There are a number of cellular telephone applications that enable travelers to download their medical records, medications, EKG, and other information so that it is accessible if needed.

LOCATING HEALTH CARE PROVIDERS AND FACILITIES ABROAD

Before going abroad, travelers should identify health care providers and facilities at their destination. This is especially true for travelers with preexisting or complicated medical issues. Travelers who require regular dialysis need to arrange appointments at an adequate clinical site. Similarly, pregnant travelers should identify reliable health facilities. More choices are generally available in urban areas than in rural or remote areas.

The following list of resources will help identify health care providers and facilities around the world. CDC does not endorse any particular provider or medical insurance company, and accreditation does not necessarily ensure a good outcome. If travelers are likely to seek health care abroad, they should be encouraged to thoroughly research health care facilities in the area.

- The Department of State (www.usembassy. gov) can help travelers locate medical services and notify friends, family, or employer of an emergency.

- The Department of State also maintains a list of travel medical insurance providers at travel.state.gov/content/passports/en/go/ health/insurance-providers.html.

- The International Society of Travel Medicine maintains a directory of health care professionals with expertise in travel medicine in more than 80 countries. Search these clinics at www.istm.org.

- The International Association for Medical Assistance to Travelers maintains a network of physicians, hospitals, and clinics that have agreed to provide care to members.

Membership is free, although donations are suggested. Search for clinics at www.iamat. org/doctors_clinics.cfm.

- The Joint Commission International (JCI) aims to improve patient safety through accreditation and certification of health care facilities. For a list of facilities accredited through JCI, see www.jointcommissioninternational.org/ JCI-Accredited-Organizations.

- Embassies and consulates in other countries, hotel doctors, and credit card companies (especially those with special privileges) may also provide information.

- A number of countries or national travel medicine societies have websites related to travel medicine that provide access to clinicians, including the following:
  - > Canada: Health Canada (www.phac-aspc. gc.ca and travel.gc.ca)
  - > Great Britain: National Travel Health Network and Centre (www.nathnac.org) and British Global and Travel Health Association (www.bgtha.org)
  - > South Africa: South African Society of Travel Medicine (www.sastm.org.za)
  - > Australia: Travel Medicine Alliance (www. travelmedicine.com.au)
  - > China: International Travel Healthcare Association (http://en.itha.org.cn)

- Travelers also may consider contracting with one of a number of private companies that provide physician services abroad as well as medical evacuations. One example is International SOS, which operates throughout the world. Provider locations and details may be found at www.internationalsos.com.

AVOID TRAVEL WHEN SICK

Travelers should evaluate their health before travel to ensure that they are healthy enough for their itinerary and should avoid travel if they become ill before or during their trip. Travelers may be reluctant to postpone or cancel a trip when ill because of their financial investment in a trip, among other factors. However, some airlines check for visibly sick passengers in the waiting area and during boarding. If a passenger looks visibly ill, the airline may prohibit that person from boarding.

Encouraging travelers, especially those with chronic or complicated health conditions, to purchase trip cancellation insurance, which will protect some or all of the investment in a trip, may increase compliance with this recommendation.

DRUGS AND OTHER PHARMACEUTICALS

The quality of drugs and medical products abroad cannot be guaranteed, as they may not meet regulated standards or could be counterfeit (see *Perspectives:* Pharmaceutical Quality & Falsified Drugs earlier in this chapter). To minimize risks associated with substandard drugs and pharmaceuticals, travelers should

- Bring with them all the medicines that they think they will need, including pain relievers and antidiarrheal medication.

- Insist that a new needle and syringe be used when receiving an injection. Travelers who know beforehand that they will require injections during their trip can bring their own injection supplies (see the Travel Health Kits section earlier in this chapter).

- Carry an epinephrine autoinjector, if needed, in carry-on luggage. Include a letter from the prescribing physician that explains the allergy and a copy of the prescription.

BLOOD SAFETY

A medical emergency abroad, such as a motor vehicle accident or trauma, could result in the need for a blood transfusion. Not all countries have accurate, reliable, and systematic screening of blood donations for infectious agents, which increases the risk of transfusion-related transmission of disease. Travelers in developing countries should receive a blood transfusion only in life-or-death situations. Although it is difficult to ensure access to safe blood, travelers can take a few measures to increase their chances of having a safe blood transfusion in the event of a medical emergency:

- If a blood transfusion is required, travelers should make every effort to ensure that the blood has been screened for transmissible diseases, including HIV. Although this is difficult to do at the point of service, travelers who plan ahead—especially those with medical conditions that might require transfusions—and locate medical services before traveling will increase their chances of obtaining higher-quality care abroad.

- Travelers may consider registering with agencies such as the Blood Care Foundation that attempt to rapidly deliver reliable blood products to members while abroad (www.bloodcare.org.uk/blood-transfusions-abroad.html).

All travelers should consider being immunized against hepatitis B virus before travel, especially those who travel frequently to developing countries, those whose itinerary indicates spending a prolonged period in developing countries, and those whose activities (such as adventure travel) put them at higher risk for serious injury.

BIBLIOGRAPHY

1. Kolars JC. Rules of the road: a consumer's guide for travelers seeking health care in foreign lands. J Travel Med. 2002 Jul-Aug;9(4):198–201.

2. World Health Organization. Medicines: spurious/falsely-labelled/falsified/counterfeit (SFFC) medicines [fact sheet no. 275]. Geneva: World Health Organization; 2012 [updated January 2016 cited 2016 Sep. 22]; Available from: http://www.who.int/mediacentre/factsheets/fs275/en/.

3. World Health Organization. Blood safety [fact sheet no. 279]. Geneva: World Health Organization; 2014 [updated July 2016 cited 2016 Sep. 22]; Available from: http://www.who.int/mediacentre/factsheets/fs279/en/.

TRAVEL INSURANCE, TRAVEL HEALTH INSURANCE, & MEDICAL EVACUATION INSURANCE

Rhett J. Stoney

Severe illness or injury abroad may result in a financial burden on travelers. Although planning for every possible contingency is impossible, travelers can reduce the cost of a medical emergency by considering the purchase of a specialized insurance policy for their trip, regardless of whether or not they have a domestic health insurance plan. There are 3 types of policies: travel insurance, travel health insurance, and medical evacuation insurance. These insurance policies can be purchased before a trip to provide coverage in the event of an illness or injury and may be of particular importance to travelers with chronic medical conditions. Basic accident or travel insurance may even be required for travelers with certain itineraries. For example, cruise ships have medical staff on board, but treatment may not be included in passengers' ticket costs. In this case, those traveling by cruise ship may want to consider a specialized insurance policy.

DOMESTIC HEALTH INSURANCE AND OVERSEAS TRAVEL

Some health insurance carriers in the United States may cover emergencies that occur while traveling abroad. Travelers should examine their coverage and itinerary to determine which medical services, if any, will be covered abroad and the level of supplemental insurance needed. The following is a list of characteristics to consider:

- Exclusions for treating exacerbations of pre-existing medical conditions

- The company's policy for "out-of-network" services

- Coverage for complications of pregnancy (or for a neonate, especially if the newborn requires intensive care)

- Exclusions for high-risk activities such as skydiving, scuba diving, and mountain climbing

- Exclusions regarding psychiatric emergencies

- Exclusions for injuries related to terrorist attacks, acts of war, or natural disasters

- Whether preauthorization is needed for treatment, hospital admission, or other services

- Whether a second opinion is required before obtaining emergency treatment

- Whether there is a 24-hour physician-backed support center

PAYING FOR HEALTH SERVICES ABROAD

Medical care abroad usually requires cash or credit card payment at the point of service, regardless of whether the traveler has insurance coverage in his or her home country. Additionally, the existence of nationalized health care services in a given destination does not ensure that nonresidents will be covered. This could result in a large out-of-pocket expenditure of perhaps thousands of dollars. A discussion of insurance options is an important part of any pretravel consultation. In addition to covering costs of treatment or medical evacuation, the travel health insurer can also assist in organizing and coordinating care and keeping relatives informed. This is especially important when the traveler is severely ill or injured and requires medical evacuation. Although all travelers should consider insurance, it is particularly important for travelers who plan extended travel outside the United States, have underlying health conditions, or plan to participate in high-risk activities on their trip, especially if the destination is remote or lacks high-quality medical facilities. Regardless of which insurance option (or options) is (are) selected for a trip, when paying out-of-pocket for care overseas, travelers should obtain copies of all bills and receipts and, if necessary, contact a US consular officer, who can assist US citizens with transferring funds from the United States.

TRAVEL INSURANCE

Travel insurance protects the financial investment in a trip, including lost baggage and trip cancellation. Travelers may be more likely to avoid travel when sick if they know their financial investment in the trip is protected. Depending on the policy, travel insurance may or may not cover medical expenses abroad, so travelers need to carefully research the coverage offered to determine if additional travel health and medical evacuation insurance is needed.

SUPPLEMENTAL TRAVEL HEALTH AND MEDICAL EVACUATION INSURANCE

Travel health insurance and medical evacuation insurance are both short-term supplemental policies that cover health care costs on a trip and are relatively inexpensive. Many commercial companies offer travel health insurance, which may be purchased separately or in conjunction with medical evacuation insurance. Frequent travelers may consider purchasing annual policies or even policies that will provide coverage for repatriation to one's home country.

Although travel health insurance will cover some health care costs abroad, the quality of care may be inadequate, and medical evacuation from a resource-poor area to a hospital where definitive care can be obtained may be necessary. The cost of evacuation can exceed $100,000. In such cases, medical evacuation insurance would cover the cost of transportation to a facility where adequate care can be provided. Medical evacuation companies may have better resources and experience in some parts of the world than others; travelers may want to ask about a company's resources in a given area, especially if planning a trip to remote destinations. The traveler should scrutinize all policies before purchase, looking for those that provide the following:

- Arrangements with hospitals to guarantee payments directly

- Assistance via a 24-hour physician-backed support center (critical for medical evacuation insurance)

- Emergency medical transport to facilities that are equivalent to those in the home country or to the home country itself (repatriation)

- Any specific medical services that may apply to their circumstances, such as coverage of high-risk activities

Even if an insurance provider is selected carefully, travelers should be aware that unexpected delays in care may still arise, especially in remote destinations. In special circumstances, travelers may be advised to postpone or cancel international trips if the health risks are too high.

FINDING AN INSURANCE PROVIDER

The following resources, although not all-inclusive, provide information about purchasing travel health and medical evacuation insurance:

- Department of State (www.travel.state.gov)

- International Association for Medical Assistance to Travelers (www.iamat.org)

- American Association of Retired Persons (www.aarp.org) (for information about Medicare supplement plans, see below)

SPECIAL CONSIDERATIONS FOR TRAVELERS WITH UNDERLYING MEDICAL CONDITIONS

Travelers with underlying medical conditions should discuss any concerns with the insurer before departure. In a study of international travelers with travel health insurance claims, only two-thirds of claims were fully met. Preexisting illness and poor documentation were the main reasons for refusal. Travelers with medical conditions should choose a medical assistance company that allows them to store their medical history before departure, so it can be accessed anywhere. Travelers should carry a letter from their health care provider listing their medical conditions and current medications (including their generic names), written in the local language if possible. Those with cardiac disease should carry a copy (paper or electronic) of their most recent ECG. They should also pack all medications in their original bottles, checking beforehand with the destination's embassy to ensure that none are considered illegal in the destination country.

SPECIAL CONSIDERATIONS FOR MEDICARE BENEFICIARIES

The Social Security Medicare program does not provide coverage for medical costs outside the United States, except in limited circumstances. Some Medigap (Medicare supplement insurance) plans may provide limited coverage for emergency care abroad. As with all travelers, Medicare beneficiaries should examine their coverage carefully and supplement it with additional travel health insurance, as needed.

CHECKLIST FOR DISCUSSING INSURANCE WITH TRAVELERS

The following checklist can guide an insurance discussion before travel.

Before travel:

- Scrutinize the traveler's domestic health insurance policy to see what medical services may or may not be covered abroad.

- Consider travel, travel health, and medical evacuation insurance.

- Locate medical services in areas that the traveler plans to visit and carry this information with them on their trip.

During travel:

- Carry copies of insurance policy identity cards, including any supplemental insurance purchased for a trip, and insurance claim forms.

- Retain copies of all bills and receipts for medical care received abroad.

BIBLIOGRAPHY

1. American Association of Retired Persons, Education and Outreach. Overview of Medicare supplemental insurance. Washington, DC: American Association of Retired Persons; 2010 [cited 2016 Mar. 8]; Available from: http://www.aarp.org/health/medicare-insurance/info-10-2008/overview_medicare_supplemental_insurance.html.

2. Centers for Medicare and Medicaid Services. Medicare coverage outside the United States. Baltimore: CMS; 2016 [cited 2016 Mar. 8]; Available from: https://www.medicare.gov/Pubs/pdf/11037.pdf.

3. Leggat PA, Carne J, Kedjarune U. Travel insurance and health. J Travel Med. 1999 Dec;6(4):243–8.

4. Leggat PA, Leggat FW. Travel insurance claims made by travelers from Australia. J Travel Med. 2002 Mar-Apr;9(2):59–65.

5. Teichman PG, Donchin Y, Kot RJ. International aeromedical evacuation. N Engl J Med. 2007 Jan 18;356(3):262–70.

6. US Department of State. Insurance Providers for Overseas Coverage. Washington, DC: US Department of State; 2016 [cited 2016 Sep. 22]; Available from: https://travel.state.gov/content/passports/en/go/health/insurance-providers.html.

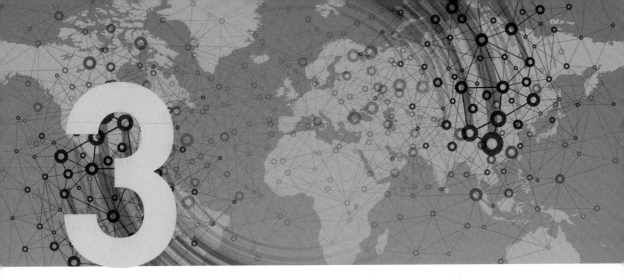

3

Infectious Diseases Related to Travel

AMEBIASIS

Jennifer R. Cope

INFECTIOUS AGENT

The protozoan parasite *Entamoeba histolytica*, possibly other *Entamoeba* spp.

TRANSMISSION

Fecal-oral route, either directly by person-to-person contact (such as by diaper-changing or sexual practices) or indirectly by eating or drinking fecally contaminated food or water.

EPIDEMIOLOGY

Amebiasis is distributed worldwide, particularly in the tropics, most commonly in areas of poor sanitation. Long-term travelers (duration >6 months) are significantly more likely than short-term travelers (duration <1 month) to develop *E. histolytica* infection. Immigrants and refugees from these areas are also at risk. People at higher risk for severe disease are those who are pregnant,

immunocompromised, or receiving corticosteroids; associations with diabetes and alcohol use have also been reported.

CLINICAL PRESENTATION

Most patients have a gradual illness onset days or weeks after infection. Symptoms include cramps, watery or bloody diarrhea, and weight loss and may last several weeks. Occasionally, the parasite may spread to other organs (extraintestinal amebiasis), most commonly the liver. Amebic liver abscesses may be asymptomatic, but most patients present with fever and right upper quadrant abdominal pain, usually in the absence of diarrhea.

DIAGNOSIS

Microscopy does not distinguish between *E. histolytica* (known to be pathogenic), *E. bangladeshi*,

E. dispar, and *E. moshkovskii*. *E. dispar* and *E. moshkovskii* have historically been considered nonpathogenic, but evidence is mounting that *E. moshkovskii* can cause illness; *E. bangladeshi* has only recently been identified, so its pathogenic potential is not well understood. More specific tests such as EIA or PCR are needed to confirm the diagnosis of *E. histolytica*. Additionally, serologic tests can help diagnose extraintestinal amebiasis.

TREATMENT

For symptomatic intestinal infection and extraintestinal disease, treatment with metronidazole or tinidazole should be followed by treatment with iodoquinol or paromomycin. Asymptomatic patients infected with *E. histolytica* should also be treated with iodoquinol or paromomycin, because they can infect others and because 4%–10% develop disease within a year if left untreated.

PREVENTION

Food and water precautions (see Chapter 2, Food & Water Precautions) and hand hygiene. Avoid fecal exposure during sexual activity.

CDC website: www.cdc.gov/parasites/amebiasis

BIBLIOGRAPHY

1. Choudhuri G, Rangan M. Amebic infection in humans. Indian J Gastroenterol. 2012 Jul;31(4):153–62.

2. Cordel H, Prendki V, Madec Y, Houze S, Paris L, Bouree P, et al. Imported amoebic liver abscess in France. PLoS Negl Trop Dis. 2013;7(8):e2333.

3. Heredia RD, Fonseca JA, Lopez MC. *Entamoeba moshkovskii* perspectives of a new agent to be considered in the diagnosis of amebiasis. Acta Trop. 2012 Sep;123(3):139–45.

4. Lachish T, Wieder-Finesod A, Schwartz E. Amebic Liver Abscess in Israeli Travelers: A Retrospective Study. Am J Trop Med Hyg. 2016 May 4;94(5):1015–9.

5. Shimokawa C, Kabir M, Taniuchi M, Mondal D, Kobayashi S, Ali IK, et al. Entamoeba moshkovskii is associated with diarrhea in infants and causes diarrhea and colitis in mice. J Infect Dis. 2012 Sep 1;206(5):744–51.

6. Ximenez C, Moran P, Rojas L, Valadez A, Gomez A, Ramiro M, et al. Novelties on amoebiasis: a neglected tropical disease. J Glob Infect Dis. 2011 Apr;3(2):166–74.

ANGIOSTRONGYLIASIS, NEUROLOGIC

LeAnne M. Fox, Francisca Abanyie

INFECTIOUS AGENT

Angiostrongylus cantonensis, rat lungworm, a nematode parasite.

TRANSMISSION

Various species of rats are the definitive hosts of the parasite, known as the rat lungworm. Rats can infect only snails and slugs, which are the intermediate hosts. Transmission to humans occurs by consuming infected snails or slugs or contaminated raw produce or vegetable juices. Infective larvae have also been found in freshwater shrimp, crabs, and frogs.

EPIDEMIOLOGY

Most described cases have occurred in Asia and the Pacific Basin (such as in parts of Thailand, Taiwan, mainland China, the Hawaiian Islands, and other Pacific Islands); however, cases have been reported in many areas of the world, including the Caribbean.

CLINICAL PRESENTATION

Incubation period is typically 1–3 weeks but ranges from 1 day to >6 weeks. *A. cantonensis* is considered the most common infectious cause of eosinophilic meningitis in humans. Common manifestations include headache, photophobia, stiff neck, nausea, vomiting, fatigue, and body aches. Abnormal skin sensations (such as tingling or painful feelings) are more common than in other types of meningitis. A low-grade fever might be noted. Symptoms are usually self-limited but may persist for weeks or months. Severe cases can be associated with paralysis, blindness, or death.

DIAGNOSIS

Typically presumptive, on the basis of clinical and epidemiologic criteria in people with otherwise unexplained eosinophilic meningitis. PCR testing of cerebrospinal fluid is available from CDC (www.cdc.gov/dpdx; 404-718-4745; parasites@cdc.gov). Serum antibody testing may be available in reference laboratories.

TREATMENT

The larvae die spontaneously and supportive care usually suffices, including analgesics for pain and corticosteroids to limit inflammation. No antihelminthic drugs have been proven to be effective in treatment.

PREVENTION

Food and water precautions, particularly:

- Avoid eating raw or undercooked snails, slugs, and other possible hosts.

- Eat raw produce, such as lettuce, only if it has been thoroughly washed or treated with bleach. Such measures might provide some protection but may not eliminate the risk.

- Wear gloves (and wash hands) if snails or slugs are handled.

CDC website: www.cdc.gov/parasites/angiostrongylus

BIBLIOGRAPHY

1. Chotmongkol V, Sawadpanitch K, Sawanyawisuth K, Louhawilai S, Limpawattana P. Treatment of eosinophilic meningitis with a combination of prednisolone and mebendazole. Am J Trop Med Hyg. 2006 Jun;74(6):1122–4.

2. Hochberg NS, Blackburn BG, Park SY, Sejvar JJ, Effler PV, Herwaldt BL. Eosinophilic meningitis attributable to *Angiostrongylus cantonensis* infection in Hawaii: clinical characteristics and potential exposures. Am J Trop Med Hyg. 2011 Oct;85(4):685–90.

3. Wang QP, Lai DH, Zhu XQ, Chen XG, Lun ZR. Human angiostrongyliasis. Lancet Infect Dis. 2008 Oct;8(10):621–30.

ANTHRAX

Kate Hendricks Walters, Rita M. Traxler, Chung K. Marston

INFECTIOUS AGENT

Aerobic, gram-positive, encapsulated, spore-forming, nonmotile, nonhemolytic, rod-shaped bacterium *Bacillus anthracis*.

TRANSMISSION

Worldwide, most *B. anthracis* is transmitted by direct contact with *B. anthracis*–infected animals, their carcasses, or contaminated products from infected animals. Such products include meat, hides, wool, or items made with those products, such as drum heads or wool clothing. Anthrax has a variety of presentations—cutaneous, gastrointestinal, injection, inhalation, and meningitis—and most are synonymous with their mode of transmission. The exception is meningitis, which may complicate any of the other types. It may also occur with no obvious portal of entry, in which case it is called primary anthrax meningitis.

Introducing spores through the skin can result in cutaneous anthrax; abrasion of the skin increases susceptibility. Eating meat from infected animals can result in gastrointestinal anthrax. Since 2000, injecting, and possibly smoking and snorting, heroin has been associated with *B. anthracis* soft-tissue infections in intravenous drug users in northern Europe. Inhaling spores aerosolized during work with contaminated materials such as hides or wool can result in inhalation anthrax.

Anthrax in humans is not generally considered to be contagious; person-to-person transmission of cutaneous anthrax has rarely been reported.

EPIDEMIOLOGY

Anthrax is a zoonotic disease that primarily affects herbivores such as cattle, sheep, goats, antelope, and deer, which become infected by ingesting contaminated vegetation, water, or soil; humans are generally incidental hosts. Anthrax is most common in agricultural regions in Central and South America, sub-Saharan Africa, Central and Southwestern Asia, and Southern and Eastern Europe. Although outbreaks occur most years in livestock and wild herbivores in the United States and Canada, human anthrax is now rare in both of these countries.

Worldwide, the most commonly reported form (95%–99%) of anthrax in humans is cutaneous anthrax. Outbreaks of cutaneous and gastrointestinal anthrax have been associated with handling infected animals and butchering and consuming meat from those animals. Most of these outbreaks are reported from endemic areas of Asia and Africa.

A single case of travel-associated anthrax has been reported. In 2006, a case of cutaneous anthrax was reported in a woman who traveled with a small group of tourists to Namibia, Botswana, and South Africa. Although she had no direct contact with animals, another group member handled 1 or more animal carcasses and shortly afterward helped her clean an abrasion on her finger, which was later the site of the anthrax lesion.

Additional cases have occurred from playing or handling drums made with contaminated goat hides that were imported from anthrax-endemic countries. Although the risk of acquiring anthrax from these drums appears to be low,

life-threatening or fatal disease is possible: cases of cutaneous (4), gastrointestinal (1), and inhalation (3) anthrax have been reported among people who have handled, played, or made drums or who have been in the same place as people participating in these activities.

Severe soft tissue infections, including cases with sepsis and systemic infection, have been reported in drug users in northern Europe and are suspected to be due to recreational use of heroin contaminated with *B. anthracis* spores. No associated cases have been identified in people who have not taken heroin. To date, no heroin has been found to be contaminated with *B. anthracis* spores.

Inhalation exposure was historically associated with the industrial processing of hides or wool (hence, "woolsorters' disease"). However, in more recent decades it has also resulted from bioterrorism. Occasional anthrax cases have occurred in the United States and elsewhere in which the exposure source remains unidentified.

CLINICAL PRESENTATION

Cutaneous anthrax usually develops 1–7 days after exposure, but incubations as long as 17 days have been reported. Before antimicrobial therapy, almost a quarter of patients with cutaneous anthrax died. The case-fatality ratio is <2% with antimicrobial therapy. Cutaneous anthrax is characterized by localized itching followed by the development of a painless papule, which turns vesicular and enlarges, ulcerates, and develops into a depressed black eschar within 7–10 days of the initial lesion. The head, neck, forearms, and hands are the most commonly affected sites. Edema usually surrounds the lesion, sometimes with secondary vesicles, hyperemia, and regional lymphadenopathy. Patients may have malaise and headache; about a third are febrile.

Gastrointestinal anthrax usually develops 1–7 days after consumption of contaminated meat; however, incubations as long as 16 days have been reported. More than half of cases die if untreated; with treatment, the case-fatality ratio is <40%. There are 2 main types, oropharyngeal and intestinal. Fever and chills are usual with either. The oropharyngeal type is characterized by severe sore throat, difficulty swallowing, swelling of the neck, and regional lymphadenopathy; airway compromise can occur. Symptoms of the intestinal type include nausea, vomiting, and diarrhea, which may be bloody; marked ascites may develop. Shock and death may occur within 2–5 days of onset.

Cases of anthrax in injection drug users usually develop within 1–4 days of exposure; more than a quarter of the confirmed cases die. Cases present with severe soft tissue infection manifested by swelling, erythema, and excessive bruising at the injection site; pain may be less than would be anticipated for the degree of swelling. In approximately a third of cases, the localized symptoms are accompanied by signs of sepsis.

Inhalation anthrax usually develops within a week after exposure, but the incubation period may be prolonged (up to 2 months). Fatality ratios before 2001 were 90%; since then, they have been 45%. Initially, most patients have constitutional symptoms such as fever, chills, and fatigue, which may be accompanied by cough, making inhalation anthrax difficult to distinguish from influenza and community-acquired pneumonia. This is often described as the prodromal period. Over the next day or so, chest pain develops in about half of patients, and nonthoracic complaints such as nausea, vomiting, headache, and diaphoresis develop in approximately one-third. Upper respiratory tract symptoms occur in only a quarter of patients, and myalgias are rare. Altered mental status or shortness of breath generally brings patients to the attention of the medical establishment and heralds the fulminant phase of illness.

Anthrax meningitis may develop from hematogenous spread of any of the clinical forms of anthrax, or it may occur alone; half of all reported cases are sequelae of cutaneous anthrax. Although anthrax meningitis is usually fatal, survival is significantly more likely if the patient receives multiple antimicrobials that include a bactericidal agent.

DIAGNOSIS

Laboratory diagnosis depends on bacterial culture and isolation of *B. anthracis*; detection of bacterial DNA, antigens, or toxins; or detection of a host immune response to *B. anthracis*. Anthrax lethal toxin can be detected in acute-phase serum, while serologic testing of host antibody responses requires acute- and convalescent-phase sera for diagnosis. Confirmatory testing, including isolate identification, antigen detection in tissues, or quantitative serology, should be performed in the United States by the state health department or Laboratory Response Network laboratories, or internationally by the relevant national reference laboratory. Guidelines for collecting and submitting clinical specimens for testing and algorithms for laboratory diagnosis can be found at www.cdc. gov/anthrax/lab-testing/index.html. Specimens for culture should be collected before initiating antimicrobial therapy. Anthrax is a nationally notifiable disease.

Diagnostic procedures for inhalation anthrax include thoracic imaging studies to detect a widened mediastinum or pleural effusion. Unless contraindicated, lumbar puncture should be performed to rule out meningitis in all patients with systemic illness.

TREATMENT

Naturally occurring localized or uncomplicated cutaneous anthrax can be treated with 7–10 days of a single oral antimicrobial agent. First-line agents include ciprofloxacin or an equivalent fluoroquinolone or doxycycline; clindamycin is an alternative, as are penicillins if the isolate is penicillin susceptible.

Treatment recommendations for systemic disease are available at wwwnc.cdc.gov/eid/article/ 20/2/13-0687_intro. Additional recommendations to prevent or treat anthrax in pregnant, postpartum, and lactating women are available at wwwnc.cdc.gov/eid/article/20/2/13-0611_intro.

PREVENTION

The CDC published updated recommendations in 2010 for preexposure use of anthrax vaccine and for postexposure management of previously unvaccinated people (www.cdc.gov/mmwr/ preview/mmwrhtml/rr5906a1.htm). Vaccination against anthrax is not recommended for travelers. To prevent anthrax, travelers should:

- Avoid direct or indirect contact with carcasses of animals in anthrax-endemic regions.

- Not eat meat from animals that were not inspected by health officials and found to be healthy at the time of slaughter.

- Not import animal products, trophies, or souvenirs from anthrax-endemic regions that are prohibited by either the CDC or the United States Department of Agriculture (USDA). A map of endemic areas can be found at www.cdc.gov/anthrax/specificgroups/travelers.html.

No tests are available to determine if animal products are free of contamination with *B. anthracis* spores. Additional information regarding import regulations may be found in the following references:

- Chapter 6, Taking Animals & Animal Products across International Borders

- USADA regulations at www.aphis.usda.gov/aphis/ourfocus/importexport
- World Organisation for Animal Health (OIE) Terrestrial Animal Health Code at www.oie.int/en/international-standard-setting/terrestrial-code/access-online

Animal-hide drum owners or players should report any unexplained fever or new skin lesions to their health care provider and describe any recent contact with animal-hide drums.

CDC website: www.cdc.gov/anthrax

BIBLIOGRAPHY

1. Bales ME, Dannenberg AL, Brachman PS, Kaufmann AF, Klatsky PC, Ashford DA. Epidemiologic response to anthrax outbreaks: field investigations, 1950–2001. Emerg Infect Dis. 2002 Oct;8(10):1163–74.

2. CDC. Anthrax contamination of Haitian goatskin products. MMWR Morb Mortal Wkly Rep. 1981 July 17;30(27):338.

3. CDC. Gastrointestinal anthrax after an animal-hide drumming event—New Hampshire and Massachusetts, 2009. MMWR Morb Mortal Wkly Rep. 2010 Jul 23;59(28):872–7.

4. Eurosurveillance editorial team. Probable human anthrax death in Scotland. Euro Surveill. 2006;11(8):E060817.2.

5. Griffith J, Blaney D, Shadomy S, Lehman M, Pesik N, Tostenson S, et al. Investigation of inhalation anthrax case, United States. Emerg Infect Dis. 2014 Feb;20(2):280–3.

6. Hanczaruk M, Reischl U, Holzmann T, Frangoulidis D, Wagner DM, Keim PS, et al. Injectional anthrax in heroin users, Europe, 2000–2012. Emerg Infect Dis. 2014 Feb;20(2):322–3.

7. Hendricks KA, Wright ME, Shadomy SV, Bradley JS, Morrow MG, Pavia AT, et al. Centers for disease control and prevention expert panel meetings on prevention and treatment of anthrax in adults. Emerg Infect Dis. 2014 Feb;20(2).

8. Meaney-Delman D, Zotti ME, Creanga AA, Misegades LK, Wako E, Treadwell TA, et al. Special considerations for prophylaxis for and treatment of anthrax in pregnant and postpartum women. Emerg Infect Dis. 2014 Feb;20(2).

9. Van den Enden E, Van Gompel A, Van Esbroeck M. Cutaneous anthrax, Belgian traveler. Emerg Infect Dis. 2006 Mar;12(3):523–5.

B VIRUS

D. Scott Schmid

INFECTIOUS AGENT

Macacine herpesvirus I, or B virus, is an enveloped, double-stranded DNA virus in the family Herpesviridae, genus *Simplexvirus*. B virus is also commonly referred to as herpes B, monkey B virus, herpesvirus simiae, and herpesvirus B.

B virus is commonly found among macaques, a genus of Old World monkeys.

TRANSMISSION

Transmission is typically caused by bites or scratches from an infected macaque but may also occur through contact with body fluids or tissues of an infected macaque. A single case of human-to-human spread has been documented, in which a woman became infected through direct contact with the lesions of her infected spouse.

EPIDEMIOLOGY

Macaques are the natural reservoir for B virus infection. No other primates are known to carry any risk of B virus infection unless they have become infected by contact with infected macaques. Although B virus infections in macaques are usually asymptomatic or cause only mild disease, approximately 70% of untreated infections in humans are fatal. People at risk for B virus infection are veterinarians, laboratory workers, and others who have close contact with Old World macaques or monkey cell cultures, but infections in humans are rare. Since B virus was identified in 1932, fewer than 50 cases of human infection have been documented.

CLINICAL PRESENTATION

Disease onset typically occurs within 1 month of exposure, although the actual incubation period can be as short as 3–7 days. The first signs of disease typically include influenza-like symptoms (fever, headache, myalgias) and sometimes vesicular lesions near the exposure site. Localized neurologic symptoms such as pain, numbness, or itching may occur near the wound site. Lymphadenitis, lymphangitis, nausea, vomiting, and abdominal pain may also occur. Spread of the infection to the central nervous system (CNS) causes acute ascending encephalomyelitis. Most patients with CNS involvement die despite antiviral therapy and supportive care, and those who survive usually suffer serious neurologic sequelae. Respiratory failure associated with ascending paralysis is the most common cause of death.

DIAGNOSIS

In the United States, diagnostic testing of human specimens is performed only at the National B Virus Resource Center at Georgia State University. Detection of viral DNA by B virus PCR from clinical specimens is the standard for diagnosis of infection. Detection of B virus–specific antibodies in serum is also diagnostic. Culture is generally unsuccessful as the virus is unlikely to remain viable during transit or after being frozen and thawed. For more information, see www2.gsu.edu/~wwwvir/index.html.

TREATMENT

For any suspected exposure, immediate first aid is crucial. The wound should be cleansed by thoroughly washing and scrubbing the area with soap, concentrated detergent solution, povidone-iodine, or chlorhexidine and water. The wound should then be irrigated with running water for 15–20 minutes. For urine splashes to the eyes, repeated flushes of the eyes should be performed for 15 minutes with sterile saline solution or water. **Specimens for diagnostic testing should not be obtained from wound sites before washing because doing so may force virus more deeply into the wound.**

Antiviral therapy is recommended as postexposure prophylaxis in high-risk exposures (see www.cdc.gov/herpesbvirus/firstaid-treatment.html). When recommended, the first choice of drug for postexposure prophylaxis is valacyclovir and an alternative is acyclovir. If B virus infection is diagnosed, treatment consists of intravenous acyclovir or ganciclovir, depending on whether CNS symptoms are present.

PREVENTION

Adhering to laboratory and animal facility protocols will reduce the risk of B virus transmission among laboratory workers. Visitors to parks and other tourist destinations (such as certain religious temples) with free-roaming macaques should avoid contact with the animals (including feeding or petting them).

CDC website: www.cdc.gov/herpesbvirus

BIBLIOGRAPHY

1. CDC. Notice to readers: occupational safety and health in the care and use of nonhuman primates. MMWR Recomm Rep. 2003;52(38):920.

2. Chosewood LC WD. Section VIII–Agent summary statements. In: Chosewood LC WD, editor. Biosafety in microbiological and biomedical laboratories. 5th ed. Washington, DC: US Department of Health and Human Services; 2009. pp. 205–8.

3. Cohen JI, Davenport DS, Stewart JA, Deitchman S, Hilliard JK, Chapman LE, et al. Recommendations for prevention of and therapy for exposure to B virus (*Cercopithecine herpesvirus* 1). Clin Infect Dis. 2002 Nov 15;35(10):1191–203.

4. Health NIfOSa. Hazard ID 5—*Cercopithicine herpesvirus* 1 (B virus) infection resulting from ocular exposure. Atlanta: CDC; 1999 [cited 2016 Sep. 21]. Available from: http://www.cdc.gov/niosh/docs/99-100/.

5. Veterinarians NAoSPH. Compendium of measure to prevent disease associated with animals in public settings, 2009. MMWR Recomm Rep. 2009;58(RR-05):1–15.

BARTONELLA INFECTIONS

Christina A. Nelson

INFECTIOUS AGENT

Gram-negative bacteria in the genus *Bartonella*. Human illness is primarily caused by *Bartonella henselae* (cat-scratch disease [CSD]), *B. quintana* (trench fever), and *B. bacilliformis* (Carrión disease). A variety of *Bartonella* spp. can cause culture-negative endocarditis; other clinical syndromes due to *Bartonella* spp. have also been reported. For example, in 2007, a newly recognized species of *Bartonella* (*B. rochalimae*) was identified in a traveler with fever and splenomegaly who had visited Peru.

TRANSMISSION

B. henselae is contracted through scratches from domestic or feral cats, particularly kittens. Direct transmission to humans by the bite of infected cat fleas is likely but has not yet been proven. *B. quintana* is transmitted by the human body louse. *B. bacilliformis* is transmitted by infected sand flies (genus *Lutzomyia*).

EPIDEMIOLOGY

CSD and trench fever are distributed worldwide. In the United States, CSD is more common in children, and the incidence peaks from August through January. Trench fever typically occurs in populations that do not have access to proper hygiene, such as refugees and the homeless. Carrión disease has limited geographic distribution; transmission occurs in the Andes Mountains at 1,000–3,000 m (3,281–9,843 ft) elevation in Peru, Colombia, and Ecuador; sporadic cases have also been reported in Bolivia, Chile, and possibly Guatemala. Most cases are reported in Peru. Short-term travelers to endemic areas are likely at low risk.

CLINICAL PRESENTATION

CSD typically manifests as a papule or pustule at the inoculation site and enlarged, tender lymph nodes that develop proximal to the inoculation site 1–3 weeks after exposure. *B. henselae* infection may also cause prolonged fever, follicular conjunctivitis, neuroretinitis, or encephalitis. Trench fever symptoms include fever, headache, transient rash, and bone pain (mainly in the shins, neck, and back).

Some *Bartonella* spp. can cause subacute endocarditis, which is often culture-negative. Bacillary angiomatosis (caused by *B. henselae* or *B. quintana*) and peliosis hepatis (caused by *B. henselae*) occur primarily in people infected with HIV. Bacillary angiomatosis may present as skin, subcutaneous, or bone lesions.

Carrión disease has 2 distinct phases: an acute phase (Oroya fever) characterized by fever, myalgia, headache, and anemia and an eruptive phase (verruga peruana) characterized by red-to-purple nodular skin lesions.

DIAGNOSIS

CSD can be diagnosed clinically in patients with typical presentation and a compatible exposure history. Serology can confirm the diagnosis, although cross-reactivity may limit interpretation in some circumstances. *B. henselae* may also be detected by PCR or culture of lymph node aspirates by using special techniques.

Trench fever can be diagnosed by serology or blood culture for *B. quintana*. PCR may also aid the diagnosis of disseminated *Bartonella* infections when performed by clinical laboratories using validated methods. Endocarditis caused by *Bartonella* spp. can be diagnosed by elevated serology of the patient and by PCR or culture of excised heart valve tissue.

Oroya fever is typically diagnosed via blood culture or direct observation of the bacilli in peripheral blood smears, though sensitivity of these methods is low. PCR and serologic testing may also aid diagnosis.

TREATMENT

Most cases of CSD eventually resolve without treatment, but a small percentage of people will develop disseminated disease with severe complications. The use of antibiotics to shorten the course of disease is debated, although azithromycin speeds the decrease in lymph node volume.

Various antibiotics are effective against *Bartonella* infections, and regimens including agents such as tetracyclines, fluoroquinolones, trimethoprim-sulfamethoxazole, rifampin, and aminoglycosides have been used. Recommended regimens and duration of treatment vary by clinical disease.

PREVENTION

Avoid rough play with cats, particularly strays and kittens, to prevent scratches. This is especially important for immunocompromised people. Wash hands promptly after handling cats. Protect against bites of sand flies and body lice (see Chapter 2, Protection against Mosquitoes, Ticks, & Other Arthropods). Flea control for cats is also important.

CDC website: www.cdc.gov/bartonella

BIBLIOGRAPHY

1. Bass JW, Freitas BC, Freitas AD, Sisler CL, Chan DS, Vincent JM, et al. Prospective randomized double blind placebo-controlled evaluation of azithromycin for treatment of cat-scratch disease. Pediatr Infect Dis J. 1998 Jun;17(6):447–52.

2. Eremeeva ME, Gerns HL, Lydy SL, Goo JS, Ryan ET, Mathew SS, et al. Bacteremia, fever, and splenomegaly caused by a newly recognized *Bartonella* species. N Engl J Med. 2007 Jun 7;356(23):2381–7.

3. Florin TA, Zaoutis TE, Zaoutis LB. Beyond cat scratch disease: widening spectrum of *Bartonella henselae* infection. Pediatrics. 2008 May;121(5):e1413–25.

4. Fournier PE, Thuny F, Richet H, Lepidi H, Casalta JP, Arzouni JP, et al. Comprehensive diagnostic strategy for blood culture-negative endocarditis: a prospective study of 819 new cases. Clin Infect Dis. 2010 Jul 15;51(2):131–40.

5. Maguina C, Gotuzzo E. Bartonellosis. New and old. Infect Dis Clin North Am. 2000 Mar;14(1):1–22, vii.

6. Rolain JM, Brouqui P, Koehler JE, Maguina C, Dolan MJ, Raoult D. Recommendations for treatment of human infections caused by *Bartonella* species. Antimicrob Agents Chemother. 2004 Jun;48(6): 1921–33.

BRUCELLOSIS

Maria E. Negron, Rebekah Tiller, Grishma A. Kharod

INFECTIOUS AGENT

Facultative, intracellular, gram-negative cocco-bacilli; known human pathogens include *Brucella abortus*, *B. melitensis*, *B. suis*, and *B. canis*.

TRANSMISSION

Most commonly through consumption of unpasteurized dairy products or undercooked meat from infected animals and direct contact with infected animals, especially those that have recently given birth. Since wildlife can be reservoirs for *Brucella* spp., hunting can be a risk for exposure as well. *Brucella* can enter the body via skin wounds, mucous membranes, or inhalation. Person-to-person transmission is rare.

EPIDEMIOLOGY

High-risk regions include the Mediterranean Basin, South and Central America, Eastern Europe, Asia, Africa, and the Middle East. In these areas, brucellosis is primarily enzootic in cattle, sheep, and goat populations, as well as feral swine.

CLINICAL PRESENTATION

Incubation period is usually 2–4 weeks (range, 5 days to 5 months). Initial presentation is non-specific, including fever, muscle aches, fatigue, headache, and night sweats. Focal infections are common and can affect most organs in the body.

DIAGNOSIS

Blood culture is the diagnostic gold standard, but is not always positive. If culture of blood, bone marrow, or other clinical specimen is performed, the laboratory must be informed that *Brucella* is suspected, as the culture takes longer to grow and laboratory personnel require additional personnel protective equipment when handling cultures. A serum agglutination test is the most common serologic approach, but other serology assays (including ELISA) and PCR have been used to make a diagnosis. Brucellosis is a nationally notifiable disease.

TREATMENT

Doxycycline, rifampin, trimethoprim-sulfamethoxazole, fluoroquinolones, aminoglycosides, and other agents have been used in various combinations for a minimum of 6–8 weeks. If bacteria localize in organs and tissues and cause focal infection, surgical drainage could be indicated. Late diagnosis or inappropriate therapy can result in chronic disease or relapse.

PREVENTION

Avoid unpasteurized dairy products and undercooked meat. Wear protective equipment when dressing or butchering wild animals potentially infected with *Brucella* spp. In clinical microbiology laboratories, if *Brucella* spp. is suspected, culture isolates should be handled under BSL-3 conditions.

CDC website: www.cdc.gov/brucellosis

BIBLIOGRAPHY

1. Al Dahouk S, Nockler K. Implications of laboratory diagnosis on brucellosis therapy. Expert Rev Anti Infect Ther. 2011 Jul;9(7):833–45.

2. Ariza J, Bosilkovski M, Cascio A, Colmenero JD, Corbel MJ, Falagas ME, et al. Perspectives for the treatment of brucellosis in the 21st century: the Ioannina recommendations. PLoS Med. 2007 Dec;4(12):e317.

3. Arnow PM, Smaron M, Ormiste V. Brucellosis in a group of travelers to Spain. JAMA. 1984 Jan 27;251(4):505–7.

4. Memish ZA, Balkhy HH. Brucellosis and international travel. J Travel Med. 2004 Jan-Feb;11(1):49–55.

5. Organization WH. Brucellosis. Geneva: World Health Organization; 2012 [cited 2016 Sep. 21]. Available from: http://www.who.int/zoonoses/diseases/brucellosis/en/.

6. Pappas G, Papadimitriou P, Akritidis N, Christou L, Tsianos EV. The new global map of human brucellosis. Lancet Infect Dis. 2006 Feb;6(2):91–9.

7. Rhodes HM, Williams DN, Hansen GT. Invasive human brucellosis infection in travelers to and immigrants from the Horn of Africa related to the consumption of raw camel milk. Travel Med Infect Dis. 2016 May-Jun;14(3):255–60.

8. Yousefi-Nooraie R, Mortaz-Hejri S, Mehrani M, Sadeghipour P. Antibiotics for treating human brucellosis. Cochrane Database Syst Rev. 2012;10:Cd007179.

CAMPYLOBACTERIOSIS

Aimee L. Geissler, Barbara E. Mahon, Collette Fitzgerald

INFECTIOUS AGENT

Infection is caused by gram-negative, spiral-shaped microaerophilic bacteria of the family Campylobacteriaceae. Most infections are caused by *Campylobacter jejuni*; at least 18 other species, including *C. coli*, also cause infection. *C. jejuni* and *C. coli* are carried normally in the intestinal tracts of many domestic and wild animals.

TRANSMISSION

The major modes of transmission include eating contaminated foods (especially undercooked chicken and foods contaminated by raw chicken), drinking contaminated water or milk (unpasteurized milk, most commonly), and having contact with animals, particularly farm animals such as cows and chickens, as well as domestic cats and dogs. *Campylobacter* can also be transmitted from person to person by the fecal-oral route.

EPIDEMIOLOGY

Campylobacter is a leading cause of bacterial diarrheal disease worldwide; in the United States, it is estimated to cause 1.3 million human illnesses every year. *Campylobacter* is the most common laboratory-confirmed enteric pathogen reported in travelers returning to the United States from every region of the world. The risk of infection is highest in travelers to Africa and South America, especially in areas with poor restaurant hygiene and inadequate sanitation. The infectious dose is small; <500 organisms can cause disease.

CLINICAL PRESENTATION

Incubation period is typically 2–4 days. Campylobacteriosis is characterized by diarrhea (frequently bloody), abdominal pain, fever, and occasionally nausea and vomiting. More severe illness can occur, including dehydration, bloodstream infection, and symptoms mimicking acute appendicitis or ulcerative colitis. People with campylobacteriosis are at increased risk for postinfectious complications, including reactive arthritis (2%–5% of patients), irritable bowel syndrome (9%–13%), and Guillain-Barré syndrome (GBS) (0.1%). *C. jejuni* is the most frequently observed antecedent bacterial infection in cases of GBS; symptoms usually begin 1–3 weeks after the onset of *Campylobacter* enteritis.

DIAGNOSIS

Diagnosis is traditionally based on isolation of the organism from stool specimens or rectal swabs by using selective media incubated under reduced oxygen tension at 42°C (107.6°F) for 72 hours. Visualization of motile and curved, spiral, or S-shaped rods by stool phase-contrast or dark-field microscopy can provide rapid presumptive evidence for *Campylobacter* enteritis. A stool specimen should be collected during the acute phase of the diarrheal illness and before antibiotic treatment is initiated. Because the organism is fastidious, a delay in transporting the specimen will affect the viability of *Campylobacter* spp. A laboratory may reject stool samples without preservative that are in transit for more than 2 hours. If transport and processing are not possible within 2 hours of stool sample collection, specimens should be placed in transport medium according to standard guidelines. Only through culture can *Campylobacter* be subtyped and tested for antimicrobial susceptibility. Rapid culture-independent diagnostic tests, including both antigen tests and nucleic acid–based tests, are becoming widely available and more commonly used. The sensitivity and specificity of stool antigen tests are variable, and in settings of low prevalence, the positive predictive value is likely to be low. Therefore, laboratories should confirm positive results of stool antigen tests by culture. Nucleic acid–based tests have recently been approved and appear to have higher sensitivity and specificity than the antigen tests. Campylobacteriosis is a nationally notifiable disease.

TREATMENT

The disease is generally self-limited, lasting a week or less. Antibiotic therapy decreases the duration of symptoms and bacterial shedding if administered early in the course of disease. Because campylobacteriosis generally cannot be distinguished from other causes of travelers' diarrhea without a diagnostic test, the use of empiric antibiotics in travelers should follow the guidelines for travelers' diarrhea.

Rates of antibiotic resistance, especially fluoroquinolone resistance, have risen sharply in the past 20 years, and high rates of resistance are now seen in many regions. Travel abroad is a risk factor for infection with resistant *Campylobacter*. Clinicians should suspect resistant infection in returning travelers with campylobacteriosis in whom empiric fluoroquinolone treatment has failed. When fluoroquinolone resistance is proven or suspected, azithromycin is usually the next choice of treatment, although resistance to macrolides has also been reported.

PREVENTION

No vaccine is available. Prevention is best achieved by adhering to standard food and water safety precautions (see Chapter 2, Food & Water Precautions) and thorough handwashing after contact with animals or environments that may be contaminated with animal feces. Antibiotic prophylaxis is not recommended.

CDC website: www.cdc.gov/foodsafety/diseases/ campylobacter

BIBLIOGRAPHY

1. Coker AO, Isokpehi RD, Thomas BN, Amisu KO, Obi CL. Human campylobacteriosis in developing countries. Emerg Infect Dis. 2002 Mar;8(3):237–44.

2. Fitzgerald C, Nachamkin I. *Campylobacter* and *Arcobacter*. In: Jorgensen JH, Pfaller MA, Carroll KC, Funke G, Landry ML, Richter SS, et al., editors. Manual of Clinical Microbiology. 11th ed. Washington, D. C.: American Society for Microbiology Press; 2015. pp. 998–1012.

3. Friedman CR, Hoekstra RM, Samuel M, Marcus R, Bender J, Shiferaw B, et al. Risk factors for sporadic *Campylobacter* infection in the United States: a case-control study in FoodNet sites. Clin Infect Dis. 2004 Apr 15;38 Suppl 3:S285–96.

4. Humphrey T, O'Brien S, Madsen M. Campylobacters as zoonotic pathogens: a food production perspective. Int J Food Microbiol. 2007 Jul 15;117(3):237–57.

5. Kassenborg HD, Smith KE, Vugia DJ, Rabatsky-Ehr T, Bates MR, Carter MA, et al. Fluoroquinolone-resistant *Campylobacter* infections: eating poultry outside of the home and foreign travel are risk factors. Clin Infect Dis. 2004 Apr 15;38 Suppl 3:S279–84.

6. Kendall ME, Crim S, Fullerton K, Han PV, Cronquist AB, Shiferaw B, et al. Travel-associated enteric infections diagnosed after return to the United States, Foodborne Diseases Active Surveillance Network (FoodNet), 2004–2009. Clin Infect Dis. 2012 Jun;54 Suppl 5:S480–7.

7. Moore JE, Barton MD, Blair IS, Corcoran D, Dooley JS, Fanning S, et al. The epidemiology of antibiotic resistance in *Campylobacter*. Microbes Infect. 2006 Jun;8(7):1955–66.

8. World Health Organization. The global view of campylobacteriosis: report of an expert consultation. Geneva: World Health Organization; 2012 [cited 2016 Sep. 21]. Available from: http://apps.who.int/iris/bitstream/10665/80751/1/9789241564601_eng.pdf?ua=1.

9. World Health Organization. WHO estimates of the global burden of foodborne diseases. Geneva: World Health Organization; 2015 [cited 2016 Sep. 22]. Available from: http://www.who.int/foodsafety/areas_work/foodborne-diseases/ferg/en/.

CHIKUNGUNYA

J. Erin Staples, Susan L. Hills, Ann M. Powers

INFECTIOUS AGENT

Chikungunya virus is a single-stranded RNA virus that belongs to the family Togaviridae, genus *Alphavirus*.

TRANSMISSION

Chikungunya virus is transmitted to humans via the bite of an infected mosquito of the *Aedes* spp., predominantly *Aedes aegypti* and *Ae. albopictus*. Nonhuman and human primates are likely the main reservoirs of the virus, and human-to-vector-to-human transmission occurs during outbreaks of the disease. Bloodborne transmission is possible; 1 case was documented in a health care worker who was stuck with a needle after drawing blood from an infected patient. Cases have also been documented among laboratory personnel handling infected blood and through aerosol exposure in the laboratory.

The risk of a person transmitting the virus to a biting mosquito or through blood is highest when the patient is viremic, usually during the first 2–6 days of illness. Maternal-fetal transmission has been documented during pregnancy; the highest risk occurs when a woman is viremic at the time of delivery. Studies have not found virus in breast milk.

EPIDEMIOLOGY

Chikungunya virus often causes large outbreaks with high attack rates, affecting one-third to three-quarters of the population in areas where the virus is circulating. Outbreaks of chikungunya have occurred in Africa, Asia, Europe, and islands in the Indian and Pacific Oceans. In late 2013, the first locally acquired cases of chikungunya were reported in the Americas on islands in the Caribbean. By the end of 2014, more than 1.1 million suspect cases of chikungunya had been reported in the Americas. Since then the virus has continued to circulate and cause disease in the Americas, Southeast Asia, Pacific Islands, and Africa.

Risk to travelers is highest in areas experiencing ongoing epidemics of the disease (for the most updated information see the Travel Health Notices section on the CDC Travelers' Health website at wwwnc.cdc.gov/travel/notices). Most epidemics occur during the tropical rainy season and abate during the dry season. However, outbreaks in Africa have occurred after periods of drought, where open water containers in close proximity to human habitation served as vector-breeding sites. Risk of infection exists throughout the day, as the primary vector, *Ae. aegypti*, aggressively bites during the daytime. *Ae. aegypti* mosquitoes bite indoors or outdoors near a dwelling. They typically breed in domestic containers that hold water, including buckets and flower pots.

Both adults and children can become infected and symptomatic with the disease. From 2010 through 2013, 110 cases of chikungunya were identified or reported among US travelers who predominantly traveled to areas with known ongoing outbreaks. Following the outbreaks in the Americas, however, >3,500 chikungunya cases have been reported from US states through the end of April 2016. Although most were in travelers, a few cases acquired locally in the continental United States were reported in 2014 and 2015. In addition, several US territories (Puerto Rico, US Virgin Islands, and American Samoa) have reported locally acquired cases from 2014–2016.

CLINICAL PRESENTATION

Approximately 3%–28% of people infected with chikungunya virus will remain asymptomatic. For people who develop symptomatic illness, the incubation period is typically 3–7 days (range, 1–12 days). Disease is most often characterized by sudden onset of high fever (temperature typically >102°F [39°C]) and joint pains. Other symptoms may include headache, myalgia, arthritis, conjunctivitis, nausea, vomiting, or a maculopapular rash. Fevers typically last from several days up to 1 week; the fever can be biphasic. Joint symptoms are often severe and can be debilitating. They usually involve multiple joints, typically bilateral and symmetric. They occur most commonly in hands and feet, but they can affect more proximal joints. Rash usually occurs after onset of fever. It typically involves the trunk and extremities but can also include the palms, soles, and face.

Abnormal laboratory findings can include thrombocytopenia, lymphopenia, and elevated creatinine and liver function tests. Rare but serious complications of the disease can occur, including myocarditis, ocular disease (uveitis, retinitis), hepatitis, acute renal disease, severe bullous lesions, and neurologic disease, such as meningoencephalitis, Guillain-Barré syndrome, myelitis, or cranial nerve palsies. Groups identified as having increased risk for more severe disease include neonates exposed intrapartum, adults >65 years of age, and people with underlying medical conditions, such as hypertension, diabetes, or heart disease.

Acute symptoms of chikungunya typically resolve in 7–10 days. Fatalities associated with infection occur but are typically rare and most commonly reported in older adults. Some patients will have a relapse of rheumatologic symptoms such as polyarthralgia, polyarthritis, tenosynovitis, or Raynaud syndrome in the months after acute illness. Studies have reported variable proportions, ranging from 5% to 80%, of patients with persistent joint pains for months or years after their illness.

Pregnant women have symptoms and outcomes similar to those of other people, and most infections that occur during pregnancy will not result in the virus being transmitted to the fetus. However, when intrapartum transmission occurs, it can result in complications for the baby, including neurologic disease, hemorrhagic symptoms, and myocardial disease. There are also rare reports of spontaneous abortions after maternal infection during the first trimester.

DIAGNOSIS

The differential diagnosis of chikungunya virus infection depends on the clinical signs and symptoms as well as where the person was suspected of being infected. Diseases that should be considered in the differential diagnosis include dengue, Zika, malaria, leptospirosis, parvovirus, enterovirus, group A *Streptococcus*, rubella, measles, adenovirus, postinfectious arthritis, rheumatologic conditions, or alphavirus infections (including Mayaro, Ross River, Barmah Forest, O'nyong-nyong, and Sindbis viruses).

Preliminary diagnosis is based on the patient's clinical features, places and dates of travel, and activities. Laboratory diagnosis is generally accomplished by testing serum to detect virus, viral nucleic acid, or virus-specific IgM and neutralizing antibodies. During the first week after onset of symptoms, chikungunya can often be diagnosed by performing viral culture or nucleic acid amplification on serum. Virus-specific IgM and neutralizing antibodies normally develop toward the end of the first week of illness. Therefore, to definitively rule out the diagnosis, convalescent-phase samples should be obtained from patients whose acute-phase samples test negative.

Testing for chikungunya virus is performed at CDC, several state health department laboratories, and several commercial laboratories. Health care providers should report suspected chikungunya cases to their state or local health departments to facilitate diagnosis and mitigate the risk of local transmission. Because chikungunya is a nationally notifiable disease, state health departments should report laboratory-confirmed cases to CDC through ArboNET, the national surveillance system for arboviral diseases.

TREATMENT

No specific antiviral treatment is available for chikungunya. Treatment is for symptoms and can include rest, fluids, and use of analgesics and antipyretics. Nonsteroidal anti-inflammatory drugs can be used to help with acute fever and pain. In dengue-endemic areas, however, acetaminophen is the preferred first-line treatment for fever and joint pain until dengue can be ruled out, to reduce the risk of hemorrhage. For patients with persistent joint pain, use of nonsteroidal anti-inflammatory drugs, corticosteroids including topical preparations, and physical therapy may help lessen the symptoms.

PREVENTION

No vaccine or preventive drug is available. The best way to prevent infection is to avoid mosquito bites (see Chapter 2, Protection against Mosquitoes, Ticks, & Other Arthropods). Travelers at increased risk for more severe disease, including travelers with underlying medical conditions and women who are late in their pregnancy (as their unborn infants are at increased risk), may consider avoiding travel to areas with ongoing outbreaks. If travel is unavoidable, emphasize the need for protective measures against mosquito bites.

CDC website: www.cdc.gov/chikungunya

BIBLIOGRAPHY

1. CDC. Geographic distribution of chikungunya virus. Atlanta: CDC; 2014 [cited 2016 Sep. 22]. Available from: http://www.cdc.gov/chikungunya/geo/index.html.

2. Lee VJ, Chow A, Zheng X, Carrasco LR, Cook AR, Lye DC, et al. Simple clinical and laboratory predictors of chikungunya versus dengue infections in adults. PLoS Negl Trop Dis. 2012;6(9):e1786.

3. Lindsey NP, Prince HE, Kosoy O, Laven J, Messenger S, Staples JE, et al. Chikungunya virus disease in travelers – United States, 2010–2013. Am J Trop Med Hyg. 2015 Jan;92(1):82–7.

4. Pan American Health Organization and CDC. Preparedness and response for chikungunya virus introduction in the Americas. Washington, DC: Pan American Health Organization; 2011 [cited 2016 Sep. 22]. Available from: http://new.paho.org/hq/index.php?option=com_content&view=article&id=3545&Itemid=2545&lang=en.

5. Rajapakse S, Rodrigo C, Rajapakse A. Atypical manifestations of chikungunya infection. Trans R Soc Trop Med Hyg. 2010 Feb;104(2):89–96.

6. Simon F, Javelle E, Cabie A, Bouquillard E, Troisgros O, Gentile G, et al. French guidelines for the management of chikungunya (acute and persistent presentations). November 2014. Med Mal Infect. 2015 Jul;45(7):243–63.

7. Staples JE, Fischer M. Chikungunya virus in the Americas—what a vectorborne pathogen can do. N Engl J Med. 2014 Sep 4;371(10):887–9.

8. Thiberville SD, Moyen N, Dupuis-Maguiraga L, Nougairede A, Gould EA, Roques P, et al. Chikungunya fever: epidemiology, clinical syndrome, pathogenesis and therapy. Antiviral Res. 2013 Sep;99(3):345–70.

9. World Health Organization. Chikungunya: case definitions for acute, atypical and chronic cases. Conclusions of an expert consultation, Managua, Nicaragua, 20-21 May 2015. Wkly Epidemiol Rec. 2015 Aug 14;90(33):410–4.

3

CHOLERA

Karen K. Wong, Erin Burdette, Eric D. Mintz

INFECTIOUS AGENT

Cholera is an acute bacterial intestinal infection caused by toxigenic *Vibrio cholerae* O-group 1 or O-group 139. Many other serogroups of *V. cholerae*, with or without the cholera toxin gene (including the nontoxigenic strains of the O1 and O139 serogroups), can cause a choleralike illness. Only toxigenic strains of serogroups O1 and O139 have caused widespread epidemics and are reportable to the World Health Organization (WHO) as "cholera." *V. cholerae* O1 is the source of an ongoing global pandemic, while the O139 serogroup remains localized to a few areas in Asia.

V. cholerae O1 has 2 biotypes, classical and El Tor, and each biotype has 2 distinct serotypes, Inaba and Ogawa. The symptoms of infection are indistinguishable, although more people infected with the El Tor biotype remain asymptomatic or have only a mild illness. Globally, most cases of cholera are caused by O1 El Tor organisms. In recent years, an El Tor variant that has characteristics of both classical and El Tor biotypes and may be more virulent than older El Tor strains has emerged in Asia

and has spread to Africa and the Caribbean. This strain is responsible for the epidemic on Hispaniola and may cause a higher proportion of severe episodes of cholera and higher death rates.

TRANSMISSION

Toxigenic *V. cholerae* O1 and O139 are free-living bacterial organisms found in fresh and brackish water, often in association with copepods or other zooplankton, shellfish, and aquatic plants. Cholera infections are most commonly acquired from drinking water in which *V. cholerae* is found naturally or into which it has been introduced from the feces of an infected person. Other common vehicles include fish and shellfish. Other foods, including produce, are less commonly implicated. Direct transmission from person to person, even to health care workers during epidemics, has been reported but is not frequent.

EPIDEMIOLOGY

Cholera is endemic in approximately 50 countries, primarily in Africa and South and Southeast Asia, and can emerge in dramatic epidemics, although most cases go unreported. In October 2010, a large cholera epidemic began in Haiti and spread to the Dominican Republic and Cuba; it is now endemic in Hispaniola, and occasional small outbreaks occur in the Dominican Republic and in Cuba. Sporadic cases associated with travel to or from cholera-affected countries continue to occur.

From 2010 through 2014, 91 cases of cholera were confirmed in the United States among people who had traveled internationally in the week before illness. Of these, 75% were associated with travel to the Caribbean, and 10% were associated with travel to India or Pakistan; other travel destinations reported included countries in Southeast Asia and West Africa. Risk of infection is highest for travelers to countries where cholera is endemic or where there is an active epidemic. The risk is increased for those who drink untreated water, do not follow handwashing recommendations, do not use latrines or other sanitation systems, or eat raw or poorly cooked food, especially seafood. Health care and response workers in cholera-affected areas, such as in an outbreak or after a disaster, may also be at increased risk of cholera. People who have low gastric acidity or those with blood type O are at higher risk of severe cholera illness. Travelers who observe safe food, water, sanitation, and handwashing recommendations while in countries affected by cholera have virtually no risk of acquiring cholera.

CLINICAL PRESENTATION

Cholera most commonly manifests as watery diarrhea in an afebrile person. Infection is often mild or asymptomatic, but it can be severe. Severe cholera is characterized by acute, profuse watery diarrhea, described as "rice-water stools," often accompanied by nausea and vomiting, and can rapidly lead to severe volume depletion. Signs and symptoms include tachycardia, loss of skin turgor, dry mucous membranes, hypotension, and thirst. Additional symptoms, including muscle cramps, are secondary to the resulting electrolyte imbalances. If untreated, rapid loss of body fluids can lead to severe dehydration, hypovolemic shock, and death within hours. With adequate and timely rehydration, case-fatality ratios (CFRs) are <1%.

DIAGNOSIS

Cholera is confirmed through culture of a stool specimen or rectal swab. Cary-Blair medium can be used for transport, and selective media such as taurocholate-tellurite-gelatin agar and thiosulfate-citrate-bile salts agar may be used for isolation and identification. Reagents for serogrouping *V. cholerae* isolates are available in state health department laboratories. Culture-independent diagnostic tests do not yield an isolate for antimicrobial susceptibility testing and subtyping and should not be used for routine diagnosis. All isolates obtained in the United States should be sent to CDC via state health department laboratories for identification and virulence testing. Cholera is a nationally notifiable disease.

TREATMENT

Rehydration is the cornerstone of cholera treatment. Oral rehydration solution and, when necessary, intravenous fluids and electrolytes, if administered in a timely manner and in adequate volumes, will reduce CFRs to <1%. Antibiotics reduce fluid requirements and duration of illness and are indicated in conjunction with aggressive hydration for severe cases and for those with moderate dehydration and ongoing fluid losses. Whenever possible, antimicrobial susceptibility testing should inform treatment choices. In most countries, doxycycline is recommended as the first-line antibiotic treatment for adults, and azithromycin is recommended for children and pregnant women. Multidrug-resistant isolates are emerging, particularly in South Asia, with resistance to quinolones, trimethoprim-sulfamethoxazole, and tetracycline. The strain from Hispaniola is also multidrug resistant; however, it is still sensitive to doxycycline and tetracycline. Zinc supplementation reduces the severity and duration of cholera and other diarrheal diseases in children living in resource-limited areas.

PREVENTION

Food and Water

Safe food and water precautions and frequent handwashing are critical in preventing cholera (see Chapter 2, Food & Water Precautions). Chemoprophylaxis is not indicated.

Vaccine

No country or territory requires vaccination against cholera as a condition for entry. CVD 103-HgR, a single-dose oral cholera vaccine (Vaxchora, PaxVax), is licensed and available in the United States. The vaccine was previously marketed under the names Orochol and Mutacol in other countries. Vaxchora was approved in June 2016 for use in adults ≥18 years of age.

INDICATIONS

The Advisory Committee on Immunization Practices (ACIP) recommends CVD 103-HgR vaccine for adult travelers (age 18–64 years) to an area of active cholera transmission. An area of active cholera transmission is defined as a province, state, or other administrative subdivision within a country with endemic or epidemic cholera caused by toxigenic *V. cholerae* O1 and includes areas with cholera activity within the last year that are prone to recurrence of cholera epidemics; it does not include areas where rare sporadic cases have been reported.

The vaccine is not routinely recommended for most travelers from the United States, as most do not visit areas with active cholera transmission.

VACCINE EFFICACY

Adults aged 18–45 years who received Vaxchora were protected against severe diarrhea after oral *V. cholerae* O1 challenge at 10 days and at 3 months after vaccination (vaccine efficacy 90% and 80%, respectively). In adults aged 46–64 years, vibriocidal antibody seroconversion rates, the best available marker for protection against cholera, were noninferior to the response seen in adults aged 18–45 years.

VACCINE ADMINISTRATION

Vaxchora is administered in a single oral dose, which consists of ingestion of the entire contents of 1 double-chambered sachet. Vaxchora should be taken at least 10 days before potential cholera exposure. Eating or drinking should be avoided for 60 minutes before and after oral ingestion of Vaxchora. Prepare and administer Vaxchora in a health care setting equipped to dispose of medical waste.

BOOSTER DOSES

The safety and efficacy of revaccination with CVD 103-HgR have not been established.

VACCINE SAFETY AND ADVERSE REACTIONS

Serious adverse events were rare among recipients of Orochol and Mutacol, the previously marketed formulation of the CVD 103-HgR vaccine. Systemic adverse events, which may include diarrhea and headache, occur at similar rates in Vaxchora recipients and nonrecipients.

PRECAUTIONS AND CONTRAINDICATIONS

Vaxchora is contraindicated in people with a history of severe allergic reaction to any ingredient of Vaxchora or to a previous dose of any cholera vaccine. A study with the older formulation of CVD 103-HgR showed that concomitant use of chloroquine decreased the immune response to the vaccine; therefore, antimalarial prophylaxis with chloroquine should begin no sooner than 10 days after administration of Vaxchora. Coadministration of mefloquine and proguanil with CVD 103-HgR did not diminish the vaccine's immunogenicity. Antibiotics may decrease the immune response to CVD 103-HgR, so vaccine should not be administered to patients who have received antibiotics in the previous 14 days.

Vaxchora is not currently licensed for use in children <18 years of age. No information is available on the use of Vaxchora during pregnancy or lactation. The safety and effectiveness of Vaxchora have not been established in immunocompromised people. There was no difference in adverse events reported among HIV-positive recipients of an older formulation of the CVD 103-HgR vaccine and those who received placebo.

Vaxchora may be shed in the stool for at least 7 days, and the vaccine strain may be transmitted to nonvaccinated close contacts. Clinicians and travelers should use caution when considering whether to use the vaccine in people with immunocompromised close contacts.

CDC website: www.cdc.gov/cholera

BIBLIOGRAPHY

1. Chen WH, Cohen MB, Kirkpatrick BD, Brady RC, Galloway D, Gurwith M, et al. Single-dose live oral cholera vaccine CVD 103-HgR protects against human experimental infection with vibrio cholerae O1 El Tor. Clin Infect Dis. 2016 Jun 1;62(11):1329–35.

2. Danzig L, editor. Vaxchora™ clinical data summary. Meeting of the Advisory Committee on Immunization Practices; 2016 February 24; Atlanta, GA.

3. Gaffga NH, Tauxe RV, Mintz ED. Cholera: a new homeland in Africa? Am J Trop Med Hyg. 2007 Oct;77(4):705–13.

4. Harris JB, Larocque RC, Charles RC, Mazumder RN, Khan AI, Bardhan PK. Cholera's western front. Lancet. 2010 Dec 11;376(9757):1961–5.

5. Harris JB, LaRocque RC, Qadri F, Ryan ET, Calderwood SB. Cholera. Lancet. 2012 Jun 30;379(9835):2466–76.

6. Kollaritsch H, Que JU, Kunz C, Wiedermann G, Herzog C, Cryz SJ, Jr. Safety and immunogenicity of live oral cholera and typhoid vaccines administered alone or in combination with antimalarial drugs, oral polio vaccine, or yellow fever vaccine. J Infect Dis. 1997 Apr;175(4):871–5.

7. Loharikar A, Newton AE, Stroika S, Freeman M, Greene KD, Parsons MB, et al. Cholera in the United States, 2001–2011: a reflection of patterns of global epidemiology and travel. Epidemiol Infect. 2015 March;143(4):695–703.

8. Schilling KA, Cartwright EJ, Stamper J, Locke M, Esposito DH, Balaban V, et al. Diarrheal illness among US residents providing medical services in Haiti during the cholera epidemic, 2010–2011. J Travel Med. 2014 Jan-Feb;21(1):55–7.

9. World Health Organization. Cholera, 2014. Wkly Epidemiol Rec. 2015 Oct 2;90(40):517–28.

COCCIDIOIDOMYCOSIS

Tom M. Chiller, Paige A. Armstrong, Orion Z. McCotter

INFECTIOUS AGENT

The fungi *Coccidioides immitis* and *C. posadasii*.

TRANSMISSION

Through inhalation of fungal conidia from the environment. Not transmitted from person to person.

EPIDEMIOLOGY

Endemic in the southwestern United States and parts of Mexico and Central and South America. Travelers are at increased risk if they participate in activities that expose them to soil disruption and outdoor dust. Outbreaks have been associated with activities such as construction, archaeological excavation, and military training exercises.

CLINICAL PRESENTATION

The incubation period is 7–21 days. Most infections (60%) are asymptomatic. Symptomatic infection ranges from primary pulmonary illness to severe disseminated disease. Primary pulmonary coccidioidomycosis is characterized by fatigue, cough, fever, shortness of breath, headache, night sweats, muscle aches, joint pain, and rash. These infections are often self-limited, and symptoms typically resolve in a few weeks to months. However, 5%–10% of people go on to develop serious or chronic lung disease, such as cavitary pneumonia, fibrosis, and bronchiectasis. In rare instances (approximately 1% of infections), dissemination to the central nervous system, joints, bones, or skin may occur.

Older people (≥65 years), people with diabetes, and people who smoke are at increased risk of developing severe pulmonary complications. People with depressed cellular immune function, pregnant women, and people of African American or Filipino descent are at increased risk of developing disseminated disease.

DIAGNOSIS

The methods most commonly used to diagnose coccidioidomycosis are serology, culture, and histopathology. EIA is a sensitive serologic method to detect IgM and IgG. Immunodiffusion and complement fixation can also detect antibodies and are often used to confirm diagnosis. Isolation of *Coccidioides* from fungal culture of respiratory specimens or tissue provides a definitive diagnosis. Microscopy of sputum or tissue can identify *Coccidioides* spherules but has low sensitivity. Coccidioidomycosis is a nationally notifiable disease.

TREATMENT

Expert opinions differ on the proper management of patients with uncomplicated primary pulmonary disease in the absence of risk factors for severe or disseminated disease. Some experts recommend no therapy since most illnesses are self-limited, whereas others advise treatment to reduce the intensity or duration of symptoms. Treatment with antifungal agents has not been proven to prevent dissemination. People at high risk for dissemination and people with the following clinical manifestations should receive antifungal therapy:

- Severe acute pulmonary disease
- Chronic pulmonary disease
- Disseminated disease

Depending on the clinical situation, azole antifungal agents or amphotericin B may be used.

PREVENTION

Limit exposure to outdoor dust in endemic areas.

CDC website: www.cdc.gov/fungal/diseases/ coccidioidomycosis

BIBLIOGRAPHY

1. Ampel NM. Coccidioidomycosis. In: Kauffman CA, Pappas PG, Sobel JD, Dismukes WE, editors. Essentials of Clinical Mycology. New York: Springer Science+Business Media, LLC; 2011. pp. 349–66.

2. Ampel NM. Coccidioidomycosis: a review of recent advances. Clin Chest Med. 2009 Jun;30(2):241–51.

3. CDC. Coccidioidomycosis in travelers returning from Mexico–Pennsylvania, 2000. MMWR. 2000;49(44):1004–6.

4. Chiller TM, Galgiani JN, Stevens DA. Coccidioidomycosis. Infect Dis Clin North Am. 2003 Mar;17(1):41–57, viii.

5. Crum NF, Lederman ER, Stafford CM, Parrish JS, Wallace MR. Coccidioidomycosis: a descriptive survey of a reemerging disease. Clinical characteristics and current controversies. Medicine (Baltimore). 2004 May;83(3):149–75.

6. Galgiani JN, Ampel NM, Blair JE, Catanzaro A, Johnson RH, Stevens DA, et al. Coccidioidomycosis. Clin Infect Dis. 2005 Nov 1;41(9):1217–23.

7. Rosenstein NE, Emery KW, Werner SB, Kao A, Johnson R, Rogers D, et al. Risk factors for severe pulmonary and disseminated coccidioidomycosis: Kern County, California, 1995–1996. Clin Infect Dis. 2001 Mar 1;32(5):708–15.

8. Thompson GR, 3rd. Pulmonary coccidioidomycosis. Semin Respir Crit Care Med. 2011 Dec;32(6):754–63.

CRYPTOSPORIDIOSIS

Michele C. Hlavsa, Lihua Xiao

INFECTIOUS AGENT

Among the many protozoan parasites in the genus *Cryptosporidium*, *Cryptosporidium hominis* and *C. parvum* cause >90% of human infections.

TRANSMISSION

Cryptosporidium is transmitted via the fecal-oral route. Its low infectious dose, prolonged survival in moist environments, protracted communicability, and extreme chlorine tolerance make *Cryptosporidium* ideally suited for transmission through drinking or recreational water (such as swimming pools) that has been contaminated with *Cryptosporidium*. Transmission can also occur through eating contaminated food, contact with infected people (for example, while providing care or during oral-anal sex) or animals, or contact with fecally contaminated surfaces.

EPIDEMIOLOGY

Cryptosporidiosis is endemic worldwide, and the highest rates are in developing countries. International travel is a risk factor for sporadic cryptosporidiosis in the United States and other industrialized nations; however, few studies have assessed the prevalence of cryptosporidiosis in travelers. One study found 2.9% prevalence of *Cryptosporidium* infection among those with travel-associated diarrhea; cryptosporidiosis was associated with travel to Asia, particularly India, and Latin America. Another study found a 6.4% prevalence of *Cryptosporidium* infection among North Americans with diarrhea associated with travel to 2 Mexican cities. This study suggests an association between cryptosporidiosis and longer length of stay.

CLINICAL PRESENTATION

Symptoms begin within 2 weeks (typically 5–7 days) after infection and are generally self-limited. The most common symptom is profuse, watery diarrhea. Other symptoms can include abdominal pain, flatulence, urgency, nausea, vomiting, and low-grade fever. In immunocompetent people, symptoms typically resolve within 2–3 weeks; patients might experience a recurrence of symptoms after a brief period of recovery and before complete symptom resolution. Clinical presentation of cryptosporidiosis in immunocompromised patients varies with level of immunosuppression, ranging from no symptoms or transient disease to relapsing or chronic diarrhea or even choleralike diarrhea, which can lead to dehydration and life-threatening wasting and malabsorption. Extraintestinal cryptosporidiosis (in the biliary or respiratory tract or rarely the pancreas) has been documented in children and immunocompromised people.

DIAGNOSIS

Tests for *Cryptosporidium* are typically not included in routine ova and parasite testing. Therefore, clinicians should specifically request testing for this parasite when *Cryptosporidium* infection is suspected. New molecular enteric panel assays generally include *Cryptosporidium* as a target pathogen. Because *Cryptosporidium* can be excreted intermittently, multiple stool collections (3 stool specimens collected on separate days) increase test sensitivity. Diagnostic techniques include microscopy with direct fluorescent antibody (considered the gold standard), EIA kits, rapid immunochromatographic cartridge assays, and microscopy with modified acid-fast staining. False-positive results might occur when using rapid immunochromatographic cartridge assays if they are not used according to the manufacturer's directions. Confirmation by microscopy might be considered.

Infections caused by the different *Cryptosporidium* species and subtypes can differ clinically. However, most *Cryptosporidium* species, all with multiple subtypes, are indistinguishable by traditional diagnostic tests. To better understand cryptosporidiosis epidemiology and track infection sources, CDC has launched CryptoNet (www.cdc.gov/parasites/crypto/cryptonet.html), which provides *Cryptosporidium* genotyping and subtyping services in collaboration with state public health agencies. CryptoNet recommends not preserving stool for *Cryptosporidium* testing in formalin because formalin impedes reliable genotyping and subtyping. Cryptosporidiosis is a nationally notifiable disease.

TREATMENT

Most immunocompetent people will recover without treatment. Nitazoxanide is approved to treat cryptosporidiosis in immunocompetent people aged ≥1 year. Nitazoxanide has not been shown to be an effective treatment of cryptosporidiosis in immunocompromised patients. However, dramatic clinical and parasitologic responses without specific treatment have been reported in these patients after the immune system has been reconstituted. Protease inhibitors might have direct anti-*Cryptosporidium* activity. Oral rehydration is the most effective supportive therapy in both immunocompetent and immunocompromised patients.

PREVENTION

Food and water precautions (see Chapter 2, Food & Water Precautions) and handwashing (www.cdc.gov/handwashing). *Cryptosporidium* is extremely tolerant to halogens (such as chlorine

3

or iodine). Water can be treated effectively by filtering with an absolute 1-μm filter or heating to a rolling boil (any water brought to a boil should be adequately disinfected; however, if fuel supplies are adequate, travelers may wish to boil for 1 minute to allow for a margin of safety). Alcohol-based hand sanitizers are not effective against the parasite.

CDC website: www.cdc.gov/parasites/crypto

BIBLIOGRAPHY

1. Cama VA, Bern C, Roberts J, Cabrera L, Sterling CR, Ortega Y, et al. *Cryptosporidium* species and subtypes and clinical manifestations in children, Peru. Emerg Infect Dis. 2008 Oct;14(10):1567–74.

2. Cartwright RY. Food and waterborne infections associated with package holidays. J Appl Microbiol. 2003;94 Suppl:12S–24S.

3. Kotloff KL, Nataro JP, Blackwelder WC, Nasrin D, Farag TH, Panchalingam S, et al. Burden and aetiology of diarrhoeal disease in infants and young children in developing countries (the Global Enteric Multicenter Study, GEMS): a prospective, case-control study. Lancet. 2013 Jul 20;382(9888):209–22.

4. Lalonde LF, Gajadhar AA. Effect of storage media, temperature, and time on preservation of *Cryptosporidium* parvum oocysts for PCR analysis. Vet Parasitol. 2009 Mar 23;160(3-4):185–9.

5. Nair P, Mohamed JA, DuPont HL, Figueroa JF, Carlin LG, Jiang ZD, et al. Epidemiology of cryptosporidiosis in North American travelers to Mexico. Am J Trop Med Hyg. 2008 Aug;79(2):210–4.

6. Pantenburg B, Cabada MM, White AC, Jr. Treatment of cryptosporidiosis. Expert Rev Anti Infect Ther. 2009 May;7(4):385–91.

7. Roy SL, DeLong SM, Stenzel SA, Shiferaw B, Roberts JM, Khalakdina A, et al. Risk factors for sporadic cryptosporidiosis among immunocompetent persons in the United States from 1999–2001. J Clin Microbiol. 2004 Jul;42(7):2944–51.

8. van Lieshout L, Roestenberg M. Clinical consequences of new diagnostic tools for intestinal parasites. Clin Microbiol Infect. 2015 Jun;21(6):520–8.

9. Weitzel T, Wichmann O, Muhlberger N, Reuter B, Hoof HD, Jelinek T. Epidemiological and clinical features of travel-associated cryptosporidiosis. Clin Microbiol Infect. 2006 Sep;12(9):921–4.

3

CUTANEOUS LARVA MIGRANS

Susan Montgomery

INFECTIOUS AGENT

Larval stages of dog and cat hookworms (usually *Ancylostoma* spp.).

TRANSMISSION

Skin contact with contaminated soil or sand.

EPIDEMIOLOGY

Most cases are reported in travelers to the Caribbean, Africa, Asia, and South America. Beaches (and sandboxes) where domestic animals may roam are a common source of infection. Infection occurs in short- as well as long-term travelers.

CLINICAL PRESENTATION

Creeping eruption usually appears 1–5 days after skin penetration, but the incubation period may be ≥1 month. Typically, a serpiginous, erythematous track appears in the skin and is associated with intense itchiness and mild swelling. Usual locations are the foot and buttocks, although any skin surface coming in contact with contaminated soil can be affected.

DIAGNOSIS

Diagnosed on the basis of characteristic skin lesions. Biopsy is not recommended.

TREATMENT

Cutaneous larva migrans is self-limiting; migrating larvae usually die after 5–6 weeks. Albendazole is very effective for treatment. Ivermectin is effective but not approved for this indication. Symptomatic treatment for frequent severe itching may be helpful.

BIBLIOGRAPHY

1. Caumes E. Treatment of cutaneous larva migrans. Clin Infect Dis. 2000 May;30(5):811–4.
2. Gillespie SH. Cutaneous larva migrans. Curr Infect Dis Rep. 2004 Feb;6(1):50–3.
3. Heukelbach J, Feldmeier H. Epidemiological and clinical characteristics of hookworm-related cutaneous larva migrans. Lancet Infect Dis. 2008 May;8(5):302–9.
4. Hochedez P, Caumes E. Hookworm-related cutaneous larva migrans. J Travel Med. 2007 Sep-Oct;14(5):326–33.
5. Lederman ER, Weld LH, Elyazar IR, von Sonnenburg F, Loutan L, Schwartz E, et al. Dermatologic conditions of the ill returned traveler: an analysis from the GeoSentinel Surveillance Network. Int J Infect Dis. 2008 Nov;12(6):593–602.

PREVENTION

Reduce contact with contaminated soil by wearing shoes and protective clothing and using barriers such as towels when seated on the ground.

CDC website: www.cdc.gov/parasites/ zoonotichookworm

CYCLOSPORIASIS

Barbara L. Herwaldt

INFECTIOUS AGENT

Cyclospora cayetanensis, a coccidian protozoan parasite.

TRANSMISSION

Ingestion of infective *Cyclospora* oocysts, such as in contaminated food or water.

EPIDEMIOLOGY

Most common in tropical and subtropical regions, where outbreaks are frequently seasonal (such as during summers and rainy season in Nepal); even short-term travelers can become infected. Outbreaks in the United States and Canada have been linked to imported fresh produce.

CLINICAL PRESENTATION

Incubation period averages 1 week (range, 2 days to >2 weeks). Onset of symptoms is often abrupt but can be gradual; some people have an influenzalike prodrome. The most common symptom is watery diarrhea, which can be profuse. Other symptoms can include anorexia, weight loss, abdominal cramps, bloating, nausea, body aches, vomiting, and low-grade fever. If untreated, the illness can last for several weeks or months, with a remitting-relapsing course.

DIAGNOSIS

Diagnosed by detecting *Cyclospora* oocysts in stool specimens. Stool examinations for ova and parasites usually do not include methods for detecting *Cyclospora* unless testing for this parasite is specifically requested. Diagnostic assistance for *Cyclospora* and other parasitic diseases is also available from CDC (www.cdc.gov/dpdx; 404-718-4745; parasites@cdc.gov). Cyclosporiasis is a nationally notifiable disease.

TREATMENT

Trimethoprim-sulfamethoxazole; no highly effective alternatives have been identified.

PREVENTION

Food and water precautions (see Chapter 2, Food & Water Precautions); disinfection with chlorine or iodine is unlikely to be effective.

BIBLIOGRAPHY

1. Abanyie F, Harvey RR, Harris JR, Wiegand RE, Gaul L, Desvignes-Kendrick M, et al. 2013 multistate outbreaks of Cyclospora cayetanensis infections associated with fresh produce: focus on the Texas investigations. Epidemiol Infect. 2015 Dec;143(16):3451–8.

2. Hall RL, Jones JL, Herwaldt BL. Surveillance for laboratory-confirmed sporadic cases of Cyclosporiasis—United States, 1997–2008. MMWR Surveill Summ. 2011 Apr 8;60(2):1–11.

3. Herwaldt BL. *Cyclospora cayetanensis*: a review, focusing on the outbreaks of cyclosporiasis in the 1990s. Clin Infect Dis. 2000 Oct;31(4):1040–57.

4. Herwaldt BL. The ongoing sage of US outbreaks of cyclosporiasis associated with imported fresh produce: what *Cyclospora cayetanensis* has taught us and what we have yet to learn. In: Institute of Medicine, editor. Addressing Foodborne Threats to Health: Policies, Practices, and Global Coordination, Workshop Summary. Washington, DC: National Academies Press; 2006. pp. 85–115, 33–40.

5. Ortega YR, Sanchez R. Update on *Cyclospora cayetanensis*, a food-borne and waterborne parasite. Clin Microbiol Rev. 2010 Jan;23(1):218–34.

6. Shlim DR. *Cyclospora cayetanensis*. Clin Lab Med. 2002 Dec;22(4):927–36.

CDC website: www.cdc.gov/parasites/ cyclosporiasis

CYSTICERCOSIS

Paul T. Cantey, Susan Montgomery

INFECTIOUS AGENT

Taenia solium, a cestode parasite.

TRANSMISSION

Ingestion of eggs, excreted by a human carrier of the adult *T. solium* tapeworm, via fecally contaminated food or through close contact with the carrier. Autoinfection is also possible. Larval cysts of *T. solium* infect brain, muscle, or other tissues. Eating undercooked pork with cysticerci results in tapeworm infection (taeniasis), not human cysticercosis.

EPIDEMIOLOGY

Common where sanitary conditions are poor and where pigs have access to human feces. Occurs globally; endemic areas include Mexico, Latin America, sub-Saharan Africa, India, and East Asia. Uncommon in travelers. Seen in immigrants from endemic regions.

CLINICAL PRESENTATION

Median latent period of 5 years (range, 1–30 years). Symptoms depend on the number, location, and stage of cysts. The most common location is brain parenchyma. Most common presentation is seizures. Other presentations include increased intracranial pressure, encephalitis, symptoms of space-occupying lesion, and hydrocephalus. Cysticercosis should be excluded in any adult with new-onset seizures who comes from an endemic area or has potential exposure to a tapeworm carrier.

DIAGNOSIS

Neuroimaging studies (CT or MRI) and confirmatory serologic testing. The most specific serologic test is the enzyme-linked immunotransfer blot, but this test may be negative in up to 30% of patients with a single parenchymal lesion.

TREATMENT

Control of symptoms is the cornerstone of therapy. Anticonvulsants, corticosteroids, or both may be indicated. For some lesions, surgical intervention may be the treatment of choice. Antiparasitic treatment (albendazole, praziquantel) should *not* be initiated in patients with heavy infections, cysticercotic encephalitis, or increased intracranial pressure, as dying cysts can cause or worsen some symptoms. In these cases, the priority is neurologic management (steroids, mannitol), neurosurgical management, or both. In the clinical setting antiparasitic treatment reduces the risk of recurrent seizures. Clinicians can consult CDC to obtain more information about diagnosis and treatment (CDC

Parasitic Diseases Inquiries: 404-718-4745 or parasites@cdc.gov).

PREVENTION

Food and water precautions (see Chapter 2, Food & Water Precautions).

CDC website: www.cdc.gov/parasites/ cysticercosis

BIBLIOGRAPHY

1. Del Brutto OH. Neurocysticercosis among international travelers to disease-endemic areas. J Travel Med. 2012 Mar-Apr;19(2):112–7.
2. Garcia HH, Del Brutto OH, Nash TE, White AC, Jr., Tsang VC, Gilman RH. New concepts in the diagnosis and management of neurocysticercosis (Taenia solium). Am J Trop Med Hyg. 2005 Jan;72(1):3–9.
3. Garcia HH, Gonzales I, Lescano AG, Bustos JA, Pretell EJ, Saavedra H, et al. Enhanced steroid dosing reduces

seizures during antiparasitic treatment for cysticercosis and early after. Epilepsia. 2014 Sep;55(9):1452–9.
4. Garcia HH, Gonzales I, Lescano AG, Bustos JA, Zimic M, Escalante D, et al. Efficacy of combined antiparasitic therapy with praziquantel and albendazole for neurocysticercosis: a double-blind, randomised controlled trial. Lancet Infect Dis. 2014 Aug;14(8):687–95.
5. Garcia HH, Gonzalez AE, Evans CA, Gilman RH, Cysticercosis Working Group in Peru. Taenia solium cysticercosis. Lancet. 2003 Aug 16;362(9383):547–56.

DENGUE

Tyler M. Sharp, Janice Perez-Padilla, Stephen H. Waterman

INFECTIOUS AGENT

Dengue, an acute febrile illness, is caused by infection with any of 4 related positive-sense, single-stranded RNA viruses of the genus *Flavivirus*, dengue viruses 1, 2, 3, or 4.

TRANSMISSION

Transmission occurs through the bite of infected *Aedes* mosquitoes, primarily *Aedes aegypti* and *Ae. albopictus*. Because of the approximately 7-day viremia in humans, bloodborne transmission is possible through exposure to infected blood, organs, or other tissues (such as bone marrow). In addition, perinatal dengue transmission occurs when the mother is infected near the time of birth, in which infection occurs via microtransfusions when the placenta is detached or through mucosal contact with mother's blood during birth. Congenital transmission has not been documented. Dengue may also be transmitted

through breast milk. There is no evidence of sexual transmission.

EPIDEMIOLOGY

Dengue is endemic throughout the tropics and subtropics and is a leading cause of febrile illness among travelers returning from Latin America, the Caribbean, and Southeast Asia, according to an analysis of data collected by the GeoSentinel Surveillance Network. Dengue occurs in >100 countries worldwide (Maps 3-1 through 3-3), including Puerto Rico, the US Virgin Islands, and US-affiliated Pacific Islands. Sporadic outbreaks with local transmission have occurred in Florida, Hawaii, and along the Texas-Mexico border. Although the geographic distribution of dengue is similar to that of malaria, dengue is more of a risk in urban and residential areas than is malaria. DengueMap (www.healthmap.org/dengue/index.php) shows up-to-date information on areas of ongoing transmission.

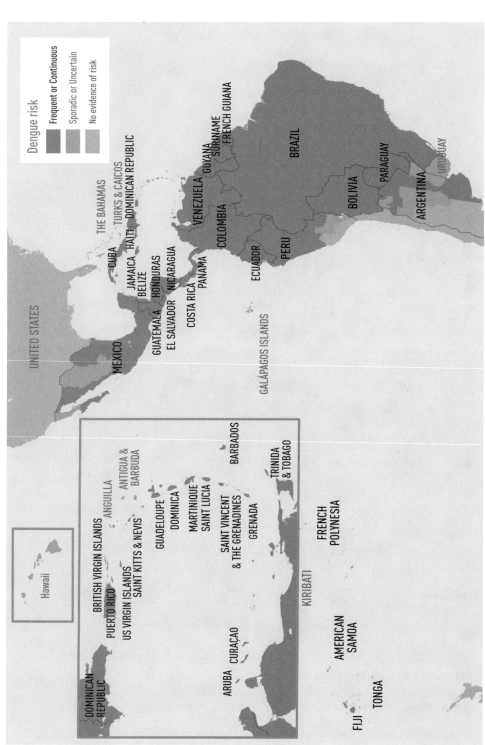

MAP 3-1. Dengue risk in the Americas and the Caribbean[1,2]

[1] Risk areas are shown on a national level except for where evidence exists of different risk levels at subnational regions. Areas that are too small to be seen on the regional maps are labeled in dark blue or light blue depending on their risk categorization.

[2] Jentes et al. Evidence-based risk assessment and communication: a new global dengue-risk map for travellers and clinicians. J Travel Med 2016 Jun 13;23(6).

Dengue risk
- Frequent or Continuous
- Sporadic or Uncertain
- No evidence of risk

3

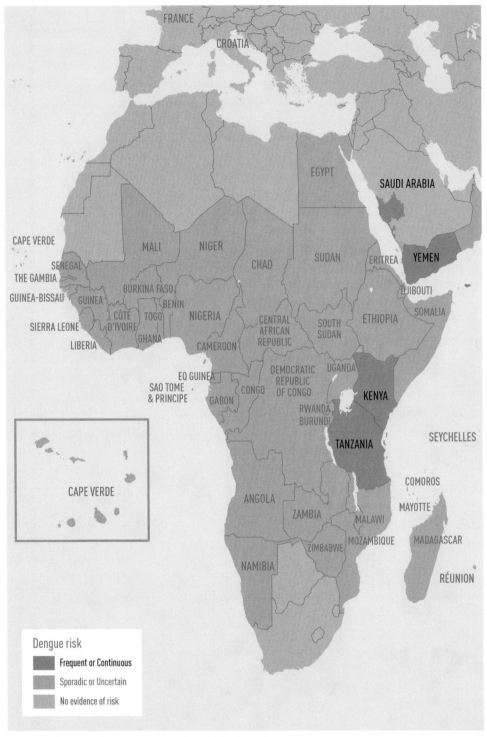

MAP 3-2. Dengue risk in Africa and the Middle East[1,2]

[1] Risk areas are shown on a national level except for where evidence exists of different risk levels at subnational regions. Areas that are too small to be seen on the regional maps are labeled in dark blue or light blue depending on their risk categorization.

[2] Jentes et al. Evidence-based risk assessment and communication: a new global dengue-risk map for travellers and clinicians. J Travel Med 2016 Jun 13;23(6).

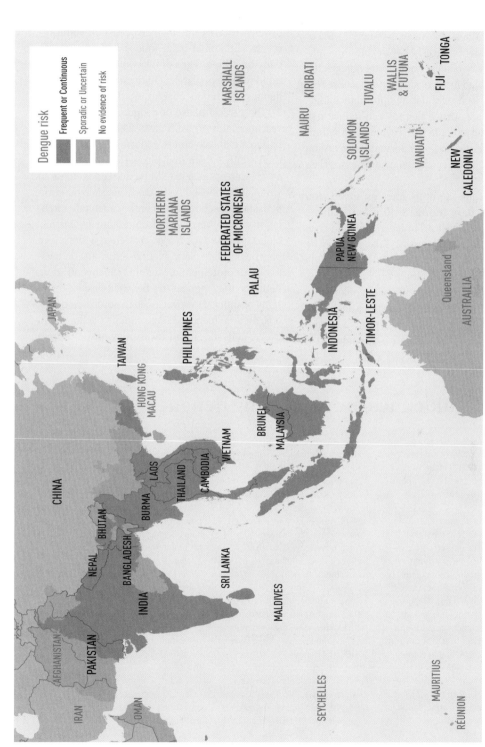

MAP 3-3. Dengue risk in Asia and Oceania[1,2]

[1] Risk areas are shown on a national level except for where evidence exists of different risk levels at subnational regions. Areas that are too small to be seen on the regional maps are labeled in dark blue or light blue depending on their risk categorization.

[2] Jentes et al. Evidence-based risk assessment and communication: a new global dengue-risk map for travellers and clinicians. J Travel Med 2016 Jun 13;23(6).

Legend — Dengue risk:
- Frequent or Continuous
- Sporadic or Uncertain
- No evidence of risk

3

CLINICAL PRESENTATION

An estimated 75% of infections are asymptomatic. Symptomatic infection (dengue) most commonly presents as a mild to moderate, nonspecific, acute, febrile illness. However, as many as 5% of all dengue patients develop severe, life-threatening disease. Early clinical findings are nonspecific but require a high index of suspicion, because recognizing early signs of shock and promptly initiating intensive supportive therapy can reduce risk of death among patients with severe dengue from 10% to <1%. See Box 3-1 for information regarding the World Health Organization guidelines for classifying dengue.

Dengue begins abruptly after an incubation period of 5–7 days (range, 3–10 days), and the course follows 3 phases: febrile, critical, and convalescent. Fever typically lasts 2–7 days and can be biphasic. Other signs and symptoms may include severe headache; retroorbital pain; muscle, joint, and bone pain; macular or maculopapular rash; and minor hemorrhagic manifestations, including petechiae, ecchymosis, purpura, epistaxis, bleeding gums, hematuria, or a positive tourniquet test result. Some patients have injected oropharynx and facial erythema in the first 24–48 hours after onset. Warning signs of progression to severe dengue occur in the late febrile phase around the time of defervescence and include persistent vomiting, severe abdominal pain, mucosal bleeding, difficulty breathing, signs of hypovolemic shock, and rapid decline in platelet count with an increase in hematocrit (hemoconcentration).

The critical phase of dengue begins at defervescence and typically lasts 24–48 hours. Most patients clinically improve during this phase, but those with substantial plasma leakage develop severe dengue as a result of a marked increase in vascular permeability. Initially, physiologic compensatory mechanisms maintain adequate circulation, which narrows pulse pressure as diastolic blood pressure increases. Patients with severe plasma leakage have pleural effusions or ascites, hypoproteinemia, and hemoconcentration. Patients may appear to be well despite early signs of shock. However, once hypotension develops, systolic blood pressure rapidly declines, and irreversible shock and death may ensue despite

BOX 3-1. Guidelines for classifying dengue

In November 2009, World Health Organization (WHO) issued a new guideline that classifies symptomatic cases as dengue or severe dengue.

Dengue is defined by a combination of ≥2 clinical findings in a febrile person who traveled to or lives in a dengue-endemic area. Clinical findings include nausea, vomiting, rash, aches and pains, a positive tourniquet test, leukopenia, and the following warning signs: abdominal pain or tenderness, persistent vomiting, clinical fluid accumulation, mucosal bleeding, lethargy, restlessness, and liver enlargement. The presence of a warning sign may predict severe dengue in a patient.

Severe dengue is defined by dengue with any of the following symptoms: severe plasma leakage leading to shock or fluid accumulation with respiratory distress; severe bleeding; or severe organ impairment such as elevated transaminases ≥1,000 IU/L, impaired consciousness, or heart impairment.

From 1975 through 2009, symptomatic dengue virus infections were classified according to the WHO guidelines as dengue fever, dengue hemorrhagic fever (DHF), and dengue shock syndrome (the most severe form of DHF). The case definition was changed to the 2009 clinical classification after reports that the case definition of DHF was both too difficult to apply in resource-limited settings and too specific, as it failed to identify a substantial proportion of severe dengue cases, including cases of hepatic failure and encephalitis. The 2009 clinical classification has been criticized for being overly inclusive, as it allows several different ways to qualify for severe dengue, and nonspecific warning signs are used as diagnostic criteria for dengue. Last, the new guidelines have been criticized because they do not define the clinical criteria for establishing severe dengue (with the exception of providing laboratory cutoff values for transaminase levels), thereby leaving severity determination up to individual clinical judgment.

resuscitation. Patients can also develop severe hemorrhagic manifestations, including hematemesis, bloody stool, melena, or menorrhagia, especially if they have prolonged shock. Uncommon manifestations include hepatitis, myocarditis, pancreatitis, and encephalitis.

As plasma leakage subsides, the patient enters the convalescent phase and begins to reabsorb extravasated intravenous fluids and pleural and abdominal effusions. As a patient's well-being improves, hemodynamic status stabilizes (although he or she may manifest bradycardia), and diuresis ensues. The patient's hematocrit stabilizes or may fall because of the dilutional effect of the reabsorbed fluid, and the white cell count usually starts to rise, followed by a recovery of platelet count. The convalescent-phase rash may desquamate and be pruritic.

Laboratory findings commonly include leucopenia, thrombocytopenia, hyponatremia, elevated aspartate aminotransferase and alanine aminotransferase, and a normal erythrocyte sedimentation rate.

Data are limited on health outcomes of dengue in pregnancy and effects of maternal infection on the developing fetus. Perinatal transmission can occur, and peripartum maternal infection may increase the likelihood of symptomatic infection in the newborn. Of the 41 perinatal transmission cases described in the literature, all developed thrombocytopenia, most had evidence of plasma leakage evidenced by ascites or pleural effusions, and fever was absent in only 2. Nearly 40% had a hemorrhagic manifestation, and one-fourth had hypotension. Symptoms in perinatally infected neonates typically present during the first week of life. Placental transfer of maternal IgG against dengue virus (from a previous maternal infection) may increase risk for severe dengue among infants infected at 6–12 months of age, when the protective effect of these antibodies wanes.

DIAGNOSIS

Clinicians should consider dengue in a patient who was in an endemic area within 2 weeks before symptom onset. Because dengue is a nationally notifiable disease, all suspected cases should be reported to the local health department. Laboratory confirmation can be made from a single acute-phase serum specimen obtained early (≤5 days after fever onset) in the illness by detecting viral genomic sequences with RT-PCR or dengue nonstructural protein 1 (NS1) antigen by immunoassay. Later in the illness (≥4 days after fever onset), IgM against dengue virus can be detected with ELISA. For patients presenting during the first week after fever onset, diagnostic testing should include a test for dengue virus (PCR or NS1) and IgM. For patients presenting >1 week after fever onset, IgM is most useful, although NS1 has been reported positive up to 12 days after fever onset (Figure 3-1). In the United States, both IgM ELISA and real-time RT-PCR are approved as in vitro diagnostic tests.

Presence of virus by RT-PCR or NS1 antigen in a single diagnostic specimen is considered laboratory confirmation of dengue in patients with a compatible clinical and travel history. IgM in a single serum sample suggests a probable recent dengue infection and should be considered diagnostic for dengue if the infection most likely occurred in a place where other potentially cross-reactive flaviviruses (such as Zika, West Nile, yellow fever, and Japanese encephalitis viruses) are not a risk. If infection is likely to have occurred in a place where other potentially cross-reactive flaviviruses circulate, both molecular and serologic diagnostic testing should be performed to detect evidence of infection with dengue and the other flaviviruses.

IgG by ELISA in a single serum sample is not useful for diagnostic testing because it remains detectable for life after a dengue infection. In addition, people infected with or vaccinated against other flaviviruses (such as yellow fever or Japanese encephalitis) may produce cross-reactive flavivirus antibodies, yielding false-positive serologic dengue diagnostic test results.

Dengue diagnostic testing (molecular and serologic) is available from several commercial reference diagnostic laboratories, state public health laboratories, and CDC (www.cdc.gov/Dengue/clinicalLab/index.html). Consultation on dengue diagnostic testing can be obtained from CDC at 787-706-2399.

TREATMENT

No specific antiviral agents exist for dengue. Patients should be advised to stay well hydrated

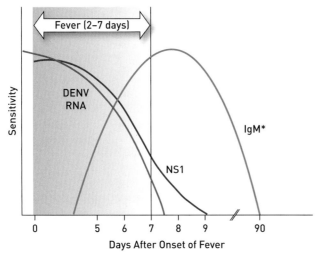

FIGURE 3-1. Relative sensitivity of detection of dengue virus nucleic acid, antigen, and IgM[1]

Abbreviations: DENV, dengue virus; NS1, nonstructural protein 1.

[1] DENV RNA and NS1 are detectable during the first week of illness. Anti-DENV IgM is detectable starting approximately 5 days after illness onset. Although most cases only have detectable IgM anti-DENV for 14–20 days after illness onset, in some cases it may be detectable for up to 90 days. Detection of anti-DENV IgG is neither sensitive nor specific in identifying patients with dengue.

and to avoid aspirin (acetylsalicylic acid), aspirin-containing drugs, and other nonsteroidal anti-inflammatory drugs (such as ibuprofen) because of their anticoagulant properties. Fever should be controlled with acetaminophen and tepid sponge baths. Febrile patients should avoid mosquito bites to reduce risk of further transmission. For those who develop severe dengue, close observation and frequent monitoring in an intensive care unit setting may be required. Prophylactic platelet transfusions in dengue patients are not beneficial and may contribute to fluid overload. Similarly, administration of corticosteroids has no demonstrated benefit and is potentially harmful to patients; corticosteroids should not be used except in the case of autoimmune-related complication (such as hemophagocytic lymphohistiocytosis or immune thrombocytopenia purpura).

PREVENTION

No vaccine is available in the United States, although 1 has been licensed for use in Mexico, the Philippines, Brazil, and Thailand. No prophylaxis is available to prevent dengue. Risk increases with duration of travel and disease incidence in the travel destination (such as during the rainy season and during epidemics). Travelers going to the tropics for any length of time should avoid mosquito bites by taking the following preventive measures:

- Select accommodations with well-screened windows and doors or air conditioning when possible. *Aedes* mosquitoes typically live indoors and are often found in dark, cool places, such as in closets, under beds, behind curtains, in bathrooms, and on porches. Travelers should be advised to use insecticides to get rid of mosquitoes in these areas.

- Wear clothing that covers the arms and legs, especially during the early morning and late afternoon, when risk of being bitten is the highest.

- Use insect repellent (see Chapter 2, Protection against Mosquitoes, Ticks, & Other Arthropods).

- For longer-term travelers, empty and clean or cover any standing water that can be mosquito-breeding sites in the local residence (such as water storage tanks or flower pots).

CDC website: www.cdc.gov/dengue

BIBLIOGRAPHY

1. Barthel A, Gourinat AC, Cazorla C, Joubert C, Dupont-Rouzeyrol M, Descloux E. Breast milk as a possible route of vertical transmission of dengue virus? Clin Infect Dis. 2013 Aug;57(3):415–7.

2. Bhatt S, Gething PW, Brady OJ, Messina JP, Farlow AW, Moyes CL, et al. The global distribution and burden of dengue. Nature. 2013 Apr 25;496(7446):504–7.

3. Guzman MG, Halstead SB, Artsob H, Buchy P, Farrar J, Gubler DJ, et al. Dengue: a continuing global threat. Nat Rev Microbiol. 2010 Dec;8(12 Suppl):S7–16.

4. Leder K, Torresi J, Libman MD, Cramer JP, Castelli F, Schlagenhauf P, et al. GeoSentinel surveillance of illness in returned travelers, 2007–2011. Ann Intern Med. 2013 Mar 19;158(6):456–68.

5. Schwartz E, Weld LH, Wilder-Smith A, von Sonnenburg F, Keystone JS, Kain KC, et al. Seasonality, annual trends, and characteristics of dengue among ill returned travelers, 1997–2006. Emerg Infect Dis. 2008 Jul;14(7):1081–8.

6. Simmons CP, Farrar JJ, van Vinh Chau N, Wills B. Dengue. N Engl J Med. 2012 Apr 12;366(15):1423–32.

7. Srikiatkhachorn A, Rothman AL, Gibbons RV, Sittisombut N, Malasit P, Ennis FA, et al. Dengue—how best to classify it. Clin Infect Dis. 2011 Sep;53(6):563–7.

8. Streit JA, Yang M, Cavanaugh JE, Polgreen PM. Upward trend in dengue incidence among hospitalized patients, United States. Emerg Infect Dis. 2011 May;17(5):914–6.

9. Tomashek KM, Margolis HS. Dengue: a potential transfusion-transmitted disease. Transfusion. 2011 Aug;51(8):1654–60.

10. World Health Organization. Dengue: guidelines for diagnosis, treatment, prevention and control. Geneva: World Health Organization; 2009.

3

DIPHTHERIA

Tejpratap S. P. Tiwari

INFECTIOUS AGENT

Toxigenic strains of *Corynebacterium diphtheriae* biotype *mitis*, *gravis*, *intermedius*, or *belfanti*.

TRANSMISSION

Person-to-person through oral or respiratory droplets, close physical contact, and rarely, by fomites. Cutaneous diphtheria is common in tropical countries, and contact with discharge from skin lesions may transmit infection in these environments.

EPIDEMIOLOGY

Endemic in many countries in Asia, the South Pacific, the Middle East, and Eastern Europe and in Haiti and the Dominican Republic; outbreaks in Indonesia, Thailand, Laos, South Africa, Sudan, and Pakistan have occurred since 2011. Respiratory and cutaneous diphtheria have been reported in travelers, though rare.

CLINICAL PRESENTATION

The incubation period is 2–5 days (range, 1–10 days). Affected anatomic sites include the mucous membrane of the upper respiratory tract (nose, pharynx, tonsils, larynx, and trachea [respiratory diphtheria]), skin (cutaneous diphtheria), or rarely, mucous membranes at other sites (eye, ear, vulva). Nasal diphtheria can be asymptomatic or mild, with a blood-tinged discharge.

Respiratory diphtheria has a gradual onset and is characterized by a mild fever (rarely >101°F [38.3°C]), sore throat, difficulty swallowing, malaise, loss of appetite, and if the larynx is involved, hoarseness. The hallmark of respiratory diphtheria is a pseudomembrane that appears within 2–3 days of illness over the mucous lining of the tonsils, pharynx, larynx, or nares and that can extend into the trachea. The pseudomembrane is firm, fleshy, grey, and adherent; it will bleed after attempts to remove or dislodge it. Fatal airway obstruction can result if the pseudomembrane extends into the larynx or trachea, or if a piece of it becomes dislodged.

DIAGNOSIS

A presumptive diagnosis is usually based on clinical features. Diagnosis is confirmed by isolating

C. diphtheriae from culture of nasal or throat swabs or membrane tissue. Diphtheria is a nationally notifiable disease.

TREATMENT

Patients with respiratory diphtheria require hospitalization to monitor response to treatment and manage complications. Equine diphtheria antitoxin (DAT) is the mainstay of treatment and is administered after specimen testing, without waiting for laboratory confirmation. In the United States, DAT is available to physicians under an investigational new drug protocol by contacting CDC at 770-488-7100.

An antibiotic (erythromycin or penicillin) should be used to eliminate the causative organisms, stop exotoxin production, and reduce communicability. Supportive care (airway, cardiac monitoring) is required. Antimicrobial prophylaxis (erythromycin or penicillin) is recommended for close contacts of patients.

PREVENTION

All travelers should be up-to-date with diphtheria toxoid vaccine before departure. After a childhood primary series and a booster dose during adolescence, routine booster doses with a diphtheria toxoid–containing vaccine given either as Td (tetanus-diphtheria) or Tdap (tetanus-diphtheria-acellular pertussis if not previously given) should be given to all adults every 10 years. This booster is particularly important for travelers who will live or work with local populations in countries where diphtheria is endemic.

CDC website: www.cdc.gov/diphtheria

BIBLIOGRAPHY

1. CDC. Fatal respiratory diphtheria in a US traveler to Haiti–Pennsylvania, 2003. MMWR Morb Mortal Wkly Rep. 2004 Jan 9;52(53):1285–6.
2. CDC. Updated recommendations for use of tetanus toxoid, reduced diphtheria toxoid and acellular pertussis (Tdap) vaccine from the Advisory Committee on Immunization Practices, 2010. MMWR Morb Mortal Wkly Rep. 2011 Jan 14;60(1):13–5.
3. Galazka A. The changing epidemiology of diphtheria in the vaccine era. J Infect Dis. 2000 Feb;181 Suppl 1:S2–9.
4. World Health Organization. Diphtheria vaccine. Wkly Epidemiol Rec. 2006 Jan 20;81(3):24–32.

EBOLA VIRUS DISEASE & MARBURG VIRUS DISEASE

Mary Choi, Barbara Knust

INFECTIOUS AGENT

The family Filoviridae includes viruses of the *Ebolavirus* and *Marburgvirus* genuses, which can cause hemorrhagic fever in humans and nonhuman primates. Five species within the genus *Ebolavirus* have been identified: *Tai Forest ebolavirus* (Taï Forest virus), *Sudan ebolavirus* (Sudan virus), *Zaire ebolavirus* (Ebola virus), *Bundibugyo ebolavirus* (Bundibugyo virus), and *Reston ebolavirus* (Reston virus). *Marburg marburgvirus* is the single species in its genus.

TRANSMISSION

Bats are the suspected reservoir species for the viruses within the genus *Ebolavirus*. Fruit bats (*Rousettus aegypticacus*) are the natural reservoirs for Marburg virus. Outbreaks occur when a person becomes infected after exposure to the reservoir species or a secondarily infected nonhuman primate or antelope species and then transmits the virus to other people in the community. In the community, Ebola virus and Marburg virus are generally transmitted by direct physical contact between unprotected skin or mucous membranes and blood or other infected body fluids of patients in the acute phase of Ebola virus disease (EVD) or Marburg virus disease (MVD) or from patients who have died from EVD or MVD. Aerosol transmission of Ebola virus in humans has not been documented.

After recovery from acute disease, the virus or its RNA persists in some specific body fluids of convalescent EVD or MVD patients. Ebola virus RNA has been detected in breast milk up to 21 days after the onset of the disease and in vaginal secretions up to 33 days after onset. Ebola virus has also been shown to persist in "immune-privileged" sites (such as the central nervous system, eye, testes). Ebola virus and Marburg virus have been cultured from ocular aqueous humor at 2 and 3 months after disease onset, respectively.

Evidence suggests that Ebola and Marbug viruses can be sexually transmitted from a male survivor to his female partner months after onset of disease. In pregnant women with EVD, there can be in utero transmission of Ebola virus to the fetus.

EPIDEMIOLOGY

People at greatest risk of EVD or MVD include family members, health care workers or others who come into direct contact with infected patients or corpses without protective equipment, people who have come into contact or close proximity to bats (visiting bat caves), and those who have handled infected primates or carcasses. Additionally, sexual partners of recent male EVD or MVD survivors may be at risk if they have had contact with virus-infected semen.

Countries where domestically acquired EVD cases have been reported and that should be considered areas where future epidemics could occur include Republic of the Congo, Côte d'Ivoire, Democratic Republic of the Congo, Gabon, Uganda, Guinea, Liberia, and Sierra Leone.

Typically, previous Ebola outbreaks had been limited in scope and geographic extent. However, in March of 2014, an outbreak of Ebola virus was detected in a rural area of Guinea near the border with Liberia and Sierra Leone. By June of 2014, cases were reported in all three countries and across many districts. The outbreak was the largest and most complex Ebola epidemic ever

reported. Additional cases occurred in Nigeria, Senegal, Mali, Spain, the United Kingdom, Italy, and the United States after infected people traveled from West Africa.

Countries with confirmed human cases of Marburg hemorrhagic fever include Uganda, Kenya, Democratic Republic of the Congo, Angola, and possibly Zimbabwe. Four cases of Marburg hemorrhagic fever have occurred in travelers visiting caves harboring bats, including Kitum cave in Kenya and Python cave in Maramagambo Forest, Uganda. Miners in the Democratic Republic of the Congo and Uganda have also acquired Marburg virus infection from working in underground mines harboring bats.

Reston virus is believed to be endemic in the Philippines but has not been shown to cause human disease.

CLINICAL PRESENTATION

The incubation period for EVD and MVD ranges from 2–21 days, although most people develop symptoms after 7–10 days. Signs and symptoms of EVD and MVD can vary but, in general, patients present with an abrupt-onset fever, weakness, myalgias, arthralgias, and headache. This is often followed by gastrointestinal symptoms including anorexia, abdominal discomfort, nausea, vomiting, and diarrhea. Conjunctival injection, rash, and hiccups have also been reported. In the West African EVD epidemic, diarrhea was severe with up to 10 L of output reported per 24 hours. Intravascular volume depletion is common and may be associated with profound electrolyte depletion, hypoprofusion, and shock. Coagulopathy is a late manifestation and can present with a petechial rash, ecchymoses, and sometimes overt bleeding (epistaxis, melena, bloody diarrhea). Hypoxia, another late manifestation, was noted in half of EVD patients (median oxygen saturation 84.5%). Laboratory abnormalities include elevations in liver enzymes, initial drop in leukocyte count, and thrombocytopenia. Because the incubation period may be as long as 21 days, patients may not develop illness until returning from travel; therefore, a thorough travel and exposure history is critical. Fatality ratios for EVD vary, ranging from 19%–90% depending on *Ebolavirus* species and the availability of medical care.

Pregnant women with EVD appear to be at high risk of spontaneous abortions, stillbirth, and pregnancy-related hemorrhage. Limited evidence suggests that the prognosis for neonates born to mothers with EVD is poor, and most die within 19 days of birth.

DIAGNOSIS

US-based clinicians should notify local health authorities immediately of any suspected cases of viral hemorrhagic fevers occurring in patients residing in the United States, or notify the CDC directly regarding any patients requiring evacuation to the United States (contact the CDC Emergency Operations Center at 770-488-7100). Personal protective equipment is indicated for any patients where EVD or MVD is suspected and includes droplet and contact precautions. Whole blood, plasma, or serum may be tested for virologic (RT-PCR, antigen detection, virus isolation) and immunologic (IgM, IgG) evidence of infection. Tissue may be tested by immunohistochemistry, RT-PCR, and virus isolation. Postmortem skin biopsies fixed in formalin and blood collected within a few hours after death by cardiac puncture can be used for diagnosis. Diagnostic testing of blood and other body fluid specimens calls for special handling procedures.

TREATMENT

Currently, there is no proven specific therapy for EVD. The mainstay of treatment is early aggressive supportive care directed at maintaining effective intravascular volume and correcting electrolyte imbalances. Several additional experimental immune therapy treatments and antivirals are currently under investigation. With aggressive supportive care, reported case-fatality ratios were 43% among EVD patients treated in West Africa and 18.5% among patients treated in the United States and Europe. EVD patients may also have concomitant malaria infection. As such, empiric use of antimalarial therapy should be considered when rapid diagnostic testing is not immediately available. In general, NSAIDs such as ibuprofen and diclofenac are not recommended due to their platelet activity.

Currently there is no FDA-approved vaccine to prevent EVD. Experimental Ebola vaccines are under development, including a recombinant vesicular stomatitis virus–based vaccine and a chimpanzee adenovirus–based vaccine. However, these investigational products are in the early stages of product development and are not yet available.

CDC website: www.cdc.gov/vhf/ebola

BIBLIOGRAPHY

1. Bah EI, Lamah MC, Fletcher T, Jacob ST, Brett-Major DM, Sall AA, et al. Clinical presentation of patients with Ebola virus disease in Conakry, Guinea. N Engl J Med. 2015 Jan 1;372(1):40–7.

2. CDC. Ebola virus disease—U.S. healthcare workers and settings—personal protective equipment. 2016 [cited 2016 Sep. 22]. Available from: http://www.cdc.gov/vhf/ebola/healthcare-us/ppe/index.html.

3. Ewer K, Rampling T, Venkatraman N, Bowyer G, Wright D, Lambe T, et al. A monovalent chimpanzee adenovirus Ebola vaccine boosted with MVA. N Engl J Med. 2016 Apr 28;374(17):1635–46.

4. Fallah M. A Cohort study of survivors of Ebola virus infection in Liberia (PREVAIL III). Conference on Retroviruses and Opportunistic Infections; February 22–25, 2016; Boston, Massachusetts.

5. Fields BN, Knipe DM, Howley PM. Fields virology. Philadelphia: Wolters Kluwer Health/Lippincott Williams & Wilkins; 2007.

6. Fowler RA, Fletcher T, Fischer WA, 2nd, Lamontagne F, Jacob S, Brett-Major D, et al. Caring for critically ill patients with Ebola virus disease. Perspectives from West Africa. Am J Respir Crit Care Med. 2014 Oct 1;190(7):733–7.

7. Osterholm MT, Moore KA, Kelley NS, Brosseau LM, Wong G, Murphy FA, et al. Transmission of Ebola viruses: what we know and what we do not know. mBio. 2015;6(2):e00137.

8. Regules JA, Beigel JH, Paolino KM, Voell J, Castellano AR, Munoz P, et al. A Recombinant vesicular stomatitis virus Ebola vaccine—preliminary report. N Engl J Med. 2015 Apr 1. DOI: http://dx.doi.org/10.1056/NEJMoa1414216

9. Uyeki TM, Mehta AK, Davey RT, Jr., Liddell AM, Wolf T, Vetter P, et al. Clinical management of Ebola virus disease in the United States and Europe. N Engl J Med. 2016 Feb 18;374(7):636–46.

10. World Health Organization. Clinical care for survivors of Ebola virus disease. 2016 [cited 2016 Apr. 11]. Available from: http://www.who.int/csr/resources/publications/ebola/guidance-survivors/en/.

ECHINOCOCCOSIS

Pedro L. Moro, Paul T. Cantey

INFECTIOUS AGENT

Larval stages of taeniid cestodes of the genus *Echinococcus*.

TRANSMISSION

Oral contact with contaminated dog feces, particularly in the course of playful and close contact between children and dogs, or through contaminated food or water.

EPIDEMIOLOGY

Echinococcus granulosus is prevalent in broad regions of Eurasia, several South American countries, North and Central America, and Africa. Foci of transmission are found in many other countries. In nonendemic countries, *E. granulosus* is typically seen among immigrants or refugees coming from endemic countries. *E. multilocularis* is endemic in the central part of Europe, parts of the Near East, Russia, the Central Asian Republics, China, northern Japan, northwestern Canada, and Alaska. *E. vogeli* is indigenous to the humid tropical forests in central and northern South America. A small number of polycystic echinococcosis cases in these areas are caused by *E. oligarthrus*.

CLINICAL PRESENTATION

Cystic Echinococcosis or Cystic Hydatid Disease

In humans, hydatid cysts of *E. granulosus* are slowly enlarging masses comparable to benign neoplasms; most human infections remain asymptomatic. Clinical manifestations are determined by the site, size, and condition of the cysts. Hydatid cysts in the liver and the lungs together account for 90% of affected localizations.

Alveolar Echinococcosis or Alveolar Hydatid Disease

The embryo of *E. multilocularis* seems to localize invariably in the liver of the intermediate host (such as wild rodents) and humans. Patients eventually die from hepatic failure, invasion of contiguous structures, or less frequently, metastases to the brain.

Polycystic Echinococcosis or Polycystic Hydatid Disease

Polycystic echinococcosis is usually caused by *E. vogeli* or *E. oligarthrus*. Relatively large cysts develop over years and are primarily found in the liver and occasionally in the thorax or abdominal cavity. Those who are symptomatic may present with a painful right hypochondrial mass, progressive jaundice, or, as in the other forms of disease, liver abscess(es).

DIAGNOSIS

A presumptive diagnosis can be made on the basis of a combination of the individual's history and imaging studies, such as an ultrasound or CT scan. Lesions may be found incidentally in an asymptomatic person. Serologic assays may also be performed, and newer ones are under development. Additional information and diagnostic assistance are available through CDC (www.cdc. gov/dpdx; 404-718-4745; parasites@cdc.gov).

TREATMENT

For cystic echinococcosis, treatment depends on cyst characteristics and cyst type. WHO has developed ultrasound criteria than can assist in determining treatment strategies. Some uncomplicated cysts do not require any treatment. Surgical removal is preferred when cysts are large (>10 cm), secondarily infected, or located in certain organs (brain, lung, or kidney). PAIR (puncture, aspiration, injection, reaspiration) is a minimally invasive technique used to treat some types of cysts in the liver and other abdominal locations. It is less risky and less expensive than surgery. Benzimidazoles (albendazole, mebendazole) should be given to prevent recurrence after surgery or PAIR. Additional percutaneous interventions are sometimes needed. Benzimidazoles may be used to treat small cysts (<5 cm). Albendazole should be given continuously, with no monthly treatment interruptions and in 2 divided doses, with a fat-rich meal to increase its bioavailability. Approximately 30% of patients treated with albendazole are cured after 3–6 months, and even higher proportions (30%–50%) demonstrate regression of cyst size and alleviation of symptoms.

Alveolar hydatid disease may require surgery and long-term albendazole but has a high case-fatality ratio. Praziquantel is used in some circumstances. Management of complex cases may require consultation with a tropical medicine specialist.

PREVENTION
Advise travelers to avoid contact with dogs or wild canids in endemic areas. Also advise them not to drink untreated water from streams, canals, lakes, or rivers and to observe food and water precautions (see Chapter 2, Food & Water Precautions).

CDC website: www.cdc.gov/parasites/ echinococcosis

BIBLIOGRAPHY

1. Brunetti E, Kern P, Vuitton DA. Expert consensus for the diagnosis and treatment of cystic and alveolar echinococcosis in humans. Acta Trop. 2010 Apr;114(1):1–16.

2. Eckert J, Gottstein B, Heath D, Liu FJ. Prevention of echinococcosis in humans and safety precautions. In: Eckert J, Gemmell MA, Meslin FX, Pawlowski ZS, editors. WHO/OIE Manual on Echinococcosis in Humans and Animals: a Public Health Problem of Global Concern. Paris: World Organization for Animal Health; 2001. pp. 238–45.

3. Mandal S, Mandal MD. Human cystic echinococcosis: epidemiologic, zoonotic, clinical, diagnostic and therapeutic aspects. Asian Pac J Trop Med. 2012 Apr;5(4):253–60.

4. McManus DP, Zhang W, Li J, Bartley PB. Echinococcosis. Lancet. 2003 Oct 18;362(9392):1295–304.

5. Moro PL, Schantz PM. Echinococcosis: historical landmarks and progress in research and control. Ann Trop Med Parasitol. 2006 Dec;100(8):703–14.

6. Stojkovic M, Rosenberger K, Kauczor HU, Junghanss T, Hosch W. Diagnosing and staging of cystic echinococcosis: how do CT and MRI perform in comparison to ultrasound? PLoS Negl Trop Dis. 2012;6(10):e1880.

ESCHERICHIA COLI, DIARRHEAGENIC

Ciara E. O'Reilly, Martha Iwamoto, Patricia M. Griffin

INFECTIOUS AGENT
Escherichia coli are gram-negative bacteria that inhabit the gastrointestinal tract. Most strains do not cause illness. Pathogenic *E. coli* are categorized into pathotypes on the basis of their virulence genes. Six pathotypes are associated with diarrhea (diarrheagenic): enterotoxigenic *E. coli* (ETEC), Shiga toxin–producing *E. coli* (STEC), enteropathogenic *E. coli* (EPEC), enteroaggregative *E. coli* (EAEC), enteroinvasive *E. coli* (EIEC), and possibly diffusely adherent *E. coli* (DAEC). Other pathotypes that are common causes of urinary tract infections, bloodstream infections, and meningitis are not covered here. Serotypes of *E. coli* are determined by surface antigens (O and H), and specific serotypes tend to cluster within specific pathotypes. Some *E. coli* have virulence factors of more than 1 pathotype. An example is the O104:H4 strain that caused an outbreak in Germany in 2011; it produced Shiga toxin and had adherence properties typical of EAEC.

STEC are also called verotoxigenic *E. coli* (VTEC), and the term enterohemorrhagic *E. coli* (EHEC) is commonly used to specify STEC strains capable of causing human illness, especially bloody diarrhea and hemolytic uremic syndrome (HUS).

TRANSMISSION

Diarrheagenic pathotypes can be passed in the feces of humans and other animals. Transmission occurs through the fecal-oral route, primarily via contaminated food or water and also through person-to-person contact and contact with animals or their environment. People constitute the main reservoir for non-STEC pathotypes that cause diarrhea in humans. The intestinal tracts of animals, especially cattle and other ruminants, are the primary reservoirs of STEC.

EPIDEMIOLOGY

Travel to less-developed countries is associated with higher risk for travelers' diarrhea, including some types of *E. coli* infection. ETEC is the most common pathotype that causes diarrhea among travelers returning from most regions. Travel-associated infections caused by non-STEC diarrheagenic *E. coli* are likely underrecognized because most clinical laboratories do not use methods that can detect them. Risk of non-STEC diarrheagenic *E. coli* infections (primarily ETEC) can be divided into 3 grades, according to the destination country:

- Low-risk countries include the United States, Canada, Australia, New Zealand, Japan, and countries in Northern and Western Europe.

- Intermediate-risk countries include those in Eastern Europe, South Africa, and some of the Caribbean islands.

- High-risk areas include most of Asia, the Middle East, Africa, Mexico, and Central and South America.

STEC infections are more commonly reported in industrialized countries than in less-developed countries. Additional information about travelers' diarrhea is available in Chapter 2, Travelers' Diarrhea.

CLINICAL PRESENTATION

Where information is available, non-STEC diarrheagenic *E. coli* infections have an incubation period ranging from 9 hours to 3 days. The median incubation period of STEC infections is 3–4 days, with a range of 1–10 days. The clinical manifestations of diarrheagenic *E. coli* vary by pathotype (Table 3-1).

DIAGNOSIS

Many patients with travel-associated *E. coli* infections, especially those with nonbloody diarrhea, as commonly occurs with ETEC infection, are likely to be managed symptomatically and are unlikely to have the diagnosis confirmed by a laboratory. Most US clinical laboratories do not use tests that can detect diarrheagenic *E. coli* other than STEC, although recently approved nucleic acid amplification tests that can detect ETEC are now available in some clinical laboratories. Testing for non-STEC pathotypes is typically done at public health laboratories and only when an outbreak of diarrheal illness of unknown origin is being investigated. In this situation, isolates may be submitted via state health departments to CDC for testing. These tests typically involve PCR testing or whole genome sequence analysis for the specific virulence genes of ETEC, EPEC, EAEC, EIEC, and DAEC.

When a decision is made to identify a cause of an acute diarrheal illness, in addition to routine culture for *Salmonella*, *Shigella*, and *Campylobacter*, the stool sample should be cultured for *E. coli* O157:H7 and simultaneously assayed for non-O157 STEC with a test that detects Shiga toxins (or the genes that encode them). For more information, see www.cdc.gov/mmwr/preview/mmwrhtml/rr5812a1.htm. All presumptive *E. coli* O157 isolates and Shiga toxin–positive specimens should be sent to a public health laboratory for further characterization. Rapid, accurate diagnosis of STEC infection is important, because early clinical management decisions can affect patient outcomes, and early detection can help prevent secondary spread.

TREATMENT

Patients with profuse diarrhea or vomiting should be rehydrated. Evidence from studies of children with STEC O157 infection indicates that early use of intravenous fluids (within the first 4 days of diarrhea onset) may decrease the

Table 3-1. Mechanism of pathogenesis and typical clinical syndrome of *Escherichia coli* pathotypes

PATHOTYPE	MECHANISM OF PATHOGENESIS	TYPICAL CLINICAL SYNDROME
ETEC	Small bowel adherence; heat-stable or heat-labile enterotoxin production	Acute watery diarrhea, afebrile, occasionally severe
EAEC	Small and large bowel adherence mediated via various adhesions and accessory proteins; enterotoxin and cytotoxin production	Watery diarrhea with mucous, occasionally bloody; can cause prolonged or persistent diarrhea in children
EPEC	Small bowel adherence and epithelial cell effacement mediated by intimin	Severe acute watery diarrhea; may be persistent; common cause of infant diarrhea in developing countries
EIEC	Mucosal invasion and inflammation of large bowel	Watery diarrhea that may progress to bloody diarrhea (dysenterylike syndrome), fever
DAEC	Diffuse adherence to epithelial cells	Watery diarrhea but pathogenicity not conclusively demonstrated
STEC	Large bowel adherence mediated via intimin; Shiga toxin 1, Shiga toxin 2 production	Watery diarrhea that progresses (often for STEC O157, less often for non-O157) to bloody diarrhea in 1–3 days; abdominal cramps and tenderness; if fever present, low-grade; hemolytic uremic syndrome complicates ≈6% of STEC O157 and ≈1% of non-O157 infections

Abbreviations: ETEC, enterotoxigenic *E. coli*; EAEC, enteroaggregative *E. coli*; EPEC, enteropathogenic *E. coli*; EIEC, enteroinvasive *E. coli*; DAEC, diffusely adherent *E. coli*; STEC, Shiga toxin–producing *E. coli*.

risk of oligoanuric renal failure. Antibiotics to treat non-STEC diarrheagenic *E. coli* include fluoroquinolones such as ciprofloxacin, macrolides such as azithromycin, and rifaximin. Clinicians treating a patient whose clinical syndrome suggests STEC infection (Table 3-1) should be aware that administering antimicrobial agents may increase the risk of HUS. Resistance to antibiotics is increasing worldwide. The decision to use an antibiotic should be carefully weighed against the severity of illness, the possibility that the pathogen is resistant, and the risk of adverse reactions, such as rash, antibiotic-associated colitis, and vaginal yeast infection. Antimotility agents should be avoided in patients with bloody diarrhea and patients with STEC infection, because these agents may increase the risk of complications, including toxic megacolon, HUS, and neurologic complications. (See Chapter 2, Travelers' Diarrhea and Chapter 7, Traveling Safely with Infants & Children for information about managing travelers' diarrhea in children.)

PREVENTION

There is no vaccine for *E. coli* infection, nor are any medications recommended for prevention. Taking antibiotics can adversely affect the intestinal microbiota and increase susceptibility to gut infections. Food and water are primary sources of *E. coli* infection, so travelers should be reminded of the importance of adhering to food and water precautions (see Chapter 2, Food & Water Precautions). People who may be exposed to livestock, especially ruminants, should be instructed about the importance of handwashing in preventing infection. Because soap and water may not be readily available in at-risk areas, travelers should consider taking hand sanitizer that contains ≥60% alcohol. During *E. coli* outbreaks, clinicians should alert people traveling to affected areas and be cognizant of possible infections among returning travelers.

CDC website: www.cdc.gov/ecoli

BIBLIOGRAPHY

1. CDC. Outbreak of *Escherichia coli* O104:H4 infections associated with sprout consumption—Europe and North America, May-July 2011. MMWR Morb Mortal Wkly Rep. 2013 Dec. 20, 2013;62(50):1029–31.

2. DuPont HL. Systematic review: the epidemiology and clinical features of travellers' diarrhoea. Aliment Pharmacol Ther. 2009 Aug;30(3):187–96.

3. Hedican EB, Medus C, Besser JM, Juni BA, Koziol B, Taylor C, et al. Characteristics of O157 versus non-O157 Shiga toxin-producing *Escherichia coli* infections in Minnesota, 2000–2006. Clin Infect Dis. 2009 Aug 1;49(3):358–64.

4. Hickey CA, Beattie TJ, Cowieson J, Miyashita Y, Strife CF, Frem JC, et al. Early volume expansion during diarrhea and relative nephroprotection during subsequent hemolytic uremic syndrome. Arch Pediatr Adolesc Med. 2011 Oct;165(10):884–9.

5. Kaper JB, Nataro JP, Mobley HL. Pathogenic *Escherichia coli*. Nat Rev Microbiol. 2004 Feb;2(2):123–40.

6. Kendall ME, Crim S, Fullerton K, Han PV, Cronquist AB, Shiferaw B, et al. Travel-associated enteric infections diagnosed after return to the United States, Foodborne Diseases Active Surveillance Network (FoodNet), 2004–2009. Clin Infect Dis. 2012 Jun;54 Suppl 5:S480–7.

7. Mintz ED. Enterotoxigenic *Escherichia coli*: outbreak surveillance and molecular testing. Clin Infect Dis. 2006 Jun 1;42(11):1518–20.

8. Ouyang-Latimer J, Jafri S, VanTassel A, Jiang ZD, Gurleen K, Rodriguez S, et al. In vitro antimicrobial susceptibility of bacterial enteropathogens isolated from international travelers to Mexico, Guatemala, and India from 2006–2008. Antimicrob Agents Chemother. 2011 Feb;55(2):874–8.

9. Shah N, DuPont HL, Ramsey DJ. Global etiology of travelers' diarrhea: systematic review from 1973 to the present. Am J Trop Med Hyg. 2009 Apr;80(4):609–14.

10. Wong CS, Mooney JC, Brandt JR, Staples AO, Jelacic S, Boster DR, et al. Risk factors for the hemolytic uremic syndrome in children infected with *Escherichia coli* O157:H7: a multivariable analysis. Clin Infect Dis. 2012 Jul;55(1):33–41.

FASCIOLIASIS

LeAnne M. Fox

INFECTIOUS AGENT

Trematode flatworms *Fasciola hepatica* and *F. gigantica*.

TRANSMISSION

Consumption of watercress or other aquatic plants contaminated with infective metacercariae or contaminated freshwater.

EPIDEMIOLOGY

Broadly distributed. The highest rates of *F. hepatica* infection have been reported from Bolivia, Peru, Egypt, Iran, Portugal, and France. *F. gigantica* has a more limited distribution (parts of Africa, the Middle East, and South and East Asia).

CLINICAL PRESENTATION

The acute phase begins 6–12 weeks after exposure and can last up to 4 months. Most infected people are asymptomatic, but findings might include marked eosinophilia, abdominal pain, intermittent high fever, weight loss, or urticaria. Within weeks to months, symptoms of the acute phase subside as worms enter the bile ducts, beginning the chronic phase. Chronically infected people in this phase may also be asymptomatic or may present with biliary colic, epigastric pain, nausea, jaundice, or pruritus. The long-term prognosis depends on the extent of the liver and biliary damage.

DIAGNOSIS

Detection of eggs in stool or duodenal or biliary aspirates. Serologic tests may be useful during the acute phase, since egg production does not start until 3–4 months after exposure. Serologic testing is available through CDC (www.cdc.gov/dpdx; 404-718-4745; parasites@cdc.gov). Radiologic examinations, including ultrasonogram and CT of the liver, can be helpful, especially during the hepatic or migratory acute phase.

TREATMENT

First-line treatment is with triclabendazole, which is not commercially available for human use in the United States; it is available to US-licensed physicians through the CDC Drug Service, under a special protocol, which requires both CDC and FDA to agree that the drug is indicated for treatment of a particular patient (404-718-4745; parasites@cdc.gov). An alternative drug is nitazoxanide. Surgical resection or endoscopic retrograde cholangiopancreatographic removal of adult flukes can be done in cases with biliary tract obstruction.

PREVENTION

Avoid eating uncooked aquatic plants, including watercress, especially from endemic grazing areas; avoid drinking untreated freshwater.

CDC website: www.cdc.gov/parasites/fasciola

BIBLIOGRAPHY

1. Garcia HH, Moro PL, Schantz PM. Zoonotic helminth infections of humans: echinococcosis, cysticercosis and fascioliasis. Curr Opin Infect Dis. 2007 Oct;20(5):489–94.

2. Mas-Coma S, Bargues MD, Valero MA. Fascioliasis and other plant-borne trematode zoonoses. Int J Parasitol. 2005 Oct;35(11-12):1255–78.

3. Rowan SE, Levi ME, Youngwerth JM, Brauer B, Everson GT, Johnson SC. The variable presentations and broadening geographic distribution of hepatic fascioliasis. Clin Gastroenterol Hepatol. 2012 Jun;10(6):598–602.

FILARIASIS, LYMPHATIC

LeAnne M. Fox

INFECTIOUS AGENT

Filarial nematodes *Wuchereria bancrofti*, *Brugia malayi*, and *B. timori*.

TRANSMISSION

Through the bite of infected *Aedes*, *Culex*, *Anopheles*, and *Mansonia* mosquitoes.

EPIDEMIOLOGY

Found in sub-Saharan Africa, Egypt, southern Asia, the western Pacific Islands, the northeastern coast of Brazil, Guyana, Haiti, and the Dominican Republic. Travelers are at low risk, although infection has been documented in long-term travelers. Most infections are seen in immigrants and refugees.

CLINICAL PRESENTATION

Most infections are asymptomatic, but lymphatic dysfunction may lead to lymphedema of the leg, scrotum, penis, arm, or breast years after infection. Acute episodes in people with lymphatic dysfunction are associated with painful swelling of an affected limb, fever, or chills due to bacterial superinfection. Tropical pulmonary eosinophilia is a potentially serious progressive lung disease that presents with nocturnal cough, wheezing, and fever, resulting from immune hyperresponsiveness to microfilariae in the pulmonary capillaries.

DIAGNOSIS

Microscopic detection of microfilariae on an appropriately timed thick blood film. Determination of serum antifilarial IgG is also a diagnostically useful test. This assay is available through the Parasitic Diseases Laboratory at the National Institutes of Health (301-496-5398) or through CDC (www.cdc.gov/dpdx; 404-718-4745; parasites@cdc.gov). Microfilariae are usually not detected in patients with tropical pulmonary eosinophilia. Diagnosis requires epidemiologic risk and filarial antibody testing.

TREATMENT

The drug of choice, diethylcarbamazine, can be obtained from CDC under an investigational new drug protocol. Patients with lymphedema and hydrocele can benefit from lymphedema management and, in the case of hydrocele, surgical repair. There is evidence that a 4- to 8- week course of doxycycline (200 mg daily) can both sterilize adult worms and improve lymphatic pathologic features.

BIBLIOGRAPHY

1. Debrah AY, Mand S, Specht S, Marfo-Debrekyei Y, Batsa L, Pfarr K, et al. Doxycycline reduces plasma VEGF-C/sVEGFR-3 and improves pathology in lymphatic filariasis. PLoS pathogens. 2006 Sep;2(9):e92.

2. Eberhard ML, Lammie PJ. Laboratory diagnosis of filariasis. Clin Lab Med. 1991 Dec;11(4):977–1010.

3. Lipner EM, Law MA, Barnett E, Keystone JS, von Sonnenburg F, Loutan L, et al. Filariasis in travelers presenting to the GeoSentinel Surveillance Network. PLoS Negl Trop Dis. 2007;1(3):e88.

4. Magill AJ, Ryan ET, Hill DR, Solomon T. Hunter's Tropical Medicine and Emerging Infectious Diseases. 9th ed. New York: Elsevier Inc.; 2013.

5. Taylor MJ, Makunde WH, McGarry HF, Turner JD, Mand S, Hoerauf A. Macrofilaricidal activity after doxycycline treatment of Wuchereria bancrofti: a double-blind, randomised placebo-controlled trial. Lancet. 2005 Jun 18-24;365(9477):2116–21.

PREVENTION

Mosquito precautions (see Chapter 2, Protection against Mosquitoes, Ticks, & Other Arthropods).

CDC website: www.cdc.gov/parasites/lymphaticfilariasis

GIARDIASIS

Kathleen E. Fullerton, Jonathan S. Yoder

INFECTIOUS AGENT

The anaerobic protozoan parasite *Giardia intestinalis* (formerly known as *G. lamblia* or *G. duodenalis*).

TRANSMISSION

Giardia is transmitted via the fecal-oral route. Its low infectious dose, protracted communicability, and moderate chlorine tolerance make *Giardia* ideally suited for transmission through drinking and recreational water. Transmission also occurs through person-to-person contact, such as caring for an infected person, through sexual contact, through eating food contaminated by infected food handlers or by contaminated water used for irrigation or washing food, and by contact with fecally contaminated surfaces.

EPIDEMIOLOGY

Giardia is endemic worldwide. *Giardia*-related acute diarrhea was a top 10 diagnosis in ill US travelers returning from the Caribbean, Middle East, Eastern Europe, Central America, South America, North Africa, sub-Saharan Africa, and South-Central Asia. The risk of infection increases with duration of travel. Backpackers or campers who drink untreated water from lakes or rivers are also more likely to be infected. *Giardia* is commonly identified in routine screening of refugees and internationally adopted children, although many are asymptomatic.

CLINICAL PRESENTATION

Many infected are asymptomatic, though if symptoms develop, they typically develop 1–2 weeks after infection and generally resolve within 2–4 weeks. Symptoms include diarrhea (often with foul-smelling, greasy stools), abdominal cramps, bloating, flatulence, fatigue, anorexia, and nausea. Usually, a patient presents with the gradual onset of 2–5 loose stools per day and gradually increasing fatigue. Sometimes upper gastrointestinal symptoms are more prominent. Weight loss may occur over time. Fever and vomiting are uncommon. Reactive arthritis, irritable bowel syndrome, and other chronic symptoms sometimes occur after infection with *Giardia* (see Chapter 5, Persistent Travelers' Diarrhea).

DIAGNOSIS

Giardia cysts or trophozoites are not consistently seen in the stools of infected patients. Diagnostic yield can be increased by examining up to 3 stool samples over several days. Direct fluorescent antibody testing is extremely sensitive and specific. Rapid immunochromatographic cartridge assays also are available but should not take the place of routine ova and parasite examination. Only molecular testing (such as PCR) can be used to identify the subtypes of *Giardia*. Retesting is only recommended if symptoms persist after treatment. Giardiasis is a nationally notifiable disease.

TREATMENT

Effective treatments include metronidazole, tinidazole, and nitazoxanide. An alternative is paromomycin. Because making a definitive diagnosis is difficult, empiric treatment can be used in patients with the appropriate history and typical symptoms.

PREVENTION

Food and water precautions (see Chapter 2, Food & Water Precautions and Water Disinfection for Travelers) and hand hygiene.

CDC website: www.cdc.gov/parasites/giardia

BIBLIOGRAPHY

1. Abramowicz M, editor. Drugs for Parasitic Infections. New Rochelle (NY): The Medical Letter, Inc.; 2013.
2. Adam EA, Yoder JS, Gould LH, Hlavsa MC, Gargano JW. Giardiasis outbreaks in the United States, 1971–2011. Epidemiol Infect. 2016 Oct;144(13):2790–801.
3. Cantey PT, Roy S, Lee B, Cronquist A, Smith K, Liang J, et al. Study of nonoutbreak giardiasis: novel findings and implications for research. Am J Med. 2011 Dec;124(12):1175 e1–8.
4. Escobedo AA, Cimerman S. Giardiasis: a pharmacotherapy review. Expert Opin Pharmacother. 2007 Aug;8(12):1885–902.
5. Hagmann SH, Han PV, Stauffer WM, Miller AO, Connor BA, Hale DC, et al. Travel-associated disease among US residents visiting US GeoSentinel clinics after return from international travel. Fam Pract. 2014 Dec;31(6):678–87.
6. Harvey K, Esposito DH, Han P, Kozarsky P, Freedman DO, Plier DA, et al. Surveillance for travel-related disease—GeoSentinel Surveillance System, United States, 1997–2011. MMWR Surveill Summ. 2013 Jul 19;62:1–23.
7. Johnston SP, Ballard MM, Beach MJ, Causer L, Wilkins PP. Evaluation of three commercial assays for detection of giardia and cryptosporidium organisms in fecal specimens. J Clin Microbiol. 2003 Feb;41(2):623–6.
8. Ross AG, Cripps AW. Enteropathogens and chronic illness in returning travelers. N Engl J Med. 2013 Aug 22;369(8):784.
9. Staat MA, Rice M, Donauer S, Mukkada S, Holloway M, Cassedy A, et al. Intestinal parasite screening in internationally adopted children: importance of multiple stool specimens. Pediatrics. 2011 Sep;128(3):e613–22.
10. Swaminathan A, Torresi J, Schlagenhauf P, Thursky K, Wilder-Smith A, Connor BA, et al. A global study of pathogens and host risk factors associated with infectious gastrointestinal disease in returned international travellers. J Infect. 2009 Jul;59(1):19–27.

HAND, FOOT, & MOUTH DISEASE

Eileen Schneider

INFECTIOUS AGENT

In the United States, coxsackievirus A16 is most commonly detected, but other enteroviruses (such as coxsackievirus A10) can cause hand, foot, and mouth disease. In the past few years, coxsackievirus A6 has been detected in outbreaks. Internationally, enterovirus 71 is a common etiologic agent.

TRANSMISSION

Person-to-person, through contact with saliva, nose and throat secretions, fluid in blisters, or stool of an infected person.

EPIDEMIOLOGY

A common illness in young children, with worldwide distribution. Recent large outbreaks have been reported in Cambodia, China, Japan, Korea, Malaysia, Singapore, Thailand, Taiwan, and Vietnam.

CLINICAL PRESENTATION

Incubation period is 4–6 days. Patients usually present with fever and malaise, followed by sore throat and the development of vesicles in the mouth and a rash, often vesicular, on the hands (palms) and feet (soles). In some cases, the rash may be more widespread. Lesions usually resolve in 1 week, but rare complications can include aseptic meningitis and encephalitis.

BIBLIOGRAPHY

1. CDC. Notes from the field: severe hand, foot, and mouth disease associated with coxsackievirus A6—Alabama, Connecticut, California, and Nevada, November 2011–February 2012. MMWR Morb Mortal Wkly Rep. 2012 Mar 30;61(12):213–4.
2. Ooi MH, Wong SC, Lewthwaite P, Cardosa MJ, Solomon T. Clinical features, diagnosis, and

management of enterovirus 71. Lancet Neurol. 2010 Nov;9(11):1097–105.
3. World Health Organization. A guide to clinical management and public health response for hand, foot and mouth disease (HFMD). Geneva: World Health Organization; 2011 [cited 2016 Sep. 23]. Available from: http://www.wpro.who.int/publications/docs/GuidancefortheclinicalmanagementofHFMD.pdf.

DIAGNOSIS

Diagnosis is most often made clinically. Laboratory testing (such as PCR) is available and is usually performed on atypical or severe cases.

TREATMENT

Supportive care.

PREVENTION

Avoiding close contact with infected people, maintaining good hand hygiene, and disinfecting potentially contaminated surfaces, including toys.

CDC website: www.cdc.gov/hand-foot-mouth

3

HELICOBACTER PYLORI

Ronnie Henry, Bradley A. Connor

INFECTIOUS AGENT

Helicobacter pylori is a small, curved, microaerophilic, gram-negative, rod-shaped bacterium.

TRANSMISSION

Believed to be mainly fecal-oral or possibly oral-oral.

EPIDEMIOLOGY

About two-thirds of the world's population is infected, but it is more common in developing countries.

CLINICAL PRESENTATION

Usually asymptomatic, but *H. pylori* is the major cause of peptic ulcer disease and gastritis worldwide, which present as gnawing or

burning epigastric pain. Less commonly, symptoms include nausea, vomiting, or loss of appetite. Infected people have a 2- to 6-fold increased risk of developing gastric cancer and mucosal-associated-lymphoid-type (MALT) lymphoma compared with their uninfected counterparts.

DIAGNOSIS

Fecal antigen assay, urea breath test, rapid urease test, or histology of biopsy specimen. A positive serology indicates present or past infection.

TREATMENT

Asymptomatic infections do not need to be treated. Patients with active duodenal or gastric ulcers should be treated if they are infected. Treatment should be determined on an individual basis. Standard treatments are clarithromycin triple therapy (proton pump inhibitor [PPI] + clarithromycin + amoxicillin or metronidazole) or bismuth quadruple therapy (PPI or H$_2$-blocker + bismuth + metronidazole + tetracycline). See www.acg.gi.org/physicians/guidelines/ManagementofHpylori.pdf.

PREVENTION
No specific recommendations.

BIBLIOGRAPHY

1. Chey WD, Wong BC. American College of Gastroenterology guideline on the management of *Helicobacter pylori* infection. Am J Gastroenterol. 2007 Aug;102(8):1808–25.

2. Lindkvist P, Wadstrom T, Giesecke J. *Helicobacter pylori* infection and foreign travel. J Infect Dis. 1995 Oct;172(4):1135–6.

3. Peterson WL, Fendrick AM, Cave DR, Peura DA, Garabedian-Ruffalo SM, Laine L. *Helicobacter pylori*-related disease: guidelines for testing and treatment. Arch Intern Med. 2000 May 8;160(9): 1285–91.

HELMINTHS, SOIL-TRANSMITTED
Christine Dubray

INFECTIOUS AGENTS
Ascaris lumbricoides (roundworm), *Ancylostoma duodenale* (hookworm), *Necator americanus* (hookworm), and *Trichuris trichiura* (whipworm) are helminths (parasitic worms) that infect the intestine and are transmitted via contaminated soil.

TRANSMISSION
Eggs are passed in feces from an infected person. Infection with roundworm and whipworm occurs when eggs in soil have become infective and are ingested. Hookworm infection (see the Cutaneous Larva Migrans section) usually occurs when larvae penetrate the skin of people walking barefoot on contaminated soil. One kind of hookworm (*Ancylostoma duodenale*) can also be transmitted when larvae are ingested.

EPIDEMIOLOGY
A large part of the world's population is infected with 1 or more of these helminths, but the prevalence is highest in tropical and subtropical countries where water supplies and sanitation are poor. Travelers to these countries should be at low risk of infection if preventive measures are taken. Infections in the United States are typically seen in immigrant and refugee populations. Since these worms do not multiply in hosts, reinfection occurs only as a result of multiple contacts with the infective stages.

CLINICAL PRESENTATION
Most infections are asymptomatic, especially when few worms are present. Pulmonary symptoms occur in a small percentage of patients when roundworm larvae pass through the lungs. Roundworm can also cause intestinal discomfort, obstruction, and impaired nutritional status. Hookworm infection can lead to anemia due to blood loss and chronic protein deficiency. Whipworm infection can cause chronic abdominal pain, diarrhea, blood loss, dysentery, and rectal prolapse. However, travelers are rarely at risk because these more severe manifestations are generally associated with high worm burdens seen in indigenous populations.

DIAGNOSIS
The standard method for diagnosing soil-transmitted helminths is by identifying eggs in a stool specimen using a microscope.

TREATMENT

The drugs most commonly used are albendazole and mebendazole. Mebendazole is available in the United States only through compounding pharmacies.

PREVENTION

Food and water precautions (see Chapter 2, Food & Water Precautions). To avoid hookworm infection, travelers should not walk barefoot in areas where hookworm is common and where there may be human fecal contamination of the soil. In general, avoid ingesting soil that may be contaminated with human feces, including where human fecal matter or wastewater is used to fertilize crops.

CDC website: www.cdc.gov/parasites/sth

BIBLIOGRAPHY

1. Bethony J, Brooker S, Albonico M, Geiger SM, Loukas A, Diemert D, et al. Soil-transmitted helminth infections: ascariasis, trichuriasis, and hookworm. Lancet. 2006 May 6;367(9521):1521–32.

2. Brooker S, Bundy DAP. Soil-transmitted helminths (geohelminths). In: Cook GC, Zumla A, editors. Manson's Tropical Diseases. 22nd ed. London: Saunders; 2009. pp. 1515–48.

3. Brooker S, Clements AC, Bundy DA. Global epidemiology, ecology and control of soil-transmitted helminth infections. Adv Parasitol. 2006;62:221–61.

HEPATITIS A

Noele P. Nelson

INFECTIOUS AGENT

Hepatitis A virus (HAV) is a nonenveloped RNA virus classified as a picornavirus. HAV can survive in the environment for prolonged periods at low pH and in freezing to moderate temperatures.

TRANSMISSION

HAV is transmitted through direct person-to-person contact (fecal-oral transmission); contaminated water, ice, or shellfish harvested from sewage-contaminated water; or from contaminated raw, inadequately cooked, or frozen fruits, vegetables, or other foods. HAV is shed in the feces of infected people. People are most infectious 1–2 weeks before the onset of clinical signs and symptoms (jaundice or elevation of liver enzymes), when the concentration of virus is highest in the stool and blood. Viral excretion and the risk of transmission diminish rapidly after liver dysfunction or symptoms appear, which is concurrent with the appearance of circulating antibodies to HAV. Infants and children can shed virus for up to 6 months after infection.

EPIDEMIOLOGY

HAV is common in areas with inadequate sanitation and limited access to clean water. In highly endemic areas (such as parts of Africa and Asia), a large proportion of adults in the population are immune to HAV, and epidemics of hepatitis A are uncommon. In areas of intermediate endemicity (such as Central and South America, Eastern Europe, and parts of Asia), childhood transmission is less frequent, more adolescents and adults are susceptible to infection, and outbreaks are common. In areas of low endemicity (such as the United States and Western Europe), infection is less common, but disease occurs among people in high-risk groups and as communitywide outbreaks.

Hepatitis A is among the most common vaccine-preventable infections acquired during travel. In the United States the most frequently identified risk factors for hepatitis A are international travel and exposure to contaminated food. Cases of travel-related hepatitis A can occur in travelers to developing countries with "standard" tourist itineraries, accommodations, and eating behaviors. Risk is highest for those who live in or visit rural areas, trek in backcountry areas, or frequently eat or drink in settings of poor sanitation. Common source food exposures are increasingly recognized as a risk for hepatitis A, and sporadic outbreaks are reported in Europe, Australia, North America, and other regions with low levels of endemic transmission.

CLINICAL PRESENTATION

The incubation period averages 28 days (range, 15–50 days). Infection can be asymptomatic or range in severity from a mild illness lasting 1–2 weeks to a severely disabling disease lasting several months. Clinical manifestations include the abrupt onset of fever, malaise, anorexia, nausea, and abdominal discomfort, followed within a few days by jaundice. The likelihood of having symptoms with HAV infection is related to the age of the infected person. In children aged <6 years, most (70%) infections are asymptomatic; jaundice is uncommon in symptomatic young children. Among older children and adults, the illness usually lasts <2 months, although approximately 10%–15% of infected people have prolonged or relapsing symptoms over a 6- to 9-month period. Severe hepatic and extrahepatic complications, including fulminant hepatitis and liver failure, are rare but more common in older adults and people with underlying liver disease. Chronic infection does not occur. The overall case-fatality ratio is 0.3%; however, the ratio is 1.8% among adults aged >50 years.

DIAGNOSIS

HAV cannot be differentiated from other types of viral hepatitis on the basis of clinical or epidemiologic features. Diagnosis requires a positive test for antibody to HAV (anti-HAV) IgM in serum, detectable from 2 weeks before the onset of symptoms to approximately 6 months afterward.

Serologic tests for total anti-HAV (IgG and IgM) are available commercially. A positive total anti-HAV result and a negative IgM anti-HAV result indicate past infection or vaccination and immunity. The presence of serum IgM anti-HAV usually indicates current or recent infection and does not distinguish between immunity from infection and vaccination. Acute hepatitis A is a nationally notifiable disease.

TREATMENT

Supportive care.

PREVENTION

Vaccination or immune globulin (IG), food and water precautions, maintaining standards of hygiene and sanitation.

Vaccine

Two monovalent hepatitis A vaccines, Vaqta (Merck & Co, Inc, Whitehouse Station, NJ) and Havrix (GlaxoSmithKline Beecham Biologicals, Rixensart, Belgium), are approved for people ≥12 months of age in a 2-dose series, and a combined hepatitis A and hepatitis B (Twinrix, GlaxoSmithKline) vaccine is approved for people ≥18 years of age in the United States (Table 3-2). The immunogenicity of the combination vaccine is equivalent to that of the monovalent hepatitis A and hepatitis B vaccines when tested after completion of the recommended schedule.

INDICATIONS FOR USE

All susceptible people traveling for any purpose, frequency, or duration to countries with high or intermediate HAV endemicity should be vaccinated or receive IG before departure. Although the Advisory Committee for Immunization Practices recommends hepatitis A vaccination for travelers, published maps may not be the best guide for determining endemicity in developing countries. Prevalence patterns of HAV infection vary among regions within a country, and missing or obsolete data present a challenge. Countries where the prevalence of HAV infection is decreasing have growing numbers of susceptible people and risk for large outbreaks of hepatitis A. In recent years, large outbreaks of hepatitis A were reported in developed countries among people who had been exposed to imported food

Table 3-2. Vaccines to prevent hepatitis A

VACCINE	TRADE NAME (MANUFACTURER)	AGE (Y)	DOSE	ROUTE	SCHEDULE	BOOSTER
Hepatitis A vaccine, inactivated	Havrix (GlaxoSmithKline)	1–18	0.5 mL (720 ELU)	IM	0, 6–12 mo	None
		≥19	1.0 mL (1,440 ELU)	IM	0, 6–12 mo	None
Hepatitis A vaccine, inactivated	Vaqta (Merck & Co., Inc.)	1–18	0.5 mL (25 U)	IM	0, 6–18 mo	None
		≥19	1.0 mL (50 U)	IM	0, 6–18 mo	None
Combined hepatitis A and B vaccine	Twinrix (GlaxoSmithKline)	≥18 (primary)	1.0 mL (720 ELU HAV + 20 µg HBsAg)	IM	0, 1, 6 mo	None
		≥18 (accelerated)	same as above	IM	0, 7, 21–30 d	12 mo

Abbreviations: ELU, ELISA units of inactivated HAV; IM, intramuscular; U, units HAV antigen; HAV, hepatitis A virus; HBsAg, hepatitis B surface antigen.

contaminated with HAV. Taking into account the complexity of interpreting hepatitis A risk maps and potential risk of foodborne hepatitis A in countries with low endemicity, some experts advise people traveling outside the United States to consider hepatitis A vaccination regardless of destination.

Vaccination is recommended for unvaccinated household members and other people who anticipate close personal contact (such as household contacts or regular babysitters) with an international adoptee from a country of high or intermediate endemicity during the 60 days after arrival of the child in the United States. The first dose of the 2-dose hepatitis A vaccine series should be administered as soon as adoption is planned, ideally ≥2 weeks before the arrival of the child (see Chapter 7, International Adoption).

VACCINE ADMINISTRATION

One dose of a monovalent hepatitis A vaccine protects most healthy people aged 1–40 years and should be administered as soon as travel is considered. The monovalent vaccine series should be completed according to the licensed schedule for long-term protection. No data on single-dose hepatitis A vaccine efficacy are available for Twinrix. An alternate, accelerated 4-dose schedule is available for Twinrix; doses can be administered at 0, 7, and 21–30 days, followed by a dose at 12 months.

Hepatitis A vaccine at the age-appropriate dose is preferred to IG for children and adults aged 1–40 years. For optimal protection, adults aged >40 years, immunocompromised people, and people with chronic liver disease or other chronic medical conditions planning to depart to an area in <2 weeks should receive the initial dose of vaccine along with IG (0.02 mL/kg) at a separate injection site.

Travelers who are aged <12 months, are allergic to a vaccine component, or who otherwise elect not to receive vaccine should receive a single dose of IG (0.02 mL/kg), which provides effective protection against HAV infection for up to 3 months. Those who do not receive vaccination and plan to travel for >3 months should receive an IG dose of 0.06 mL/kg, which must be repeated if the duration of travel is >5 months. IG can be repeated every 6 months thereafter if the traveler remains in a high-risk setting, though hepatitis A vaccination should be encouraged if not contraindicated.

Although vaccinating an immune traveler is not contraindicated and does not increase the risk for adverse effects, screening for total anti-HAV before travel can be useful in some circumstances to determine susceptibility and eliminate unnecessary vaccination. Postvaccination testing for serologic response is not indicated.

OTHER VACCINE CONSIDERATIONS

Using vaccine according to the licensed schedule is preferable. An interrupted series does not need to be restarted. More than 95% of vaccinated people develop levels of anti-HAV that correlate with protection 1 month after the first dose. Given their similar immunogenicity, a series that has been started with one brand of hepatitis A monovalent vaccine may be completed with another brand of monovalent vaccine. For children and adults who complete the primary series, booster doses of vaccine are not recommended.

VACCINE SAFETY AND ADVERSE REACTIONS

Among adults, the most frequently reported side effects after hepatitis A vaccination are tenderness or pain at the injection site (56%–67%) and headache (14%–16%). Among children (11–25 months of age), the most common reported side effects are pain or tenderness at the injection site (32%–37%) and redness (21%–29%). No serious adverse events in children or adults have been reported that could be attributed definitively to the vaccine; no increase in serious adverse events has been identified among vaccinated people compared with baseline rates.

PRECAUTIONS AND CONTRAINDICATIONS

Hepatitis A–containing vaccines should not be administered to travelers with a history of hypersensitivity to any vaccine component, including neomycin. Twinrix should not be administered to people with a history of hypersensitivity to yeast. The tip caps of prefilled syringes of Havrix and Twinrix and the vial stopper, syringe plunger stopper, and tip caps of Vaqta may contain dry natural rubber, which may cause allergic reactions in latex-sensitive people. Because hepatitis A vaccine consists of inactivated virus and hepatitis B vaccine consists of a recombinant protein, no special precautions are needed for vaccination of immunocompromised travelers. Providers should check precautions and contraindications before administering IG.

PREGNANCY

The safety of hepatitis A vaccine for pregnant women has not been determined. However, because hepatitis A vaccine is produced from inactivated HAV, the theoretical risk to either the pregnant woman or the developing fetus is thought to be low. A recent review of the Vaccine Adverse Event Reporting System did not identify any concerning patterns of adverse events in pregnant women or their infants after hepatitis A vaccination (Havrix, Vaqta) or hepatitis A and B combined vaccination (Twinrix) during pregnancy. The risk of vaccination should be weighed against the risk of hepatitis A among female travelers who might be at high risk for exposure to HAV.

Postexposure Prophylaxis

Travelers who are exposed to HAV and who have not received hepatitis A vaccine previously should be administered 1 dose of monovalent hepatitis A vaccine or IG (0.02 mL/kg) as soon as possible, ideally within 2 weeks of exposure. The efficacy of IG or vaccine when administered >2 weeks after exposure has not been established. The relative efficacy of vaccine is comparable to IG for postexposure prophylaxis among people aged 1–40 years.

For healthy people aged 1–40 years, a dose of monovalent hepatitis A vaccine is recommended. For people aged >40 years, IG is preferred, but vaccine can be used if IG is unavailable. IG is recommended for children aged <12 months, people who are immunocompromised, people who have chronic liver disease, and people for whom vaccine is contraindicated. Twinrix is not approved for postexposure prophylaxis. More detailed information can be found in the Advisory Committee on Immunization Practices recommendations at www.cdc.gov/mmwr/preview/mmwrhtml/mm5641a3.htm.

CDC website: www.cdc.gov/hepatitis/HAV

3

BIBLIOGRAPHY

1. Averhoff FM, Khudyakov Y, NP N. Vaccines. 7th ed. Philadelphia: Saunders Elsevier; 2016.

2. CDC. Update: Prevention of hepatitis A after exposure to hepatitis A virus and in international travelers. Updated recommendations of the Advisory Committee on Immunization Practices (ACIP). MMWR Morb Mortal Wkly Rep. 2007 Oct 19;56(41):1080–4.

3. CDC. Updated recommendations from the Advisory Committee on Immunization Practices (ACIP) for use of hepatitis A vaccine in close contacts of newly arriving international adoptees. MMWR Morb Mortal Wkly Rep. 2009 Sep 18;58(36):1006–7.

4. CDC. Viral Hepatitis Surveillance—United States, 2013 [cited 2016 Sep. 23]. Available from: http://www.cdc.gov/hepatitis/statistics/2013surveillance/pdfs/2013hepsurveillancerpt.pdf.

5. Collier MG, Khudyakov YE, Selvage D, Adams-Cameron M, Epson E, Cronquist A, et al. Outbreak of hepatitis A in the USA associated with frozen pomegranate arils imported from Turkey: an epidemiological case study. Lancet Infect Dis. 2014 Oct;14(10):976–81.

6. Fiore AE, Wasley A, Bell BP. Prevention of hepatitis A through active or passive immunization: recommendations of the Advisory Committee on Immunization Practices (ACIP). MMWR Recomm Rep. 2006 May 19;55(RR-7):1–23.

7. Mohd Hanafiah K, Jacobsen KH, Wiersma ST. Challenges to mapping the health risk of hepatitis A virus infection. Int J Health Geogr. 2011;10:57.

8. Moro PL, Museru OI, Niu M, Lewis P, Broder K. Reports to the Vaccine Adverse Event Reporting System after hepatitis A and hepatitis AB vaccines in pregnant women. Am J Obstet Gynecol. 2014 Jun;210(6):561.e1–6.

9. Mutsch M, Spicher VM, Gut C, Steffen R. Hepatitis A virus infections in travelers, 1988–2004. Clin Infect Dis. 2006 Feb 15;42(4):490–7.

10. Nelson NP, Murphy TV. Hepatitis A: the changing epidemiology of hepatitis A. Clin Liver Dis. 2013 Dec 20;2(6):227–30.

3

HEPATITIS B

Francisco Averhoff

INFECTIOUS AGENT

Hepatitis B virus (HBV), a small, circular, partially double-stranded DNA virus in the family Hepadnaviridae.

TRANSMISSION

HBV is transmitted by contact with contaminated blood, blood products, and other body fluids (such as semen). Examples of exposures associated with transmission that travelers may encounter include poor infection control during medical or dental procedures, receipt of blood products, injection drug use, tattooing or acupuncture, and unprotected sex.

EPIDEMIOLOGY

An estimated 248 million people have chronic HBV infection globally. Although accurate data are lacking from many countries, Map 3-4 shows the estimated prevalence of chronic HBV infection by country. No data are available to show the specific risk to travelers; however, published reports of travelers acquiring hepatitis B are rare, and the risk for travelers who do not have high-risk behaviors or exposures is low. The risk for HBV infection may be higher in countries where the prevalence of chronic HBV infection is high or intermediate; expatriates, missionaries, and long-term development workers may be at increased risk for HBV infection in such countries. All travelers should be aware of how HBV is transmitted and take measures to minimize their exposures.

CLINICAL PRESENTATION

HBV infection primarily affects the liver. Typically, the incubation period for hepatitis B is 90 days (range, 60–150 days). The typical signs and symptoms of acute infection include malaise, fatigue, anorexia, nausea, vomiting, abdominal pain, and jaundice. In some cases, skin rashes, joint pain, and arthritis may occur. Among people aged ≥5 years, 30%–50% will develop signs and symptoms. In

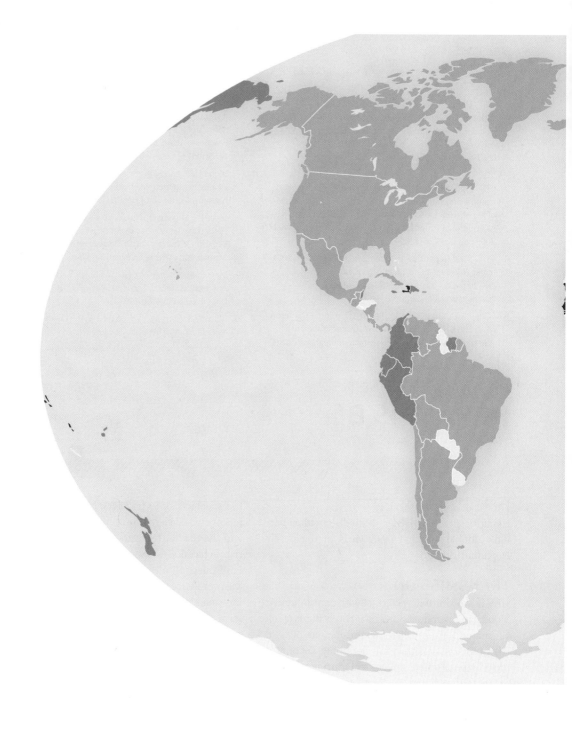

MAP 3-4. **Prevalence of hepatitis B virus infection**[1]

[1] Disease data source: Schweitzer A, Horn J, Mikolajczyk R, Krause G, Ott J. Estimations of worldwide prevalence of chronic hepatitis B virus infection: a systematic review of data published between 1965 and 2013. The Lancet. 2015 Jul 28; 386(10003):1546–1555.

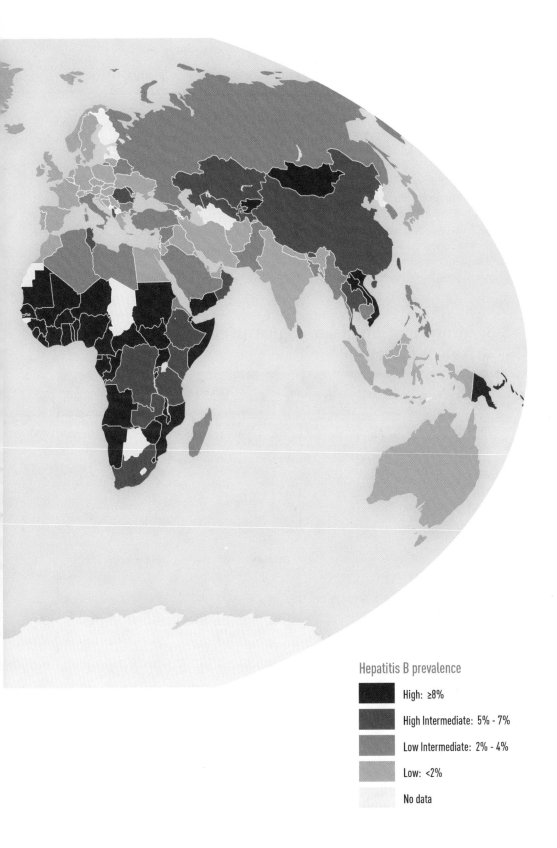

Hepatitis B prevalence

■	High: ≥8%
■	High Intermediate: 5% - 7%
■	Low Intermediate: 2% - 4%
■	Low: <2%
□	No data

children aged <5 years and immunocompromised adults, HBV infection is typically asymptomatic, but it can be asymptomatic at any age among healthy people. The overall case-fatality ratio of acute hepatitis B is approximately 1%.

Acute hepatitis B progresses to chronic HBV infection in 30%–90% of people infected as infants or young children and in <5% of people infected during adolescence or adulthood. Chronic infection with HBV may result in chronic liver disease, including cirrhosis, liver cancer, and death. People infected with HBV are susceptible to infection with hepatitis D virus; coinfection increases the risk of fulminant hepatitis and rapidly progressive liver disease.

DIAGNOSIS

Serologic markers specific for hepatitis B are necessary to diagnose HBV infection and to identify the stage of infection (Table 3-3). These markers can differentiate between acute, resolving, and chronic infection. Hepatitis B is a nationally notifiable disease.

TREATMENT

No specific treatment is available for acute hepatitis B; however, supportive treatment, including hospitalization, may be indicated for some people with severe clinical manifestations. Antiviral drugs are approved and available to treat chronic HBV infection and prevent progression of disease.

Table 3-3. Interpretation of serologic test results for hepatitis B virus infection[1]

SEROLOGIC MARKER				INTERPRETATION
HBSAG[2]	TOTAL ANTI-HBC	IGM ANTI-HBC	ANTI-HBS	
–	–	–	–	Never infected
+	–	–	–	Early acute infection; transient (≤18 days) after vaccination
+	+	+	–	Acute infection
–	+	+	+ or –	Acute resolving infection
–	+	–	+	Recovered from past infection and immune
+	+	–	–	Chronic infection
–	+	–	–	False positive (susceptible); past infection; occult infection[3]; or passive transfer of anti-HBc to infant born to HBsAg-positive mother
–	–	–	+	Immune if concentration is ≥10 mIU/mL after vaccine series completion; passive transfer after hepatitis B immune globulin administration

Abbreviations: HBsAg, hepatitis B surface antigen; anti-HBc, antibody to hepatitis B core antigen; anti-HBs, antibody to hepatitis B surface antigen.
[1] From: CDC. A comprehensive immunization strategy to eliminate transmission of hepatitis B virus infection in the United States: recommendations of the Advisory Committee on Immunization Practices (ACIP). Part II: immunization of adults. MMWR Recomm Rep. 2006 Dec 8;55(RR-16):1–33.
[2] To ensure that an HBsAg-positive test result is not a false positive, samples with reactive HBsAg results should be tested with a licensed neutralizing confirmatory test, if recommended in the manufacturer's prescribing information.
[3] People positive only for anti-HBc are unlikely to be infectious except under unusual circumstances in which they are the source for direct percutaneous exposure of susceptible recipients to large quantities of virus (such as blood transfusion or organ transplant).

PREVENTION

Vaccine

INDICATIONS FOR USE

Hepatitis B vaccination should be administered to all unvaccinated people traveling to areas with intermediate to high prevalence of chronic HBV infection (HBV surface antigen prevalence ≥2%). Complete vaccination information and recommendations for the United States are available at www.cdc.gov/vaccines/vpd-vac/hepb/default.htm. Vaccination to prevent hepatitis B may be considered for all international travelers, regardless of destination, depending on the traveler's behavioral risk. However, the vaccine should be considered for all nonimmune travelers since it is often difficult to assess risk during the pretravel consultation or even in the primary care setting.

VACCINE ADMINISTRATION

Hepatitis B vaccine (Table 3-4) is usually administered as a 3-dose series on a 0-, 1-, 6-month schedule to achieve immunity. The second dose should be given ≥1 month after the first dose; the third dose should be given ≥2 months after the second dose and ≥4 months after the first dose. The third dose should not be administered before age 24 weeks. Four doses of hepatitis B vaccine can be administered when a combination vaccine containing hepatitis B is administered after the birth dose. Postexposure prophylaxis with hepatitis B immune globulin (HBIG) administered in conjunction with hepatitis B vaccine, as well as hepatitis B vaccine alone, is effective in preventing transmission after exposure to HBV.

Exceptions to this schedule are available with specific licensed products in the United States; Recombivax HB (Merck & Co.) is licensed for a 2-dose schedule for children aged 11–15 years, and Engerix-B (GlaxoSmithKline) is licensed for a 4-dose schedule, with the first 3 doses within 2 months and a booster at 12 months (doses at 0, 1, 2, and 12 months). Combination vaccines including hepatitis B are available for children, and a combination hepatitis A and hepatitis B vaccine, Twinrix (GlaxoSmithKline), is also licensed in the United States. Consult the prescribing information when administering alternate schedules and formulations. Vaccination series begun with one brand may be completed with another brand. Protection from the primary vaccination series is robust, and >95% of healthy people achieve immunity with the 3-dose series. Serologic testing and booster vaccination are not recommended before travel for immunocompetent adults who have been previously vaccinated.

SPECIAL SITUATIONS

Ideally, hepatitis B vaccination should begin ≥6 months before travel so the full vaccine series can be completed before departure. Because some protection is provided by 1 or 2 doses, the vaccine series should be initiated, if indicated, even if it cannot be completed before departure. Optimal protection, however, is not conferred until after the final vaccine dose is received, and travelers should be advised to complete the vaccine series. An approved accelerated vaccination schedule can be used for people traveling on short notice who face imminent exposure or for emergency responders to disaster areas. The accelerated vaccination schedule calls for vaccine doses administered at days 0, 7, and 21–30; a booster should be administered at 12 months to promote long-term immunity. A combined hepatitis A and hepatitis B vaccine can also be used on the same 3-dose schedule (0, 7, and 21–30 days), with a booster at 12 months.

VACCINE SAFETY AND ADVERSE REACTIONS

Hepatitis B vaccines are safe for people of all ages. Pain at the injection site (3%–29%) and fever (temperature >99.9°F [37.7°C]; 1%–6%) are the most frequently reported side effects among vaccine recipients. Hepatitis B vaccines should not be administered to people with a history of hypersensitivity to any vaccine component, including yeast. The vaccine contains a recombinant protein (hepatitis B surface antigen) that is noninfectious.

Limited data indicate no apparent risk of adverse events to the mother or the developing fetus when hepatitis B vaccine is administered to pregnant women. HBV infection affecting a pregnant woman can result in serious disease for the mother and chronic infection for the newborn. Neither pregnancy nor lactation should be considered a contraindication for vaccination.

Table 3-4. Vaccines to prevent hepatitis B

VACCINE	TRADE NAME (MANUFACTURER)	AGE (Y)	DOSE	ROUTE	SCHEDULE	BOOSTER
Hepatitis B vaccine, recombinant[1]	Engerix-B (GlaxoSmithKline)	0–19 (primary)	0.5 mL (10 µg HBsAg)	IM	0, 1, 6 mo	None
		0–10 (accelerated)	0.5 mL (10 µg HBsAg)	IM	0, 1, 2 mo	12 mo
		11–19 (accelerated)	1.0 mL (20 µg HBsAg)	IM	0, 1, 2 mo	12 mo
		≥20 (primary)	1.0 mL (20 µg HBsAg)	IM	0, 1, 6 mo	None
		≥20 (accelerated)	1.0 mL (20 µg HBsAg)	IM	0, 1, 2 mo	12 mo
Hepatitis B vaccine, recombinant[1]	Recombivax HB (Merck & Co., Inc.)	0–19 (primary)	0.5 mL (5 µg HBsAg)	IM	0, 1, 6 mo	None
		11–15 (adolescent accelerated)	1.0 mL (10 µg HBsAg)	IM	0, 4–6 mo	None
		≥20 (primary)	1.0 mL (10 µg HBsAg)	IM	0, 1, 6 mo	None
Combined hepatitis A and B vaccine	Twinrix (GlaxoSmithKline)	≥18 (primary)	1.0 mL (720 ELU HAV + 20 µg HBsAg)	IM	0, 1, 6 mo	None
		≥18 (accelerated)	same as above	IM	0, 7, 21–30 d	12 mo

Abbreviations: HBsAg, hepatitis B surface antigen; IM, intramuscular; ELU, ELISA units of inactivated HAV; HAV, hepatitis A virus.
[1] Consult the prescribing information for differences in dosing for hemodialysis and other immunocompromised patients.

3

Personal Protection Measures

As part of the pretravel education process, all travelers should be counseled and given information about the risks for hepatitis B and other bloodborne pathogens from contaminated equipment or items used during medical, dental, or cosmetic procedures; blood products; injection drug use; any activities or procedures that involve piercing the skin or mucosa; or unprotected sexual activity. When seeking medical or dental care or cosmetic procedures (such as tattooing or piercing), travelers should be alert to the use of equipment that has not been adequately sterilized or disinfected, reuse of contaminated equipment, and unsafe injecting practices (such as reuse of disposable needles and syringes). HBV and other bloodborne pathogens can be transmitted if tools are not sterile or if personnel do not follow proper infection control procedures. Travelers should consider the health risks when receiving medical or dental care overseas; information may be available from the US embassy. The health risks should be strongly considered when deciding to obtain a tattoo or body piercing in areas where adequate sterilization or disinfection procedures might not be available or practiced.

CDC website: www.cdc.gov/hepatitis/HBV

BIBLIOGRAPHY

1. CDC. A comprehensive immunization strategy to eliminate transmission of hepatitis B virus infection in the United States: recommendations of the Advisory Committee on Immunization Practices (ACIP) part 1: immunization of infants, children, and adolescents. MMWR Recomm Rep. 2005 Dec 23;54(RR-16):1–31.

2. CDC. A comprehensive immunization strategy to eliminate transmission of hepatitis B virus infection in the United States: recommendations of the Advisory Committee on Immunization Practices (ACIP) Part II: immunization of adults. MMWR Recomm Rep. 2006 Dec 8;55(RR-16):1–33.

3. CDC. Updated US Public Health Service guidelines for the management of occupational exposures to HBV, HCV, and HIV and recommendations for post-exposure prophylaxis. MMWR Recomm Rep. 2001 Jun 29;50(RR-11):1–42.

4. Mariano A, Mele A, Tosti ME, Parlato A, Gallo G, Ragni P, et al. Role of beauty treatment in the spread of parenterally transmitted hepatitis viruses in Italy. J Med Virol. 2004 Oct;74(2):216–20.

5. Pepin J, Abou Chakra CN, Pepin E, Nault V, Valiquette L. Evolution of the global burden of viral infections from unsafe medical injections, 2000–2010. PLoS One. 2014;9(6):e99677.

6. Sagliocca L, Stroffolini T, Amoroso P, Manzillo G, Ferrigno L, Converti F, et al. Risk factors for acute hepatitis B: a case-control study. J Viral Hepat. 1997 Jan;4(1):63–6.

7. Schweitzer A, Horn J, Mikolajczyk RT, Krause G, Ott JJ. Estimations of worldwide prevalence of chronic hepatitis B virus infection: a systematic review of data published between 1965 and 2013. Lancet. 2015 Oct 17;386(10003):1546–55.

8. Terrault NA, Bzowej NH, Chang KM, Hwang JP, Jonas MM, Murad MH. AASLD guidelines for treatment of chronic hepatitis B. Hepatology. 2016 Jan;63(1):261–83.

HEPATITIS C

Deborah Holtzman

INFECTIOUS AGENT

Hepatitis C virus (HCV), a spherical, enveloped, positive-strand RNA virus.

TRANSMISSION

Transmission of HCV is bloodborne and most often involves exposure to contaminated needles or syringes or receipt of blood or blood products that have not been screened for HCV. Although infrequent, HCV can be transmitted through other procedures that involve blood exposure, such as tattooing, during sexual contact, or perinatally from mother to child.

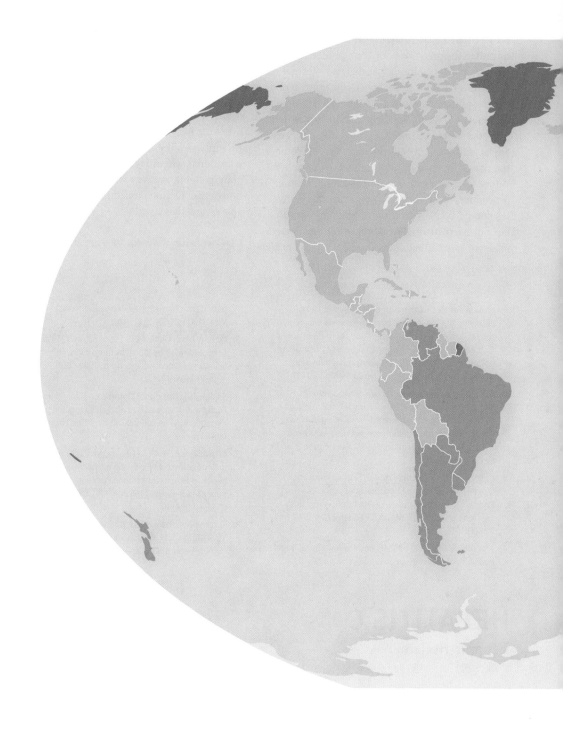

MAP 3-5. Prevalence of hepatitis C virus infection[1]

[1] Disease data source: Gower et al. Global epidemiology and genotype distribution of the hepatitis C virus infection. J Hepatol. 2014 Nov;61(1 Suppl):S45–57. doi: 10.1016/j.jhep.2014.07.027. Epub 2014 Jul 30.

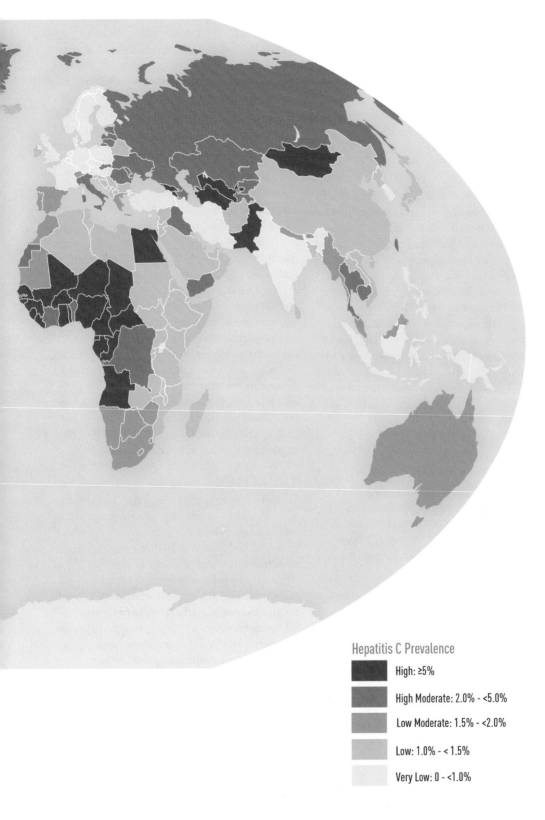

3

Hepatitis C Prevalence

- High: ≥5%
- High Moderate: 2.0% - <5.0%
- Low Moderate: 1.5% - <2.0%
- Low: 1.0% - < 1.5%
- Very Low: 0 - <1.0%

EPIDEMIOLOGY

Globally, an estimated 130–150 million people are living with HCV infection (chronically infected), and more than 700,000 were estimated to have died from HCV-related liver disease in 2013. Although the quality of epidemiologic data varies widely across countries and regions, the most recent global estimates indicate that the prevalence of HCV infection is <1.5% in many developed countries, including the United States (Map 3-5). The prevalence is higher (≥1.5%) in several countries in Latin America, Eastern Europe and the former Soviet Union, and certain countries in Africa, the Middle East, and Asia; the prevalence is reported to be highest (approximately 10%) in Egypt. The most frequent current mode of transmission in the United States and most developed countries is through sharing drug-injection equipment. In countries where HCV is more common (≥1.5% prevalence), the predominant mode of transmission is from unsafe injections and other health care exposures where infection control practices are poor. Travelers' risk for contracting HCV infection is generally low, but they should exercise caution, as the following activities can result in blood exposure:

- Receiving blood transfusions that have not been screened for HCV

- Having medical or dental procedures

- Activities such as acupuncture, tattooing, being shaved, or injection drug use in which equipment has not been adequately sterilized or disinfected or in which contaminated equipment is reused

- Working in health care fields (medical, dental, or laboratory) that entail direct exposure to human blood

CLINICAL PRESENTATION

HCV is a major cause of cirrhosis and hepatocellular cancer and is the leading reason for liver transplantation in the United States. Most people (80%) with acute HCV infection have no symptoms. If symptoms occur, they may include loss of appetite, abdominal pain, fatigue, nausea, dark urine, and jaundice. Of those infected, as many as 75% will remain infected unless treated with antiviral medications. For people who develop chronic HCV infection, the most common symptom is fatigue. Cirrhosis develops in approximately 10%–20% of people after 20 years of chronic infection. This progression is often clinically silent, and evidence of liver disease may not occur until late in the course of the disease. HCV testing is required for diagnosis. However, testing is not routinely provided in many countries, and most HCV-infected people are unaware of their infection.

DIAGNOSIS

Two major types of tests are available: IgG assays for HCV antibodies and nucleic acid amplification testing to detect HCV RNA in blood (viremia). Assays for IgM, to detect early or acute infection, are not available. Approximately 70%–75% of people who seroconvert to anti-HCV, indicative of acute infection, will progress to chronic infection and persistent viremia. Because a positive HCV antibody test cannot discriminate between someone who was previously infected but resolved or cleared the infection and someone with current infection, it is essential that HCV RNA testing follow a positive HCV antibody test to identify people with current (chronic) HCV infection. Hepatitis C is a nationally notifiable disease.

TREATMENT

Treatment for hepatitis C continues to evolve rapidly. Since 2014, several new all-oral direct-acting antiviral agents have been approved for use both in the United States and other countries. These new treatment regimens are of short duration (typically 12 weeks) with few side effects and cure rates exceeding 90% for those who complete treatment. However, the effectiveness of these antiviral therapies differs to some extent by genotype. Travelers who think they may have been exposed should see their health care provider upon return and get tested for HCV, and if found to have evidence of infection, be referred for care and evaluated for treatment, including genotyping as appropriate. Other drugs and therapeutic combinations in development show promise of further improvements in therapy for HCV infection. The most up-to-date treatment guidelines and information can be found at www.hcvguidelines.org.

PREVENTION

No vaccine is available to prevent HCV infection, nor does immune globulin provide protection. Before traveling, people should check with their health care providers to understand the potential risk of infection and any precautions they should take. When seeking medical or dental care, travelers should be alert to the use of medical, surgical, or dental equipment that has not been adequately sterilized or disinfected; reuse of contaminated equipment; and unsafe injection practices (such as reuse of disposable needles and syringes). HCV and other bloodborne pathogens can be transmitted if instruments are not sterile or the clinician does not follow other proper infection-control procedures (washing hands, using latex gloves, and cleaning and disinfecting surfaces and instruments). In some parts of the world, such as parts of sub-Saharan Africa, blood donors may not be screened for HCV. Travelers should be advised to consider the health risks if they are thinking about getting a tattoo or body piercing or having a medical procedure in areas where adequate sterilization or disinfection procedures might not be practiced. Travelers should be advised to seek testing for HCV upon return if they received blood transfusions or sustained other blood exposures for which they could not assess the risks.

CDC website: www.cdc.gov/hepatitis/HCV

BIBLIOGRAPHY

1. American Association for Study of Liver Diseases (AASLD), Infectious Diseases Society of America (IDSA). Recommendations for testing, managing, and treating hepatitis C. [updated 2014 Aug 11; cited 2016 Sep. 23]. Available from: http://www.hcvguidelines.org/.

2. Averhoff FM, Glass N, Holtzman D. Global burden of hepatitis C: considerations for healthcare providers in the United States. Clin Infect Dis. 2012 Jul;55 Suppl 1: S10–5.

3. CDC. Testing for HCV infection: an update of guidance for clinicians and laboratorians. MMWR Morb Mortal Wkly Rep. 2013 May 10;62(18):362–5.

4. GBD 2013 Mortality and Causes of Death Collaborators. Global, regional, and national age-sex specific all-cause and cause-specific mortality for 240 causes of death, 1990–2013: a systematic analysis for the Global Burden of Disease Study 2013. Lancet. 2015 Jan 10; 385(9963):117–71.

5. Gower E, Estes C, Blach S, Razavi-Shearer K, Razavi H. Global epidemiology and genotype distribution of the hepatitis C virus infection. J Hepatol. 2014 Nov; 61(1 Suppl):S45–57.

6. Messina JP, Humphreys I, Flaxman A, Brown A, Cooke GS, Pybus OG, et al. Global distribution and prevalence of hepatitis C virus genotypes. Hepatology. 2015 Jan;61(1):77–87.

7. Smith DB, Bukh J, Kuiken C, Muerhoff AS, Rice CM, Stapleton JT, et al. Expanded classification of hepatitis C virus into 7 genotypes and 67 subtypes: updated criteria and genotype assignment web resource. Hepatology. 2014 Jan;59(1):318–27.

8. Ward JW, Mermin JH. Simple, effective, but out of reach? Public health implications of HCV drugs. N Engl J Med. 2015 Dec 31;373(27):2678–80.

9. Westbrook RH, Dusheiko G. Natural history of hepatitis C. J Hepatol. 2014 Nov;61(1 Suppl):S58–68.

10. World Health Organization. Hepatitis C. 2015 [updated July 2015; cited 2016 Sep. 23]. Available from: http://www.who.int/mediacentre/factsheets/fs164_apr2014/en/.

3

HEPATITIS E

Eyasu H. Teshale

INFECTIOUS AGENT

Infection is caused by hepatitis E virus (HEV), a single-stranded, single-serotype, RNA virus belonging to the Hepeviridae family. Four HEV genotypes are known to cause human disease. HEV genotype 3 causes hepatitis E in developed countries, whereas genotypes 1, 2, and 4 are associated with illness in developing countries. HEV genotype 1 and to some extent genotype 2 are associated with large waterborne outbreaks.

TRANSMISSION

HEV genotype 1 is transmitted primarily by the fecal-oral route. In regions with poor sanitation and limited access to safe drinking water, epidemics and interepidemic occurrences of hepatitis E are largely waterborne. In developing countries transmission to fetuses and neonates by women infected during pregnancy is common. In Japan and Europe, sporadic disease can be zoonotic and foodborne, associated with eating meat and offal (including liver) of deer, boars, and pigs and is mainly caused by HEV genotype 3. In France, disease can be acquired from eating *figatellu*, a sausage delicacy prepared from raw pig liver. A hepatitis E outbreak on a cruise ship was associated with consumption of shellfish. Transmission from blood transfusion is rare. Rare symptomatic disease is observed in the United States, but its mode of transmission is generally unknown.

EPIDEMIOLOGY

Waterborne outbreaks (which can be large, often involving hundreds to thousands of people) have occurred in South and Central Asia, tropical East Asia, Africa, and Central America. In outbreak-prone areas, interepidemic disease is sporadically encountered. Sporadic disease also occurs in regions that are not prone to outbreaks, such as the Middle East, temperate East Asia (including China), North and South America, and Europe (Map 3-6).

During outbreaks of hepatitis E, clinical attack rates are highest in young adults aged 15–49 years.

In outbreak-prone areas, pregnant women—whether infected sporadically or during an epidemic—are at risk of their HEV infection progressing to liver failure and death. Miscarriages and neonatal deaths are common complications of HEV infection. In areas that are not prone to outbreaks, symptomatic disease is observed most frequently in adults aged >50 years. HEV genotype 3 infection acquired by people who are immunosuppressed, particularly recipients of solid-organ allografts, may progress to chronic infection.

People living in the United States are at highest risk of HEV infection when they travel to areas where epidemics have occurred. When traveling in Japan and Europe, eating raw or inadequately cooked venison, boar meat, pig liver, pig meat, or food products derived from these is a risk factor for infection.

CLINICAL PRESENTATION

The incubation period of HEV infection is 2–9 weeks (mean 6 weeks). Signs and symptoms of acute hepatitis E include jaundice, fever, loss of appetite, abdominal pain, and lethargy. Infection with HEV genotype 3, common in developed countries, is generally asymptomatic but can progress to chronic infection in rare cases, whereas genotypes 1, 2, and 4 result only in acute infection. For most people, HEV infection and disease is self-limited. Pregnant women with genotype 1, 2, or 4 infection (especially those infected during the third trimester) may present with or progress to liver failure, and their fetuses are at risk of spontaneous abortion and premature delivery. To date, there is no evidence that HEV genotype 3 is associated with severe outcome in pregnant women. People with preexisting liver disease may undergo further hepatic decompensation with HEV infection. Recipients of solid organ transplants tend to have no symptoms associated with acute and chronic HEV infection, but progressive liver injury can result when infected with HEV genotype 3.

DIAGNOSIS

The diagnosis of acute hepatitis E is established by detecting anti-HEV IgM in serum. Detecting HEV RNA in serum or stools further confirms the serologic diagnosis but is seldom required. Longerterm, serial detection of HEV RNA in serum or stools, regardless of the HEV antibody serostatus, suggests chronic HEV infection. No diagnostic test for HEV has been approved by the Food and Drug Administration.

TREATMENT

Treatment is supportive. Oral ribavirin has been used to treat chronic hepatitis E in solid-organ transplant recipients.

PREVENTION

No vaccine is available for prevention. Travelers should avoid drinking unboiled or unchlorinated water and beverages that contain unboiled water or ice. Travelers should eat only thoroughly cooked food, including seafood, meat, offal, and products derived from these (see Chapter 2, Food & Water Precautions).

CDC website: www.cdc.gov/hepatitis/HEV

BIBLIOGRAPHY

1. Kamar N, Izopet J, Tripon S, Bismuth M, Hillaire S, Dumortier J, et al. Ribavirin for chronic hepatitis E virus infection in transplant recipients. N Engl J Med. 2014 Mar 20;370(12):1111–20.
2. Khuroo MS, Khuroo MS. Hepatitis E: an emerging global disease—from discovery towards control and cure. J Viral Hepat. 2016 Feb;23(2):68–79.
3. Krawczynski K. Hepatitis E virus. Semin Liver Dis. 2013 Feb;33(1):1–93.
4. Riveiro-Barciela M, Minguez B, Girones R, Rodriguez-Frias F, Quer J, Buti M. Phylogenetic demonstration of hepatitis E infection transmitted by pork meat ingestion. Journal of clinical gastroenterology. 2015 Feb;49(2):165–8.

HISTOPLASMOSIS

Brendan R. Jackson, Tom M. Chiller

INFECTIOUS AGENT

Histoplasma capsulatum, a dimorphic fungus that grows as a mold in soil and as a yeast in animal and human hosts.

TRANSMISSION

Through inhalation of spores (conidia) from soil (often soil contaminated with bat guano or bird droppings); not transmitted from person to person.

EPIDEMIOLOGY

Distributed worldwide, except in Antarctica, but most often associated with river valleys. Activities that expose people to soil disruption or areas where bats live and birds roost, such as construction, excavation, demolition, farming, gardening, and caving, can increase risk of histoplasmosis. Outbreaks have been reported associated with travel to many countries in Central and South America, most often associated with visiting caves.

CLINICAL PRESENTATION

Incubation period is typically 3–17 days for acute disease. Ninety percent of infections are asymptomatic or result in a mild influenzalike illness. Some infections may cause acute pulmonary histoplasmosis, manifested by high fever, headache, nonproductive cough, chills, weakness, pleuritic chest pain, and fatigue. Most people spontaneously recover 2–3 weeks after onset of symptoms, although fatigue may persist longer. High-dose exposure can lead to severe pulmonary disease. Dissemination, especially to the gastrointestinal tract and central nervous system, can occur in people who are immunocompromised.

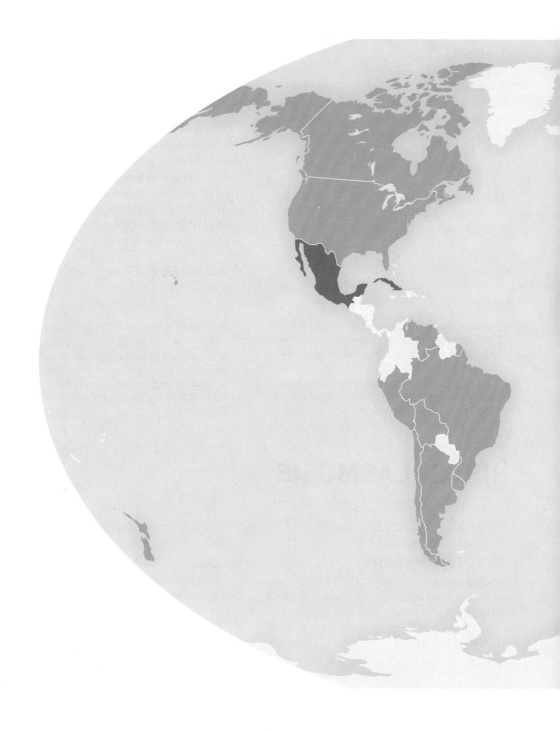

MAP 3-6. Hepatitis E endemic countries[1]

[1] Disease data adapted from: World Health Organization. The Global Prevalence of Hepatitis E Virus Infection and Susceptibility: A Systematic Review. (WHO/IVB/10.14). 2010 (Accessed Aug 13, 2016). Available from: http://apps.who.int iris/bitstream/10665/70513/1/WHO_IVB_10.14_eng.pdf.

[2] Defined as waterborne outbreaks or confirmed Hepatitis E virus infection ≥25% of sporadic non-A, non-B hepatitis.

[3] Defined as confirmed Hepatitis E virus infection in <25% of sporadic non-A, non-B hepatitis.

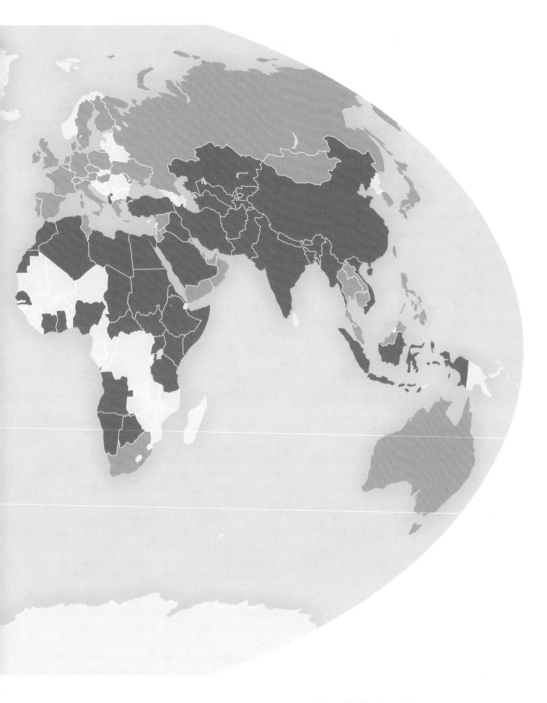

Hepatitis E endemicity

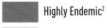 Highly Endemic[2]

Endemic[3]

Not Endemic or Endemicity Unknown

3

DIAGNOSIS

Several methods are available to diagnose histoplasmosis.

- Culture of *H. capsulatum* from bone marrow, blood, sputum, and tissue specimens is the definitive method but may take weeks to grow.

- Demonstration of the typical intracellular yeast forms in tissue by microscopic examination strongly supports the diagnosis of histoplasmosis when clinical, epidemiologic, and other laboratory studies are compatible. Molecular diagnostics, such as PCR on tissue specimens, are increasingly available to support microscopic findings.

- EIA on urine, serum, plasma, bronchoalveolar lavage, or cerebrospinal fluid is a rapid diagnostic test commercially available in the United States.

- Antibody tests are available for histoplasmosis. Testing a single serum specimen can aid in diagnosis, but testing serial specimens offers greater specificity (detection of seroconversion and increases in antibody titer).

- Other endemic mycoses (such as blastomycosis, paracoccidioidomycosis, and penicilliosis) can lead to false-positive EIA and antibody tests for *H. capsulatum*.

TREATMENT

Treatment is not usually indicated for immunocompetent people with acute, localized pulmonary infection. People with more extensive disease or persistent symptoms beyond 1 month are generally treated with an azole drug, such as itraconazole, for mild to moderate illness or amphotericin B for severe infection.

PREVENTION

People at increased risk for severe disease should avoid high-risk areas, such as bat-inhabited caves.

CDC website: www.cdc.gov/fungal/diseases/histoplasmosis

BIBLIOGRAPHY

1. CDC. Outbreak of histoplasmosis among travelers returning from El Salvador—Pennsylvania and Virginia, 2008. MMWR Morb Mortal Wkly Rep. 2008 Dec 19;57(50):1349–53.

2. Hage CA, Azar MM, Bahr N, Loyd J, Wheat LJ. Histoplasmosis: up-to-date evidence-based approach to diagnosis and management. Semin Respir Crit Care Med. 2015 Oct;36(5):729–45.

3. Kauffman CA. Histoplasmosis: a clinical and laboratory update. Clin Microbiol Rev. 2007 Jan;20(1):115–32.

4. Morgan J, Cano MV, Feikin DR, Phelan M, Monroy OV, Morales PK, et al. A large outbreak of histoplasmosis among American travelers associated with a hotel in Acapulco, Mexico, spring 2001. Am J Trop Med Hyg. 2003 Dec;69(6):663–9.

5. Weinberg M, Weeks J, Lance-Parker S, Traeger M, Wiersma S, Phan Q, et al. Severe histoplasmosis in travelers to Nicaragua. Emerg Infect Dis. 2003 Oct;9(10):1322–5.

6. Wheat LJ. Histoplasmosis: a review for clinicians from non-endemic areas. Mycoses. 2006 Jul;49(4):274–82.

HIV INFECTION

Philip J. Peters, John T. Brooks

INFECTIOUS AGENT

HIV, an enveloped positive-strand RNA virus in the Retroviridae family.

TRANSMISSION

HIV can be transmitted through sexual contact, needle- or syringe-sharing, unsafe medical injection or blood transfusion, and organ or tissue transplantation. It can also be transmitted from mother to child during pregnancy, at birth, and postpartum through breastfeeding. HIV may be transmitted occupationally to health care workers who are exposed to blood and other potentially infectious bodily fluids via percutaneous injury or splash exposures to mucous membranes or nonintact skin (see Chapter 8, Health Care Workers).

EPIDEMIOLOGY

HIV infection occurs worldwide. As of the end of 2014, an estimated 37 million people were living with HIV infection. Although sub-Saharan Africa has experienced a substantial decline in the number of new infections annually, from 2.3 million in 2000 to 1.4 million in 2014 (a 41% decline), it remains the most affected part of the world (25.8 million cases or 70% of all people living with HIV infection). Although the reported adult HIV prevalence in many regions of the world is low, certain populations are disproportionately affected, such as sex workers, people who inject drugs, men who have sex with men, transgender people, and prisoners. Sex workers are particularly vulnerable; the prevalence among sex workers is 12 times as high as in the general population.

The risk of HIV infection for international travelers is generally low, although the risk is determined less by geographic destination and more by behaviors such as injection drug use and unprotected sex. Travelers who might undergo medical procedures in low-income countries, whether scheduled or in an emergency, should be aware that the blood supply (and organs and tissues used for transplantation) might not be adequately screened, increasing the risk of HIV transmission, and that HIV can be transmitted by unsafe medical injection practices (reusing needles, syringes, or single-dose medication vials).

CLINICAL PRESENTATION

HIV infection is a chronic disease characterized by ongoing viral replication and a gradual exhaustion and destruction of CD4 T lymphocytes. As the CD4 cell count declines, an HIV-infected person's susceptibility to opportunistic infections and infection-related malignancies increases. An estimated 40%–90% of people experience symptoms during acute HIV infection, which often presents as an infectious mononucleosislike or influenzalike syndrome, but the clinical features can be highly variable. Symptoms typically begin a median of 10 days after HIV infection and can include fever, maculopapular rash, arthralgia,

myalgia, malaise, lymphadenopathy, oral ulcers, pharyngitis, and weight loss. The presence of fever and rash has the best positive predictive value. Unfortunately, acute symptomatic HIV infection is rarely diagnosed by health care providers, as its symptoms are often attributed to other viral infections or secondary syphilis.

DIAGNOSIS

Any traveler who reports risk behaviors for HIV infection, suspects that she or he may have been exposed to HIV, or has symptoms that could be consistent with HIV infection should be tested. HIV can be diagnosed with laboratory-based or point-of-care assays that detect anti-HIV antibodies, HIV p24 antigen, or HIV-1 RNA. In the United States, the recommended laboratory-based screening test for HIV is a combination antigen/antibody assay that detects antibodies against HIV as well as p24 antigen. The combination antigen/antibody assay becomes reactive approximately 2–3 weeks after HIV infection. It is estimated that 99% of people will develop a reactive combination antigen/antibody result within 6 weeks of infection, but in rare cases, it can take up to 6 months to develop a reactive test result. Point-of-care HIV antibody tests performed on oral fluid (instead of blood) have been associated with a lower sensitivity during early HIV infection. The earliest time after exposure that HIV infection can be diagnosed is approximately 9 days, when HIV-1 RNA becomes detectable in blood. Any person with unknown HIV status who is diagnosed with an AIDS-defining illness, such as *Pneumocystis* pneumonia, should be tested for HIV. For further information on HIV testing, travelers should talk to their health care provider, or identify an HIV testing site near them by visiting the National HIV Testing Resources website at www.hivtest.org or call CDC-INFO toll-free at 800-CDC-INFO (800-232-4636) or 888-232-6348 (TTY). Both of these resources are confidential.

TREATMENT

Prompt medical care and effective treatment with antiretrovirals can partially reverse HIV-induced damage to the immune system and prolong life. Effective treatment also substantially reduces the risk of HIV transmission to others.

US guidelines recommend that all people diagnosed with HIV infection be offered treatment for their own health and to prevent transmission to others. Detailed information on specific treatments is available from the Department of Health and Human Services AIDSinfo (www.aidsinfo.nih.gov). Travelers may contact AIDSinfo toll-free at 800-448-0440 (English or Spanish) or 888-480-3739 (TTY).

PREVENTION

Although no vaccine can prevent HIV infection, travel medicine clinicians have several HIV prevention options available.

Education

Travelers should be advised that they are at risk if they:

- Have sexual contact (heterosexual or homosexual) with an infected person or a person whose HIV infection status is unknown.

- Use or allow the use of contaminated, unsterilized syringes or needles for any injections or other procedures that pierce the skin, including acupuncture, use of illicit drugs, steroid or vitamin injections, medical or dental procedures, ear or body piercing, or tattooing.

- Receive infected blood, blood components, or clotting factor concentrates. HIV infection by this route is rare in facilities where donated blood and plasma are screened for HIV.

- Work in a health care setting. Typically, exposures occur as a result of percutaneous exposure to contaminated sharps, including needles, lancets, scalpels, and broken glass (from capillary or test tubes). See Chapter 8, Health Care Workers.

Risk Reduction

To reduce their risk of acquiring HIV, travelers should:

- Avoid sexual encounters with people who are infected with HIV, whose HIV infection status is unknown, or who are at high risk for HIV infection, such as people who inject drugs, sex workers (both male and female), and other people with multiple sexual partners.

- Use condoms consistently and correctly, especially if engaging in vaginal, anal, or oral sex with a person who is HIV infected or whose HIV status is unknown.

- Avoid injecting drugs.

- Avoid sharing needles or other devices that can puncture skin.

- Avoid, if possible, blood transfusions or use of clotting factor concentrates and exposure to nonsterile injections and other invasive medical equipment.

- Ensure that if traveling for purposes of medical treatment (see Chapter 2, Medical Tourism), the blood and blood products used in the facility where the traveler will be treated are screened for HIV, and that such facilities exercise proper infection control practices.

Condoms

People who are sensitive to latex should use condoms made of polyurethane or other synthetic materials (not lambskin) and should carry their own supply of male or female condoms. If no condom is available, travelers should abstain from sex with people who are HIV-infected or whose HIV status is unknown. Barrier methods other than condoms do not prevent HIV transmission. Spermicides alone are also not effective. The widely used spermicide nonoxynol-9 can increase the risk of HIV transmission and should not be used.

Preexposure Prophylaxis

Preexposure prophylaxis (or PrEP) is highly effective in preventing HIV infection. PrEP consists of 2 oral antiretroviral medications (tenofovir and emtricitabine), coformulated as a single pill (Truvada) that is taken once daily. Daily PrEP can lower the risk of HIV infection from sex by as much as 90% or injection drug use by as much as 70% and is indicated for people at substantial risk for HIV infection. Detailed information is available from CDC (www.cdc.gov/hiv/risk/prep). Travelers who may have sex with people who are infected with HIV or who are at high risk for HIV infection and travelers who may inject drugs should discuss PrEP with their primary care and travel medicine providers. Travelers taking PrEP should carry proper documentation and be aware that some countries (see below for further information) may deny entry to people with evidence of HIV infection, which PrEP medications might mistakenly indicate to customs officials.

Sterile Syringes and Needles

Syringes and needles used to draw blood or administer injections should be sterile, single use, disposable, and prepackaged in a sealed container. If possible, travelers should avoid receiving medications from multidose vials, which may have become contaminated by used needles. Travelers with diabetes, hemophilia, or other conditions that necessitate routine or frequent injections should be advised to carry a supply of medication, syringes and needles, and disinfectant swabs sufficient to last their entire stay abroad. These travelers should request documentation of the medical necessity for traveling with these items (a letter from a licensed health care provider) to avoid having them confiscated, such as by inspection personnel at ports of entry (see Chapter 2, Travel Health Kits for more information about traveling with medications).

Postexposure Prophylaxis

Travelers who will be working in a medical setting (such as a nurse volunteer drawing blood or medical missionary performing surgeries) may have contact with HIV-infected or potentially infected biological materials. Detailed advice regarding management of postexposure prophylaxis in the occupational setting is found in Chapter 8, Health Care Workers. General recommendations on postexposure prophylaxis include the following:

- People who have been exposed to HIV in a nonoccupational setting (through sex or needle sharing) should seek immediate medical consultation to consider postexposure prophylaxis.

- Postexposure prophylaxis for potential exposure to HIV as a result of mass-casualty events is generally not warranted, except in special circumstances (for example, a blast injury in a facility that contained a large archive of HIV-infected blood specimens).

- Clinicians seeking advice on postexposure prophylaxis can call the US National HIV/AIDS Clinicians' Consultation Center PEPline toll-free at 888-448-4911 (www.nccc.ucsf.edu).

HIV TESTING REQUIREMENTS FOR US TRAVELERS ENTERING FOREIGN COUNTRIES

International travelers should be advised that some countries screen incoming travelers for HIV infection and may deny entry to people with AIDS or evidence of HIV infection. These countries usually screen only people planning extended visits, such as for work or study. People intending to visit a country for an extended stay should review that country's policies and requirements. This information is usually available from the consular officials of the individual nations. Information about entry and exit requirements compiled by the Department of State can be found by country at http://travel.state.gov/content/passports/en/country.html.

CDC website: www.cdc.gov/hiv

BIBLIOGRAPHY

1. CDC. Preexposure prophylaxis for the prevention of HIV in the United States: a clinical practice guideline. Atlanta 2014 [cited 216 Sep. 23]. Available from: http://www.cdc.gov/hiv/pdf/PrEPguidelines2014.pdf.

2. CDC. Preexposure prophylaxis for the prevention of HIV in the United States: clinical providers' supplement. Atlanta2014 [cited 2016 Sep. 23]. Available from: http://www.cdc.gov/hiv/pdf/PrEPProviderSupplement2014.pdf.

3. Joint United Nations Programme on HIV/AIDS (UNAIDS). Global report: UNAIDS report on the global AIDS epidemic 2013. Geneva: UNAIDS; 2013 [cited 2016 Sep. 23]. Available from: http://www.unaids.org/en/media/unaids/contentassets/documents/epidemiology/2013/gr2013/UNAIDS_Global_Report_2013_en.pdf.

4. Kuhar DT, Henderson DK, Struble KA, Heneine W, Thomas V, Cheever LW, et al. Updated US Public Health Service guidelines for the management of occupational

exposures to human immunodeficiency virus and recommendations for postexposure prophylaxis. Infect Control Hosp Epidemiol. 2013 Sep;34(9):875–92.

5. Rice B, Gilbart VL, Lawrence J, Smith R, Kall M, Delpech V. Safe travels? HIV transmission among Britons travelling abroad. HIV Med. 2012 May;13(5):315–7.

6. Smith DK, Grohskopf LA, Black RJ, Auerbach JD, Veronese F, Struble KA, et al. Antiretroviral postexposure prophylaxis after sexual, injection-drug use, or other nonoccupational exposure to HIV in the United States: recommendations from the US Department of Health and Human Services. MMWR Recomm Rep. 2005 Jan 21;54(RR-2):1–20.

INFLUENZA

Grace Appiah, Joseph Bresee

INFECTIOUS AGENT

Influenza is caused by infection of the respiratory tract with influenza viruses, RNA viruses of the *Orthomyxovirus* genus. Influenza viruses are classified into 3 types: A, B, and C. Only virus types A and B commonly cause illness in humans. Influenza A viruses are further classified into subtypes based on 2 surface proteins, hemagglutinin (HA) and neuraminidase (NA). Although 3 types and subtypes of influenza virus cocirculate in humans worldwide (influenza A [H1N1], A [H3N2], and influenza B viruses), the distribution of these viruses varies from year to year and between geographic areas and time of year. Information about circulating viruses in various regions can be found via CDC (www.cdc.gov/flu/weekly) or the World Health Organization (www.who.int/topics/influenza/en). Avian and swine influenza viruses can occasionally infect and cause disease in humans, usually associated with close exposure to infected animal populations. Notably, avian influenza A (H5N1) and A (H7N9) have led to sporadic human cases in recent years, and swine-origin A (H3N2) variant viruses have been associated with disease in humans in the United States.

TRANSMISSION

Influenza viruses spread from person to person, primarily through respiratory droplet transmission (such as when an infected person coughs or sneezes near a susceptible person). Transmission via large-particle droplets requires close proximity between the source and the recipient, because droplets generally travel only short distances (approximately 6 feet or less) through the air, before settling onto surfaces. Indirect (fomite) transmission can also occur, such as when a person touches a virus-contaminated surface and then touches his or her face. Airborne transmission via small-particle aerosols in the vicinity of the infectious person also occurs.

Most adults who are ill with influenza shed the virus in the upper respiratory tract and are infectious from the day before symptom onset to approximately 5–7 days after symptom onset. Infectiousness is highest within 3 days of illness onset and is correlated with fever. Children and those who are immunocompromised or severely ill may shed influenza virus for 10 days or more after the onset of symptoms. Seasonal influenza viruses have rarely been detected from nonrespiratory sources such as stool or blood.

EPIDEMIOLOGY

Seasonal Influenza

Influenza circulation varies geographically. The risk of exposure to influenza during travel depends on the time of year and destination. In temperate regions, influenza typically circulates at higher levels during colder winter months: October to May in the Northern Hemisphere and April to September in the Southern Hemisphere. In many tropical or subtropical regions, influenza can occur throughout the year.

Influenza is typically most common in children, especially in school-aged children. Rates of severe illness and death are typically highest among people aged ≥65, children <2 years, and people of any age who have underlying medical conditions that place them at increased risk for complications of influenza. Children aged <2 years have rates of influenza-associated hospitalizations that are as high as those in the elderly, although with much lower death rates. CDC estimates that from 1976 through 2006, annual influenza-associated deaths in the United States ranged from a low of approximately 3,000 people to a high of approximately 49,000 people; approximately 80%–90% of these deaths occurred among people aged ≥65 years.

Zoonotic Influenza

Influenza B viruses circulate widely only among humans, although influenza A viruses circulate among many animal populations. The primary reservoir for influenza A viruses is wild waterfowl and other wild birds, but viruses are common in swine populations as well. Influenza A viruses can also infect other animal species, such as poultry, cats, dogs, horses, sea lions, and bats.

Human infections with animal-origin influenza A viruses are uncommon. In the United States, human influenza illnesses caused by swine-origin influenza A viruses (called "variant" influenza virus infections and denoted with the letter "v") have been sporadically identified. In 2012, 309 cases (and 1 death) of human illnesses caused by influenza A (H3N2v) viruses were identified. In the summer of 2013, 19 human cases were identified in 5 states. Most illnesses caused by H3N2v have occurred after direct or indirect contact with an infected pig, often among exhibitors or visitors to agricultural fairs. Limited person-to-person transmission has occurred with this virus. The severity of illness has been similar to that seen with seasonal influenza.

Although avian influenza viruses do not commonly infect humans, disease resulting from these viruses has been reported. From 1997 through March 2016, 850 human illnesses caused by avian influenza A (H5N1) virus were reported globally, approximately 53% of which were fatal. Most disease from H5N1 has occurred after direct or close contact with sick or dead infected poultry. H5N1 is widespread among poultry in some countries in Asia and the Middle East and is considered to be endemic among poultry in 6 countries: Bangladesh, China, Egypt, India (West Bengal), Indonesia, and Vietnam (Map 3-7). Egypt, Indonesia, and Cambodia have accounted for 71% of reported infections in humans globally. Instances of limited, nonsustained human-to-human transmission of H5N1 virus have been reported. In the United States, since December 2014, highly pathogenic avian influenza (HPAI) H5 infections have been detected in backyard and commercial poultry from 21 states. Although no human HPAI H5 infections have been reported in the United States, surveillance in domestic birds is ongoing given the low but continued risk of transmission to humans.

Avian influenza A (H7N9) virus emerged in China in 2013, and as of March 2016, has caused 767 confirmed human illnesses. Most cases have been identified in mainland China, but several cases associated with exposure in mainland China and subsequent travel have been identified in Malaysia, Taiwan, and Hong Kong. In 2014, Canada reported the first imported H7N9 case in North America. Most of the people with illness caused by H7N9 had exposure to infected poultry or contaminated environments, and the virus has been found in poultry and environmental samples collected in China. A small proportion of human H7N9 illnesses has been mild, but most patients have developed severe respiratory illness, and 38% have died.

Although rare, human infections with other avian influenza A viruses, including H7N2, H7N3, H7N7, H9N2, and H10N8, have been reported in recent years. In the United States, 2 infections with H7N2 virus were reported in humans in 2002 and 2003, both of whom recovered.

CLINICAL PRESENTATION

Uncomplicated influenza illness is characterized by the abrupt onset of signs and symptoms that include fever, muscle aches, headache, malaise, nonproductive cough, sore throat, vomiting, and rhinitis. Less commonly, rashes have been associated with influenza infection. Illness without fever can occur, especially in the elderly. Children

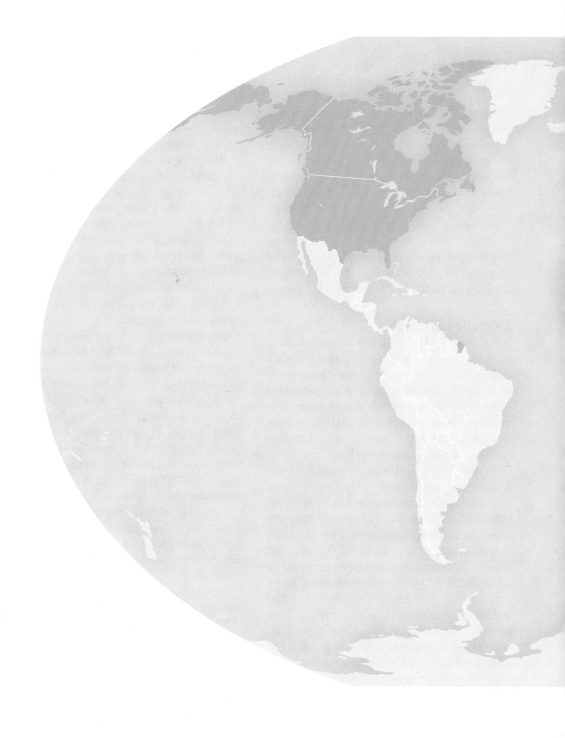

MAP 3-7. Distribution of highly pathogenic avian influenza A (H5N1) virus

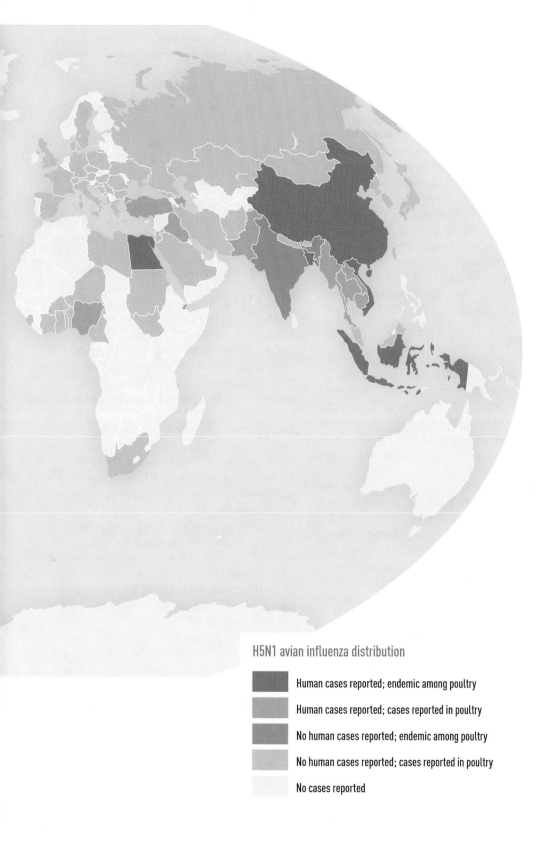

3

H5N1 avian influenza distribution

Human cases reported; endemic among poultry

Human cases reported; cases reported in poultry

No human cases reported; endemic among poultry

No human cases reported; cases reported in poultry

No cases reported

are more likely than adults to also experience nausea, vomiting, or diarrhea when ill with influenza. Physical findings are predominantly localized to the respiratory tract and include nasal discharge, pharyngeal inflammation without exudates, and occasionally rales on chest auscultation. The incubation period is usually 1–4 days after exposure. Influenza illness typically resolves within 1 week for most previously healthy children and adults who do not receive antiviral medication, although cough and malaise can persist for >2 weeks, especially in the elderly. Complications of influenza virus infection include primary influenza viral pneumonia, secondary bacterial pneumonia, parotitis, exacerbation of underlying medical conditions (such as pulmonary and cardiac disease), encephalopathy, myocarditis, myositis, and coinfections with other viral or bacterial pathogens.

DIAGNOSIS

Influenza can be difficult to distinguish from respiratory illnesses caused by other pathogens on the basis of signs and symptoms alone. The positive predictive value of clinical signs and symptoms for influenzalike illness (fever with either cough or sore throat) for laboratory-confirmed influenza virus infection is 30%–88%, depending on the level of influenza activity.

Diagnostic tests available for influenza include viral culture, rapid influenza diagnostic tests (RIDTs), immunofluorescence assays, and RT-PCR. Most patients with clinical illness consistent with uncomplicated influenza in an area where influenza viruses are circulating do not require diagnostic testing for clinical management. Patients who should be considered for influenza diagnostic testing include the following:

- Hospitalized patients with suspected influenza

- Patients for whom a diagnosis of influenza will inform decisions regarding clinical care, including patients who do not improve on antiviral therapy and those with medical conditions that place them at high risk of complications

- Patients for whom results of influenza testing would affect infection control or management

of close contacts, including other patients, such as in institutional outbreaks or other settings (cruise ships or tour groups, for example)

The sensitivity of RIDTs varies but is substantially lower than for RT-PCR or viral culture. The sensitivity of RIDTs to detect animal-origin influenza viruses, including avian influenza viruses, can vary by test type and virus subtype. Therefore, a negative RIDT result does not rule out influenza virus infection, and health care providers should not rely on a negative RIDT result to make decisions about treatment. The decision to start antiviral treatment should not be delayed while waiting for results of confirmatory laboratory testing.

TREATMENT

Early antiviral treatment can shorten the duration of fever and other symptoms and reduce the risk of complications from influenza. Antiviral treatment is recommended as early as possible for any patient with confirmed or suspected influenza who is hospitalized; has severe, complicated, or progressive illness; or is at a higher risk for influenza-associated complications (www.cdc.gov/flu/professionals/antivirals/summary-clinicians.htm). Antiviral treatment can also be considered for any previously healthy patient with confirmed or suspected influenza not at high risk of complications.

Treatment is most effective if it can be initiated within 48 hours of illness onset. For hospitalized patients, those with severe illness, or those at higher risk of complications, antiviral therapy may still be beneficial if started >48 hours after illness onset. Three FDA-approved antiviral agents are recommended for the treatment and prophylaxis of influenza: oral oseltamivir (Tamiflu, Genentech), inhaled zanamivir (Relenza, GlaxoSmithKline), and intravenous (IV) peramivir (Rapivab, BioCryst Pharmaceuticals).

All 3 antiviral medications are neuraminidase inhibitors that have activity against both influenza A and B viruses. Oseltamivir is approved for treatment in children aged ≥14 days and for prophylaxis of patients aged ≥1 year. Oseltamivir is the preferred agent to treat patients with severe or complicated influenza illness who are able to

3

tolerate oral medications. Zanamivir is approved to treat those aged ≥7 years and for prophylaxis in those aged ≥5 years. Inhaled zanamivir is not recommended for use in people with underlying chronic respiratory disease. Peramivir is approved to treat those aged ≥18 years and is indicated for use in patients unable to tolerate or absorb oral antiviral therapy (Table 3-5). Two other medications, amantadine and rimantadine, are not recommended for treatment or prophylaxis of influenza because of widespread viral resistance among circulating influenza A viruses. Amantadine and rimantadine are not active against influenza B viruses.

For severely ill hospitalized patients, IV peramivir or IV zanamivir (an investigational product) should be considered for those who cannot tolerate or absorb oral oseltamivir. IV zanamivir should be considered for severely ill patients with known or suspected oseltamivir/peramivir-resistant virus infection. IV zanimivir is available only under an approved emergency investigational new drug request in hospitalized patients with severe influenza.

People at increased risk for complications of influenza should discuss antiviral treatment and prophylaxis with their health care provider before travel to areas where influenza activity is occurring. CDC recommends antiviral treatment for human infection with avian or swine influenza viruses.

PREVENTION

Vaccine

AVAILABLE VACCINE PRODUCTS AND INDICATIONS FOR USE

In the United States, annual influenza vaccination is recommended for those aged ≥6 months and is the most effective way to prevent influenza and its complications. Several influenza vaccines are approved for use in the United States (www.cdc.gov/flu/protect/vaccine/vaccines.htm) and can be grouped into categories: inactivated influenza vaccine (IIV), live attenuated influenza vaccine (LAIV), and recombinant influenza vaccine (RIV). However, for the 2016–2017 influenza season, CDC has recommended that LAIV not be used following analyses that indicated lower effectiveness

of the vaccine compared with inactivated vaccine. (For updates and the following season recommendations, providers should access http://www.cdc.gov/flu/protect/vaccine/index.htm.) For people for whom more than 1 type of vaccine is indicated, there is no preference for any particular category. During their first influenza season, children aged 6 months through 8 years require 2 doses of influenza vaccine (given ≥4 weeks apart) to induce sufficient immune response.

IIV can be administered by intramuscular injection, transdermally via needle-free jet injector, or intradermal injection depending on the product. IIVs are labeled for use in people aged ≥6 months, but specific age indications vary by manufacturer and product; label instructions should be followed. High-dose IIV and adjuvanted IIV vaccines, which may elicit higher levels of antibodies than standard-dose vaccines, are available for people aged ≥65 years. RIV is labeled for use in people aged ≥18 years.

Influenza vaccine composition can be trivalent, protecting against 3 different influenza viruses (2 influenza subtype A and 1 type influenza B), or quadrivalent, with protection against 4 different influenza viruses (2 influenza subtype A and 2 influenza type B strains). Quadrivalent vaccine includes a representative strain from 2 antigenically distinct influenza B lineages, Yamagata and Victoria.

Any traveler, including people at high risk for complications of influenza, who did not receive influenza vaccine during the preceding fall or winter and wants to reduce the risk for influenza infection should consider influenza vaccination ≥2 weeks before departure if he or she plans to travel to the tropics, with organized tourist groups at any time of year, or to the Southern Hemisphere from April through September.

No information is available about the benefits of revaccinating people before summer travel who were vaccinated during the preceding fall, and revaccination is not recommended. People at higher risk for influenza complications should consult with their health care provider to discuss the risk for influenza or other travel-related diseases before traveling during the summer.

Seasonal influenza vaccines are not expected to provide protection against human infection

Table 3-5. Recommended dosage and duration of antiviral medications for treatment and prophylaxis of influenza A and B

ANTIVIRAL AGENT	USE	CHILDREN	ADULTS
Oseltamivir (Tamiflu)	Treatment (5 days)	**If child is <1 year old**[1]: 3 mg/kg/dose twice daily[2,3] **If ≥1 year old, dose varies by child's weight:** ≤15 kg, the dose is 30 mg twice a day. >15–23 kg, the dose is 45 mg twice a day. >23–40 kg, the dose is 60 mg twice a day. >40 kg, the dose is 75 mg twice a day.	75 mg twice daily
	Prophylaxis (7 days)	**If child is <3 months old:** use of oseltamivir for prophylaxis is not recommended unless situation is judged critical because data in this age group are limited. **If child is ≥3 months and <1 year old**[1]: 3 mg/kg/dose once daily.[2] **If ≥1 year old, dose varies by child's weight:** ≤15 kg, the dose is 30 mg once a day. >15–23 kg, the dose is 45 mg once a day. >23–40 kg, the dose is 60 mg once a day. >40 kg, the dose is 75 mg once a day.	75 mg once daily
Zanamivir[4] (Relenza)	Treatment (5 days)	10 mg (two 5-mg inhalations) twice daily **(FDA approved and recommended for use in children ≥7 years)**	10 mg (two 5-mg inhalations) twice daily
	Prophylaxis (7 days)	10 mg (two 5-mg inhalations) once daily[4] **(FDA approved for and recommended for use in children ≥5 years)**	10 mg (two 5-mg inhalations) once daily
Peramivir[5] (Rapivab)	Treatment (1 day)	No FDA approval for use in children	600 mg dose via IV infusion for 15–30 minutes[5]

[1] Oral oseltamivir is approved by the FDA for treatment of acute uncomplicated influenza with twice-daily dosing in people aged ≥14 days and for prophylaxis with once-daily dosing in people aged ≥1 year. Although not part of the FDA-approved indications, use of oral oseltamivir for treatment of influenza in infants <14 days old, and for prophylaxis in infants 3 months to 1 year of age, is recommended by CDC and the American Academy of Pediatrics.

[2] This is the FDA-approved oral oseltamivir treatment dose for infants aged ≥14 days and <1 year old and provides oseltamivir exposure in children similar to that achieved by the approved dose of 75 mg orally twice daily for adults, as shown in 2 studies of oseltamivir pharmacokinetics in children. The American Academy of Pediatrics (AAP) recommended an oseltamivir treatment dose of 3.5 mg/kg orally twice daily for infants aged 9–11 months for the 2015–2016 season. It is unknown whether this higher dose will improve efficacy or prevent the development of antiviral resistance. However, there is no evidence that the 3.5 mg/kg dose is harmful or causes more adverse events to infants in this age group. The AAP also recommended an oseltamivir treatment dose of 3 mg/kg orally twice daily for term infants aged 0–8 months for the 2015–2016 season.

[3] Current weight-based dosing recommendations are not appropriate for premature infants. Premature infants might have slower clearance of oral oseltamivir because of immature renal function, and doses recommended for full-term infants might lead to very high drug concentrations in this age group. CDC recommends dosing as also recommended by the American Academy of Pediatrics: 1.0 mg/kg/dose, orally, twice daily, for those <38 weeks postmenstrual age; 1.5 mg/kg/dose, orally, twice daily, for those 38–40 weeks postmenstrual age; 3.0 mg/kg/dose, orally, twice daily, for those >40 weeks postmenstrual age.

[4] Inhaled zanamivir is approved to treat acute uncomplicated influenza with twice-daily dosing in people aged ≥7 years and for prophylaxis with once-daily dosing in people aged ≥5 years.

[5] Intravenous peramivir is FDA approved and recommended for treatment in adults ≥18 years. If used to treat hospitalized patients, a minimum of 5 days of IV peramivir should be given (not a single dose as is recommended for outpatients with uncomplicated illness).

with animal-origin influenza viruses, including avian influenza A (H5N1 and H7N9) viruses.

VACCINE SAFETY AND ADVERSE REACTIONS

INACTIVATED INFLUENZA VACCINE (IIV)

The most frequent side effects of vaccination with intramuscular and intradermal IIV in adults are soreness and redness at the vaccination site. These local injection-site reactions are slightly more common with vaccine administered intradermally, with needle-free jet injection and with high-dose IIV. They generally are mild and rarely interfere with the ability to conduct usual activities. Fever, malaise, myalgia, headache, and other systemic symptoms sometimes occur after vaccination; these may be more frequent in people with no previous exposure to the influenza virus antigens in the vaccine (such as young children) and are generally short-lived.

Guillain-Barré syndrome (GBS) was associated with the 1976 swine influenza vaccine, with an increased risk of 1 additional case of GBS per 100,000 people vaccinated. None of the studies of influenza vaccines other than the 1976 influenza vaccine have demonstrated a risk of GBS of similar magnitude. Currently, the estimated risk for vaccine-related GBS is low, approximately 1 additional case per 1 million people vaccinated.

LIVE ATTENUATED INFLUENZA VACCINE (LAIV)

The most frequent side effects of LAIV reported in healthy adults include minor upper respiratory symptoms, runny nose, and sore throat, which are generally well tolerated. Some children and adolescents have reported fever, vomiting, myalgia, and wheezing. These symptoms, particularly fever, are more often associated with the first administered LAIV dose and are self-limited.

Although LAIV is licensed for people aged 2–49 years, CDC recommended that LAIV not be used during the 2016–2017 season following analyses that indicated lower effectiveness of LAIV compared with IIV. (Recommendations for subsequent seasons may be found at www.cdc.gov/flu/protect/vaccine/index.htm.) Children aged 2–4 years who have a history of wheezing in the past year or who have a diagnosis of asthma should not receive LAIV. Children and adults aged 2–49 years who have conditions that increase the risk of severe influenza, including pregnancy and

immunocompromising conditions, should receive IIV or RIV and not LAIV. Caretakers of severely immunocompromised people should also not receive LAIV or should avoid contact with such people for 7 days after receipt of LAIV to decrease the risk of live virus transmission.

RECOMBINANT INFLUENZA VACCINE (RIV)

The first RIV was licensed in the United States in January 2013. Limited postmarketing safety data are available, but prelicensure safety data indicate that the most common reactions were headache, fatigue, and myalgia. RIV is not indicated for people <18 years.

PRECAUTIONS AND CONTRAINDICATIONS

Influenza vaccine is contraindicated in people who have had a previous severe allergic reaction to influenza vaccine, regardless of which vaccine component was responsible for the reaction. Immediate hypersensitivity reactions (such as hives, angioedema, allergic asthma, and systemic anaphylaxis) rarely occur after influenza vaccination. These reactions likely result from hypersensitivity to vaccine components, one of which is residual egg protein. Vaccine options are available for people with a history of egg allergy who have experienced only hives after exposure to egg, people with a history of severe reaction to egg, and people with no known history of egg allergy but who are suspected of being egg-allergic; these are outlined at www.cdc.gov/flu/professionals/vaccination/vax-summary.htm#egg-allergy.

Personal Protection Measures

Measures that may help prevent influenza virus infection and other infections during travel include avoiding close contact with sick people and washing hands often with soap and water (where soap and a safe source of water are not available, use of an alcohol-based hand sanitizer containing ≥60% alcohol is recommended). If you are ill, you can help prevent the spread of illness to others by covering your nose and mouth when coughing and sneezing and avoiding close contact with others during the illness.

The best way to prevent infection with animal-origin influenza viruses, including H5N1 and H7N9, is to follow standard travel safety precautions: follow good hand hygiene and food safety practices and avoid contact with sources of exposure. Most human infections with avian influenza viruses have occurred after direct or close contact with infected poultry. In countries where avian influenza virus outbreaks are occurring, travelers or those living abroad should avoid markets and farms where live animals are sold or raised, avoid contact with sick or dead animals, not eat undercooked or raw animal products (including eggs), and not eat or drink foods or beverages that contain animal blood.

CDC website: www.cdc.gov/flu

BIBLIOGRAPHY

1. CDC. Evaluation of 11 commercially available rapid influenza diagnostic tests—United States, 2011–2012. MMWR Morb Mortal Wkly Rep. 2012 Nov 2;61(43):873–6.

2. CDC. Prevention and control of influenza with vaccines: recommendations of the Advisory Committee on Immunization Practices, United States, 2015–16 Influenza Season. MMWR Morb Mortal Wkly Rep. 2015 Aug 7;64(30):818–25.

3. Committee on Infectious Diseases AAoP. Recommendations for prevention and control of influenza in children, 2015–2016. Pediatrics. 2015 Oct;136(4):792–808.

4. Donnelly CA, Finelli L, Cauchemez S, Olsen SJ, Doshi S, Jackson ML, et al. Serial intervals and the temporal distribution of secondary infections within households of 2009 pandemic influenza A (H1N1): implications for influenza control recommendations. Clin Infect Dis. 2011 Jan 1;52 Suppl 1:S123–30.

5. Jhung MA, Epperson S, Biggerstaff M, Allen D, Balish A, Barnes N, et al. Outbreak of variant influenza A(H3N2) virus in the United States. Clin Infect Dis. 2013 Dec;57(12):1703–12.

6. Li Q, Zhou L, Zhou M, Chen Z, Li F, Wu H, et al. Epidemiology of human infections with avian influenza A(H7N9) virus in China. N Engl J Med. 2014 Feb 6;370(6):520–32.

7. McGeer A, Green KA, Plevneshi A, Shigayeva A, Siddiqi N, Raboud J, et al. Antiviral therapy and outcomes of influenza requiring hospitalization in Ontario, Canada. Clin Infect Dis. 2007 Dec 15;45(12):1568–75.

8. Pabbaraju K, Tellier R, Wong S, Li Y, Bastien N, Tang JW, et al. Full-genome analysis of avian influenza A(H5N1) virus from a human, North America, 2013. Emerg Infect Dis. 2014 May;20(5):887–91.

9. Reed C, Chaves SS, Daily Kirley P, Emerson R, Aragon D, Hancock EB, et al. Estimating influenza disease burden from population-based surveillance data in the United States. PLoS One. 2015;10(3):e0118369.

10. Siston AM, Rasmussen SA, Honein MA, Fry AM, Seib K, Callaghan WM, et al. Pandemic 2009 influenza A(H1N1) virus illness among pregnant women in the United States. JAMA. 2010 Apr 21;303(15):1517–25.

11. Writing Committee of the WHO Consultation on Clinical Aspects of Pandemic Influenza. Clinical aspects of pandemic 2009 influenza A (H1N1) virus infection. N Engl J Med. 2010 May 6;362(18):1708–19.

JAPANESE ENCEPHALITIS

Susan L. Hills, Ingrid B. Rabe, Marc Fischer

INFECTIOUS AGENT

Japanese encephalitis (JE) virus is a single-stranded RNA virus that belongs to the genus *Flavivirus* and is closely related to West Nile and Saint Louis encephalitis viruses.

TRANSMISSION

JE virus is transmitted to humans through the bite of an infected mosquito, primarily *Culex* species. The virus is maintained in an enzootic cycle between mosquitoes and amplifying vertebrate hosts, primarily pigs and wading birds. Humans are incidental or dead-end hosts, because they usually do not develop a level or duration of viremia sufficient to infect mosquitoes.

EPIDEMIOLOGY

JE virus is the most common vaccine-preventable cause of encephalitis in Asia, occurring throughout most of Asia and parts of the western Pacific

(Map 3-8). Local transmission of JE virus has not been detected in Africa, Europe, or the Americas. Transmission principally occurs in rural agricultural areas, often associated with rice cultivation and flood irrigation. In some areas of Asia, these ecologic conditions may occur near, or occasionally within, urban centers. In temperate areas of Asia, transmission is seasonal, and human disease usually peaks in summer and fall. In the subtropics and tropics, seasonal transmission varies with monsoon rains and irrigation practices and may be prolonged or even occur year-round.

In endemic countries, where adults have acquired immunity through natural infection, JE is primarily a disease of children. However, travel-associated JE can occur among people of any age. For most travelers to Asia, the risk for JE is extremely low but varies based on destination, duration, season, and activities.

From 1973 through 2015, 79 JE cases among travelers or expatriates from nonendemic countries were published or reported to CDC. From the time a JE vaccine became available in the United States in 1993, through 2015, only 10 JE cases among US travelers were reported to CDC.

The overall incidence of JE among people from nonendemic countries traveling to Asia is estimated to be <1 case per 1 million travelers. However, expatriates and travelers who stay for prolonged periods in rural areas with active JE virus transmission are likely at similar risk as the susceptible resident population (5–50 cases per 100,000 children per year). Travelers on even brief trips might be at increased risk if they have extensive outdoor or nighttime exposure in rural areas during periods of active transmission. Short-term (<1 month) travelers whose visits are restricted to major urban areas are at minimal risk for JE. In some endemic areas, although there are few human cases among residents because of natural immunity among older people or vaccination, JE virus is still maintained locally in an enzootic cycle between animals and mosquitoes. Therefore, susceptible visitors may be at risk for infection.

CLINICAL PRESENTATION

Most human infections with JE virus are asymptomatic; <1% of people infected with JE virus develop clinical disease. Acute encephalitis is the most commonly recognized clinical manifestation of JE virus infection. Milder forms of disease, such as aseptic meningitis or undifferentiated febrile illness, can also occur. The incubation period is 5–15 days. Illness usually begins with sudden onset of fever, headache, and vomiting. Mental status changes, focal neurologic deficits, generalized weakness, and movement disorders may develop over the next few days. The classical description of JE includes a parkinsonian syndrome with mask-like facies, tremor, cogwheel rigidity, and choreoathetoid movements. Acute flaccid paralysis, with clinical and pathological features similar to those of poliomyelitis, has also been associated with JE virus infection. Seizures are common, especially among children. The case-fatality ratio is approximately 20%–30%. Among survivors, 30%–50% have serious neurologic, cognitive, or psychiatric sequelae.

Common clinical laboratory findings include moderate leukocytosis, mild anemia, and hyponatremia. Cerebrospinal fluid (CSF) typically has a mild to moderate pleocytosis with a lymphocytic predominance, slightly elevated protein, and normal ratio of CSF to plasma glucose.

DIAGNOSIS

JE should be suspected in a patient with evidence of a neurologic infection (such as encephalitis, meningitis, or acute flaccid paralysis) who has recently traveled to or resided in an endemic country in Asia or the western Pacific. Laboratory diagnosis of JE virus infection should be performed by using a JE virus–specific IgM-capture ELISA on CSF or serum. JE virus–specific IgM can be measured in the CSF of most patients by 4 days after onset of symptoms and in serum by 7 days after onset. Plaque reduction neutralization tests can be performed to confirm the presence of JE virus–specific neutralizing antibodies and discriminate between cross-reacting antibodies from closely related flaviviruses (such as dengue and West Nile viruses). A ≥4-fold rise in JE virus–specific neutralizing antibodies between acute- and convalescent-phase serum specimens may be used to confirm recent infection. Vaccination history, date of onset of symptoms, and information regarding other flaviviruses known to circulate in

3

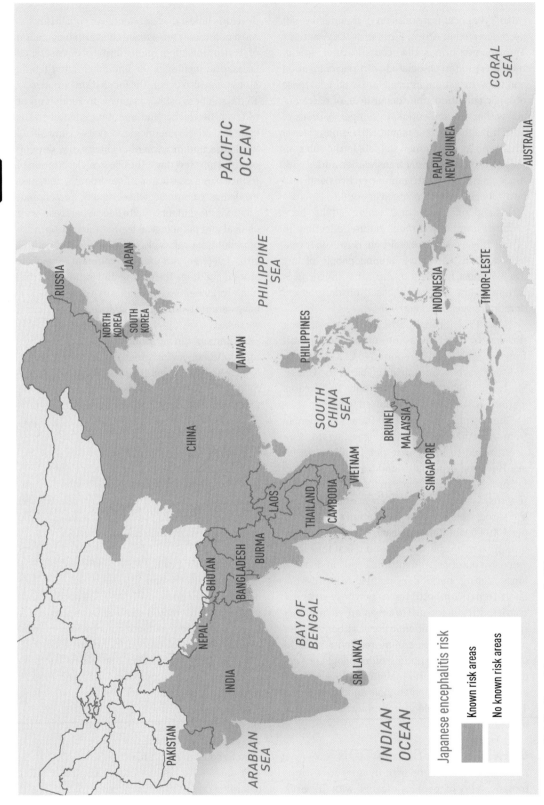

MAP 3-8. Distribution of Japanese encephalitis

Japanese encephalitis risk

■ Known risk areas

□ No known risk areas

the geographic area that may cross-react in serologic assays need to be considered when interpreting results.

Humans have low levels of transient viremia and usually have neutralizing antibodies by the time distinctive clinical symptoms are recognized. Virus isolation and nucleic-acid amplification tests are insensitive in detecting JE virus or viral RNA in blood or CSF and should not be used for ruling out a diagnosis of JE. Clinicians should contact their state or local health department or CDC at 970-221-6400 for assistance with diagnostic testing.

TREATMENT

There is no specific antiviral treatment for JE; therapy consists of supportive care and management of complications.

PREVENTION

Personal Protection Measures

The best way to prevent mosquitoborne diseases, including JE, is to avoid mosquito bites (see Chapter 2, Protection against Mosquitoes, Ticks, & Other Arthropods).

Vaccine

One JE vaccine is licensed and available in the United States—an inactivated Vero cell culture–derived vaccine, Ixiaro (Table 3-6). Ixiaro is manufactured by Valneva Scotland Limited and distributed in the United States by VaxServe (a Sanofi Pasteur company). It was approved in March 2009 for use in people aged ≥17 years and in May 2013 for use in children aged 2 months through 16 years. Other inactivated and live attenuated JE vaccines are manufactured and used in other countries but are not licensed for use in the United States.

INDICATIONS FOR USE OF JE VACCINE FOR TRAVELERS

When making recommendations regarding the use of JE vaccine for travelers, clinicians must weigh the overall low risk of travel-associated JE, the high rate of death and disability when JE occurs, the low probability of serious adverse events after immunization, and the cost of the vaccine. Evaluation of a traveler's risk should take into account the planned itinerary, including travel location, duration, activities, and seasonal patterns of disease in the areas to be visited (Table 3-7). The data in the table should be interpreted cautiously, because JE virus transmission activity varies within countries and from year to year.

The Advisory Committee on Immunization Practices recommends JE vaccine for travelers who plan to spend ≥1 month in endemic areas during the JE virus transmission season. This includes long-term travelers, recurrent travelers, or expatriates who will be based in urban areas but are likely to visit endemic rural or agricultural areas during a high-risk period of JE virus transmission. Vaccine should also be considered for the following:

- Short-term (<1 month) travelers to endemic areas during the JE virus transmission season, if they plan to travel outside an urban area and their activities will increase the risk of JE

Table 3-6. Vaccine to prevent Japanese encephalitis (JE)

VACCINE	TRADE NAME (MANUFACTURER)	AGE	DOSE	ROUTE	SCHEDULE	BOOSTER[1]
JE vaccine, inactivated	Ixiaro (Valneva)	≥17 y	0.5 mL	IM	0, 28 d	>1 y after primary series
		3–16 y	0.5 mL	IM	0, 28 d	Awaiting FDA assessment
		2 mo–2 y	0.25 mL	IM	0, 28 d	Awaiting FDA assessment

Abbreviations: IM, intramuscular; FDA, US Food and Drug Administration
[1] If potential for JE virus exposure continues.

Table 3-7. Risk for Japanese encephalitis (JE), by country[1]

COUNTRY	AFFECTED AREAS	TRANSMISSION SEASON	COMMENTS
Australia	Outer Torres Strait islands	December–May; all human cases reported February–April	1 human case reported from north Queensland mainland
Bangladesh	Presumed widespread	Most human cases reported May–October	Sentinel surveillance has identified human cases in Chittagong, Dhaka, Khulna, Rajshahi, Ranjpur, and Sylhet Divisions; highest incidence reported from Rajshahi Division; outbreak reported from Tangail District, Dhaka Division, in 1977
Bhutan	Very rare reports; probably endemic in nonmountainous areas	No data	Proximity to other endemic areas and presence of vectors suggests virus transmission is likely
Brunei	Presumed transmission in many areas in the country	Unknown; presumed year-round	Outbreak with laboratory-confirmed cases occurred in October–December 2013
Burma (Myanmar)	Limited data; presumed to be endemic countrywide	Unknown; most human cases reported May–October	Outbreaks of human disease documented in Shan and Rakhine States; antibodies documented in animals and humans in other areas
Cambodia	Presumed to be endemic countrywide	Year-round with peak season May–October	Sentinel surveillance has identified human cases in at least 15 of 23 provinces, including Phnom Penh, Takeo, Kampong Cham, Battambang, Svay Rieng, and Siem Reap; 1 case reported in 2010 in a traveler who visited Phnom Penh and Angkor Wat/Siem Reap only
China	Human cases reported from all provinces except Xizang (Tibet), Xinjiang, and Qinghai; JE virus isolated from mosquitoes in Tibet	Most human cases reported June–October	Highest rates reported from Guizhou, Shaanxi, Sichuan, and Yunnan Provinces, and Chongqing City; vaccine not routinely recommended for travel limited to Beijing, Shanghai, Hong Kong City/Kowloon, Macau, or other major cities

3

India	Human cases reported from all states except Dadra, Daman, Diu, Gujarat, Himachal Pradesh, Jammu and Kashmir, Lakshadweep, Meghalaya, Nagar Haveli, Punjab, Rajasthan, and Sikkim	Most human cases reported May–October, especially in northern India; the season may be extended or year-round in some areas, especially in southern India	Highest rates of human disease reported from the states of Andhra Pradesh, Assam, Bihar, Goa, Haryana, Karnataka, Kerala, Tamil Nadu, Uttar Pradesh, and West Bengal
Indonesia	Presumed to be endemic countrywide	Year-round; peak season varies by island	Sentinel surveillance has identified human cases in Bali, Kalimantan, Java, Nusa Tenggara, Papua, and Sumatra; several traveler cases reported in recent years from Bali
Japan[2]	Rare sporadic human cases on all islands except Hokkaido; enzootic activity ongoing	Most human cases reported July–October	Large number of human cases reported until JE vaccination program introduced in late 1960s; most recent small outbreak reported from Chugoku district in 2002; enzootic transmission without human cases observed on Hokkaido; vaccine not routinely recommended for travel limited to Tokyo or other major cities
Korea, North	Limited data; presumed to be endemic countrywide	No data; proximity to South Korea suggests peak season is likely to be May–October	
Korea, South[2]	Rare sporadic human cases countrywide; enzootic activity ongoing	Most human cases reported May–October	Large number of human cases reported until routine JE vaccination program introduced in mid-1980s; last major outbreak reported in 1982; vaccine not routinely recommended for travel limited to Seoul or other major cities
Laos	Limited data; presumed to be endemic countrywide	Year-round, with peak season June–September	Sentinel surveillance has identified human cases in north, central, and southern Laos
Malaysia	Endemic in Sarawak; sporadic cases reported from all other states	Year-round; in Sarawak, peak season October–December	Most human cases reported from Sarawak; vaccine not routinely recommended for travel limited to Kuala Lumpur or other major cities

(continued)

Table 3-7. Risk for Japanese encephalitis (JE), by country[1] (continued)

COUNTRY	AFFECTED AREAS	TRANSMISSION SEASON	COMMENTS
Nepal	Endemic in southern lowlands (Terai); cases also reported from hill and mountain districts, including the Kathmandu valley	Most human cases reported June–October	Highest rates of human disease reported from western Terai districts, including Banke, Bardiya, Dang, and Kailali; vaccine not routinely recommended for those trekking in high-altitude areas
Pakistan	Limited data; human cases reported from around Karachi	Unknown	
Papua New Guinea	Limited data; probably widespread	Unknown; probably year-round	Sporadic human cases reported from Western Province; serologic evidence of disease from Gulf and Southern Highland Provinces; a case of JE was reported from near Port Moresby in 2004
Philippines	Human, animal, and mosquito studies have indicated transmission in 32 provinces located in all regions of the country; presumed to be endemic countrywide	Year-round with peak season April–August	Several traveler cases recently reported
Russia	Rare human cases reported from the Far Eastern maritime areas south of Khabarovsk	Most human cases reported July–September	Vaccine not routinely recommended
Singapore	Rare sporadic human cases reported	Year-round	Vaccine not routinely recommended
Sri Lanka	Endemic countrywide except in mountainous areas	Year-round with variable peaks based on monsoon rains	Highest rates of human disease reported from Anuradhapura, Gampaha, Kurunegala, Polonnaruwa, and Puttalam districts

3

Taiwan[2]	Rare sporadic human cases islandwide	Most human cases reported May–October	Large number of human cases reported until routine JE vaccination introduced in 1968; vaccine not routinely recommended for travel limited to Taipei or other major cities
Thailand	Endemic countrywide; seasonal epidemics in the northern provinces	Year-round with peak season May–October, especially in the north	Highest rates of human disease reported from the Chiang Mai Valley; several cases reported recently in travelers who visited resort or coastal areas of southern Thailand
Timor-Leste	Sporadic human cases reported; presumed to be endemic countrywide	No data; cases reported year-round in neighboring West Timor	
Vietnam	Endemic countrywide; seasonal epidemics in the northern provinces	Year-round with peak season May–October, especially in the north	Highest rates of disease in the northern provinces around Hanoi and northwestern and northeastern provinces bordering China
Western Pacific Islands	Outbreaks of human disease reported in Guam in 1947–1948 and Saipan in 1990	Unknown; most human cases reported October–March	Outbreaks likely followed introduction of virus, with enzootic cycle not sustained; vaccine not recommended

[1] Data are based on published reports and personal correspondence. Risk assessments should be performed cautiously, because risk can vary within areas and from year to year, and surveillance data regarding human cases and JE virus transmission are incomplete.

[2] In some endemic areas, human cases among residents are limited because of natural immunity among older people or vaccination. However, because JE virus is maintained in an enzootic cycle between animals and mosquitoes, susceptible visitors to these areas still may be at risk for infection.

3

virus exposure. Examples of higher-risk activities or itineraries include 1) spending substantial time outdoors in rural or agricultural areas, especially during the evening or night; 2) participating in extensive outdoor activities (such as camping, hiking, trekking, biking, fishing, hunting, or farming); and 3) staying in accommodations without air conditioning, screens, or bed nets.

- Travelers to an area with an ongoing JE outbreak.
- Travelers to endemic areas who are uncertain of specific destinations, activities, or duration of travel.

JE vaccine is not recommended for short-term travelers whose visits will be restricted to urban areas or times outside a well-defined JE virus transmission season.

VACCINE EFFICACY AND IMMUNOGENICITY

There are no efficacy data for Ixiaro. The vaccine was licensed in the United States on the basis of its ability to induce JE virus neutralizing antibodies as a surrogate for protection, as well as safety evaluations in almost 5,000 adults. In pivotal immunogenicity studies, 96% of adults and 100% of children aged 2 months through 17 years developed protective neutralizing antibodies at 28 days after receiving a primary immunization series of 2 doses administered 28 days apart. Among adults aged ≥65 years, 65% are seroprotected at 42 days after the 2-dose primary series.

A study in adults on persistence of protective neutralizing antibodies after a primary 2-dose series of Ixiaro showed that at 5 years postvaccination, 82% of subjects were seroprotected. However, the study was conducted in areas where tickborne encephalitis (TBE) vaccine is available. In a subgroup analysis, seroprotection rates at 24–60 months in the TBE vaccine group ranged from 94%–100%, compared with 64%–72% in the group in which TBE vaccine was not administered. TBE vaccine is not available in the United States; therefore, JE seroprotection rates for US travelers are likely to be most similar to the rates in the group not administered TBE vaccine.

One observational study investigated long-term protection following a booster dose of Ixiaro

in adults. After a booster dose administered at 15 months, 96% of subjects were still seroprotected approximately 6 years later.

There are limited data on duration of seroprotection and need for a booster dose in children. In a study conducted among children from non-endemic countries, 89% were seroprotected at 3 years after a primary 2-dose series of Ixiaro. This rate was higher than that in a comparative adult study. In a study conducted among children in a JE-endemic country, 90% of children were seroprotected at 36 months after the primary series. Seroprotection rates were variable by age group, but at least 81% of children in each age group were seroprotected.

An accelerated primary series of 2 doses of Ixiaro administered 7 days apart has been studied in adults aged 18–65 years. In the accelerated schedule group, 99% of adults were seroprotected, compared with 100% of adults in the standard schedule group. The accelerated primary series was noninferior to the conventional dosing schedule. An accelerated schedule (administered on days 0 and 7) has been licensed for use in Europe.

VACCINE ADMINISTRATION

The primary immunization schedule for Ixiaro is 2 doses administered intramuscularly on days 0 and 28 (Table 3-6). For children aged 2 months through 2 years, each dose is 0.25 mL, and for adults and children aged ≥3 years, each dose is 0.5 mL. To administer a 0.25-mL dose, health care providers must expel and discard half of the volume from the 0.5-mL prefilled syringe by pushing the plunger stopper up to the edge of the red line on the syringe barrel before injection. The 2-dose series should be completed ≥1 week before travel.

BOOSTER DOSES

For adults, if the primary series of Ixiaro was administered >1 year previously, a booster dose should be given before potential reexposure or if there is a continued risk for JE virus infection. Data on the response to a booster dose administered ≥2 years after the primary series are not available.

There are limited data on the use of Ixiaro as a booster dose after a primary series with the mouse brain–derived inactivated JE vaccine. Two studies have been conducted, 1 in US military personnel and the other at 2 travel clinics in Europe. Both studies demonstrated that in adults who had previously received at least a primary series of mouse brain–derived inactivated JE vaccine, a single dose of Ixiaro adequately boosted neutralizing antibody levels and provided at least short-term protection. In addition, seroprotective titers against both vaccine virus strains persisted in all participants who could be followed up at 2 years in the European study (N = 18). However, additional data are needed on the duration of protection after a single dose of Ixiaro in prior recipients of a mouse brain–derived vaccine. Until those data are available, people who have received JE-Vax, the mouse brain–derived vaccine formerly used in the United States, and require further vaccination against JE virus, should receive a 2-dose primary series of Ixiaro.

VACCINE SAFETY AND ADVERSE REACTIONS

Local symptoms of pain and tenderness were the most commonly reported symptoms in a safety study with 1,993 adult participants who received 2 doses of Ixiaro. Headache, myalgia, fatigue, and an influenzalike illness were each reported at a rate of >10%. In children, fever was the most commonly reported systemic reaction in studies.

PRECAUTIONS AND CONTRAINDICATIONS

A severe allergic reaction after a previous dose of Ixiaro or any other JE vaccine, or to any component of Ixiaro, is a contraindication to administration of Ixiaro. Ixiaro contains protamine sulfate, a compound known to cause hypersensitivity reactions in some people. No studies of Ixiaro in pregnant women have been conducted. Therefore, administration of Ixiaro to pregnant women usually should be deferred. However, pregnant women who must travel to an area where risk for JE virus infection is high should be vaccinated when the theoretical risk of immunization is outweighed by the risk of infection.

CDC website: www.cdc.gov/japaneseencephalitis

BIBLIOGRAPHY

1. CDC. Recommendations for use of a booster dose of inactivated Vero cell culture-derived Japanese encephalitis vaccine: advisory committee on immunization practices, 2011. MMWR Morb Mortal Wkly Rep. 2011 May 27;60(20):661–3.

2. CDC. Use of Japanese encephalitis vaccine in children: recommendations of the advisory committee on immunization practices, 2013. MMWR Morb Mortal Wkly Rep. 2013 Nov 15;62(45):898–900.

3. Fischer M, Lindsey N, Staples JE, Hills S. Japanese encephalitis vaccines: recommendations of the Advisory Committee on Immunization Practices (ACIP). MMWR Recomm Rep. 2010 Mar 12;59(Rr-1):1–27.

4. Hills SL, Griggs AC, Fischer M. Japanese encephalitis in travelers from non-endemic countries, 1973–2008. Am J Trop Med Hyg. 2010 May;82(5):930–6.

5. Jelinek T, Burchard GD, Dieckmann S, Buhler S, Paulke-Korinek M, Nothdurft HD, et al. Short-Term immunogenicity and safety of an accelerated pre-exposure prophylaxis regimen with Japanese encephalitis vaccine in combination with a rabies vaccine: a phase III, multicenter, observer-blind study. J Travel Med. 2015 Jul-Aug;22(4):225–31.

6. Paulke-Korinek M, Kollaritsch H, Kundi M, Zwazl I, Seidl-Friedrich C, Jelinek T. Persistence of antibodies six years after booster vaccination with inactivated vaccine against Japanese encephalitis. Vaccine. 2015 Jul 9;33(30):3600–4.

7. Rabe IB, Miller ER, Fischer M, Hills SL. Adverse events following vaccination with an inactivated, Vero cell culture-derived Japanese encephalitis vaccine in the United States, 2009–2012. Vaccine. 2015 Jan 29;33(5):708–12.

8. Schuller E, Klingler A, Dubischar-Kastner K, Dewasthaly S, Muller Z. Safety profile of the Vero cell-derived Japanese encephalitis virus (JEV) vaccine IXIARO((R)). Vaccine. 2011 Nov 3;29(47):8669–76.

9. Tauber E, Kollaritsch H, von Sonnenburg F, Lademann M, Jilma B, Firbas C, et al. Randomized, double-blind, placebo-controlled phase 3 trial of the safety and tolerability of IC51, an inactivated Japanese encephalitis vaccine. J Infect Dis. 2008 Aug 15;198(4):493–9.

LEGIONELLOSIS (LEGIONNAIRES' DISEASE & PONTIAC FEVER)

Preeta K. Kutty, Laurel E. Garrison

INFECTIOUS AGENT

Gram-negative bacteria of the genus *Legionella*. Most cases of legionellosis are caused by *Legionella pneumophila*, but all species of *Legionella* can cause disease.

TRANSMISSION

Inhalation of a water aerosol containing the bacteria. The bacterium grows in warm freshwater environments. A single episode of possible person-to-person transmission of Legionnaires' disease has been reported.

EPIDEMIOLOGY

Legionellae are ubiquitous worldwide. Disease occurs after exposure to aquatic settings that promote bacterial growth—the aquatic environment is somewhat stagnant, the water is warm (77°F–108°F [25°C–42°C]), and the water must be aerosolized so that the bacteria can be inhaled into the lungs. These 3 conditions are met almost exclusively in developed or industrialized settings. Disease does not occur in association with natural freshwater settings such as waterfalls, lakes, or streams.

Legionellosis has been reported worldwide. The largest outbreak (449 confirmed cases) ever reported was traced to a cooling tower on the roof of a city hospital in Murcia, Spain, in 2001. Travel-associated outbreaks are commonly recognized.

Despite the presence of *Legionella* bacteria in many aquatic environments, the risk of developing legionellosis for most people is low. Travelers who are exposed to aerosolized, warm water containing *Legionella* are at risk for infection. Travelers who are aged >50 years, are current or former smokers, have chronic lung conditions, or are immunocompromised are at higher risk. Many outbreaks have been associated with exposure to cruise ships, hotels, and resorts. Exposures can occur when a person is in or near a whirlpool spa, showering in a hotel, standing near a decorative fountain, or touring in cities with buildings that have cooling towers. Patients often do not recall specific water exposures, as they frequently occur during normal activities.

CLINICAL PRESENTATION

Legionnaires' disease typically presents with pneumonia, which usually requires hospitalization and can be fatal in 10%–15% of cases. Symptom onset occurs 2–10 days after exposure; rarely up to 19 days. In outbreak settings, <5% of people exposed to the source of the outbreak develop Legionnaires' disease.

Pontiac fever is milder than Legionnaires' disease and presents as an influenzalike illness, with fever, headache, and muscle aches, but no signs of pneumonia. Pontiac fever can affect healthy people, as well as those with underlying illnesses, and symptoms occur within 72 hours of exposure. Nearly all patients fully recover. Up to 95% of people exposed in outbreak settings can develop symptoms of Pontiac fever.

DIAGNOSIS

Isolation of *Legionella* from respiratory secretions, lung tissue, pleural fluid, or a normally sterile site is an important method for diagnosis of Legionnaires' disease. Clinical isolates are often necessary to interpret the findings of an investigation through comparison with isolates obtained from environmental sources. Because of differences in mechanism of disease, *Legionella* cannot be isolated in people who have Pontiac fever.

The most used diagnostic method is the *Legionella* urinary antigen assay. However, the assay can only detect *L. pneumophila* serogroup 1, the most common cause of legionellosis. Paired serology showing a 4-fold rise in antibody

3

titer between acute- and convalescent-phase specimens also confirms the diagnosis. A single antibody titer of any level is not diagnostic of legionellosis. Other diagnostic tests include direct fluorescent antibody and PCR. Legionellosis is a nationally notifiable disease.

TREATMENT

For travelers with suspected Legionnaires' disease, specific antibiotic treatment is necessary and should be administered promptly while diagnostic tests are being processed. Appropriate antibiotics include fluoroquinolones and macrolides. Treatment may be necessary for up to 3 weeks. In severe cases, patients may have prolonged stays in intensive care units. Consultation with an infectious disease specialist is advised. Pontiac fever is a self-limited illness that requires supportive care only; antibiotics have no benefit.

PREVENTION

There is no vaccine for legionellosis, and antibiotic prophylaxis is not effective. Travelers at increased risk for infection, such as the elderly or those with immunocompromising conditions such as cancer or diabetes, may choose to avoid high-risk areas, such as whirlpool spas. If exposure cannot be avoided, travelers should be advised to seek medical attention promptly if they develop symptoms of Legionnaires' disease or Pontiac fever.

CDC website: www.cdc.gov/legionella

BIBLIOGRAPHY

1. Beer KD, Gargano JW, Roberts VA, Reses HE, Hill VR, Garrison LE, et al. Outbreaks associated with environmental and undetermined water exposures—United States, 2011–2012. MMWR Morb Mortal Wkly Rep. 2015 Aug 14;64(31):849–51.

2. Burnsed LJ, Hicks LA, Smithee LM, Fields BS, Bradley KK, Pascoe N, et al. A large, travel-associated outbreak of legionellosis among hotel guests: utility of the urine antigen assay in confirming Pontiac fever. Clin Infect Dis. 2007 Jan 15;44(2):222–8.

3. CDC. Legionellosis—United States, 2000–2009. MMWR Morb Mortal Wkly Rep. 2011 Aug 19;60(32):1083–6.

4. CDC. Surveillance for travel-associated Legionnaires disease—United States, 2005–2006. MMWR Morb Mortal Wkly Rep. 2007 Dec 7;56(48):1261–3.

5. Correia AM, Ferreira JS, Borges V, Nunes A, Gomes B, Capucho R, et al. Probable person-to-person transmission of Legionnaires' disease. N Engl J Med. 2016 Feb 4;374(5):497–8.

6. de Jong B, Payne Hallstrom L, Robesyn E, Ursut D, Zucs P, Eldsnet. Travel-associated Legionnaires' disease in Europe, 2010. Euro Surveill. 2013;18(23):1–8.

7. Garcia-Fulgueiras A, Navarro C, Fenoll D, Garcia J, Gonzalez-Diego P, Jimenez-Bunuales T, et al. Legionnaires' disease outbreak in Murcia, Spain. Emerg Infect Dis. 2003 Aug;9(8):915–21.

8. Guyard C, Low DE. *Legionella* infections and travel associated legionellosis. Travel Med Infect Dis. 2011 Jul;9(4):176–86.

9. Mouchtouri VA, Rudge JW. Legionnaires' disease in hotels and passenger ships: a systematic review of evidence, sources, and contributing factors. J Travel Med. 2015 Sep-Oct;22(5):325–37.

10. Silk BJ, Moore MR, Bergtholdt M, Gorwitz RJ, Kozak NA, Tha MM, et al. Eight years of Legionnaires' disease transmission in travellers to a condominium complex in Las Vegas, Nevada. Epidemiol Infect. 2012 Nov;140(11):1993–2002.

LEISHMANIASIS, CUTANEOUS

Barbara L. Herwaldt, Alan J. Magill

Leishmaniasis is a parasitic disease found in parts of the tropics, subtropics, and southern Europe. Leishmaniasis has several different forms. This section focuses on cutaneous leishmaniasis (CL), the most common form, both in general and in travelers.

INFECTIOUS AGENT

Leishmaniasis is caused by obligate intracellular protozoan parasites; approximately 20 *Leishmania* species cause CL.

TRANSMISSION

CL is transmitted through the bite of an infected female phlebotomine sand fly. CL also can occur after accidental occupational (laboratory) exposures to *Leishmania* parasites.

EPIDEMIOLOGY

In the Old World (Eastern Hemisphere), CL is found in parts of the Middle East, Asia (particularly southwest and central Asia), Africa (particularly the tropical region and North Africa), and southern Europe. In the New World (Western Hemisphere), CL is found in parts of Mexico, Central America, and South America. Occasional cases have been reported in Texas and Oklahoma. CL is not found in Chile, Uruguay, or Canada. Overall, CL is found in focal areas of >90 countries.

The geographic distribution of cases of CL evaluated in countries such as the United States reflects travel and immigration patterns. Although Old World CL is more common overall than New World CL, more than 60% of the CL cases diagnosed in US civilians have been acquired in Latin America, including popular tourist destinations such as Costa Rica. Cases in US service personnel have reflected military activities (such as in Afghanistan and Iraq). CL is usually more common in rural than urban areas, but it is found in some periurban and urban areas (such as in Kabul, Afghanistan). The ecologic settings range from rainforests to arid regions.

The risk is highest from dusk to dawn because sand flies typically feed (bite) at night and during twilight hours. Although sand flies are less active during the hottest time of the day, they may bite if they are disturbed (for example, if hikers brush against tree trunks or other sites where sand flies are resting). Vector activity can easily be overlooked: sand flies do not make noise, they are small (approximately one-third the size of mosquitoes), and their bites might not be noticed.

Examples of types of travelers who might have an increased risk for CL include ecotourists, adventure travelers, bird watchers, Peace Corps volunteers, missionaries, military personnel, construction workers, and people who do research outdoors at night or twilight. However, even short-term travelers in leishmaniasis-endemic areas have developed CL.

CLINICAL PRESENTATION

CL is characterized by skin lesions (open or closed sores), which typically develop within several weeks or months after exposure. In some people, the sores first appear months or years later, in the context of trauma (such as skin wounds or surgery). The sores can change in size and appearance over time. They typically progress from small papules to nodular plaques, and often lead to open sores with a raised border and central crater (ulcer), which can be covered with scales or crust. The lesions usually are painless but can be painful, particularly if open sores become infected with bacteria. Satellite lesions, regional lymphadenopathy, and nodular lymphangitis can be noted. The sores usually heal eventually, even without treatment. However, they can last for months or years and typically result in scarring.

A potential concern applies to some of the *Leishmania* species in South and Central America: some parasites might spread from the skin to the mucosal surfaces of the nose or mouth and cause sores there. This form of leishmaniasis, mucosal leishmaniasis (ML), might not be noticed until years after the original skin sores appear to have healed. Although ML is uncommon, it has occurred in travelers and expatriates whose cases of CL were not treated or were inadequately treated. The initial clinical manifestations typically involve the nose (chronic stuffiness, bleeding, and inflamed mucosa or sores) and less often the mouth; in advanced cases, ulcerative destruction of the nose, mouth, pharynx, and larynx can be noted (such as perforation of the nasal septum).

DIAGNOSIS

Clinicians should consider CL in people with chronic (nonhealing) skin lesions who have been in areas where leishmaniasis is found. Laboratory confirmation of the diagnosis is achieved by detecting *Leishmania* parasites (or DNA) in infected tissue, through light-microscopic examination of stained specimens, culture techniques, or molecular methods.

CDC can assist in all aspects of the diagnostic evaluation. Identification of the *Leishmania* species can be important, particularly if >1 species is found where the patient traveled and if the species can have different clinical and prognostic implications. Serologic testing generally is not useful for CL but can provide supportive evidence for the diagnosis of ML.

For consultative services, contact CDC Parasitic Diseases Inquiries (404-718-4745; parasites@cdc.gov).

TREATMENT

Decisions about whether and how to treat CL should be individualized, including whether to use a systemic (oral or parenteral) medication rather than a local or topical approach. All cases of ML should be treated with systemic therapy. Clinicians may consult with CDC staff about the relative merits of various approaches to treat CL and ML (see the Diagnosis section above for contact information). The response to a particular regimen may vary not only among *Leishmania* species but also for the same species in different geographic regions.

The oral agent miltefosine is FDA-approved to treat CL caused by 3 New World species in the *Viannia* subgenus [*Leishmania* (*V.*) *braziliensis, L. (V.) panamensis*, and *L. (V.) guyanensis*] as well as for ML caused by *L. (V.) braziliensis* in adults and adolescents ≥12 years of age who weigh ≥30 kg and are not pregnant or breastfeeding during therapy or for 5 months thereafter. Miltefosine is available in the United States via www.profounda.com.

Various parenteral options (such as liposomal amphotericin B) are commercially available, although not FDA-approved to treat CL or ML. The pentavalent antimonial compound sodium stibogluconate (Pentostam) is available to US-licensed physicians through the CDC Drug Service (404-639-3670) for intravenous or intramuscular administration under an investigational new drug protocol (see www.cdc.gov/laboratory/drugservice/index.html).

PREVENTION

No vaccines or drugs to prevent infection are available. Preventive measures are aimed at reducing contact with sand flies by using personal protective measures (see Chapter 2, Protection against Mosquitoes, Ticks, & Other Arthropods). Travelers should be advised to:

- Avoid outdoor activities, to the extent possible, especially from dusk to dawn, when sand flies generally are the most active.

- Wear protective clothing and apply insect repellent to exposed skin and under the edges of clothing, such as sleeves and pant legs, according to the manufacturer's instructions.

- Sleep in air-conditioned or well-screened areas. Spraying the quarters with insecticide might provide some protection. Fans or ventilators might inhibit the movement of sand flies, which are weak fliers.

Sand flies are so small (approximately 2–3 mm, less than one-eighth of an inch) that they can pass through the holes in ordinary bed nets. Although closely woven nets are available, they may be uncomfortable in hot climates. The effectiveness of bed nets can be enhanced by treatment with a pyrethroid-containing insecticide. The same treatment can be applied to window screens, curtains, bed sheets, and clothing.

CDC website: www.cdc.gov/parasites/ leishmaniasis

BIBLIOGRAPHY

1. Aronson N, Herwaldt BL, Libman M, Pearson R, Lopez-Velez R, Weina P, et al. Diagnosis and treatment of leishmaniasis: clinical practice guidelines by the Infectious Diseases Society of America (IDSA) and the American Society of Tropical Medicine and Hygiene (ASTMH). Clin Infect Dis. 2016 In press.

2. Blum J, Buffet P, Visser L, Harms G, Bailey MS, Caumes E, et al. LeishMan recommendations for treatment of cutaneous and mucosal leishmaniasis in travelers, 2014. J Travel Med. 2014 Mar-Apr;21(2):116–29.

3. Blum J, Lockwood DN, Visser L, Harms G, Bailey MS, Caumes E, et al. Local or systemic treatment for New World cutaneous leishmaniasis? Re-evaluating the evidence for the risk of mucosal leishmaniasis. Int Health. 2012 Sep;4(3):153–63.

4. Hodiamont CJ, Kager PA, Bart A, de Vries HJ, van Thiel PP, Leenstra T, et al. Species-directed therapy for leishmaniasis in returning travellers: a comprehensive guide. PLoS Negl Trop Dis. 2014 May;8(5):e2832.

5. Magill AJ. Cutaneous leishmaniasis in the returning traveler. Infect Dis Clin North Am. 2005 Mar;19(1):x–xi, 241–66.

6. Murray HW. Leishmaniasis in the United States: treatment in 2012. Am J Trop Med Hyg. 2012 Mar;86(3):434–40.

7. Schwartz E, Hatz C, Blum J. New world cutaneous leishmaniasis in travellers. Lancet Infect Dis. 2006 Jun;6(6):342–9.

8. World Health Organization. Control of the leishmaniases. Geneva: World Health Organization; 2010 [cited 2016 Sep. 23]. Available from: http://whqlibdoc.who.int/trs/WHO_TRS_949_eng.pdf.

LEISHMANIASIS, VISCERAL

Barbara L. Herwaldt, Alan J. Magill

Leishmaniasis is a parasitic disease found in parts of the tropics, subtropics, and southern Europe. Leishmaniasis has several different forms. This section focuses on visceral leishmaniasis (VL), which affects some of the internal organs of the body (such as the spleen, liver, and bone marrow).

INFECTIOUS AGENT

VL is caused by obligate intracellular protozoan parasites, particularly by the species *Leishmania donovani* and *L. infantum-chagasi*.

TRANSMISSION

VL is predominantly transmitted through the bite of an infected female phlebotomine sand fly, although congenital and parenteral transmission (through blood transfusions and needle sharing) have been reported.

EPIDEMIOLOGY

VL is usually more common in rural than urban areas, but it is found in some periurban areas (such as in northeastern Brazil). In the Old World (Eastern Hemisphere), VL is found in parts of Asia (particularly the Indian subcontinent and southwest and central Asia), the Middle East, Africa (particularly East Africa), and southern Europe. In the New World (Western Hemisphere), most cases occur in Brazil; some cases occur in scattered foci elsewhere in Latin America. Overall, VL is found in focal areas of >60 countries. Most (>90%) of the world's cases of VL occur in the Indian subcontinent (India and Bangladesh; also Nepal), East Africa (Sudan, South Sudan, and Ethiopia), and Brazil; none of the affected areas in these 7 countries are common destinations for tourists from the United States.

The geographic distribution of cases of VL evaluated in countries such as the United States reflects travel and immigration patterns. VL is uncommon in US travelers and expatriates. Occasional cases have been diagnosed in short-term travelers (tourists) to southern Europe and also in longer-term travelers (such as expatriates and deployed soldiers) to the Mediterranean region and other areas where VL is found.

CLINICAL PRESENTATION

Among symptomatic people, the incubation period typically ranges from weeks to months.

The onset of illness can be abrupt or gradual. Stereotypical manifestations of VL include fever, weight loss, hepatosplenomegaly (especially splenomegaly), and pancytopenia (anemia, leukopenia, and thrombocytopenia). If untreated, severe (advanced) cases of VL typically are fatal. Latent infection can become clinically manifest years to decades after exposure in people who become immunocompromised for other medical reasons (such as HIV infection, immunosuppressive therapy, or biologic immunomodulatory therapy).

DIAGNOSIS

Clinicians should consider VL in people with a relevant travel history (even in the distant past) and a persistent, unexplained febrile illness, especially if accompanied by other suggestive manifestations (such as splenomegaly and pancytopenia). Laboratory confirmation of the diagnosis is achieved by detecting *Leishmania* parasites (or DNA) in infected tissue (such as in bone marrow, liver, lymph node, or blood), through light-microscopic examination of stained specimens, culture techniques, or molecular methods. Serologic testing can provide supportive evidence for the diagnosis.

CDC can assist in all aspects of the diagnostic evaluation, including species identification. For consultative services, contact CDC Parasitic Diseases Inquiries (404-718-4745; parasites@cdc.gov) or see www.cdc.gov/dpdx.

TREATMENT

Infected travelers should be advised to consult an infectious disease or tropical medicine specialist. Therapy for VL should be individualized with expert consultation. The relative merits of various approaches can be discussed with CDC staff (see the Diagnosis section above for contact information).

Liposomal amphotericin B (AmBisome) is approved by the Food and Drug Administration (FDA) to treat VL and generally constitutes the drug of choice for US patients. The oral agent miltefosine is FDA approved to treat VL in patients who are infected with *L. donovani*, are ≥12 years of age, weigh ≥30 kg, and are not pregnant or breastfeeding during therapy or for 5 months thereafter; the drug is available in the United States via www.profounda.com. The pentavalent antimonial compound sodium stibogluconate (Pentostam) is available to US-licensed physicians through the CDC Drug Service (404-639-3670) for parenteral administration under an investigational new drug protocol (see www.cdc.gov/laboratory/drugservice/index.html).

PREVENTION

No vaccines or drugs to prevent infection are available. Preventive measures are aimed at reducing contact with sand flies (see Chapter 2, Protection against Mosquitoes, Ticks, & Other Arthropods; and Prevention in the previous section, Cutaneous Leishmaniasis). Preventive measures include minimizing outdoor activities, to the extent possible, especially from dusk to dawn, when sand flies generally are the most active; wearing protective clothing; applying insect repellent to exposed skin; using bed nets treated with a pyrethroid-containing insecticide; and spraying dwellings with residual-action insecticides.

CDC website: www.cdc.gov/parasites/leishmaniasis

BIBLIOGRAPHY

1. Aronson N, Herwaldt BL, Libman M, Pearson R, Lopez-Velez R, Weina P, et al. Diagnosis and treatment of leishmaniasis: clinical practice guidelines by the Infectious Diseases Society of America (IDSA) and the American Society of Tropical Medicine and Hygiene (ASTMH). Clin Infect Dis. 2016 In press.

2. Fletcher K, Issa R, Lockwood DN. Visceral leishmaniasis and immunocompromise as a risk factor for the development of visceral leishmaniasis: a changing pattern at the hospital for tropical diseases, London. PLoS One. 2015;10(4):e0121418.

3. Murray HW. Leishmaniasis in the United States: treatment in 2012. Am J Trop Med Hyg. 2012 Mar;86(3):434–40.

4. Myles O, Wortmann GW, Cummings JF, Barthel RV, Patel S, Crum-Cianflone NF, et al. Visceral leishmaniasis: clinical observations in 4 US army soldiers deployed to Afghanistan or Iraq, 2002–2004. Arch Intern Med. 2007 Sep 24;167(17):1899–901.

5. Pavli A, Maltezou HC. Leishmaniasis, an emerging infection in travelers. Int J Infect Dis. 2010 Dec;14(12):e1032–9.

6. van Griensven J, Carrillo E, Lopez-Velez R, Lynen L, Moreno J. Leishmaniasis in immunosuppressed individuals. Clin Microbiol Infect. 2014 Apr;20(4):286–99.

7. World Health Organization. Control of the leishmaniases. Geneva: World Health Organization; 2010 [cited 2016 Sep. 23]. Available from: http://whqlibdoc.who.int/trs/WHO_TRS_949_eng.pdf.

LEPTOSPIROSIS

Renee L. Galloway, Robyn A. Stoddard, Ilana J. Schafer

INFECTIOUS AGENT

Obligate aerobic, gram-negative spirochete bacteria in the genus *Leptospira*.

TRANSMISSION

The infection route is through abrasions or cuts in the skin, or through the conjunctiva and mucous membranes. Humans may be infected by direct contact with urine or reproductive fluids from infected animals. Indirect infection can occur through contact with contaminated water or wet soil or consuming contaminated food or water. Infection rarely occurs through animal bites or human-to-human contact.

EPIDEMIOLOGY

Leptospirosis has worldwide distribution; incidence is higher in tropical climates, and the estimated worldwide annual incidence is >1 million cases. Regions with the estimated highest morbidity include South and Southeast Asia, Oceania, the Caribbean, parts of sub-Saharan Africa, and parts of Latin America. Outbreaks can occur after heavy rainfall or flooding in endemic areas, especially in urban areas of developing countries, where housing conditions and sanitation are poor. Outbreaks of leptospirosis have occurred in the United States after flooding in Hawaii and Puerto Rico. Travelers participating in recreational freshwater activities, such as swimming or boating, are at increased risk, particularly after heavy rainfall or flooding and after prolonged immersion in, or swallowing, contaminated water.

CLINICAL PRESENTATION

The incubation period is 2–30 days, and illness usually occurs 5–14 days after exposure. While most infections are thought to be asymptomatic, clinical illness can present as a self-limiting acute febrile illness, estimated to occur in approximately 90% of clinical infections, or as a severe, potentially fatal illness with multiorgan dysfunction in 5%–10% of patients. In patients who progress to severe disease, the illness can be biphasic, with a temporary decrease in fever between phases. The acute, septicemic phase (approximately 7 days) presents as an acute febrile illness with symptoms including headache (can be severe and include retroorbital pain and photophobia), chills, myalgia (characteristically involving the calves and lower back), conjunctival suffusion (characteristic of leptospirosis but not occurring in all cases), nausea, vomiting, diarrhea, abdominal pain, cough, and rarely, a skin rash. The second or immune phase is characterized by antibody production and the presence of leptospires in the urine. In patients who progress to severe disease, symptoms can include jaundice, renal failure, hemorrhage, aseptic meningitis, cardiac arrhythmias, pulmonary insufficiency, and hemodynamic collapse. The classically described syndrome, Weil disease, consists of renal and liver failure and has a case-fatality ratio of 5%–15%. Severe pulmonary hemorrhagic syndrome is a rare but severe form of leptospirosis that can have a case-fatality ratio >50%. Poor prognostic indicators include older age and development of altered mental status, respiratory insufficiency, or oliguria.

DIAGNOSIS

Diagnosis of leptospirosis is usually based on serology; microscopic agglutination test is the gold standard and can only be performed at certain reference laboratories. Culture is insensitive, but detection of the organism in blood or cerebrospinal fluid (for patients with meningitis) using real-time PCR can provide a more timely diagnosis during the acute, septicemic phase. Various serologic screening tests are available, including ELISA and multiple rapid diagnostic tests; positive screening tests should be confirmed with the microscopic agglutination test. Leptospirosis is a nationally notifiable disease.

TREATMENT

Early antimicrobial therapy can be effective in decreasing the severity and duration of leptospirosis and should be initiated early, without waiting for confirmatory test results, if leptospirosis is suspected. For patients with mild symptoms, doxycycline is a drug of choice (100 mg orally, twice daily) but is not recommended for pregnant women or children aged <8 years; alternative options include ampicillin and amoxicillin. Intravenous penicillin (1.5 MU every 6 hours) is a drug of choice for patients with severe leptospirosis, and ceftriaxone was shown to be equally effective. Patients with severe leptospirosis may require hospitalization and supportive therapy, including intravenous hydration and electrolyte supplementation, dialysis in the case of oliguric renal failure, and mechanical ventilation in the case of respiratory failure.

PREVENTION

No vaccine is available in the United States. Travelers who might be at an increased risk for infection should be educated on exposure risks and advised to consider preventive measures such as chemoprophylaxis; wearing protective clothing, especially footwear; and covering cuts and abrasions with occlusive dressings. Limited studies have shown that chemoprophylaxis with doxycycline (200 mg orally, weekly), begun 1–2 days before and continuing through the period of exposure, might be effective in preventing clinical disease in adults and could be considered for people at high risk and with short-term exposures. The best way to prevent infection is to avoid exposure: travelers should avoid contact with potentially contaminated bodies of water, walking in flood waters, and contact with potentially infected animals or their body fluids.

CDC website: www.cdc.gov/leptospirosis

BIBLIOGRAPHY

1. Costa F, Hagan JE, Calcagno J, Kane M, Torgerson P, Martinez-Silveira MS, et al. Global Morbidity and Mortality of Leptospirosis: A Systematic Review. PLoS Negl Trop Dis. 2015;9(9):e0003898.

2. Galloway RL, Hoffmaster AR. Optimization of LipL32 PCR assay for increased sensitivity in diagnosing leptospirosis. Diagnostic microbiology and infectious disease. 2015 Jul;82(3):199–200.

3. Haake DA, Dundoo M, Cader R, Kubak BM, Hartskeerl RA, Sejvar JJ, et al. Leptospirosis, water sports, and chemoprophylaxis. Clin Infect Dis. 2002 May 1;34(9):e40–3.

4. Haake DA, Levett PN. Leptospira Species (Leptospirosis). In: Bennett JE, Dolin R, Blaser MJ, editors. Principles and Practice of Infectious Diseases. 8th ed. Philadelphia, PA: Saunders 2015. p. 2714–20.

5. Haake DA, Levett PN. Leptospirosis in humans. Current topics in microbiology and immunology. 2015;387:65–97.

6. Jensenius M, Han PV, Schlagenhauf P, Schwartz E, Parola P, Castelli F, et al. Acute and potentially life-threatening tropical diseases in western travelers—a GeoSentinel multicenter study, 1996–2011. Am J Trop Med Hyg. 2013 Feb;88(2):397–404.

7. Pappas G, Cascio A. Optimal treatment of leptospirosis: queries and projections. Int J Antimicrob Agents. 2006 Dec;28(6):491–6.

8. Picardeau M, Bertherat E, Jancloes M, Skouloudis AN, Durski K, Hartskeerl RA. Rapid tests for diagnosis of leptospirosis: current tools and emerging technologies. Diagnostic microbiology and infectious disease. 2014 Jan;78(1):1–8.

9. van de Werve C, Perignon A, Jaureguiberry S, Bricaire F, Bourhy P, Caumes E. Travel-related leptospirosis: a series of 15 imported cases. J Travel Med. 2013 Jul-Aug;20(4):228–31.

LYME DISEASE

Paul S. Mead

3

INFECTIOUS AGENT

Spirochetes belonging to the *Borrelia burgdorferi* sensu lato complex, including *B. afzelii*, *B. burgdorferi* sensu stricto, and *B. garinii*.

TRANSMISSION

Through the bite of *Ixodes* ticks; infected people are often unaware that they have been bitten.

EPIDEMIOLOGY

In Europe, endemic from southern Scandinavia into the northern Mediterranean countries of Italy, Spain, and Greece and east from the British Isles into central Russia. Incidence is highest in central and Eastern European countries. In Asia, infected ticks occur from western Russia through Mongolia, northeastern China, and in Japan; however, human infection appears to be uncommon in most of these areas. In North America, highly endemic areas are the northeastern and north-central United States. Transmission has not been documented in the tropics. Lyme disease is occasionally reported in travelers returning to other countries from the United States and should be considered in those with consistent symptoms and a history of hiking or camping.

CLINICAL PRESENTATION

Incubation period is typically 3–30 days. Approximately 80% of people infected with *B. burgdorferi* develop a characteristic rash, erythema migrans (EM), within 30 days of exposure. EM is a red, expanding rash, with or without central clearing, that is often accompanied by symptoms of fatigue, fever, headache, mild stiff neck, arthralgia, or myalgia. Within days or weeks, infection can spread to other parts of the body, causing more serious neurologic conditions (meningitis, radiculopathy, and facial palsy) or cardiac abnormalities (myocarditis with atrioventricular heart block). Untreated, infection can progress over a period of months to cause monoarticular or oligoarticular arthritis, peripheral neuropathy, or encephalopathy. These long-term sequelae can be typically observed over a number of months, ranging from 1 week to a few years.

DIAGNOSIS

Observation of an EM rash with a history of recent travel to an endemic area (with or without history of tick bite) is sufficient. For patients with evidence of disseminated infection (musculoskeletal, neurologic, or cardiac manifestations), 2-tiered serologic testing, consisting of an ELISA/IFA and confirmatory Western blot, is recommended. Patients suspected of acquiring Lyme disease overseas should be tested by using a C6-based ELISA, as other serologic tests may not detect infection with European species of *Borrelia*. Lyme disease is nationally notifiable.

TREATMENT

Most patients can be treated with either oral doxycycline or intravenous ceftriaxone (see http://cid.oxfordjournals.org/content/43/9/1089.full). Diagnosis and management are sometimes controversial and should be managed by those who have experience with this disease.

PREVENTION

Avoid tick habitats, use insect repellent on exposed skin and clothing, and carefully check every day for attached ticks. Minimize areas of exposed skin by wearing long-sleeved shirts, long pants, and closed shoes; tucking shirts in and tucking pants into socks may also reduce risk (see Chapter 2, Protection against Mosquitoes, Ticks, & Other Arthropods).

CDC website: www.cdc.gov/lyme

BIBLIOGRAPHY

1. Hao Q, Hou X, Geng Z, Wan K. Distribution of *Borrelia burgdorferi* sensu lato in China. J Clin Microbiol. 2011 Feb;49(2):647–50.

2. Hubalek Z. Epidemiology of lyme borreliosis. Curr Probl Dermatol. 2009;37:31–50.

3. Masuzawa T. Terrestrial distribution of the Lyme borreliosis agent *Borrelia burgdorferi* sensu lato in East Asia. Jpn J Infect Dis. 2004 Dec;57(6):229–35.

4. O'Connell S. Lyme borreliosis: current issues in diagnosis and management. Curr Opin Infect Dis. 2010 Jun;23(3):231–5.

5. Stanek G, Strle F. Lyme disease: European perspective. Infect Dis Clin North Am. 2008 Jun;22(2):327–39.

6. Steere AC. Lyme disease. N Engl J Med. 2001 Jul 12;345(2):115–25.

7. Wormser GP, Dattwyler RJ, Shapiro ED, Halperin JJ, Steere AC, Klempner MS, et al. The clinical assessment, treatment, and prevention of Lyme disease, human granulocytic anaplasmosis, and babesiosis: clinical practice guidelines by the Infectious Diseases Society of America. Clin Infect Dis. 2006 Nov 1;43(9):1089–134.

3

MALARIA

Paul M. Arguin, Kathrine R. Tan

INFECTIOUS AGENT

Malaria in humans is caused by protozoan parasites of the genus *Plasmodium: Plasmodium falciparum, P. vivax, P. ovale,* or *P. malariae*. In addition, *P. knowlesi*, a parasite of Old World (Eastern Hemisphere) monkeys, has been documented as a cause of human infections and some deaths in Southeast Asia.

TRANSMISSION

All species are transmitted by the bite of an infective female *Anopheles* mosquito. Occasionally, transmission occurs by blood transfusion, organ transplantation, needle sharing, or congenitally from mother to fetus.

EPIDEMIOLOGY

Malaria is a major international public health problem, causing an estimated 214 million infections worldwide and 438,000 deaths in 2015, according to the World Health Organization (WHO) World Malaria Report 2015. Although these numbers are decreasing, the numbers of cases of malaria in travelers has been increasing. On average, 29 additional cases have been reported in the United States each year since 1973. Despite the apparent progress in reducing the global prevalence of malaria, many areas remain malaria endemic, and the use of prevention measures by travelers is still inadequate. Information about malaria transmission in specific countries (see Yellow Fever & Malaria Information, by Country later in this chapter) is derived from various sources, including WHO. The information presented herein was accurate at the time of publication; however, factors that can change rapidly and from year to year (such as local weather conditions, mosquito vector density, and prevalence of infection) can markedly affect local malaria transmission patterns. Updated information may be found on the CDC website at www.cdc.gov/malaria.

Malaria transmission occurs in large areas of Africa, Latin America, parts of the Caribbean, Asia (including South Asia, Southeast Asia, and the Middle East), Eastern Europe, and the South Pacific (Maps 3-9 and 3-10).

The risk for acquiring malaria differs substantially from traveler to traveler and from region to region, even within a single country. This variability is a function of the intensity of transmission within the various regions and the itinerary, duration, season, and type of travel. In 2013, >1,700 cases of malaria (including 10 deaths) diagnosed in the United States and its territories were reported to CDC. Of these, 82% were acquired in Africa, 11% in Asia, 6% in the Caribbean and the Americas, and 1% in Oceania.

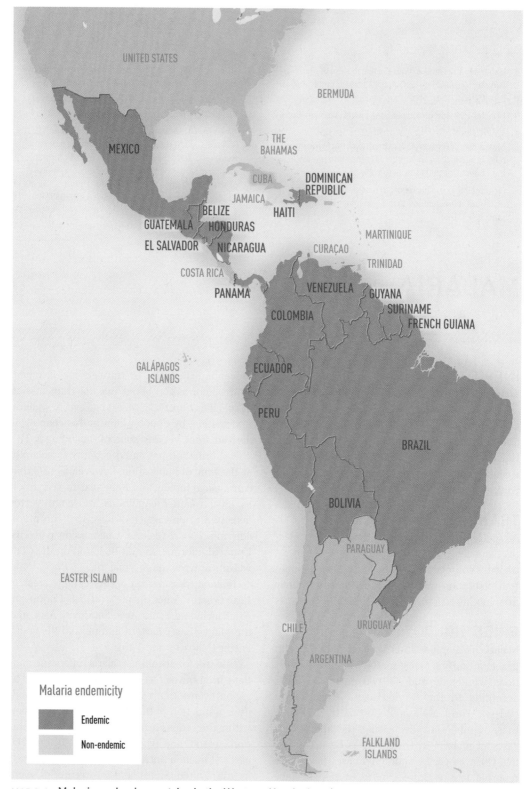

MAP 3-9. Malaria-endemic countries in the Western Hemisphere[1]

[1] In this map, countries with areas endemic for malaria are shaded completely even if transmission occurs only in a small part of the country. For more specific within-country malaria transmission information, see the Yellow Fever & Malaria Information, by Country section in this chapter.

CLINICAL PRESENTATION

Malaria is characterized by fever and influenza-like symptoms, including chills, headache, myalgias, and malaise; these symptoms can occur at intervals. Uncomplicated disease may be associated with anemia and jaundice. In severe disease, seizures, mental confusion, kidney failure, acute respiratory distress syndrome, coma, and death may occur. Malaria symptoms can develop as early as 7 days (usually ≥14 days) after initial exposure in a malaria-endemic area and as late as several months or more after departure. Suspected or confirmed malaria, especially *P. falciparum*, is a medical emergency, requiring urgent intervention as clinical deterioration can occur rapidly and unpredictably. See Box 3-2 detailing some clinical highlights for malaria.

DIAGNOSIS

Travelers who have symptoms of malaria should seek medical evaluation **as soon as possible**. Clinicians should consider malaria in any patient with a febrile illness who has recently returned from a malaria-endemic country. Malaria is a nationally notifiable disease.

Smear microscopy remains the gold standard for malaria diagnosis. Microscopy can also be used to determine the species of malaria parasite, identify the parasite life-cycle stages present, and quantify the parasitemia—all of which are necessary for providing the most appropriate treatment. Microscopy results should ideally be available within a few hours. It is an unacceptable practice to send these tests to an offsite laboratory or batch them for results to be provided days later.

3

BOX 3-2. Clinical highlights for malaria

- Overdose of antimalarial drugs, particularly chloroquine, can be fatal. Medication should be stored in childproof containers out of the reach of infants and children.
- Chemoprophylaxis can be started earlier if there are particular concerns about tolerating a medication. For example, mefloquine can be started 3–4 weeks in advance to allow potential adverse events to occur before travel. If unacceptable side effects develop, there would be time to change the medication before the traveler's departure.
- The drugs used for antimalarial chemoprophylaxis are generally well tolerated. However, side effects can occur. Minor side effects usually do not require stopping the drug. Travelers who have serious side effects should see a clinician who can determine if their symptoms are related to the medicine and make a medication change.

- In comparison with drugs with short half-lives, which are taken daily, drugs with longer half-lives, which are taken weekly, offer the advantage of a wider margin of error if the traveler is late with a dose. For example, if a traveler is 1–2 days late with a weekly drug, prophylactic blood levels can remain adequate; if the traveler is 1–2 days late with a daily drug, protective blood levels are less likely to be maintained.
- In those who are G6PD deficient, primaquine can cause hemolysis, which can be fatal. Be sure to document a normal G6PD level before prescribing primaquine.
- Travelers should be informed that malaria could be fatal if treatment is delayed. Medical help should be sought promptly if malaria is suspected, and a blood sample should be taken and examined for malaria parasites on 1 or more occasions.

- Travelers should also be informed that malaria could be fatal even when treated, which is why it is always preferable to prevent malaria cases rather than rely on treating infections after they occur.
- Malaria smear results or a rapid diagnostic test must be available immediately (within a few hours). Sending specimens to offsite laboratories where results are not available for extended periods of time (days) is not acceptable. If a patient has an illness suggestive of severe malaria and a compatible travel history in an area where malaria transmission occurs, it is advisable to start treatment as soon as possible, even before the diagnosis is established. CDC recommendations for malaria treatment can be found at www.cdc.gov/malaria/diagnosis_treatment/index.html.

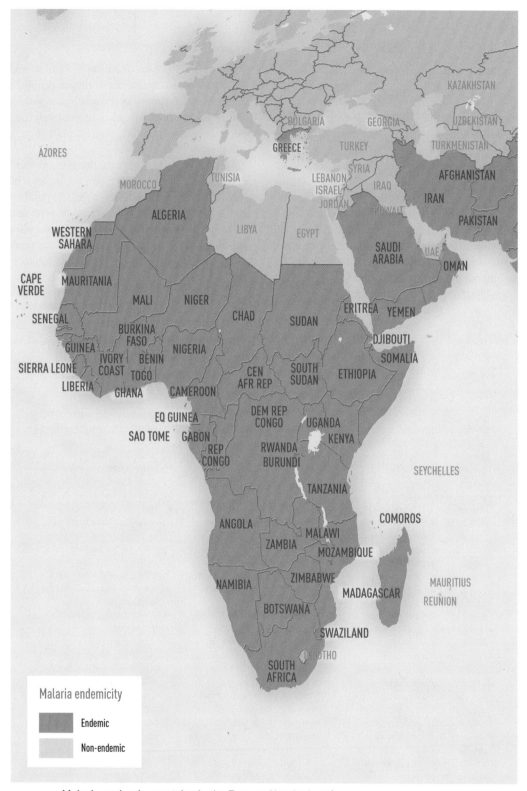

MAP 3-10. Malaria-endemic countries in the Eastern Hemisphere[1]

[1] In this map, countries with areas endemic for malaria are shaded completely even if transmission occurs only in a small part of the country. For more specific within-country malaria transmission information, see the Yellow Fever & Malaria Information, by Country section in this chapter.

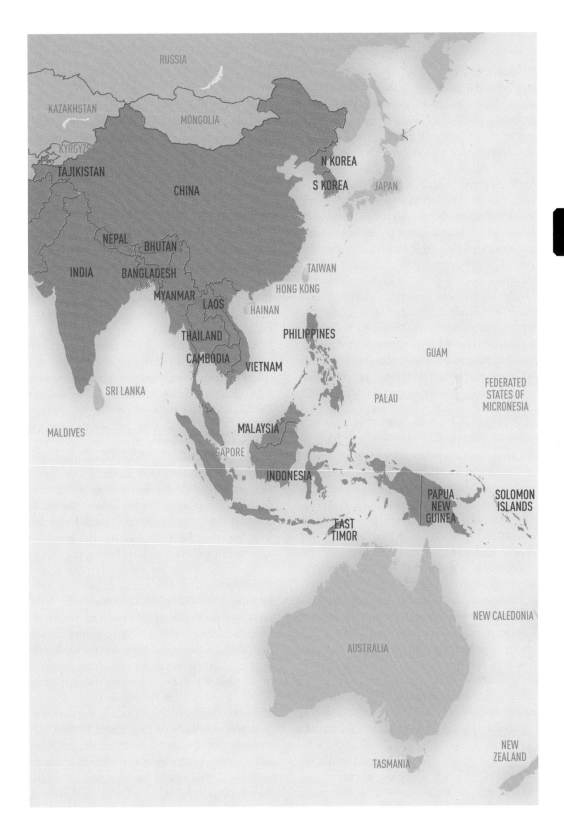

Various test kits are available to detect antigens derived from malaria parasites. Such immunologic (immunochromatographic) tests most often use a dipstick or cassette format and provide results in 2–15 minutes. These rapid diagnostic tests (RDTs) offer a useful alternative to microscopy in situations where reliable microscopic diagnosis is not immediately available. Although RDTs can detect malaria antigens within minutes, most cannot distinguish between all 5 of the species that affect humans, they are less sensitive than expert microscopy or PCR for diagnosis, they cannot quantify parasitemia, and many will persist with a positive result for days or weeks after an infection has been treated and cleared. In addition, CDC recommends that positive and negative RDT results always be confirmed by microscopy in US health care settings. Although confirmation does not have to occur simultaneously with the RDT, the information from microscopy, including the actual presence of malaria parasites, the species, life-cycle stages (asexual vs sexual blood-stage forms), and parasitemia will be most useful if it is available as soon as possible. The Food and Drug Administration (FDA) has approved 1 RDT for use in the United States by hospital and commercial laboratories, not by individual clinicians or by patients themselves. This RDT is called BinaxNOW Malaria test. Laboratories that do not provide in-house on-the-spot microscopy services should maintain a stock of malaria RDTs so that they will be able to perform malaria diagnostic testing when needed.

PCR tests are also available for detecting malaria parasites. Although these tests are more sensitive than routine microscopy, results are not usually available as quickly as microscopy results should be, thus limiting the utility of this test for acute diagnosis. PCR testing is most useful for definitively identifying the species of malaria parasite and detecting mixed infections. Species confirmation by PCR is available at the CDC malaria laboratory.

In sub-Saharan Africa, clinical overdiagnosis and the rate of false-positive microscopy for malaria may be high. Travelers to this region should be warned they may be diagnosed with malaria incorrectly, even though they are taking a reliable antimalarial regimen. In such cases, acutely ill travelers should be advised to seek the best available medical services and follow the treatment offered locally (except the use of halofantrine, which is not recommended; see below) but *not* to stop their chemoprophylaxis regimen.

TREATMENT

Malaria can be treated effectively early in the course of the disease, but delay of therapy can have serious or even fatal consequences. Travelers who have symptoms of malaria should be advised to seek medical evaluation **as soon as possible**. Specific treatment options depend on the species of malaria, the likelihood of drug resistance (based on where the infection was acquired), the age of the patient, pregnancy status, and the severity of infection.

Detailed CDC recommendations for malaria treatment can be found at www.cdc.gov/malaria/diagnosis_treatment/treatment.html. Clinicians who require assistance with the diagnosis or treatment of malaria should call the CDC Malaria Hotline (770-488-7788 or toll-free at 855-856-4713) from 9 AM to 5 PM Eastern Time. After hours or on weekends and holidays, clinicians requiring assistance should call the CDC Emergency Operations Center at 770-488-7100 and ask the operator to page the person on call for the Malaria Branch. In addition, it is advisable to consult with a clinician who has specialized travel or tropical medicine expertise or with an infectious disease physician.

Medications that are not used in the United States for the treatment of malaria, such as halofantrine, are widely available overseas. CDC does not recommend halofantrine for treatment because of cardiac adverse events, including deaths, which have been documented after treatment. These adverse events have occurred in people with and without preexisting cardiac problems and both in the presence and absence of other antimalarial drugs (such as mefloquine).

Travelers who reject the advice to take prophylaxis, who choose a suboptimal drug regimen (such as chloroquine in an area with chloroquine-resistant *P. falciparum*), or who require a less-than-optimal drug regimen for medical reasons are at increased risk for acquiring malaria and needing prompt treatment while overseas. In addition, some travelers who are taking effective

3

BOX 3-3. What is a reliable supply?

A reliable supply is a complete course of an approved malaria treatment regimen obtained in the United States before travel. A reliable supply:

- Is not counterfeit or substandard
- Will not interact adversely with the patient's other medicines, including chemoprophylaxis

- Will not deplete local resources in the destination country

prophylaxis but who will be in remote areas may decide, in consultation with their travel health provider, to take along a reliable supply of a full course of an approved malaria treatment regimen (see Box 3-3 for a definition of *reliable supply*). In the event that they are diagnosed with malaria, they will have immediate access to this treatment regimen, which if acquired in the United States is unlikely to be counterfeit and will not deplete local resources. In rare instances when access to medical care is not available and the traveler develops a febrile illness consistent with malaria, the reliable supply medication can be self-administered presumptively. **Travelers should be advised that this self-treatment of a possible malarial infection is only a temporary measure and that prompt medical evaluation is imperative.**

Two malaria treatment regimens available in the United States can be prescribed as a reliable supply: atovaquone-proguanil and artemether-lumefantrine. The use of the same or related drugs that have been taken for prophylaxis is not recommended to treat malaria. For example, atovaquone-proguanil may be used as a reliable supply medication by travelers not taking atovaquone-proguanil for prophylaxis. See Table 3-8 for the dosing recommendation.

PREVENTION

The goal of these malaria prevention guidelines is to prevent malaria caused by all species, not only *P. falciparum*. These guidelines apply to both short-term and long-term travelers. Malaria prevention consists of a combination of mosquito avoidance measures and chemoprophylaxis. Although efficacious, the recommended interventions are not 100% effective.

Preventing malaria involves striking a balance between ensuring that all people at risk for infection use the recommended prevention measures, while preventing rare occurrences of adverse effects of these interventions among people using them unnecessarily. An individual risk assessment should be conducted for every traveler, taking into account not only the destination country but also the detailed itinerary, including specific cities, types of accommodation, season, and style of travel. In addition, conditions such as pregnancy or antimalarial drug resistance at the destination may modify the risk assessment.

Depending on the level of risk, it may be appropriate to recommend no specific interventions, mosquito avoidance measures only, or mosquito avoidance measures plus chemoprophylaxis. For areas of intense transmission, such as West Africa, exposure for even short periods of time can result in transmission, so travelers to this area should be considered at high risk for infection. Malaria transmission is not distributed homogeneously throughout all countries. Some destinations have malaria transmission occurring only in certain areas. If travelers are going to high-transmission areas during peak transmission times, even though the country as a whole may have relatively low malaria transmission, they may be at high risk for infection while there.

Geography is just a part of determining a traveler's risk for infection. Risk can differ substantially for different travelers as their behaviors and circumstances differ. For example, travelers staying in air-conditioned hotels may be at lower risk than backpackers or adventure travelers. Similarly, long-term residents living in screened and air-conditioned housing are less likely to be exposed

Table 3-8. Reliable supply regimens for the treatment of malaria

DRUG[1]	ADULT DOSE	PEDIATRIC DOSE	COMMENTS
ATOVAQUONE-PROGUANIL The adult tablet contains 250 mg atovaquone and 100 mg proguanil. The pediatric tablet contains 62.5 mg atovaquone and 25 mg proguanil.	4 adult tablets, orally as a single daily dose for 3 consecutive days	Daily dose to be taken for 3 consecutive days: 5–8 kg: 2 pediatric tablets 9–10 kg: 3 pediatric tablets 11–20 kg: 1 adult tablet 21–30 kg: 2 adult tablets 31–40 kg: 3 adult tablets >41 kg: 4 adult tablets	Contraindicated in people with severe renal impairment (creatinine clearance <30 mL/min) Not recommended for people on atovaquone-proguanil prophylaxis Not recommended for children weighing <5 kg, pregnant women, and women breastfeeding infants weighing <5 kg
ARTEMETHER-LUMEFANTRINE One tablet contains 20 mg artemether and 120 mg lumefantrine.	A 3-day treatment schedule with a total of 6 oral doses is recommended for both adult and pediatric patients based on weight. The patient should receive the initial dose, followed by the second dose 8 hours later, then 1 dose twice per day for the following 2 days. 5 to <15 kg: 1 tablet per dose 15 to <25 kg: 2 tablets per dose 25 to <35 kg: 3 tablets per dose ≥35 kg: 4 tablets per dose	Not for people on mefloquine prophylaxis Not recommended for children weighing <5 kg, pregnant women, and women breastfeeding infants weighing <5 kg

[1] If used for presumptive self-treatment, medical care should be sought as soon as possible.

than are people living without such amenities. The highest risk is associated with first- and second-generation immigrants living in non-endemic countries who return to their countries of origin to visit friends and relatives (VFRs). VFR travelers often consider themselves to be at no risk, because they grew up in a malarious country and consider themselves immune. However, acquired immunity is lost quickly, and VFRs should be considered to have the same risk as other nonimmune travelers (see Chapter 8, Immigrants Returning Home to Visit Friends & Relatives [VFRs]). Travelers should also be reminded that even if a person has had malaria before, he or she can get it again, and preventive measures are still necessary.

Mosquito Avoidance Measures

Because of the nocturnal feeding habits of *Anopheles* mosquitoes, malaria transmission occurs primarily between dusk and dawn. Contact with mosquitoes can be reduced by remaining in well-screened areas, using mosquito bed nets (preferably insecticide-treated nets), using an effective insecticide spray in living and sleeping areas during evening and nighttime hours, and wearing clothes that cover most of the body.

All travelers should use an effective mosquito repellent (see Chapter 2, Protection against Mosquitoes, Ticks, & Other Arthropods). Repellents should be applied to exposed parts of the skin when mosquitoes are likely to be present. If travelers are also wearing sunscreen, sunscreen should be applied first and insect repellent second. In addition to using a topical insect repellent, a permethrin-containing product may be applied to bed nets and clothing for additional protection against mosquitoes.

Chemoprophylaxis

All recommended primary chemoprophylaxis regimens involve taking a medicine before, during, and after travel to an area with malaria. Beginning the drug before travel allows the antimalarial agent to be in the blood before the traveler is exposed to malaria parasites. In choosing a chemoprophylaxis regimen before travel, the traveler and the travel health provider should consider several factors. The travel itinerary should be reviewed in detail and compared with information on where malaria transmission occurs within a given country, to determine whether the traveler will be traveling in a part of the country where malaria occurs and if antimalarial drug resistance has been reported in that location (see the Yellow Fever & Malaria Information, by Country section later in this chapter). Additional factors to consider are the patient's other medical conditions, medications being taken (to assess potential drug interactions), the cost of the medicines, and the potential side effects. Table 3-9 lists some of the

Table 3-9. Considerations when choosing a drug for malaria prophylaxis

DRUG	REASONS TO CONSIDER USE OF THIS DRUG	REASONS TO CONSIDER AVOIDING USE OF THIS DRUG
Atovaquone-proguanil	• Good for last-minute travelers because the drug is started 1–2 days before travel. • Some people prefer to take a daily medicine. • Good choice for shorter trips because the traveler takes the medicine for only 7 days after traveling rather than 4 weeks. • Well tolerated—side effects uncommon. • Pediatric tablets are available and may be more convenient.	• Cannot be used by women who are pregnant or breastfeeding a child that weighs <5 kg. • Cannot be taken by people with severe renal impairment. • Tends to be more expensive than some of the other options (especially for long trips). • Some people (including children) would rather not take a medicine every day.
Chloroquine	• Some people would rather take medicine weekly. • Good choice for long trips because it is taken only weekly. • Some people are already taking hydroxychloroquine chronically for rheumatologic conditions; in those instances, they may not have to take an additional medicine. • Can be used in all trimesters of pregnancy.	• Cannot be used in areas with chloroquine or mefloquine resistance. • May exacerbate psoriasis. • Some people would rather not take a weekly medication. • For short trips, some people would rather not take medication for 4 weeks after travel. • Not a good choice for last-minute travelers, because drug needs to be started 1–2 weeks before travel.
Doxycycline	• Some people prefer to take a daily medicine. • Good for last-minute travelers because the drug is started 1–2 days before travel. • Tends to be the least expensive antimalarial. • People who are already taking doxycycline chronically to prevent acne do not have to take an additional medicine. • Doxycycline also can prevent some additional infections (such as rickettsial infections and leptospirosis), so it may be preferred by people planning to hike, camp, and swim in fresh water.	• Cannot be used by pregnant women and children aged <8 years. • Some people would rather not take a medicine every day. • For short trips, some people would rather not take medication for 4 weeks after travel. • Women prone to getting vaginal yeast infections when taking antibiotics may prefer taking a different medicine. • People may want to avoid the increased risk of sun sensitivity. • Some people are concerned about the potential of getting an upset stomach from doxycycline.

(continued)

Table 3-9. Considerations when choosing a drug for malaria prophylaxis (continued)

DRUG	REASONS TO CONSIDER USE OF THIS DRUG	REASONS TO CONSIDER AVOIDING USE OF THIS DRUG
Mefloquine	• Some people would rather take medicine weekly. • Good choice for long trips because it is taken only weekly. • Can be used in all trimesters of pregnancy.	• Cannot be used in areas with mefloquine resistance. • Cannot be used in patients with certain psychiatric conditions. • Cannot be used in patients with a seizure disorder. • Not recommended for people with cardiac conduction abnormalities. • Not a good choice for last-minute travelers because drug needs to be started ≥2 weeks before travel. • Some people would rather not take a weekly medication. • For short trips, some people would rather not take medication for 4 weeks after travel.
Primaquine	• It is the most effective medicine for preventing *P. vivax*, so it is a good choice for travel to places with >90% *P. vivax*. • Good choice for shorter trips because the traveler takes the medicine for 7 days after traveling rather than 4 weeks. • Good for last-minute travelers because the drug is started 1–2 days before travel. • Some people prefer to take a daily medicine.	• Cannot be used in patients with G6PD deficiency. • Cannot be used in patients who have not been tested for G6PD deficiency. • There are costs and delays associated with getting a G6PD test; however, it only has to be done once. Once a normal G6PD level is verified and documented, the test does not have to be repeated the next time primaquine is considered. • Cannot be used by pregnant women. • Cannot be used by women who are breastfeeding, unless the infant has also been tested for G6PD deficiency. • Some people (including children) would rather not take a medicine every day. • Some people are concerned about the potential of getting an upset stomach from primaquine.

benefits and limitations of medicines used for malaria chemoprophylaxis; additional information about choosing a malaria chemoprophylaxis regimen can be found at www.cdc.gov/malaria/travelers/drugs.html.

The resistance of *P. falciparum* to chloroquine has been confirmed in all areas with *P. falciparum* malaria except the Caribbean, Central America west of the Panama Canal, and some countries in the Middle East. In addition, resistance to sulfadoxine-pyrimethamine is widespread in the Amazon River Basin area of South America, much of Southeast Asia, other parts of Asia, and in large parts of Africa. Resistance to mefloquine has been confirmed on the borders of Thailand with Burma (Myanmar) and Cambodia, in the western provinces of Cambodia, in the eastern states of Burma on the border between Burma and China, along the borders of Laos and Burma, the adjacent parts of the Thailand–Cambodia border, and in southern Vietnam. The resistance of *P. vivax* to chloroquine has been confirmed in Papua New Guinea and Indonesia.

In addition to primary prophylaxis, presumptive antirelapse therapy (also known as terminal prophylaxis) uses a medication toward the end of the exposure period (or immediately thereafter) to prevent relapses or delayed-onset clinical presentations of malaria caused by hypnozoites (dormant liver stages) of *P. vivax* or *P. ovale*. Because most malarious areas of the world (except the Caribbean) have at least 1 species of relapsing malaria, travelers to these areas have some risk for acquiring either *P. vivax* or *P. ovale*, although the actual risk for an individual traveler is difficult to define. Presumptive antirelapse therapy is generally indicated only for people who have had prolonged exposure in malaria-endemic areas (such as missionaries, military personnel, or Peace Corps volunteers).

The medications recommended for chemoprophylaxis of malaria may also be available at overseas destinations. However, combinations of these medications and additional drugs that are not recommended may be commonly prescribed and used in other countries. Travelers should be strongly discouraged from obtaining chemoprophylaxis medications while abroad. The quality of these products is not known; they may not be protective and could be dangerous. These medications may have been produced by substandard manufacturing practices, may be counterfeit, or may contain contaminants. Additional information on this topic can be found in Chapter 2, *Perspectives*: Pharmaceutical Quality & Falsified Drugs, and on the FDA website (www.fda.gov/Drugs/ResourcesForYou/Consumers/BuyingUsingMedicineSafely/BuyingMedicinefromOutsidetheUnitedStates/default.htm).

MEDICATIONS USED FOR CHEMOPROPHYLAXIS

ATOVAQUONE-PROGUANIL

Atovaquone-proguanil is a fixed combination of the drugs atovaquone and proguanil. Prophylaxis should begin 1–2 days before travel to malarious areas and should be taken daily, at the same time each day, while in the malarious areas, and daily for 7 days after leaving the areas (see Table 3-10 for recommended dosages). Atovaquone-proguanil is well tolerated, and side effects are rare. The most common adverse effects reported in people using atovaquone-proguanil for prophylaxis or treatment are abdominal pain, nausea, vomiting, and headache. Atovaquone-proguanil is not

recommended for prophylaxis in children weighing <5 kg (11 lb), pregnant women, or patients with severe renal impairment (creatinine clearance <30 mL/min). Proguanil may increase the effect of warfarin, so international normalized ratio monitoring or dosage adjustment may be needed.

CHLOROQUINE AND HYDROXYCHLOROQUINE

Chloroquine phosphate or hydroxychloroquine sulfate can be used for prevention of malaria only in destinations where chloroquine resistance is not present (see Maps 3-9 and 3-10 and the Yellow Fever & Malaria Information, by Country section later in this chapter). Prophylaxis should begin 1–2 weeks before travel to malarious areas. It should be continued by taking the drug once a week, on the same day of the week, during travel in malarious areas and for 4 weeks after a traveler leaves these areas (see Table 3-10 for recommended dosages). Reported side effects include gastrointestinal disturbance, headache, dizziness, blurred vision, insomnia, and pruritus, but generally these effects do not require that the drug be discontinued. High doses of chloroquine, such as those used to treat rheumatoid arthritis, have been associated with retinopathy; this serious side effect appears to be extremely unlikely when chloroquine is used for routine weekly malaria prophylaxis. Chloroquine and related compounds have been reported to exacerbate psoriasis. People who experience uncomfortable side effects after taking chloroquine may tolerate the drug better by taking it with meals. As an alternative, the related compound hydroxychloroquine sulfate may be better tolerated.

DOXYCYCLINE

Doxycycline prophylaxis should begin 1–2 days before travel to malarious areas. It should be continued once a day, at the same time each day, during travel in malarious areas and daily for 4 weeks after the traveler leaves such areas. Insufficient data exist on the antimalarial prophylactic efficacy of related compounds such as minocycline (commonly prescribed for the treatment of acne). People on a long-term regimen of minocycline who need malaria prophylaxis should stop taking minocycline 1–2 days before

Table 3-10. Drugs used in the prophylaxis of malaria

DRUG	USAGE	ADULT DOSE	PEDIATRIC DOSE	COMMENTS
Atovaquone-proguanil	Prophylaxis in all areas	Adult tablets contain 250 mg atovaquone and 100 mg proguanil hydrochloride. 1 adult tablet orally, daily	Pediatric tablets contain 62.5 mg atovaquone and 25 mg proguanil hydrochloride. • 5–8 kg: 1/2 pediatric tablet daily • 8–10 kg: 3/4 pediatric tablet daily • 10–20 kg: 1 pediatric tablet daily • 20–30 kg: 2 pediatric tablets daily • 30–40 kg: 3 pediatric tablets daily • 40 kg: 1 adult tablet daily	Begin 1–2 days before travel to malarious areas. Take daily at the same time each day while in the malarious area and for 7 days after leaving such areas. Contraindicated in people with severe renal impairment (creatinine clearance <30 mL/min). Atovaquone-proguanil should be taken with food or a milky drink. Not recommended for prophylaxis for children weighing <5 kg, pregnant women, and women breastfeeding infants weighing <5 kg. Partial tablet doses may need to be prepared by a pharmacist and dispensed in individual capsules, as described in the text.
Chloroquine phosphate	Prophylaxis only in areas with chloroquine-sensitive malaria	300 mg base (500 mg salt) orally, once/week	5 mg/kg base (8.3 mg/kg salt) orally, once/week, up to a maximum adult dose of 300 mg base	Begin 1–2 weeks before travel to malarious areas. Take weekly on the same day of the week while in the malarious area and for 4 weeks after leaving such areas. May exacerbate psoriasis.
Doxycycline	Prophylaxis in all areas	100 mg orally, daily	≥8 years of age: 2.2 mg/kg up to adult dose of 100 mg/day	Begin 1–2 days before travel to malarious areas. Take daily at the same time each day while in the malarious area and for 4 weeks after leaving such areas. Contraindicated in children aged <8 years and pregnant women.
Hydroxychloroquine sulfate	An alternative to chloroquine for prophylaxis only in areas with chloroquine-sensitive malaria	310 mg base (400 mg salt) orally, once/week	5 mg/kg base (6.5 mg/kg salt) orally, once/week, up to a maximum adult dose of 310 mg base	Begin 1–2 weeks before travel to malarious areas. Take weekly on the same day of the week while in the malarious area and for 4 weeks after leaving such areas.

3

Drug	Use	Adult dose	Pediatric dose	Comments
Mefloquine	Prophylaxis in areas with mefloquine-sensitive malaria	228 mg base (250 mg salt) orally, once/week	≤9 kg: 4.6 mg/kg base (5 mg/kg salt) orally, once/week >9–19 kg: 1/4 tablet once/week >19–30 kg: 1/2 tablet once/week >30–45 kg: 3/4 tablet once/week >45 kg: 1 tablet once/week	Begin ≥2 weeks before travel to malarious areas. Take weekly on the same day of the week while in the malarious area and for 4 weeks after leaving such areas. Contraindicated in people allergic to mefloquine or related compounds (quinine, quinidine) and in people with active depression, a recent history of depression, generalized anxiety disorder, psychosis, schizophrenia, other major psychiatric disorders, or seizures. Use with caution in people with psychiatric disturbances or a previous history of depression. Not recommended for people with cardiac conduction abnormalities.
Primaquine[1]	Prophylaxis for short-duration travel to areas with principally P. vivax Used for presumptive antirelapse therapy (terminal prophylaxis) to decrease the risk for relapses of P. vivax and P. ovale	30 mg base (52.6 mg salt) orally, daily 30 mg base (52.6 mg salt) orally, daily for 14 days after departure from the malarious area	0.5 mg/kg base (0.8 mg/kg salt) up to adult dose orally, daily 0.5 mg/kg base (0.8 mg/kg salt) up to adult dose orally, daily for 14 days after departure from the malarious area	Begin 1–2 days before travel to malarious areas. Take daily at the same time each day while in the malarious area and for 7 days after leaving such areas. Contraindicated in people with G6PD deficiency. Also contraindicated during pregnancy and lactation, unless the infant being breastfed has a documented normal G6PD level. Indicated for people who have had prolonged exposure to P. vivax, P. ovale, or both. Contraindicated in people with G6PD deficiency. Also contraindicated during pregnancy and lactation, unless the infant being breastfed has a documented normal G6PD level.

[1] All people who take primaquine should have a documented normal G6PD level before starting the medication.

travel and start doxycycline instead. Minocycline can be restarted after the full course of doxycycline is completed (see Table 3-10 for recommended dosages).

Doxycycline can cause photosensitivity, usually manifested as an exaggerated sunburn reaction. The risk for such a reaction can be minimized by avoiding prolonged, direct exposure to the sun and by using sunscreen. In addition, doxycycline use is associated with an increased frequency of vaginal yeast infections. Gastrointestinal side effects (nausea or vomiting) may be minimized by taking the drug with a meal or by specifically prescribing doxycycline monohydrate or the enteric-coated doxycycline hyclate, rather than the generic doxycycline hyclate, which is often less expensive. To reduce the risk for esophagitis, travelers should be advised to swallow the medicine with sufficient fluids and not to take doxycycline before going to bed. Doxycycline is contraindicated in people with an allergy to tetracyclines, during pregnancy, and in infants and children aged <8 years. Vaccination with the oral typhoid vaccine Ty21a should be delayed for ≥24 hours after taking a dose of doxycycline.

MEFLOQUINE

Mefloquine prophylaxis should begin ≥2 weeks before travel to malarious areas. It should be continued once a week, on the same day of the week, during travel in malarious areas and for 4 weeks after a traveler leaves such areas (see Table 3-10 for recommended dosages). Mefloquine has been associated with rare but serious adverse reactions (such as psychoses or seizures) at prophylactic doses; these reactions are more frequent with the higher doses used for treatment. Other side effects that have occurred in chemoprophylaxis studies include gastrointestinal disturbance, headache, insomnia, abnormal dreams, visual disturbances, depression, anxiety disorder, and dizziness. Other more severe neuropsychiatric disorders occasionally reported during postmarketing surveillance include sensory and motor neuropathies (including paresthesia, tremor, and ataxia), agitation or restlessness, mood changes, panic attacks, forgetfulness, confusion, hallucinations, aggression, paranoia, and encephalopathy. On occasion, psychiatric symptoms have been

reported to continue long after mefloquine has been stopped. FDA also includes a boxed warning about rare reports of persistent dizziness after mefloquine use. Mefloquine is contraindicated for use by travelers with a known hypersensitivity to mefloquine or related compounds (such as quinine or quinidine) and in people with active depression, a recent history of depression, generalized anxiety disorder, psychosis, schizophrenia, other major psychiatric disorders, or seizures. It should be used with caution in people with psychiatric disturbances or a history of depression. A review of available data suggests that mefloquine may be used safely in people concurrently on β-blockers, if they have no underlying arrhythmia. However, mefloquine is not recommended for people with cardiac conduction abnormalities. Any traveler receiving a prescription for mefloquine must also receive a copy of the FDA medication guide, which can be found at www.accessdata.fda.gov/drugsatfda_docs/label/2008/019591s023lbl.pdf.

PRIMAQUINE

Primaquine phosphate has 2 distinct uses for malaria prevention: primary prophylaxis in areas with primarily *P. vivax* and presumptive antirelapse therapy (terminal prophylaxis).

When taken for primary prophylaxis, primaquine should be taken 1–2 days before travel to malarious areas, daily, at the same time each day, while in the malarious areas, and daily for 7 days after leaving the areas (see Table 3-10 for recommended dosages). Primary prophylaxis with primaquine obviates the need for presumptive antirelapse therapy.

When used for presumptive antirelapse therapy, primaquine is administered for 14 days after the traveler has left a malarious area. When chloroquine, doxycycline, or mefloquine is used for primary prophylaxis, primaquine is usually taken during the last 2 weeks of postexposure prophylaxis. When atovaquone-proguanil is used for prophylaxis, primaquine may be taken during the final 7 days of atovaquone-proguanil, and then for an additional 7 days. Primaquine should be given concurrently with the primary prophylaxis medication. However, if that is not feasible, the primaquine course should still be administered after the primary prophylaxis medication has been completed.

The most common adverse event in people with normal G6PD levels is gastrointestinal upset if primaquine is taken on an empty stomach. This problem is minimized or eliminated if primaquine is taken with food. In G6PD-deficient people, primaquine can cause hemolysis that can be fatal. **Before primaquine is used, G6PD deficiency MUST be ruled out by laboratory testing.**

TRAVEL TO AREAS WITH LIMITED MALARIA TRANSMISSION

For destinations where malaria cases occur sporadically and risk for infection to travelers is assessed as being low, CDC recommends that travelers use mosquito avoidance measures only, and no chemoprophylaxis should be prescribed (see the Yellow Fever & Malaria Information, by Country section later in this chapter).

TRAVEL TO AREAS WITH MAINLY *P. VIVAX* MALARIA

For destinations where the main species of malaria present is *P. vivax*, in addition to mosquito avoidance measures, primaquine is a good choice for primary prophylaxis for travelers who are not G6PD deficient. Its use for this indication is considered off-label in the United States. The predominant species of malaria and the recommended chemoprophylaxis medicines are listed in the Yellow Fever & Malaria Information, by Country section later in this chapter. For people unable to take primaquine, other drugs can be used as described below, depending on the presence of antimalarial drug resistance.

TRAVEL TO AREAS WITH CHLOROQUINE-SENSITIVE MALARIA

For destinations where chloroquine-sensitive malaria is present, in addition to mosquito avoidance measures, the many effective chemoprophylaxis options include chloroquine, atovaquone-proguanil, doxycycline, mefloquine, and in some instances, primaquine for travelers who are not G6PD deficient. Longer-term travelers may prefer the convenience of weekly chloroquine, while shorter-term travelers may prefer the shorter course of atovaquone-proguanil or primaquine.

TRAVEL TO AREAS WITH CHLOROQUINE-RESISTANT MALARIA

For destinations where chloroquine-resistant malaria is present, in addition to mosquito avoidance measures, chemoprophylaxis options are atovaquone-proguanil, doxycycline, and mefloquine.

TRAVEL TO AREAS WITH MEFLOQUINE-RESISTANT MALARIA

For destinations where mefloquine-resistant malaria is present, in addition to mosquito avoidance measures, chemoprophylaxis options are either atovaquone-proguanil or doxycycline.

CHEMOPROPHYLAXIS FOR INFANTS, CHILDREN, AND ADOLESCENTS

Infants of any age or weight or children and adolescents of any age can contract malaria. Therefore, all children traveling to malaria-endemic areas should use the recommended prevention measures, which often include taking an antimalarial drug. In the United States, antimalarial drugs are available only in oral formulations and may taste bitter. Pediatric doses should be carefully calculated according to body weight but should never exceed adult dose. Pharmacists can pulverize tablets and prepare gelatin capsules for each measured dose. If the child is unable to swallow the capsules or tablets, parents should prepare the child's dose of medication by breaking open the gelatin capsule and mixing the drug with a small amount of something sweet, such as applesauce, chocolate syrup, or jelly, to ensure the entire dose is delivered to the child. Giving the dose on a full stomach may minimize stomach upset and vomiting.

Chloroquine and mefloquine are options for use in infants and children of all ages and weights, depending on drug resistance at their destination. Primaquine can be used for children who are not G6PD deficient traveling to areas with principally *P. vivax*. Doxycycline may be used for children who are aged ≥8 years. Atovaquone-proguanil may be used for prophylaxis for infants and children weighing ≥5 kg (11 lb). Prophylactic dosing for children weighing <11 kg (24 lb) constitutes off-label use in the United States. Pediatric dosing regimens are contained in Table 3-10.

CHEMOPROPHYLAXIS DURING PREGNANCY AND BREASTFEEDING

Malaria infection in pregnant women can be more severe than in non-pregnant women. Malaria increases the risk for adverse pregnancy outcomes, including prematurity, spontaneous abortion, and stillbirth. For these reasons, and because no chemoprophylaxis regimen is completely effective, women who are pregnant or likely to become pregnant should be advised to avoid travel to areas with malaria transmission if possible (see Chapter 8, Pregnant Travelers). If travel to a malarious area cannot be deferred, use of an effective chemoprophylaxis regimen is essential.

Pregnant women traveling to areas where chloroquine-resistant *P. falciparum* has not been reported may take chloroquine prophylaxis. Chloroquine has not been found to have any harmful effects on the fetus when used in the recommended doses for malaria prophylaxis; therefore, pregnancy is not a contraindication for malaria prophylaxis with chloroquine phosphate or hydroxychloroquine sulfate.

For travel to areas where chloroquine resistance is present, mefloquine is the only medication recommended for malaria chemoprophylaxis during pregnancy. In 2011, the FDA reviewed available data for mefloquine use during pregnancy and reclassified it from category C (animal reproduction studies have shown an adverse effect on the fetus and there are no adequate and well-controlled studies in humans, but potential benefits may warrant use of the drug in pregnant women despite potential risks) to category B (animal reproduction studies have failed to demonstrate a risk to the fetus and there are no adequate and well-controlled studies in pregnant women).

Experts are investigating ways to examine the safety of atovaquone-proguanil use during pregnancy. Proguanil has been used for decades in pregnant women; however, until such time as these data are fully evaluated, atovaquone-proguanil is not recommended for use during pregnancy. Doxycycline is contraindicated for malaria prophylaxis during pregnancy because of the risk for adverse effects seen with tetracycline, a related drug, on the fetus, which include discoloration and dysplasia of the teeth and inhibition of bone growth. Primaquine should not be used during pregnancy because the drug may be passed transplacentally to a G6PD-deficient fetus and cause hemolytic anemia in utero.

Women planning to become pregnant may use the same medications that are recommended for use during pregnancy. CDC does not recommend that women planning pregnancy wait a specific period of time after the use of malaria chemoprophylaxis medicines before becoming pregnant. However, if women or their health care providers wish to decrease the amount of antimalarial drug in the body before conception, Table 3-11 provides information on the half-lives of the recommended

Table 3-11. Half-lives of malaria chemoprophylaxis drugs

DRUG	HALF-LIFE
Atovaquone	2–3 days
Chloroquine	1–2 months
Doxycycline	15–24 hours
Hydroxychloroquine	1–2 months
Mefloquine	2–4 weeks
Primaquine	4–7 hours
Proguanil	12–25 hours

malara chemoprophylaxis medicines. After 2, 4, and 6 half-lives, approximately 25%, 6%, and 2% respectively, of the drug remain in the body.

Very small amounts of antimalarial drugs are excreted in the breast milk of lactating women. Because the quantity of antimalarial drugs transferred in breast milk is insufficient to provide adequate protection against malaria, infants who require chemoprophylaxis must receive the recommended dosages of antimalarial drugs listed in Table 3-10. Because chloroquine and mefloquine may be safely prescribed to infants, it is also safe for infants to be exposed to the small amounts excreted in breast milk. Although data are very limited about the use of doxycycline in lactating women, most experts consider the theoretical possibility of adverse events to the infant to be remote.

Although no information is available on the amount of primaquine that enters human breast milk, the mother and infant should be tested for G6PD deficiency before primaquine is given to a woman who is breastfeeding. Because data are not yet available on the safety of atovaquone-proguanil prophylaxis in infants weighing <5 kg (11 lb), CDC does not recommend it to prevent malaria in women breastfeeding infants weighing <5 kg. However, it can be used to treat women who are breastfeeding infants of any weight when the potential benefit outweighs the potential risk to the infant (such as treating a breastfeeding woman who has acquired *P. falciparum* malaria in an area of multidrug-resistant strains and who cannot tolerate other treatment options).

CHOOSING A DRUG TO PREVENT MALARIA

Recommendations for drugs to prevent malaria differ by country of travel and can be found in the Yellow Fever & Malaria Information, by Country section later in this chapter. Recommended drugs for each country are listed in alphabetical order and have comparable efficacy in that country. No antimalarial drug is 100% protective; therefore, prophylaxis must be combined with the use of personal protective measures (such as insect repellent, long sleeves, long pants, sleeping in a mosquito-free setting or using an insecticide-treated bed net). When several different drugs are recommended for an area, Table 3-9 may help in the decision-making process.

CHANGING MEDICATIONS AS A RESULT OF SIDE EFFECTS DURING CHEMOPROPHYLAXIS

Medications recommended for prophylaxis against malaria have different modes of action that affect the parasites at different stages of the life cycle. Thus, if the medication needs to be changed because of side effects before a full course has been completed, there are some special considerations (see Table 3-12).

BLOOD DONATION AFTER TRAVEL TO MALARIOUS AREAS

People who have been in an area where malaria transmission occurs should be deferred from donating blood in the United States for a period of time after returning from the malarious area to prevent transmission of malaria through blood transfusion (Table 3-13).

Risk assessments may differ between travel health providers and blood banks. A travel health provider advising a traveler going to a country with relatively low malaria transmission for a short period of time and engaging in low-risk behaviors may choose insect avoidance only and no chemoprophylaxis for the traveler. However, upon the traveler's return, a blood bank may still choose to defer that traveler for 1 year because of the travel to an area where transmission occurs.

CDC website: www.cdc.gov/malaria

Table 3-12. Changing medications as a result of side effects during chemoprophylaxis

DRUG BEING STOPPED	DRUG BEING STARTED	COMMENTS
Mefloquine	Doxycycline	Begin doxycycline, continue daily while in malaria-endemic area, and continue for 4 weeks after leaving malaria-endemic area.
	Atovaquone-proguanil	• If the switch occurs ≥3 weeks before departure from the endemic area, atovaquone-proguanil should be taken daily for the rest of the stay in the endemic area and for 1 week thereafter. • If the switch occurs <3 weeks before departure from the endemic area, atovaquone-proguanil should be taken daily for 4 weeks after the switch. • If the switch occurs after departure from the endemic area, atovaquone-proguanil should be taken daily until 4 weeks after the date of departure.
	Chloroquine	Not recommended
	Primaquine	This switch would be unlikely as primaquine is only recommended for primary prophylaxis in areas with mainly *P. vivax* for people with normal G6PD activity. Should that be the case, begin primaquine, continue daily while in malaria-endemic area, and continue for 7 days after leaving malaria-endemic area.
Doxycycline	Mefloquine	Not recommended
	Atovaquone-proguanil	• If the switch occurs ≥3 weeks before departure from the endemic area, atovaquone-proguanil should be taken daily for the rest of the stay in the endemic area and for 1 week thereafter. • If the switch occurs <3 weeks before departure from the endemic area, atovaquone-proguanil should be taken daily for 4 weeks after the switch. • If the switch occurs after departure from the endemic area, atovaquone-proguanil should be taken daily until 4 weeks after the date of departure.
	Chloroquine	Not recommended
	Primaquine	This switch would be unlikely as primaquine is only recommended for primary prophylaxis in areas with mainly *P. vivax* for people with normal G6PD activity. Should that be the case, begin primaquine, continue daily while in malaria-endemic area, and continue for 7 days after leaving malaria-endemic area.
Atovaquone-proguanil	Doxycycline	Begin doxycycline, continue daily while in malaria-endemic area, and continue for 4 weeks after leaving malaria-endemic area.
	Mefloquine	Not recommended
	Chloroquine	Not recommended
	Primaquine	This switch would be unlikely as primaquine is only recommended for primary prophylaxis in areas with mainly *P. vivax* for people with normal G6PD activity. Should that be the case, begin primaquine, continue daily while in malaria-endemic area, and continue for 7 days after leaving malaria-endemic area.

3

Table 3-12. Changing medications as a result of side effects during chemoprophylaxis (continued)

DRUG BEING STOPPED	DRUG BEING STARTED	COMMENTS
Chloroquine	Doxycycline	Begin doxycycline, continue daily while in malaria-endemic area, and continue for 4 weeks after leaving malaria-endemic area.
	Atovaquone-proguanil	• If the switch occurs ≥3 weeks before departure from the endemic area, atovaquone-proguanil should be taken daily for the rest of the stay in the endemic area and for 1 week thereafter. • If the switch occurs <3 weeks before departure from the endemic area, atovaquone-proguanil should be taken daily for 4 weeks after the switch. • If the switch occurs following departure from the endemic area, atovaquone-proguanil should be taken daily until 4 weeks after the date of departure.
	Mefloquine	Not recommended
	Primaquine	Primaquine is only recommended for primary prophylaxis in areas with mainly *P. vivax* for people with normal G6PD activity. Should that be the case, begin primaquine, continue daily while in malaria-endemic area, and continue for 7 days after leaving malaria-endemic area.
Primaquine	Doxycycline	Begin doxycycline, continue daily while in malaria-endemic area, and continue for 4 weeks after leaving malaria-endemic area.
	Atovaquone-proguanil	Begin atovaquone-proguanil, continue daily while in malaria-endemic area, and continue for 7 days after leaving malaria-endemic area.
	Chloroquine	Not recommended
	Mefloquine	Not recommended

Table 3-13. Food and Drug Administration recommendations for deferring blood donation in people returning from malarious areas

GROUP	BLOOD DONATION DEFERRAL
Travelers to malaria-endemic areas	May not donate blood for 1 year after travel.
Former residents of malaria-endemic areas	May not donate blood for 3 years after departing. If they return to a malaria-endemic area within that 3-year period, they are deferred for an additional 3 years.
People diagnosed with malaria	May not donate for 3 years after treatment.

BIBLIOGRAPHY

1. Boggild AK, Parise ME, Lewis LS, Kain KC. Atovaquone-proguanil: report from the CDC expert meeting on malaria chemoprophylaxis (II). Am J Trop Med Hyg. 2007 Feb;76(2):208–23.

2. CDC. Malaria Surveillance—United States, 2013. MMWR Surveill Summ. 2016 Mar 4;65(2):1–22.

3. Fradin MS, Day JF. Comparative efficacy of insect repellents against mosquito bites. N Engl J Med. 2002 Jul 4;347(1):13–8.

4. Hill DR, Baird JK, Parise ME, Lewis LS, Ryan ET, Magill AJ. Primaquine: report from CDC expert meeting on malaria chemoprophylaxis I. Am J Trop Med Hyg. 2006 Sep;75(3):402–15.

5. Leder K, Black J, O'Brien D, Greenwood Z, Kain KC, Schwartz E, et al. Malaria in travelers: a review of the GeoSentinel surveillance network. Clin Infect Dis. 2004 Oct 15;39(8):1104–12.

6. Newman RD, Parise ME, Barber AM, Steketee RW. Malaria-related deaths among US travelers, 1963–2001. Ann Intern Med. 2004 Oct 5;141(7):547–55.

7. Steinhardt LC, Magill AJ, Arguin PM. Review: Malaria chemoprophylaxis for travelers to Latin America. Am J Trop Med Hyg. 2011 Dec;85(6):1015–24.

8. Tan KR, Magill AJ, Parise ME, Arguin PM. Doxycycline for malaria chemoprophylaxis and treatment: report from the CDC expert meeting on malaria chemoprophylaxis. Am J Trop Med Hyg. 2011 Apr;84(4):517–31.

3

...for the record

A HISTORY OF MALARIA CHEMOPROPHYLAXIS

Paul M. Arguin, Alan J. Magill

Among the many dreaded fevers that plague man, "marsh fever" was distinguished by its periodicity, enlarged spleen, and pattern of attacking those exposed to wet, warm, boggy areas. In the mid-1700s, it became broadly known by its Italian name, *mal'aria* ("bad air"), referring to bad or foul air emanating from swampy lands. The discovery and development of drugs to treat and prevent malaria have been driven for centuries by the desire and need to protect travelers, military personnel, explorers, and the commercial interests of imperial powers when they went into the malaria-endemic tropics.

Historical Milestones in Antimalarial Chemoprophylaxis

- 1620s: Jesuit missionaries living in Peru learned of the healing power of powdered bark, often known as "Jesuits' bark," from the cinchona trees growing in the high forests of Peru and Bolivia.

- 1820: French chemists isolated quinine, the most active compound in cinchona bark, which allowed for quinine's expanded availability and use.

- 1854: The Scottish surgeon William Balfour Baikie gave 6–8 grains (1 grain = 65 mg) of quinine, half in the morning and half in the evening, dissolved in sherry, to all the ship's crew during a 118-day expedition up the river Benue in modern-day Nigeria. No men died. This unprecedented accomplishment gradually led to acceptance that malaria could be prevented by chemoprophylaxis.

- 1861: Quinine first saw widespread use as a prophylactic agent in the American Civil War when both the Union and Confederate Armies, plagued with malaria, used massive quantities to prevent the disease.

- 1880: A French military physician working in Algeria, Alphonse Laveran, discovered parasites in the blood of a French soldier. The identification of the infectious agent and its life cycle was an essential step in opening the way to the development of effective prophylactic agents.

- 1914–1918: During World War I, both Allied and Axis militaries suffered terribly from malaria. German armies were denied access to quinine, as most was held by a monopoly of Dutch growers on the island of Java.

- 1920s: German chemists pursued a synthetic route to new antimalarial drugs to circumvent the Dutch monopoly, achieving spectacular success with the introduction of pamaquine and mepacrine during the 1930s.

- 1941: With America's entry into World War II, trade between the United States and Germany ceased, and mepacrine was no longer available to the Allies.

- 1942: Japanese armies overran the Dutch cinchona plantations on Java, cutting off the supply of quinine and leaving the Allies with no source for antimalarial drugs.

- 1943: American scientists quickly devised a manufacturing process for mepacrine, and the drug was given as a treatment and as a prophylactic under the name Atabrine. Meanwhile, the Allies, especially the Americans, launched the largest antimalarial drug discovery and development program the world had seen. By 1945, several new antimalarial drugs had been introduced, including chloroquine and proguanil. Chloroquine went on to assume a role both in prophylaxis for travelers and as a treatment drug for endemic areas.

- 1959: Chloroquine-resistant *Plasmodium falciparum* malaria was first reported.

- 1965: Large-scale American military involvement began in South Vietnam, reaching almost 200,000 soldiers by the end of 1965. Chloroquine-resistant malaria caused illness and death in US forces.

- 1967: A second massive US government–sponsored antimalarial drug discovery effort centered at the Walter Reed Army Institute of Research began and led to the discovery of mefloquine.

- 1971: During studies of volunteers with experimentally induced malaria infections, it was observed that tetracycline, administered to treat intercurrent bacterial infections, appeared to exert blood schizontocidal activity against chloroquine-resistant *P. falciparum*. A few additional studies were performed with tetracycline, doxycycline, and minocycline, but no formal development of the drug as an antimalarial was pursued.

- 1977: Although it was not yet available in the United States, CDC recommended sulfadoxine-pyrimethamine as an alternative for primary prophylaxis.

- Early 1980s: The Wellcome Research Laboratories developed atovaquone as an antimalarial drug. Clinical trials in uncomplicated *P. falciparum* malaria as monotherapy were disappointing, with early treatment failures due to the emergence of atovaquone-resistant parasites. However, combining atovaquone with proguanil led to an efficacious combination therapy.

- 1982: The fixed combination of pyrimethamine and sulfadoxine (Fansidar) became available in the United States. CDC recommended a combined regimen of chloroquine and Fansidar to prevent chloroquine-resistant *P. falciparum*.

- 1985: CDC added cautionary language to the recommendation for pyrimethamine-sulfadoxine use as weekly malaria chemoprophylaxis resulted in fatal cases of Stevens-Johnson syndrome. CDC added doxycycline as an alternative regimen for antimalarial prophylaxis.

- 1986: CDC removed amodiaquine as a

recommended alternative for malaria prevention.

- Late 1980s: The US Army conducted several field and human challenge clinical trials demonstrating the efficacy of doxycycline as malaria prophylaxis.

- 1987: CDC added chloroquine-proguanil as an alternative regimen for malaria prevention.

- 1988: Although it was not yet available in the United States, CDC recommended mefloquine as an alternative regimen for primary malaria prophylaxis.

- 1989: The Food and Drug Administration (FDA) approved mefloquine (Lariam).

- 1990: Pyrimethamine-sulfadoxine was removed as a recommended alternative for primary chemoprophylaxis. Mefloquine was recommended as the drug of choice to prevent malaria in areas with chloroquine-resistant P. falciparum.

- 1992: Pfizer, at the request of FDA, submitted a supplemental new drug application for doxycycline for malaria chemoprophylaxis.

- 2000: Combination of fixed dose atovaquone-proguanil (Malarone) was approved by FDA.

- 2001–2002: CDC added atovaquone-proguanil as an alternative regimen for malaria chemoprophylaxis and removed chloroquine-progaunil as a recommended alternative.

- 2003–2004: CDC listed atovaquone-proguanil, doxycycline, and mefloquine as equally recommended first-line options to prevent malaria. A recommendation for primary prophylaxis with primaquine in "special situations" was also added.

- 2010: CDC added that primary prophylaxis with primaquine was recommended for areas with mainly P. vivax.

- 2014: CDC added recommendations for carrying a "reliable supply."

The 3 largest antimalarial drug development efforts of modern times occurred during and after major conflicts of the 20th century—World War I, World War II, and the Vietnam War. The modern history of developing drugs to prevent malaria grew almost entirely from the need to protect military personnel and keep them healthy to conduct combat operations in malaria-endemic areas. Those massive government-funded efforts produced the drugs now used to keep modern civilian travelers safe from the sickness and death that mark malaria's march through time.

BIBLIOGRAPHY

1. Greenwood D. Conflicts of interest: the genesis of synthetic antimalarial agents in peace and war. J Antimicrob Chemother. 1995 Nov;36(5):857–72.

2. Kitchen LW, Vaughn DW, Skillman DR. Role of US military research programs in the development of US Food and Drug Administration—approved antimalarial drugs. Clin Infect Dis. 2006 Jul 1;43(1):67–71.

3. Smith DC. Quinine and fever: The development of the effective dosage. J Hist Med Allied Sci. 1976 Jul;31(3):343–67.

4. Smith DC, Sanford LB. Laveran's germ: the reception and use of a medical discovery. Am J Trop Med Hyg. 1985 Jan;34(1):2–20.

5. Sweeney AW. Wartime research on malaria chemotherapy. Parassitologia. 2000 Jun;42(1-2):33–45.

MEASLES (RUBEOLA)

Paul A. Gastañaduy, James L. Goodson

INFECTIOUS AGENT

Measles virus is a member of the genus *Morbillivirus* of the family Paramyxoviridae.

TRANSMISSION

Measles is transmitted from person to person primarily by the airborne route as aerosolized droplet nuclei. Infected people are usually contagious from 4 days before until 4 days after rash onset. Measles is among the most contagious viral diseases known; secondary attack rates are ≥90% in susceptible household and institutional contacts. Humans are the only natural host for sustaining measles virus transmission, which makes global eradication of measles feasible.

EPIDEMIOLOGY

The number of reported measles cases in the United States has declined from nearly 900,000 annually in the early 1940s to 37–667 cases annually from 2001 through 2015. As a result of high vaccination coverage and better measles control in the Americas, in 2000, measles in the United States was declared eliminated (defined as the absence of endemic measles virus transmission in a defined geographic area for ≥12 months in the presence of a well-performing surveillance system). In 2002, indigenous measles virus circulation was interrupted in the entire Western Hemisphere. However, measles virus continues to be imported into the region from other parts of the world, and recent outbreaks resulting from measles virus importations highlight the challenges faced in maintaining elimination. Globally, in 2014, the annual reported measles incidence was 40 cases per million population. Given the large global incidence and high communicability of the disease, travelers may be exposed to the virus in almost any country they visit, particularly those outside the Western Hemisphere, where measles is endemic or where large outbreaks are occurring. In recent years, measles has been imported into the United States from frequently visited countries, including the United Kingdom, France, Germany, India, and the Philippines, where large outbreaks have been reported. Most measles cases imported into the United States have come from unvaccinated US residents who became infected while traveling abroad, became symptomatic after returning to the United States, and in some cases infected others in their communities, causing outbreaks. Additional information on global measles control efforts is available on the Measles & Rubella Initiative website at www.measlesrubellainitiative.org.

CLINICAL PRESENTATION

The incubation period ranges from 7 to 21 days from exposure to onset of fever; rash usually appears about 14 days after exposure. Symptoms include prodromal fever that can rise as high as 105°F (40.6°C), conjunctivitis, coryza (runny nose), cough, and small spots with white or bluish-white centers on an erythematous base on the buccal mucosa (Koplik spots). A characteristic red, blotchy (maculopapular) rash appears on the third to seventh day after the prodromal symptoms appear. The rash begins on the face, becomes generalized, and lasts 4–7 days. Common complications include diarrhea (8%), middle ear infection (7%–9%), and pneumonia (1%–6%). Encephalitis, which can result in permanent brain damage, occurs in approximately 1 per 1,000–2,000 cases of measles. The risk of serious complications and death is highest for children aged ≤5 years and adults aged ≥20 years. It is also higher in populations with poor nutritional status.

Subacute sclerosing panencephalitis (SSPE), a rare but serious degenerative central nervous system disease caused by a persistent infection with a defective measles virus, is estimated to occur in 4–11 per 100,000 cases. However, among people who became infected with measles during the 1989–1991 measles resurgence in the United States, the estimated risk of SSPE was 22 per

100,000 reported measles cases. SSPE is manifested by mental and motor deterioration that starts an average of 7–10 years after measles virus infection (most frequently in children who were infected at age <2 years), progressing to coma and death.

DIAGNOSIS

Laboratory criteria for diagnosis include any of the following: a positive serologic test for measles IgM, IgG seroconversion or a significant rise in measles IgG level by any standard serologic assay, isolation of measles virus, or detection of measles virus RNA by RT-PCR.

A clinical case of measles illness is characterized by all of the following:

- Generalized maculopapular rash lasting ≥3 days

- Temperature of ≥101°F (38.3°C)

- Cough, coryza, or conjunctivitis

A confirmed case is one with an acute febrile rash illness with laboratory confirmation or direct epidemiologic linkage to a laboratory confirmed case. In a laboratory-confirmed case, the temperature does not need to reach ≥101°F (38.3°C) and the rash does not need to last ≥3 days.

Measles is a nationally notifiable disease.

TREATMENT

Treatment is supportive. The World Health Organization recommends vitamin A for all children with acute measles, regardless of their country of residence, to reduce the risk of complications. Vitamin A is administered once a day for 2 days at the following doses:

- 50,000 IU for infants aged <6 months

- 100,000 IU for infants aged 6–11 months

- 200,000 IU for children aged ≥12 months

An additional (third) age-specific dose of vitamin A should be given 2–4 weeks later to children with clinical signs and symptoms of vitamin A deficiency. Parenteral and oral formulations of vitamin A are available in the United States.

PREVENTION

Measles has been preventable since 1963 through vaccination. People who do not have evidence of measles immunity should be considered at risk for measles, particularly during international travel. Acceptable presumptive evidence of immunity to measles for international travelers includes meeting any of the following criteria:

- Documentation of age-appropriate vaccination with a live measles-containing vaccine (MMR or MMRV):
  > For infants aged 6–11 months, documented administration of 1 dose of MMR or MMRV
  > For people aged ≥12 months, 2 doses of MMR or MMRV (the first dose should be administered at age ≥12 months; the second dose should be administered no earlier than 28 days after the first dose)

- Laboratory evidence of immunity

- Laboratory confirmation of disease

- Birth before 1957

Vaccine

Measles vaccine contains live, attenuated measles virus. In the United States, it is available only in combination formulations, such as measles-mumps-rubella (MMR) and measles-mumps-rubella-varicella (MMRV) vaccines. MMRV vaccine is licensed for children aged 12 months to 12 years and may be used in place of MMR vaccine if vaccination for measles, mumps, rubella, and varicella is needed.

International travelers, including people traveling to industrialized countries, who do not have presumptive evidence of measles immunity and who have no contraindications to MMR or MMRV, should receive MMR or MMRV before travel according to the following guidelines:

- Infants aged 6–11 months should receive 1 MMR dose. Infants vaccinated before age 12 months must be revaccinated on or after the first birthday with 2 doses of MMR or MMRV separated by ≥28 days. MMRV is not licensed for children aged <12 months.

- Preschool and school-age children (aged ≥12 months) should be given 2 MMR or MMRV doses separated by ≥28 days.

- Adults born in or after 1957 should be given 2 MMR or MMRV doses separated by ≥28 days.

One dose of MMR or MMRV is approximately 85% effective when administered at age 9 months and 93% effective when administered at age ≥1 year. Vaccine effectiveness of 2 doses is 97%.

Measles-containing vaccine and immune globulin (IG) may be effective as postexposure prophylaxis. MMR or MMRV, if administered within 72 hours after initial exposure to measles virus, may provide some protection. If the exposure does not result in infection, the vaccine should induce protection against subsequent measles virus infection. IG can be used to prevent or mitigate measles in a susceptible person when administered within 6 days of exposure. However, any immunity conferred is temporary unless modified or typical measles occurs, and the person should receive MMR or MMRV 6 months after intramuscularly administered IG or 8 months after intravenously administered IG, provided the person is then aged ≥12 months and the vaccine is not otherwise contraindicated.

VACCINE SAFETY AND ADVERSE REACTIONS

In rare circumstances, MMR vaccination has been associated with the following adverse events:

- Anaphylaxis (approximately 1–3.5 occurrences per million doses administered)

- Thrombocytopenia (a rate of 1 case in every 25,000 doses during the 6 weeks after immunization)

- Febrile seizures (The risk of febrile seizures is approximately 25–33 cases for every 100,000 doses of MMR vaccine administered, but overall, the rate of febrile seizure after measles-containing vaccine is much lower than the rate with measles disease.)

- Joint symptoms (Arthralgia develops among approximately 25% of nonimmune postpubertal women from the rubella component of the MMR vaccination. Approximately 10% have acute arthritislike signs and symptoms

that generally persist for 1 day to 3 weeks and rarely recur. Chronic joint symptoms are rare, if they occur at all.)

Evidence does not support a causal link between MMR vaccination and any of the following: hearing loss, retinopathy, optic neuritis, ocular palsies, Guillain-Barré syndrome, cerebellar ataxia, Crohn's disease, or autism. A published report on MMR vaccination and inflammatory bowel disease and pervasive developmental disorders (such as autism) has never been replicated by other studies and has subsequently been widely discredited and retracted by the journal.

CONTRAINDICATIONS AND PRECAUTIONS

CONTRAINDICATIONS

Allergy—People with severe allergy (hives, swelling of the mouth or throat, difficulty breathing, hypotension, and shock) to gelatin or neomycin, or who have had a severe allergic reaction to a prior dose of MMR or MMRV vaccine, should not be revaccinated. MMR or MMRV vaccine may be administered to people who are allergic to eggs without prior routine skin testing or the use of special protocols.

Pregnancy—MMR vaccines should not be administered to pregnant women or those attempting to become pregnant. Because of the theoretical risk to the fetus when the mother receives a live virus vaccine, women should be counseled to avoid becoming pregnant for 28 days after receipt of MMR vaccine.

Immunosuppression—Enhanced replication of live vaccine viruses can occur in people who have immune deficiency disorders. Death related to vaccine-associated measles virus infection has been reported among severely immunocompromised people. Therefore, severely immunosuppressed people should not be vaccinated with MMR or MMRV vaccine (for a thorough discussion of recommendations for immunocompromised travelers, see Chapter 8, Immunocompromised Travelers):

- People with leukemia in remission, and off chemotherapy, who were not immune to measles when diagnosed with leukemia, may receive MMR vaccine. At least 3 months should elapse after termination of chemotherapy before administration of the first dose.

- MMR vaccination is recommended for all people aged ≥12 months with HIV infection who do not have evidence of measles, rubella, and mumps immunity or evidence of severe immunosuppression. The assessment of severe immunosuppression can be on the basis of CD4 values (count or percentage); absence of severe immunosuppression is defined as CD4 percentages ≥15% for ≥6 months at any age or CD4 count ≥200 cells/mm³ for ≥6 months for people aged >5 years.

- People who have received high-dose corticosteroid therapy (in general, considered to be ≥20 mg prednisone or equivalent daily or on alternate days for an interval of ≥14 days) should avoid vaccination with MMR or MMRV for ≥1 month after cessation of steroid therapy. Corticosteroid therapy usually is not a contraindication when administration is short term (<14 days) or a low to moderate dose (<20 mg of prednisone or equivalent per day).

- Other immunosuppressive therapy: in general, MMR or MMRV vaccine should be withheld for ≥3 months after cessation of the immunosuppressive therapy and remission of the underlying disease. This interval is based on the assumptions that the immune response will have been restored in 3 months and the underlying disease for which the therapy was given remains in remission.

PRECAUTIONS

Thrombocytopenia—The benefits of primary immunization are usually greater than the potential risks of thrombocytopenia. However, avoiding a subsequent dose of MMR or MMRV vaccine may be prudent if an episode of thrombocytopenia occurred within approximately 6 weeks after a previous dose of vaccine.

Personal or family history of seizures of any etiology—Compared with administration of separate MMR and varicella vaccines at the same visit, use of MMRV vaccine is associated with a higher risk for fever and febrile seizures 5–12 days after the first dose among children aged 12–23 months. Approximately 1 additional febrile seizure occurs for every 2,300–2,600 MMRV vaccine doses administered. Use of separate MMR and varicella vaccines avoids this increased risk for fever and febrile seizures.

CDC website: www.cdc.gov/measles

BIBLIOGRVAPHY

1. American Academy of Pediatrics. Measles. In: Pickering LK, editor. Red Book: 2015 Report of the Committee on Infectious Diseases. 30th ed. Elk Grove Village, IL: American Academy of Pediatrics; 2015. pp. 535–47.

2. Bellini WJ, Rota JS, Lowe LE, Katz RS, Dyken PR, Zaki SR, et al. Subacute sclerosing panencephalitis: more cases of this fatal disease are prevented by measles immunization than was previously recognized. J Infect Dis. 2005 Nov 15;192(10):1686–93.

3. CDC. General recommendations on immunization—recommendations of the Advisory Committee on Immunization Practices (ACIP). MMWR Recomm Rep. 2011;60(RR-02):1–60.

4. CDC. Prevention of measles, rubella, congenital rubella syndrome, and mumps, 2013: summary recommendations of the Advisory Committee on Immunization Practices (ACIP). MMWR Recomm Rep. 2013 Jun 14;62(RR-04):1–34.

5. Measles & Rubella Initiative [Internet]. Washington, DC: Amercian Red Cross; 2014 [cited 2016 Sep. 25]. Available from: http://www.measlesrubellainitiative.org.

6. National Notifiable Diseases Surveillance System. Measles (rubeola): 2013 case definition. Atlanta: CDC; 2013 [cited 2016 Sep. 25]. Available from: http://wwwn.cdc.gov/NNDSS/script/casedef.aspx?CondYrID=908&DatePub=1/1/2013.

7. Perry RT, Halsey NA. The clinical significance of measles: a review. J Infect Dis. 2004 May 1;189 Suppl 1:S4–16.

8. Perry RT, Murray JS, Gacic-Dobo M, Dabbagh A, Mulders MN, Strebel PM, et al. Progress toward regional measles elimination—worldwide, 2000–2014. MMWR Morb Mortal Wkly Rep. 2015 Nov 13;64(44):1246–51.

9. World Health Organization. Measles [fact sheet no. 286]. Geneva: World Health Organization; 2014 [cited 2016 Sep. 25]. Available from: http://www.who.int/mediacentre/factsheets/fs286/en.

3

MELIOIDOSIS

David D. Blaney, Jay E. Gee

INFECTIOUS AGENT

Burkholderia pseudomallei, a saprophytic gram-negative bacillus, is the causative agent of melioidosis. The bacteria are found in soil and water, widely distributed in tropical and subtropical countries.

TRANSMISSION

Through subcutaneous inoculation, ingestion, or inhalation; person-to-person transmission is extremely rare but may occur through contact with the blood or body fluids of an infected person.

EPIDEMIOLOGY

Melioidosis is endemic in Southeast Asia, Papua New Guinea, much of the Indian subcontinent, southern China, Hong Kong, and Taiwan and is considered highly endemic in northeast Thailand, Malaysia, Singapore, and northern Australia. Sporadic cases have been reported among residents of or travelers to Aruba, Colombia, Costa Rica, El Salvador, Guatemala, Guadeloupe, Honduras, Martinique, Mexico, Panama, Venezuela, and many other countries in the Americas, as well as Puerto Rico. In northeastern Brazil, clusters of melioidosis have been reported. The true extent of the distribution of the bacteria remains unknown and is considered under-reported or unrecognized in many tropical and subtropical areas. The risk is highest for adventure travelers, ecotourists, military personnel, construction and resource extraction workers, and other people whose contact with contaminated soil or water may expose them to the bacteria; infections have been reported in people who have spent less than a week in an endemic area. Cases, especially presenting as pneumonias, are often associated with periods of high rainfall such as during typhoons or the monsoon season. Risk factors for invasive melioidosis include diabetes, excessive alcohol use, chronic renal disease, chronic lung disease (such as associated with cystic fibrosis or chronic obstructive pulmonary disease), thalassemia, and malignancy or other non-HIV-related immune suppression.

CLINICAL PRESENTATION

Incubation period is generally 1–21 days; with a high inoculum, symptoms can develop in a few hours. Melioidosis may also remain latent for months or years before symptoms develop. Melioidosis may occur as a subclinical infection, localized infection (such as cutaneous abscess), pneumonia, meningoencephalitis, sepsis, or chronic suppurative infection. The latter may mimic tuberculosis, with fever, weight loss, productive cough, and upper lobe infiltrate, with or without cavitation. More than 50% of cases present with pneumonia.

DIAGNOSIS

Culture of *B. pseudomallei* from blood, sputum, pus, urine, synovial fluid, peritoneal fluid, or pericardial fluid is diagnostic. Indirect hemagglutination assay is a widely used serologic test but is not considered confirmatory. Diagnostic assistance is available through CDC (http://www.cdc.gov/ncezid/dhcpp/bacterial_special/zoonoses_lab.html).

TREATMENT

Intravenous ceftazidime, or meropenem for severe cases with sepsis, is typically used for initial treatment, for a minimum of 14 days; depending on presentation and response to therapy, this initial treatment may be extended for up to 8 weeks. This is usually followed by months of eradication treatment with an oral agent such as trimethoprim-sulfamethoxazole. Relapse may be seen, especially in patients who received a shorter-than-recommended course of therapy.

PREVENTION

Travelers should use personal protective equipment such as waterproof boots and gloves to protect against contact with soil and water in endemic areas and thoroughly clean skin

lacerations, abrasions, or burns that have been contaminated with soil or surface water.

CDC website: www.cdc.gov/melioidosis

BIBLIOGRAPHY

1. Benoit TJ, Blaney DD, Doker TJ, Gee JE, Elrod MG, Rolim DB, et al. A review of melioidosis cases in the Americas. Am J Trop Med Hyg. 2015 Dec;93(6):1134–9.

2. Currie BJ. Melioidosis: evolving concepts in epidemiology, pathogenesis, and treatment. Semin Respir Crit Care Med. 2015 Feb;36(1):111–25.

3. Currie BJ, Dance DA, Cheng AC. The global distribution of *Burkholderia pseudomallei* and melioidosis: an update. Trans R Soc Trop Med Hyg. 2008 Dec;102 Suppl 1:S1–4.

4. Limmathurotsakul D, Golding N, Dance DA, Messina JP, Pigott DM, Moyes CL, et al. Predicted global distribution

of *Burkholderia pseudomallei* and burden of melioidosis. Nat Microbiol. 2016;1:15008.

5. Limmathurotsakul D, Kanoksil M, Wuthiekanun V, Kitphati R, deStavola B, Day NP, et al. Activities of daily living associated with acquisition of melioidosis in northeast Thailand: a matched case-control study. PLoS Negl Trop Dis. 2013;7(2):e2072.

6. O'Sullivan BP, Torres B, Conidi G, Smole S, Gauthier C, Stauffer KE, et al. *Burkholderia pseudomallei* infection in a child with cystic fibrosis: acquisition in the Western Hemisphere. Chest. 2011 Jul;140(1):239–42.

7. Wiersinga WJ, Currie BJ, Peacock SJ. Melioidosis. N Engl J Med. 2012 Sep 13;367(11):1035–44.

3

MENINGOCOCCAL DISEASE

Jessica R. MacNeil, Sarah A. Meyer

INFECTIOUS AGENT

Neisseria meningitidis is a gram-negative diplococcus. Meningococci are classified into serogroups on the basis of the composition of the capsular polysaccharide. The 6 major meningococcal serogroups associated with disease are A, B, C, W, X, and Y.

TRANSMISSION

Person-to-person transmission occurs by close contact with respiratory secretions of a person with meningococcal disease or asymptomatic carriage of *N. meningitidis*. Asymptomatic carriage is transient, affecting an estimated 5%–10% of the population at any given time.

EPIDEMIOLOGY

N. meningitidis is found worldwide, but the highest incidence occurs in the "meningitis belt" of sub-Saharan Africa (Map 3-11). Meningococcal disease is hyperendemic in this region, and periodic

epidemics during the dry season (December–June) reach up to 1,000 cases per 100,000 population. By contrast, rates of disease in the United States, Europe, Australia, and South America range from 0.15 to 3 cases per 100,000 population per year.

Although meningococcal outbreaks can occur anywhere in the world, they are most common in the African meningitis belt, and large-scale epidemics occur every 5–12 years. Historically, outbreaks in the meningitis belt were primarily due to serogroup A. However, with the introduction of a monovalent serogroup A meningococcal conjugate vaccine [MenAfriVac] in the region starting in 2010, recent meningococcal outbreaks have primarily been due to serogroups C and W, although serogroup X outbreaks are also reported.

Outside the meningitis belt, infants and adolescents have the highest rates of disease. In meningitis belt countries, high rates of disease are seen in people up to age 30 years but are highest in

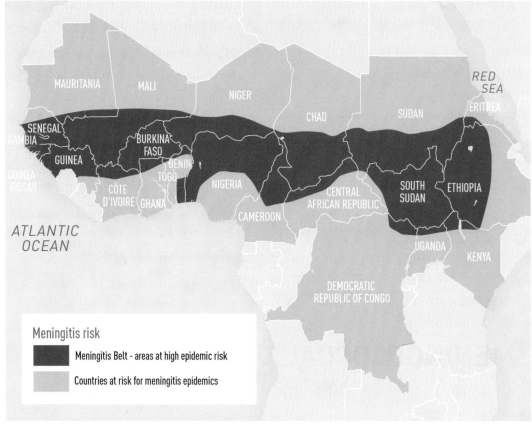

MAP 3-11. **Areas with frequent epidemics of meningococcal meningitis**[1]

[1] Disease data source: World Health Organization. International Travel and Health. Geneva, Switzerland: 2012.

children and adolescents aged 5–14 years. Risk for travelers is highest in people visiting meningitis belt countries who have prolonged contact with local populations during an epidemic. The Hajj pilgrimage to Saudi Arabia has also been associated with outbreaks of meningococcal disease in returning pilgrims and their contacts.

CLINICAL PRESENTATION

Meningococcal disease generally occurs 1–10 days after exposure and presents as meningitis in ≥50% of cases. Meningococcal meningitis is characterized by sudden onset of headache, fever, and stiffness of the neck, sometimes accompanied by nausea, vomiting, photophobia, or altered mental status. Up to 20% of people with meningococcal disease present with meningococcal sepsis, known as meningococcemia. Meningococcemia

is characterized by an abrupt onset of fever and a petechial or purpuric rash. The rash may progress to purpura fulminans. Meningococcemia often involves hypotension, acute adrenal hemorrhage, and multiorgan failure. Among infants and children aged <2 years, meningococcal disease may have nonspecific symptoms. Neck stiffness, usually seen in people with meningitis, may be absent in this age group. The case-fatality ratio of meningococcal disease is 10%–15%.

DIAGNOSIS

Early diagnosis and treatment are critical. A lumbar puncture should be done to examine the cerebrospinal fluid (CSF) and perform a Gram stain. If possible, the lumbar puncture should be done before starting antibiotic therapy to ensure that bacteria, if present, can be cultured from CSF.

Diagnosis is generally made by isolating *N. meningitidis* from blood or CSF through culture, by detecting meningococcal antigen in CSF by latex agglutination, or by evidence of *N. meningitidis* DNA by PCR.

The signs and symptoms of meningococcal meningitis are similar to those of other causes of bacterial meningitis, such as *Haemophilus influenzae* and *Streptococcus pneumoniae*. The causative organism should be identified so that the correct antibiotics can be used for treatment and prophylaxis. Meningococcal disease is nationally notifiable.

TREATMENT

Meningococcal disease is potentially fatal and should always be viewed as a medical emergency. Antibiotic treatment must be started early in the course of the disease, and empirically prior to the diagnostic test results. Several antibiotic choices are available, including third-generation cephalosporins.

PREVENTION

Vaccine

Six meningococcal vaccines are licensed in the United States. Refer to Table 3-14 for more information about available meningococcal vaccines. Approximately 7–10 days are required after vaccination for the development of protective antibody levels.

ROUTINE IMMUNIZATION

The Advisory Committee on Immunization Practices (ACIP) recommends routine administration of a quadrivalent meningococcal conjugate vaccine (MenACWY) for all people aged 11–18 years. A single dose of vaccine should be administered at age 11 or 12 years, and a booster dose should be administered at age 16 years. Routine immunization with MenACWY is not recommended for other age groups in the United States, with the exception of people at increased risk for meningococcal disease. Those at increased risk for meningococcal disease include people who have a persistent complement component deficiency (C3, C5-9, properdin, factor D, or factor H or people who are taking eculizumab [Soliris]),

people who have functional or anatomic asplenia, or people with HIV. Vaccine, product, number of doses, and booster dose recommendations are based on age and risk factor and are described in detail for each risk group in the 2013 ACIP Meningococcal Disease Recommendations (www.cdc.gov/mmwr/preview/mmwrhtml/rr6202a1.htm).

Adolescents and young adults aged 16–23 years may also be vaccinated with a serogroup B meningococcal (MenB) vaccine to provide short-term protection against most strains of serogroup B meningococcal disease. The preferred age for MenB vaccination is 16 through 18 years. ACIP also recommends routine use of MenB vaccine for people aged ≥10 years who are at increased risk for meningococcal disease, including people who have persistent complement component deficiency and people who have functional or anatomic asplenia.

IMMUNIZATION FOR TRAVELERS

ACIP recommends that travelers who visit or reside in parts of sub-Saharan Africa known as the "meningitis belt" (see Map 3-11) during the dry season (December–June) receive vaccination with a quadrivalent (serogroup A, C, W, or Y) meningococcal vaccine before travel. The preferred vaccine for people aged 2 months through 55 years and meningococcal vaccine-nonnaïve people aged ≥56 years is MenACWY, and MPSV4 is preferred for meningococcal vaccine-naïve people aged ≥56 years. Advisories for travelers to other countries are issued when outbreaks of meningococcal disease are recognized (see the CDC Travelers' Health website at www.cdc.gov/travel).

For infants aged <9 months, MenACWY-CRM (Menveo) is the only licensed vaccine that protects against serogroups A and W and therefore should be used for travelers in this age group. In children initiating vaccination at 2 months of age, MenACWY-CRM should be administered as a 4-dose series at 2, 4, 6, and 12 months of age. In children initiating vaccination at 7–23 months of age, MenACWY-CRM should be administered as a 2-dose series, with the second dose administered at ≥12 months of age and ≥3 months after the first dose, although it can be administered as early as

Table 3-14. Meningococcal vaccines licensed in the United States

VACCINE	TRADE NAME (MANUFACTURER)	AGE	DOSE	ROUTE	INTERVAL BETWEEN DOSES	BOOSTER
Meningococcal (serogroups A, C, W, and Y) polysaccharide diphtheria toxoid conjugate vaccine (MenACWY-D)[1]	Menactra (Sanofi Pasteur)	9–23 mo 2–55 y	0.5 mL 0.5 mL	IM IM	0, 3 mo 1 dose[2]	If at continued risk[3]
Meningococcal (serogroups A, C, W, and Y) oligosaccharide diphtheria CRM$_{197}$ conjugate vaccine (MenACWY-CRM)[1]	Menveo (GSK)	2–12 mo 7–23 mo 2–55 y	0.5 mL 0.5 mL 0.5 mL	IM IM IM	0, 2, 4, 10–13 mo 0, 3 mo (2nd dose administered in 2nd year of life) 1 dose[2]	If at continued risk[3]
Meningococcal (serogroups C and Y) and *Haemophilus influenzae* type B polysaccharide tetanus toxoid conjugated vaccine[4]	MenHibrix (GSK)	6 wk–18 mo	0.5 mL	IM	0, 2, 4, 10–13 mo	If at continued risk[3]
Meningococcal (serogroups A, C, W, and Y) polysaccharide vaccine (MPSV4)	Menomune (Sanofi Pasteur)	≥2 y	0.5 mL	SC	1 dose	See footnote[5]
Meningococcal serogroup B vaccine (MenB-FHbp)	Trumenba (Pfizer)	10–25 y	0.5 mL	IM	0, 2, 6 mo[6]	None
Meningococcal serogroup B vaccine (MenB-4C)	Bexsero (GSK)	10–25 y	0.5 mL	IM	0, ≥1 mo	None

Abbreviations: IM, intramuscular; SC, subcutaneous.

[1] If an infant is receiving the vaccine before travel, 2 doses may be administered as early as 8 weeks apart.

[2] For people with HIV, anatomic or functional asplenia, and people with persistent complement component deficiencies (C3, C5-9, properdin, factor D, and factor H or people taking eculizumab [Soliris]) should receive a 2-dose primary series 8–12 weeks apart.

[3] Revaccination with meningococcal conjugate vaccine (MenACWY-D or MenACWY-CRM) is recommended after 3 years for children who received their last dose at <7 years of age. Revaccination with meningococcal conjugate vaccine is recommended after 5 years for people who received their last dose at ≥7 years of age, and every 5 years thereafter for people who are at continued risk.

[4] Infants and children who received HibMenCY-TT and are traveling to areas with high endemic rates of meningococcal disease such as the African meningitis belt are not protected against serogroups A and W and should receive a quadrivalent meningococcal vaccine before travel.

[5] If multiple doses are anticipated in people aged ≥56 years, such as those traveling or living to areas with hyperendemic or epidemic meningococcal disease, MenACWY vaccine should be used instead of MPSV4. Additionally, people who have previously received MenACWY vaccine before the age of 56 should receive boosters of MenACWY if they remain at risk.

[6] In April 2016, FDA approved updates to the prescribing information for MenB-FHbp to allow for the administration of either a 3-dose schedule (0, 1–2, 6 months) or a 2-dose schedule (0, 6 months). The 3-dose schedule is preferred for groups at increased risk where more rapid protection is desired.

8 weeks after the first dose before travel. For travelers initiating vaccination at ≥9 months, either MenACWY-CRM or MenACWY-D (Menactra) may be used. For travelers 9–23 months of age who receive MenACWY-D, 2 doses should be administered, with the second dose administered at ≥3 months after the first dose, although it can be administered as early as 8 weeks after the first dose before travel. Infants and children who received Hib-MenCY-TT (MenHibrix) are not protected against serogroups A and W and should receive a quadrivalent vaccine before travel.

For most people aged 2–55 years, 1 dose of a MenACWY vaccine (MenACWY-CRM or MenACWY-D) is recommended before travel. Additional dosing instructions for people with HIV, asplenia, or persistent complement component deficiencies are available in the 2013 ACIP Meningococcal Disease Recommendations (www.cdc.gov/mmwr/preview/mmwrhtml/rr6202a1.htm).

Because MenACWY vaccine is not licensed for use in adults aged ≥56 years, MPSV4 is recommended for people aged ≥56 years who have never previously been vaccinated with MenACWY. However, for people aged ≥56 years who were previously vaccinated with MenACWY or for whom multiple doses are anticipated, MenACWY is preferred. Additionally, in the event that MPSV4 is not available, MenACWY may be administered to any person aged ≥56 years.

Travelers to the Kingdom of Saudi Arabia (KSA) for Umrah or Hajj are required to provide documentation of quadrivalent vaccine at least 10 days and no more than 3 years before arrival for polysaccharide vaccine and no more than 8 years before arrival for conjugate vaccine (see www.moh.gov.sa/en/Hajj/Pages/HealthRegulations.aspx). ACIP recommendations for adult travelers are to receive a booster dose if it has been ≥5 years since the previous MenACWY dose. Current visa requirements should be confirmed with the KSA embassy. Although the KSA Ministry of Health currently advises against travel to Hajj for pregnant women or children, these groups should receive meningococcal vaccination according to licensed indications for their age if they travel.

International travelers at risk for meningococcal disease who were previously vaccinated with a quadrivalent vaccine should receive a booster dose: for children who received their last dose at <7 years of age, a booster dose of MenACWY should be administered after 3 years and repeated every 5 years thereafter if they live in or travel to a hyperendemic areas. For people who received their last dose at ≥7 years of age, a booster dose should be administered after 5 years and every 5 years thereafter if they live in or travel to a hyperendemic area.

A monovalent serogroup A meningococcal conjugate vaccine (MenAfriVac) has progressively been introduced into meningitis belt countries since 2010 through mass vaccination campaigns. This vaccine is not available in the United States for travelers and is not recommended instead of the quadrivalent vaccines (MenACWY or MPSV4) for travelers who will be living in meningitis belt countries as it does not protect against serogroups C, W, and Y.

MenB vaccine is not recommended for people who live in or travel to meningitis belt countries, as serogroup B disease is extremely rare in this region. MenB vaccine is not routinely recommended for travel to other regions of the world unless an outbreak of serogroup B disease has been reported. Although MenB vaccine is not licensed in the United States for children <10 years of age. Some European countries have recently introduced MenB vaccine as a routine immunization for infants. Infants who will be living in these countries may consider MenB vaccination according to the routine infant immunization recommendations of that country.

VACCINE SAFETY AND ADVERSE REACTIONS

Low-grade fevers and local reactions, such as injection site pain, arm swelling, and pain that limits movement of the injected arm, are side effects seen after both conjugate and polysaccharide quadrivalent meningococcal vaccines but occur more commonly after conjugate vaccine. Symptoms are generally mild to moderate and resolve within 48–72 hours. Severe adverse events, such as high fever, chills, joint pain, rash, or seizures are rare (<5% of vaccinees) with either type of vaccine.

Although no clinical trials of meningococcal vaccines have been conducted in pregnant or lactating women, postlicensure safety data have not identified any serious safety concerns to the mother or fetus. Pregnancy or lactation should not preclude vaccination with MenACWY or MPSV4 if indicated.

PRECAUTIONS AND CONTRAINDICATIONS

People with moderate or severe acute illness should defer vaccination until their condition improves. Vaccination is contraindicated for people who have a severe allergic reaction to any component of the vaccines. All meningococcal vaccines are inactivated and may be given to immunosuppressed people.

Antibiotic Chemoprophylaxis

In the United States and most industrialized countries, antibiotic chemoprophylaxis is recommended for close contacts of a patient with invasive meningococcal disease to prevent secondary cases. Chemoprophylaxis ideally should be initiated within 24 hours after the index patient is identified; prophylaxis given >2 weeks after exposure has little value. Antibiotics used for prophylaxis include ciprofloxacin, rifampin, and ceftriaxone. Ceftriaxone is recommended for pregnant women.

CDC website: www.cdc.gov/meningococcal

BIBLIOGRAPHY

1. American Academy of Pediatrics. Meningococcal infections. In: Kimberlin DW, Brady MT, Jackson M, Long SS, editors. Red Book: 2015 Report of the Committee on Infectious Diseases. 30th ed. Elk Grove Village, IL: American Academy of Pediatrics; 2015. pp. 547–58.

2. CDC. Prevention and control of meningococcal disease: recommendations of the Advisory Committee on Immunization Practices (ACIP). MMWR Morb Mortal Wkly Rep. 2013;62(2):1–28.

3. Folaranmi T, Rubin L, Martin SW, Patel M, MacNeil JR. Use of serogroup B meningococcal vaccines in persons aged >/=10 years at increased risk for serogroup B meningococcal disease: recommendations of the Advisory Committee on Immunization Practices, 2015. MMWR Morb Mortal Wkly Rep. 2015 Jun 12;64(22):608–12.

4. Greenwood B. Manson Lecture. Meningococcal meningitis in Africa. Trans R Soc Trop Med Hyg. 1999 Jul-Aug;93(4):341–53.

5. Halperin SA, Bettinger JA, Greenwood B, Harrison LH, Jelfs J, Ladhani SN, et al. The changing and dynamic epidemiology of meningococcal disease. Vaccine. 2012 May 30;30 Suppl 2:B26–36.

6. MacNeil JR, Rubin L, Folaranmi T, Ortega-Sanchez IR, Patel M, Martin SW. Use of serogroup B meningococcal vaccines in adolescents and young adults: recommendations of the Advisory Committee on Immunization Practices, 2015. MMWR Morb Mortal Wkly Rep. 2015 Oct 23;64(41):1171–6.

7. Rosenstein NE, Perkins BA, Stephens DS, Popovic T, Hughes JM. Meningococcal disease. N Engl J Med. 2001 May 3;344(18):1378–88.

8. Stephens DS, Greenwood B, Brandtzaeg P. Epidemic meningitis, meningococcaemia, and *Neisseria meningitidis.* Lancet. 2007 Jun 30;369(9580):2196–210.

9. Wilder-Smith A. Meningococcal disease: risk for international travellers and vaccine strategies. Travel Med Infect Dis. 2008 Jul;6(4):182–6.

10. World Health Organization. Meningitis control in countries of the African meningitis belt, 2015. Wkly Epidemiol Rec. 2016 Apr 22;91(16):209–16.

MIDDLE EAST RESPIRATORY SYNDROME (MERS)

John T. Watson, Susan I. Gerber

INFECTIOUS AGENT

The MERS coronavirus, a single-stranded, positive-sense RNA virus that belongs to the family Coronaviridae, genus *Betacoronavirus*.

TRANSMISSION

Transmission dynamics are not well understood. The MERS coronavirus is genetically similar to bat coronaviruses and has been detected in camels in North Africa and the Arabian Peninsula. Although exposure to dromedary camels is a risk factor for MERS, little is known about the specific exposures that result in primary human cases. Evidence suggests that MERS can be spread from person to person among close contacts, resulting in outbreaks in families and in health care settings. Sustained community transmission of MERS has not been shown.

EPIDEMIOLOGY

MERS coronavirus is an emerging novel coronavirus that causes severe acute respiratory illness, and approximately 40% of confirmed cases have been fatal. MERS was first reported in September 2012, but illnesses with onsets as early as April 2012 were subsequently documented. The risk is ongoing in the area of the Arabian Peninsula. Index cases have lived in or recently traveled to Iran, Jordan, Kuwait, Lebanon, Oman, Qatar, Saudi Arabia, United Arab Emirates, or Yemen. MERS has also been identified in travelers from these countries returning to North America, Europe, Asia, and North Africa.

CLINICAL PRESENTATION

MERS is associated with severe acute respiratory failure, multiple organ dysfunction, and high mortality, although the spectrum of illness and clinical course are not fully defined. Mild or asymptomatic cases have been documented among contacts of cases. For people who develop symptomatic illness, the incubation period is approximately 2–14 days; median incubation period is slightly more than 5 days. Disease is most often characterized by fever, cough, and shortness of breath. Other symptoms may include chills, sore throat, myalgia, arthralgia, diarrhea, and vomiting. Initial nonspecific symptoms can progress to pneumonia. Chest radiographs have shown variable pulmonary involvement.

In addition to acute and often severe respiratory compromise, serious complications of MERS include cardiovascular collapse and acute renal injury. Abnormal laboratory findings can include thrombocytopenia, lymphopenia, and elevated liver function tests. Older age and comorbidities are associated with poor outcomes.

DIAGNOSIS

Several diagnostic assays have been developed to detect acute infection with MERS coronavirus, including real-time RT-PCR. Lower respiratory specimens (sputum, bronchoalveolar lavage, endotracheal aspirates) are the priority respiratory specimens for testing, although upper and lower respiratory, stool, and serum specimens should also be collected if possible. To increase the likelihood of detecting the virus, multiple specimens from these sites should be collected over the course of the illness. In the United States, most state laboratories are approved to test for MERS by using CDC's RT-PCR assay. Testing should be coordinated through state and local health departments and CDC.

In coordination with state and local health departments, health care providers should evaluate patients for MERS if they develop fever and pneumonia or acute respiratory distress syndrome within 14 days after traveling from countries in or near the Arabian Peninsula or have had close contact with a recent traveler from this area who has fever and acute respiratory illness.

TREATMENT

No specific antiviral treatment is available. Treatment is limited to supportive care. Standard, contact, and airborne infection control precautions are recommended for hospitalized patients with known or suspected MERS.

PREVENTION

No vaccine or preventive drug is available. CDC recommends that travelers practice general hygiene precautions such as frequent handwashing; avoiding touching the eyes, nose, and mouth; and avoiding contact with sick people. The World Health Organization (WHO) considers certain groups to be at high risk for severe MERS, including people with diabetes, kidney failure, chronic lung disease, or immunocompromised people. WHO recommends that these groups take additional precautions: avoid contact with camels, do not drink raw camel milk or raw camel urine, and do not eat undercooked meat, particularly camel meat. For more information, see www.who.int/csr/disease/coronavirus_infections/faq/en.

CDC website: www.cdc.gov/coronavirus/mers

BIBLIOGRAPHY

1. Arabi YM, Arifi AA, Balkhy HH, Najm H, Aldawood AS, Ghabashi A, et al. Clinical course and outcomes of critically ill patients with Middle East respiratory syndrome coronavirus infection. Ann Intern Med. 2014 Mar 18;160(6):389–97.

2. CDC. Interim infection prevention and control recommendations for hospitalized patients with Middle East respiratory syndrome coronavirus (MERS-CoV). [updated 2015 June; cited 2016 Sep. 25]. Available from: http://www.cdc.gov/coronavirus/mers/infection-prevention-control.html.

3. Memish ZA, Zumla AI, Al-Hakeem RF, Al-Rabeeah AA, Stephens GM. Family cluster of Middle East respiratory syndrome coronavirus infections. N Engl J Med. 2013 Jun 27;368(26):2487–94.

4. Oboho IK, Tomczyk SM, Al-Asmari AM, Banjar AA, Al-Mugti H, Aloraini MS, et al. 2014 MERS-CoV outbreak in Jeddah—a link to health care facilities. N Engl J Med. 2015 Feb 26;372(9):846–54.

5. World Health Organization. Coronavirus infections. [cited 2016 Sep. 25]. Available from: http://www.who.int/csr/disease/coronavirus_infections/en/.

6. Zumla A, Hui DS, Perlman S. Middle East respiratory syndrome. Lancet. 2015 Sep 5;386(9997):995–1007.

MUMPS

Cristina V. Cardemil, Nakia S. Clemmons

INFECTIOUS AGENT

An enveloped, negative-strand RNA virus (a paramyxovirus) of the genus *Rubulavirus*.

TRANSMISSION

By respiratory droplets, saliva, or contact with contaminated fomites.

EPIDEMIOLOGY

Endemic in many countries throughout the world. In 2014, mumps-containing vaccine was routinely used in 121 countries worldwide. The risk of exposure among travelers is high in many countries, including industrialized countries.

CLINICAL PRESENTATION

Incubation period is 16–18 days (range, 12–25 days). Mumps is an acute systemic illness which classically presents with unilateral or bilateral swelling of the parotid glands. Onset of illness is usually nonspecific, with symptoms of fever, headache, malaise, myalgia, and anorexia; however, infections may be asymptomatic. Complications may occur such as orchitis, hearing loss, aseptic meningitis, encephalitis, and pancreatitis.

DIAGNOSIS

Usually clinical, defined as illness with acute onset of unilateral or bilateral tender, self-limited swelling of the parotid glands, other salivary glands, or both, lasting ≥2 days, and without other apparent cause. Laboratory confirmation of mumps involves detection of nucleic acid by RT-PCR or virus isolation by culture. For further information on laboratory testing, see www.cdc. gov/mumps/lab/index.html. Mumps is a nationally notifiable disease.

TREATMENT
Supportive care is the mainstay of treatment.

PREVENTION
Before departure from the United States, travelers aged ≥12 months who do not have acceptable evidence of mumps immunity (as documented by 2 doses of live mumps virus vaccine, laboratory evidence of immunity, laboratory confirmation of disease, or birth before 1957) should be vaccinated with 2 doses of measles-mumps-rubella (MMR) vaccine ≥28 days apart. There is no recommendation for vaccination against mumps for infants aged <12 months before international travel; however, infants aged 6–11 months should receive 1 dose of MMR vaccine before departure to protect against measles.

CDC website: www.cdc.gov/mumps

BIBLIOGRAPHY

1. CDC. Manual for the surveillance of vaccine-preventable diseases. Atlanta: CDC; 2012 [cited 2016 Sep. 25]. Available from: http://www.cdc.gov/vaccines/pubs/surv-manual/index.html.

2. CDC. Prevention of measles, rubella, congenital rubella syndrome, and mumps, 2013: summary recommendations of the Advisory Committee on Immunization Practices (ACIP). MMWR Recomm Rep. 2013 Jun 14;62(RR-04):1–34.

3. CDC. Update: mumps outbreak—New York and New Jersey, June 2009–January 2010. MMWR Morb Mortal Wkly Rep. 2010 Feb 12;59(5):125–9.

4. Dayan GH, Quinlisk MP, Parker AA, Barskey AE, Harris ML, Schwartz JM, et al. Recent resurgence of mumps in the United States. N Engl J Med. 2008 Apr 10;358(15):1580–9.

5. World Health Organization. Immunization, vaccines and biologicals: mumps. 2015 [updated 5 Aug 2015; cited 2016 Sep. 25]. Available from: http://www.who.int/immunization/monitoring_surveillance/burden/vpd/surveillance_type/passive/mumps/en/.

NOROVIRUS
Aron J. Hall, Ben Lopman

INFECTIOUS AGENT
Norovirus infection is caused by nonenveloped, single-stranded RNA viruses of the genus *Norovirus*, which have also been referred to as "Norwalk-like viruses," Norwalk viruses, and small round-structured viruses. Norovirus is a cause of viral gastroenteritis, sometimes referred to as "stomach flu"; however, there is no biologic association with influenza or influenza viruses.

TRANSMISSION
Transmission occurs primarily through the fecal-oral route, either through direct person-to-person contact or indirectly via contaminated food or water. Norovirus is also spread through aerosols of vomitus and contaminated environmental surfaces and objects.

EPIDEMIOLOGY
Norovirus infections are common throughout the world, and globally most children will have experienced ≥1 infection by the age of 5 years. Norovirus infections can occur year round, but in temperate climates, norovirus activity peaks during the winter. Noroviruses are common in both developing and developed countries. In the

United States, norovirus is the leading cause of medically attended gastroenteritis in young children and of outbreaks of gastroenteritis; it is estimated to cause 19–21 million illnesses a year and approximately 50% of all foodborne disease outbreaks.

Norovirus is a cause of travelers' diarrhea; prevalence ranges from 3% to 17% of travelers returning with diarrhea. However, coinfection and asymptomatic infection with norovirus are common, so focused studies are needed to determine exactly how frequently norovirus is the cause of disease. Risk for infection is present anywhere food is prepared in an unsanitary manner and may become contaminated, or where drinking water is inadequately treated. Of particular risk are "ready-to-eat" cold foods, such as sandwiches and salads. Raw shellfish, especially oysters, are also a frequent source of infection, because virus from contaminated water concentrates in the gut of these filter feeders. Contaminated ice has also been implicated in outbreaks.

Norovirus outbreaks frequently occur in settings where people live in close quarters and can easily infect each other, such as hotels, cruise ships, camps, dormitories, and hospitals. Viral contamination of inanimate objects or environmental surfaces (fomites) may persist during and after outbreaks and be a source of infection. On cruise ships, for instance, such environmental contamination has caused recurrent norovirus outbreaks on successive cruises with newly boarded passengers. Transmission of norovirus on airplanes has been reported during both domestic and international flights and likely results from contamination of lavatories or from symptomatic passengers in the cabin.

CLINICAL PRESENTATION

Infected people usually have an acute onset of vomiting with nonbloody diarrhea. The incubation period is 12–48 hours. Other symptoms include abdominal cramps, nausea, and sometimes a low-grade fever. Illness is generally self-limited, and full recovery can be expected in 1–3 days for most patients. In some cases, dehydration, especially in patients who are very young or elderly, may require medical attention.

DIAGNOSIS

Norovirus infection is generally diagnosed based on symptoms. Norovirus diagnostic testing is not widely available to guide clinical management of individual patients, but laboratory testing is used during outbreak investigations by public health agencies. Norovirus diagnostic testing is usually not available in developing countries.

The most common diagnostic test used at state public health laboratories and CDC is RT-PCR, which rapidly and reliably detects the virus in stool specimens. Several commercial EIAs are also available to detect the virus in stool specimens. The specificity and sensitivity of these assays are poor compared with RT-PCR.

TREATMENT

Supportive care is the mainstay of treatment of norovirus disease, especially oral or intravenous rehydration. Antimotility agents should be avoided in children aged <3 years but may be a useful adjunct to rehydration in older children and adults. Antiemetic agents should generally be reserved for adults. Antibiotics are not useful in treating patients with norovirus disease.

PREVENTION

No vaccine is currently available, although vaccine development efforts are advancing. Noroviruses are common and highly contagious, but the risk for infection can be minimized by frequent and proper handwashing and avoiding possibly contaminated food and water. Washing hands with soap and water for at least 20 seconds is considered the most effective way to reduce norovirus contamination; alcohol-based hand sanitizers might be useful between handwashings but should not be considered a substitute for soap and water.

In addition to handwashing, measures to prevent transmission of noroviruses between people traveling together include carefully cleaning up fecal material or vomit and disinfecting contaminated surfaces and toilet areas. Products should be approved by the Environmental Protection Agency for norovirus disinfection; alternatively,

3

a solution of domestic bleach (5–25 tablespoons bleach per gallon of water) may be used. Soiled articles of clothing should be washed at the maximum available cycle length and machine-dried at high heat.

To help prevent the spread of noroviruses, ill people may be isolated on cruise ships and in institutional settings.

CDC website: www.cdc.gov/norovirus

BIBLIOGRAPHY

1. Ajami NJ, Kavanagh OV, Ramani S, Crawford SE, Atmar RL, Jiang ZD, et al. Seroepidemiology of norovirus-associated travelers' diarrhea. J Travel Med. 2014 Jan-Feb;21(1):6–11.

2. Aliabadi N, Lopman BA, Parashar UD, Hall AJ. Progress toward norovirus vaccines: considerations for further development and implementation in potential target populations. Expert Rev Vaccines. 2015;14(9):1241–53.

3. Apelt N, Hartberger C, Campe H, Loscher T. The prevalence of norovirus in returning international travelers with diarrhea. BMC Infect Dis. 2010;10:131.

4. Atmar RL, Bernstein DI, Harro CD, Al-Ibrahim MS, Chen WH, Ferreira J, et al. Norovirus vaccine against experimental human Norwalk virus illness. N Engl J Med. 2011 Dec 8;365(23):2178–87.

5. Hall AJ, Eisenbart VG, Etingue AL, Gould LH, Lopman BA, Parashar UD. Epidemiology of foodborne norovirus outbreaks, United States, 2001–2008. Emerg Infect Dis. 2012 Oct;18(10):1566–73.

6. Hall AJ, Lopman BA, Payne DC, Patel MM, Gastanaduy PA, Vinje J, et al. Norovirus disease in the United States. Emerg Infect Dis. 2013 Aug;19(8):1198–205.

7. Hall AJ, Vinjé J, Lopman B, Park GW, Yen C, Gregoricus N, et al. Updated norovirus outbreak management and disease prevention guidelines. MMWR Recomm Rep. 2011 Mar 4;60(RR-3):1–18.

8. Koo HL, Ajami NJ, Jiang ZD, Neill FH, Atmar RL, Ericsson CD, et al. Noroviruses as a cause of diarrhea in travelers to Guatemala, India, and Mexico. J Clin Microbiol. 2010 May;48(5):1673–6.

9. Patel MM, Widdowson MA, Glass RI, Akazawa K, Vinje J, Parashar UD. Systematic literature review of role of noroviruses in sporadic gastroenteritis. Emerg Infect Dis. 2008 Aug;14(8):1224–31.

10. Thornley CN, Emslie NA, Sprott TW, Greening GE, Rapana JP. Recurring norovirus transmission on an airplane. Clin Infect Dis. 2011 Sep;53(6):515–20.

ONCHOCERCIASIS (RIVER BLINDNESS)

Paul T. Cantey

INFECTIOUS AGENT

Onchocerca volvulus, a filarial nematode.

TRANSMISSION

Through female blackflies (genus *Simulium*), which typically bite during the day and breed near rapidly flowing rivers and streams.

EPIDEMIOLOGY

Endemic in much of sub-Saharan Africa. Small endemic foci are also present in the Arabian Peninsula (Yemen) and in the Americas (Brazil and Venezuela). Foci center around blackfly breeding sites, which are located near rapidly flowing water. Most infections, outside those in endemic populations, occur in expatriate groups, such as missionaries, field scientists, and Peace Corps volunteers, though infection may sometimes occur in short-term travelers (<31 days).

CLINICAL PRESENTATION

Highly pruritic, papular dermatitis; subcutaneous nodules; lymphadenitis; and ocular lesions, which can progress to visual loss and blindness. Symptoms begin after patent infections are established, which may take 18 months. Symptoms in travelers are primarily dermatologic (rash and pruritus) and may occur years after departure from endemic areas. Nodules are more common in endemic populations.

DIAGNOSIS

Presence of microfilariae in superficial skin shavings or punch biopsy, adult worms in histologic sections of excised nodules, or characteristic eye lesions. Serologic testing is most useful for detecting infection when microfilariae are not identifiable. Determination of serum antifilarial antibody is available through the National Institutes of Health (301-496-5398) or CDC (www.cdc.gov/dpdx; 404-718-4745; parasites @cdc.gov).

TREATMENT

Ivermectin is the drug of choice. Repeated annual or semiannual doses may be required to control symptoms, as the drug kills the microfilariae but not the adult worms. Some experts recommend treating patients with 1 dose of ivermectin followed by 6 weeks of doxycycline to kill *Wolbachia*, an endosymbiotic rickettsialike bacterium that appears to be required for the survival of the *O. volvulus* adult worm and for embryogenesis. Diethylcarbamazine is contraindicated in onchocerciasis, because it has been associated with severe and fatal posttreatment reactions. An expert in tropical medicine should be consulted to help manage these patients.

PREVENTION

Avoid blackfly habitats (fast-flowing rivers and streams) and use protection measures against biting insects (see Chapter 2, Protection against Mosquitoes, Ticks, & Other Arthropods).

CDC website: www.cdc.gov/parasites/onchocerciasis

BIBLIOGRAPHY

1. Hoerauf A. Filariasis: new drugs and new opportunities for lymphatic filariasis and onchocerciasis. Curr Opin Infect Dis. 2008 Dec;21(6):673–81.

2. Klion AD. Filarial infections in travelers and immigrants. Curr Infect Dis Rep. 2008 Mar;10(1):50–7.

3. Lipner EM, Law MA, Barnett E, Keystone JS, von Sonnenburg F, Loutan L, et al. Filariasis in travelers presenting to the GeoSentinel Surveillance Network. PLoS Negl Trop Dis. 2007;1(3):e88.

4. McCarthy JS, Ottesen EA, Nutman TB. Onchocerciasis in endemic and nonendemic populations: differences in clinical presentation and immunologic findings. J Infect Dis. 1994 Sep;170(3):736–41.

5. Tielsch JM, Beeche A. Impact of ivermectin on illness and disability associated with onchocerciasis. Trop Med Int Health. 2004 Apr;9(4):A45–56.

6. WHO Expert Committee. Onchocerciasis and its control. Report of a WHO Expert Committee on Onchocerciasis Control. World Health Organ Tech Rep Ser. 1995;852:1–104.

PERTUSSIS

Tami H. Skoff, Jennifer L. Liang

INFECTIOUS AGENT

Fastidious gram-negative coccobacillus *Bordetella pertussis*.

TRANSMISSION

Person-to-person transmission via aerosolized respiratory droplets or by direct contact with respiratory secretions.

EPIDEMIOLOGY

Pertussis is endemic worldwide, even in areas with high vaccination rates. In recent years, pertussis has resurged in a number of countries with successful vaccination programs, especially countries that have transitioned from whole-cell pertussis vaccine formulations to acellular pertussis preparations, including the United States. In 2012,

>48,000 cases of pertussis were reported nationally, the largest number in the United States since 1955. Disease rates are highest among young children in countries where vaccination coverage is low, which is primarily in the developing world. In developed countries, the reported incidence of pertussis is highest among infants too young to be vaccinated.

Immunity from childhood vaccination and natural disease wanes with time; therefore, adolescents and adults who have not received a tetanus-diphtheria-pertussis (Tdap) booster vaccination can become infected or reinfected. US travelers are not at increased risk for disease specifically because of international travel, but they are at risk if they come in close contact with infected people. Infants, especially those who are too young to be protected by a complete vaccination series, are at highest risk for severe illness and death from pertussis.

CLINICAL PRESENTATION

In classic disease, mild upper respiratory tract symptoms begin 7–10 days (range, 6–21 days) after exposure, followed by a cough that becomes paroxysmal. Coughing paroxysms can vary in frequency and are often followed by vomiting. Fever is absent or minimal. The clinical case definition for pertussis includes cough for ≥2 weeks with paroxysms, whoop, or posttussive vomiting.

Disease in infants aged <6 months can be atypical, with a short catarrhal stage, gagging, gasping, or apnea as early manifestations. Among infants aged <2 months, the case-fatality ratio is approximately 1%. Recently immunized children who develop disease may have mild cough illness; older children and adults may have prolonged cough with or without paroxysms. The cough gradually wanes over several weeks to months.

DIAGNOSIS

Factors such as prior vaccination status, stage of disease, antibiotic use, specimen collection and transport conditions, and use of nonstandardized tests may affect the sensitivity, specificity, and interpretation of available diagnostic tests for *B. pertussis*. CDC guidelines for the laboratory confirmation of pertussis cases include culture and PCR (when the above clinical case definition

is met); serology and direct fluorescent antibody tests are not confirmatory tests included in the current case definition for reporting purposes. Pertussis is a nationally notifiable disease.

TREATMENT

Macrolide antibiotics (azithromycin, clarithromycin, and erythromycin) are recommended to treat pertussis in people aged ≥1 month; for infants aged <1 month, azithromycin is the preferred antibiotic. Antimicrobial therapy with a macrolide antibiotic administered <3 weeks after cough onset can limit transmission to others. Postexposure prophylaxis is recommended for all household contacts of cases and for people at high risk of developing severe disease (such as infants and women in the third trimester of pregnancy) or those who will have contact with a person at high risk of severe illness. The recommended agents and dosing regimens for prophylaxis are the same as for the treatment of pertussis.

PREVENTION

Vaccine

Travelers should be up-to-date with pertussis vaccinations before departure. Multiple pertussis vaccines are available in the United States for infants and children, and 2 vaccines are available for adolescents and adults. A complete listing of licensed vaccines can be found at www.fda.gov/BiologicsBloodVaccines/Vaccines/ApprovedProducts/ucm093833.htm.

INFANTS AND CHILDREN

In the United States, all infants and children should receive 5 doses of acellular pertussis vaccine in combination with diphtheria and tetanus toxoids (DTaP) at ages 2, 4, 6, and 15–18 months and 4–6 years. An accelerated schedule of doses may be used to complete the DTaP series.

Children aged 7–10 years who are not fully vaccinated against pertussis and for whom no contraindication to pertussis vaccine exists should receive a single dose of tetanus toxoid, reduced diphtheria toxoid, and acellular pertussis vaccine (Tdap) to provide protection against pertussis. If additional doses of tetanus and diphtheria toxoid-containing vaccines are needed, then they should be vaccinated according to catch-up guidance, with Tdap preferred as the first dose (www.cdc.gov/vaccines/schedules/hcp/imz/catchup.html).

ADOLESCENTS AND ADULTS

Adolescents aged 11–18 years who have completed the recommended childhood DTwP/DTaP vaccination series and who have not previously received Tdap and adults aged ≥19 years who have not previously received Tdap should receive a single dose of Tdap instead of tetanus and diphtheria toxoids (Td) vaccine for booster immunization against tetanus, diphtheria, and pertussis. To provide pertussis protection before travel, Tdap can be given regardless of the interval from the last Td, except to people for whom pertussis vaccination is contraindicated or for people who have previously received Tdap. Adolescents and adults who have never been immunized against pertussis, tetanus, or diphtheria; who have incomplete immunization; or whose immunity is uncertain should follow the catch-up schedule established for Td/Tdap.

PREGNANT WOMEN

Women should have a dose of Tdap during *each* pregnancy, irrespective of her history of receiving Tdap. Although Tdap may be given at any time during pregnancy, to maximize the maternal antibody response and passive antibody transfer to the infant, optimal timing for Tdap administration is at 27–36 weeks' gestation.

CDC website: www.cdc.gov/pertussis

BIBLIOGRAPHY

1. Acosta AM, DeBolt C, Tasslimi A, Lewis M, Stewart LK, Misegades LK, et al. Tdap vaccine effectiveness in adolescents during the 2012 Washington State pertussis epidemic. Pediatrics. 2015 Jun;135(6):981–9.

2. American Academy of Pediatrics. Pertussis (whooping cough). In: Pickering LK, editor. Red Book: 2012 Report of the Committee on Infectious Diseases. 29th ed. Elk Grove Village, IL: American Academy of Pediatrics; 2012. pp. 553–66.

3. Broder KR, Cortese MM, Iskander JK, Kretsinger K, Slade BA, Brown KH, et al. Preventing tetanus, diphtheria, and pertussis among adolescents: use of tetanus toxoid, reduced diphtheria toxoid and acellular pertussis vaccines. Recommendations of the Advisory Committee on Immunization Practices (ACIP). MMWR Recomm Rep. 2006 Dec 15;55(RR-17):1–33.

4. CDC. Pertussis (whooping cough) postexposure antimicrobial prophylaxis. [cited 2016 Sep. 25]. Available from: http://www.cdc.gov/pertussis/outbreaks/pep.html.

5. CDC. Updated recommendations for use of tetanus toxoid, reduced diphtheria toxoid and acellular pertussis (Tdap) vaccine from the Advisory Committee on Immunization Practices, 2010. MMWR Morb Mortal Wkly Rep. 2011 Jan 14;60(1):13–5.

6. CDC. Updated recommendations for use of tetanus toxoid, reduced diphtheria toxoid, and acellular pertussis vaccine (Tdap) in pregnant women--Advisory Committee on Immunization Practices (ACIP), 2012. MMWR Morb Mortal Wkly Rep. 2013;62(7):131–5.

7. Edwards KM, Decker MD. Pertussis vaccines. In: Plotkin SA, Orenstein WA, Offit PA, editors. Vaccines. 6th ed. Philadelphia: Saunders Elsevier; 2012. p. 447–92.

8. Misegades LK, Winter K, Harriman K, Talarico J, Messonnier NE, Clark TA, et al. Association of childhood pertussis with receipt of 5 doses of pertussis vaccine by time since last vaccine dose, California, 2010. Jama. 2012 Nov 28;308(20):2126–32.

9. Tan T, Dalby T, Forsyth K, Halperin SA, Heininger U, Hozbor D, et al. Pertussis across the globe: recent epidemiologic trends from 2000 to 2013. Pediatr Infect Dis J. 2015 Sep;34(9):e222–32.

10. Tiwari T, Murphy TV, Moran J. Recommended antimicrobial agents for the treatment and postexposure prophylaxis of pertussis: 2005 CDC Guidelines. MMWR Recomm Rep. 2005 Dec 9;54(RR-14):1–16.

3

PINWORM (ENTEROBIASIS, OXYURIASIS, THREADWORM)

Christine Dubray

INFECTIOUS AGENT

The intestinal nematode (roundworm) *Enterobius vermicularis*.

TRANSMISSION

Egg transmission occurs by the fecal-oral route, either directly or indirectly via contaminated hands or objects such as clothes, toys, and bedding.

EPIDEMIOLOGY

Pinworm is endemic worldwide and commonly clusters within families. Those most likely to be infected with pinworm are school-age children, people who take care of infected children, and people who are institutionalized. Travelers are at risk if staying in crowded conditions with infected people.

CLINICAL PRESENTATION

Incubation period is usually 1–2 months, but successive reinfections may be needed before symptoms appear. The most common symptom is an itchy anal region, which can disturb sleep. Adult worms can migrate from the anal area to other sites, including the vulva, vagina, and urethra. Secondary bacterial infection can occur from skin irritation.

DIAGNOSIS

The first option is to look for adult worms near the anus 2–3 hours after the infected person is asleep. The second option is microscopic identification of worm eggs collected by touching transparent tape to the anal area when the person first awakens in the morning. This method should be conducted on 3 consecutive mornings and before washing.

The third option is microscopic examination of samples taken from under fingernails; samples should be taken before handwashing. Examining stool samples is not recommended because pinworm eggs are sparse.

TREATMENT

Drugs of choice are mebendazole, albendazole, or pyrantel pamoate (which is available without prescription). Mebendazole is available in the United States only through compounding pharmacies. Each is given as a single dose and repeated in 2 weeks. In households where >1 member is infected or where repeated, symptomatic infections occur, all household members should be treated at the same time. For children younger than 2 years of age, in whom experience with these drugs is limited, risks and benefits should be considered by a physician before drug administration. Infected people should also bathe in the morning and change underwear and bedclothes frequently. Infected people should also practice personal hygiene measures such as washing hands before eating or preparing food, keeping fingernails short, not scratching the perianal region, and not biting nails.

PREVENTION

Hand hygiene is the most effective method of prevention. Bed linen and underclothing of infected children should be changed first thing in the morning. They should not be shaken (to avoid contaminating the environment), and should be laundered promptly in hot water and followed by a hot dryer to kill any eggs that may be there.

CDC website: www.cdc.gov/parasites/pinworm

BIBLIOGRAPHY

1. American Academy of Pediatrics. Pinworm infection (*Enterobius vermicularis*). In: Kimberlin DW, editor. Red Book: 2015 Report of the Committee on Infectious Diseases. 30h ed. Elk Grove Village, IL: American Academy of Pediatrics; 2015. pp. 621–2.

2. American Public Health Association. Enterobiasis. In: Heyman DL, editor. Control of Communicable Diseases Manual. 19th ed. Washington, DC: American Public Health Association; 2008. pp. 223–5.

3. Kucik CJ, Martin GL, Sortor BV. Common intestinal parasites. Am Fam Physician. 2004 Mar 1;69(5):1161–8.

3 | PLAGUE (BUBONIC, PNEUMONIC, SEPTICEMIC)

Paul S. Mead

INFECTIOUS AGENT

The gram-negative bacterium *Yersinia pestis*.

TRANSMISSION

Usually through the bite of infected rodent fleas. Less common exposures include handling infected animal tissues (hunters, wildlife personnel), inhalation of infectious droplets from cats or dogs with plague, and, rarely, contact with a pneumonic plague patient.

EPIDEMIOLOGY

Endemic in rural areas in central and southern Africa (especially eastern Democratic Republic of Congo, northwestern Uganda, and Madagascar), central Asia and the Indian subcontinent, the northeastern part of South America, and parts of the southwestern United States. Overall risk to travelers is low.

CLINICAL PRESENTATION

Incubation period is typically 1–6 days. Symptoms and signs of the 3 clinical presentations of plague illness are as follows:

- Bubonic (most common)—rapid onset of fever; painful, swollen, and tender lymph nodes, usually inguinal, axillary, or cervical

- Pneumonic—high fever, overwhelming pneumonia, cough, bloody sputum, chills

- Septicemic—fever, prostration, hemorrhagic or thrombotic phenomena, progressing to acral gangrene

DIAGNOSIS

Y. pestis can be isolated from bubo aspirates, blood cultures, or sputum culture if pneumonic. Diagnosis can be confirmed in public health laboratories by culture or serologic tests for the *Y. pestis* F1 antigen. Plague is a nationally notifiable disease.

TREATMENT

Parenteral antibiotic therapy with streptomycin or gentamicin appears to be equally effective. Levofloxacin and ciprofloxacin have been approved by the Food and Drug Administration for treatment based on animal studies. Second-line agents include doxycycline, tetracycline, and chloramphenicol.

PREVENTION

Reduce contact with fleas and potentially infected rodents and other wildlife. No plague vaccine is available for commercial use in the United States.

CDC website: www.cdc.gov/plague

BIBLIOGRAPHY

1. Neerinckx S, Bertherat E, Leirs H. Human plague occurrences in Africa: an overview from 1877 to 2008. Trans R Soc Trop Med Hyg. 2010 Feb;104(2):97–103.

2. Perry RD, Fetherston JD. *Yersinia pestis*--etiologic agent of plague. Clin Microbiol Rev. 1997 Jan;10(1):35–66.

3. World Health Organization. Human plague: review of regional morbidity and mortality, 2004–2009. Wkly Epidemiol Rec. 2009 Feb 5;85(6):40–5.

PNEUMOCOCCAL DISEASE

Fernanda C. Lessa

3

INFECTIOUS AGENT

The gram-positive coccus *Streptococcus pneumoniae*.

TRANSMISSION

Person to person through close contact via respiratory droplets.

EPIDEMIOLOGY

Streptococcus pneumoniae is the most common bacterial cause of community-acquired pneumonia worldwide. Disease incidence is higher in developing than in industrialized countries. Risk is highest in young children, the elderly, and those with chronic illnesses or immune suppression.

CLINICAL PRESENTATION

The major clinical syndromes of pneumococcal disease are pneumonia, bacteremia, and meningitis. Pneumococcal pneumonia classically presents with sudden onset of fever and malaise, pleuritic chest pain, cough with purulent or blood-tinged sputum, or dyspnea. In the elderly, fever, shortness of breath, or altered mental status may be the initial symptoms. Pneumococcal meningitis is less common than pneumonia, and symptoms may include headache, lethargy, vomiting, irritability, fever, stiff neck, and seizures. People with cochlear implants are at increased risk of pneumococcal meningitis.

DIAGNOSIS

Isolation of *S. pneumoniae* from blood or other normally sterile body sites such as pleural fluid or cerebral spinal fluid (CSF). Tests are also available to detect pneumococcal antigen in body fluids.

A urinary antigen test for *S. pneumoniae* is commercially available, simple to use, and has reasonable specificity to detect pneumococcal pneumonia in adults, making it a useful addition for diagnostic evaluation. Pneumococcal pneumonia may be suspected if a sputum specimen contains gram-positive diplococci, polymorphonuclear leukocytes, and few epithelial cells. Gram-positive diplococci on staining of CSF may indicate pneumococcal meningitis. High white blood cell counts should raise suspicion for bacterial infection.

TREATMENT

Therapy depends on the syndrome, but patients who present with community-acquired pneumonia should be empirically treated for pneumococcal infection. Pneumococcal bacteria are resistant to ≥1 antibiotic in 30% of severe cases, although level and type of resistance varies among locations.

For pneumonia, current clinical practice guidelines recommend amoxicillin for children (http://pediatrics.aappublications.org/content/128/6/e1677) and macrolides (such as azithromycin) or doxycline for adults (www.idsociety.org/IDSA_Practice_Guidelines) in outpatient settings. In patients requiring hospitalization, the initial treatment might include a broad-spectrum cephalosporin and often vancomycin until antibiotic susceptibility results are available.

Patients with presumptive pneumococcal meningitis by CSF staining should be treated with a broad-spectrum cephalosporin plus vancomycin until susceptibility results are available.

PREVENTION

The 13-valent pneumococcal conjugate vaccine (PCV13) provides protection against the 13 serotypes responsible for most severe illness. PCV13 has been part of the US infant immunization schedule since 2010 and is also recommended for all adults aged ≥65 years and some adults aged 19–64 with immunocompromising conditions. A 23-valent pneumococcal polysaccharide vaccine (PPSV23) is recommended for all adults aged ≥65 years and people aged 2–64 years with underlying medical conditions. The intervals between PCV13 and PPSV23 given in series differ by age and risk group (see www.cdc.gov/vaccines/hcp/acip-recs/vacc-specific/pneumo.html). PCV13 and PPSV23 should not be coadministered. Adults aged ≥65 years who are immunocompetent should receive PPSV23 ≥1 year after PCV13, while those with immunocompromising conditions should receive PPSV23 ≥8 weeks after PCV13.

CDC website: www.cdc.gov/pneumococcal/index.html

BIBLIOGRAPHY

1. CDC. Intervals between PCV13 and PPSV23 vaccines: recommendations of the Advisory Committee on Immunization Practices (ACIP). MMWR Morb Mortal Wkly Rep. 2015 Sep 4;64(34):944–7.

2. CDC. Licensure of a 13-valent pneumococcal conjugate vaccine (PCV13) and recommendations for use among children--Advisory Committee on Immunization Practices (ACIP), 2010. MMWR Morb Mortal Wkly Rep. 2010 Mar 12;59(9):258–61.

3. CDC. Use of 13-valent pneumococcal conjugate vaccine and 23-valent pneumococcal polysaccharide vaccine among adults aged >/=65 years: recommendations of the Advisory Committee on Immunization Practices (ACIP). MMWR Morb Mortal Wkly Rep. 2014 Sep 19;63(37):822–5.

4. CDC. Use of 13-valent pneumococcal conjugate vaccine and 23-valent pneumococcal polysaccharide vaccine among children aged 6-18 years with immunocompromising conditions: recommendations of the Advisory Committee on Immunization Practices (ACIP). MMWR Morb Mortal Wkly Rep. 2013 June 28, 2013;62(25):521–4.

5. Rudan I, O'Brien KL, Nair H, Liu L, Theodoratou E, Qazi S, et al. Epidemiology and etiology of childhood pneumonia in 2010: estimates of incidence, severe morbidity, mortality, underlying risk factors and causative pathogens for 192 countries. J Glob Health. 2013 Jun;3(1):010401.

POLIOMYELITIS

James P. Alexander, Manisha Patel, Steven G. F. Wassilak

INFECTIOUS AGENT

Poliovirus (genus *Enterovirus*) types 1, 2, and 3. Polioviruses are small (27–30 nm), nonenveloped viruses with capsids enclosing a single-stranded, positive-sense RNA genome about 7,500 nucleotides long. Most of the properties of polioviruses are shared with the other enteroviruses.

TRANSMISSION

Fecal-oral or oral transmission. Acute infection involves the oropharynx, gastrointestinal tract, and occasionally the central nervous system.

EPIDEMIOLOGY

Before a vaccine was available, infection with poliovirus was common worldwide, with seasonal peaks and epidemics in the summer and fall in temperate areas. The incidence of poliomyelitis in the United States declined rapidly after the licensure of inactivated polio vaccine (IPV) in 1955 and live oral polio vaccine (OPV) in the 1960s. The last cases of indigenously acquired polio in the United States occurred in 1979. The Global Polio Eradication Initiative (GPEI) subsequently eliminated polio in the Americas, where the last wild poliovirus (WPV)–associated polio case was detected in 1991. In January 2000, a change in vaccination policy in the United States from use of live OPV to exclusive use of IPV eliminated the 8–10 vaccine-associated paralytic poliomyelitis (VAPP) cases that had occurred annually since the introduction of OPV in the 1960s.

GPEI has built upon the success in the Americas and made great progress in eradicating WPVs, reducing the number of reported polio cases worldwide by more than 99% since the mid-1980s. As of April 2016, WPV circulation has never been interrupted in only 2 countries: Afghanistan and Pakistan. Because of polio eradication efforts, the number of countries where travelers are at risk for polio has decreased dramatically. The last documented case of WPV-associated paralysis in a US resident traveling abroad occurred in 1986 in a 29-year-old vaccinated adult who had been traveling in South and Southeast Asia. In 2005, an unvaccinated US adult traveling abroad acquired VAPP after contact with an infant recently vaccinated with OPV.

In spite of progress made in eradicating WPVs globally, polio-free countries remain at risk for imported WPV cases and outbreaks, and travelers to some countries are at risk for exposure to WPV. During 2003–2013, northern Nigeria served as a reservoir for the spread of WPV into 26 previously polio-free countries, many of which were part of a "WPV importation belt" extending across sub-Saharan Africa from the west coast to the Horn of Africa in the east. With the intensification of polio eradication activities in Nigeria and neighboring countries during 2012–2014, outbreaks were controlled and endemic transmission in Nigeria was interrupted. From 2012 through early 2014, imported WPV from Pakistan was found in some sewage samples taken in Egypt, Israel, and the West Bank and Gaza (without any identified polio cases) and caused outbreaks in Iraq and Syria—all of which were controlled by July 2015. In addition to these risks, travelers are also at risk for contracting polio from cases and outbreaks of vaccine-derived poliovirus (VDPV), which can develop and circulate in areas with low vaccination coverage where OPV is used.

For additional information on the status of polio eradication efforts, countries or areas with active WPV or VDPV circulation, and vaccine recommendations, consult the travel notices on the CDC Travelers' Health website (www.cdc.gov/travel) or the GPEI website (www.polioeradication.org).

CLINICAL PRESENTATION

Clinical manifestations of poliovirus infection range from asymptomatic (most infections) to symptomatic, including acute flaccid paralysis of a single limb to quadriplegia, respiratory failure, and rarely, death.

DIAGNOSIS

The diagnosis is made by identifying poliovirus in clinical specimens (usually stool) obtained from an acutely ill patient. Poliovirus may be detected by cell culture followed by identification using plaque reduction neutralization tests or PCR. Poliovirus may also be identified by direct nucleic acid amplification from stool specimens followed by genomic sequencing to confirm the genotype and determine the likely geographic origin. Shedding in fecal specimens can be intermittent, but usually poliovirus can be detected for up to 4 weeks after onset of illness. During the first 3–10 days of the illness, poliovirus can also be detected from oropharyngeal specimens. Poliovirus is rarely detected in the blood or cerebrospinal fluid. Polio is a nationally notifiable disease.

TREATMENT

Only treatment for symptoms is available, ranging from pain and fever relief to intubation and mechanical ventilation for patients with respiratory insufficiency.

PREVENTION

Vaccine

RECOMMENDATIONS FOR HEALTH PROTECTION

In the United States, infants and children should be vaccinated against polio as part of a routine immunization series (see Infants and Children below). Polio vaccination is recommended for all travelers to countries with WPV or VDPV circulation. Countries are considered to have WPV or VDPV circulation if they have evidence during the previous 12 months of ongoing endemic circulation (WPV only), a polio outbreak, or environmental evidence (through sewage sampling) of WPV or VDPV circulation. For additional information on countries with WPV or VDPV circulation and vaccine recommendations, consult the travel notices on the CDC Travelers' Health website (www.cdc.gov/travel) or the weekly update of reported WPV and VDPV cases at the GPEI website (www.polioeradication.org/Dataandmonitoring/Poliothisweek.aspx).

Before traveling to areas that have WPV or VDPV circulation, travelers should ensure that they have completed the recommended age-appropriate polio vaccine series and that adults have received a single lifetime IPV booster dose. In addition, CDC recommends a single lifetime IPV booster dose for certain adult travelers to some countries that border areas with WPV circulation. These recommendations are based on evidence of historical cross-border transmission. These recommendations apply only to travelers with a high risk of exposure to someone with imported WPV infection. These travelers would include those working in health care settings, refugee camps, or other humanitarian aid settings. Since the situation is dynamic, refer to the CDC Travelers' Health website destination pages for the most up-to-date polio vaccine recommendations (wwwnc.cdc. gov/travel/destinations/list).

To eliminate the risk for VAPP, IPV has been the only polio vaccine available in the United States since 2000; however, OPV continues to be used in many countries and for global polio eradication activities. For complete information on recommendations for poliomyelitis vaccination, consult the Advisory Committee on Immunization Practices recommendations website (www.cdc. gov/vaccines/hcp/acip-recs/vacc-specific/polio. html) and the World Health Organization position paper on poliovirus vaccines (www.who.int/wer/2016/wer9112/en).

COUNTRY REQUIREMENTS

In May 2014, the World Health Organization (WHO) declared the international spread of polio to be a public health emergency of international concern under the authority of the International Health Regulations (2005). To prevent further spread of disease, WHO issued temporary polio vaccine recommendations for long-term travelers (staying >4 weeks) and residents departing from countries with WPV transmission ("exporting WPV" or "infected with WPV"). In November 2015, these recommendations were extended to long-term travelers (staying >4 weeks) and

residents departing from countries with VDPV transmission ("infected with VDPV"). Clinicians should be aware that long-term travelers and residents may be required to show proof of polio vaccination when departing from these countries. All polio vaccination administration should be documented on an International Certificate of Vaccination or Prophylaxis (ICVP). The polio vaccine must be received between 4 weeks and 12 months before the date of departure from the polio-affected country. Country requirements may change, so clinicians should check for updates on the CDC Travelers' Health website. Refer to the Clinical Update: Interim CDC Guidance for Travel to and from Countries Affected by the New Polio Vaccine Requirements (wwwnc.cdc.gov/travel/news-announcements/polio-guidance-new-requirements) for a list of affected countries, guidance on meeting the vaccination requirements, and instructions on how to order and fill out the ICVP.

INFANTS AND CHILDREN

In the United States, all infants and children should receive 4 doses of IPV at ages 2, 4, and 6–18 months and 4–6 years. The final dose should be administered at age ≥4 years, regardless of the number of previous doses, and should be given ≥6 months after the previous dose. A fourth dose in the routine IPV series is not necessary if the third dose was administered at age ≥4 years and ≥6 months after the previous dose. If the routine series cannot be administered within the recommended intervals before protection is needed, the following alternatives are recommended:

- The first dose should be given to infants at age ≥6 weeks.

- The second and third doses should be administered ≥4 weeks after the previous doses.

- The minimum interval between the third and fourth doses is 6 months.

If the age-appropriate series is not completed before departure, the remaining IPV doses to complete a full series should be administered when feasible, at the intervals recommended above.

ADULTS

Adults who are traveling to areas where WPV or VDPV is actively circulating and who are unvaccinated, incompletely vaccinated, or whose vaccination status is unknown should receive a series of 3 doses: 2 doses of IPV administered at an interval of 4–8 weeks; a third dose should be administered 6–12 months after the second. If 3 doses of IPV cannot be administered within the recommended intervals before protection is needed, the following alternatives are recommended:

- If >8 weeks is available before protection is needed, 3 doses of IPV should be administered ≥4 weeks apart.

- If <8 weeks but >4 weeks is available before protection is needed, 2 doses of IPV should be administered ≥4 weeks apart.

- If <4 weeks is available before protection is needed, a single dose of IPV is recommended.

If <3 doses are administered, the remaining IPV doses to complete a 3-dose series should be administered when feasible, at the intervals recommended above, if the person remains at increased risk for poliovirus exposure.

Adults who have completed a routine series of polio vaccine are considered to have lifelong immunity to poliomyelitis, but data on duration of immunity are lacking. As a precaution, adults (≥18 years of age) who are traveling to areas where WPV or VDPV is actively circulating and who have received a routine series with either IPV or OPV in childhood should receive another dose of IPV before departure. For adults, available data do not indicate the need for more than a single life-time booster dose with IPV.

INTERNATIONAL ADOPTION OF CHILDREN

The international adoption of children from countries or areas where WPV or VDPV is actively circulating is a special situation. International adoptees might not have completed a primary vaccination series against polio and might not have received a dose of polio vaccine before departure. Thus, there is a small risk that they might be infected with WPV or VDPV and remain infectious upon entry into the United States and potentially transmit to US household members and caregivers. So, as a measure of prudence, the polio vaccination status of all household members and caregivers of international adoptees whose origin is a country with active WPV or VDPV circulation should be assessed before the entry of the child into the United States. Those who are unvaccinated, incompletely vaccinated, or whose vaccination status is unknown should be brought up-to-date. Adults who have completed the primary series should consider a one-time booster of IPV as well.

VACCINE SAFETY AND ADVERSE REACTIONS

Minor local reactions (pain and redness) can occur after IPV administration. No serious adverse reactions to IPV have been documented. IPV should not be administered to people who have experienced a severe allergic reaction (such as anaphylaxis) after a previous dose of IPV or after receiving streptomycin, polymyxin B, or neomycin, which IPV contains in trace amounts; hypersensitivity reactions can occur after IPV administration among people sensitive to these 3 antibiotics.

PREGNANCY AND BREASTFEEDING

If a pregnant woman is unvaccinated or incompletely vaccinated and requires immediate protection against polio because of planned travel to a country or area where WPV or VDPV is actively circulating, IPV can be administered as recommended for adults. Breastfeeding is not a contraindication to administration of polio vaccine to an infant or mother.

PRECAUTIONS AND CONTRAINDICATIONS

IPV may be administered to people with diarrhea. Minor upper respiratory illnesses with or without fever, mild to moderate local reactions to a previous dose of IPV, current antimicrobial therapy, and the convalescent phase of acute illness are not contraindications for vaccination.

IMMUNOSUPPRESSION

IPV may be administered safely to immunocompromised travelers and their household contacts. Although a protective immune response cannot be ensured, IPV might confer some protection to the immunocompromised person. People with certain primary immunodeficiency diseases should not be given OPV and should avoid contact with excreted OPV virus (such as exposure to a child vaccinated with OPV in the previous 6 weeks); however, this situation no longer occurs in the United States unless a child receives OPV overseas.

CDC website: www.cdc.gov/polio

BIBLIOGRAPHY

1. CDC. Immunization schedules. Atlanta: CDC; 2016 [cited 2016 Sep. 25]. Available from: http://www.cdc.gov/vaccines/schedules/index.html.

2. CDC. Progress toward polio eradication—worldwide, 2014–2015. MMWR Morb Mortal Wkly Rep. 2015 May 22;64(19):527–31.

3. CDC. Progress toward poliomyelitis eradication—Nigeria, January 2014–July 2015. MMWR Morb Mortal Wkly Rep. 2015 Aug 21;64(32):878–82.

4. CDC. Update on vaccine-derived polioviruses—worldwide, January 2014–March 2015. MMWR Morb Mortal Wkly Rep. 2015 Jun 19;64(23):640–6.

5. CDC. Updated recommendations of the Advisory Committee on Immunization Practices (ACIP) regarding routine poliovirus vaccination. MMWR Morb Mortal Wkly Rep. 2009 Aug 7;58(30):829–30.

6. Prevots DR, Burr RK, Sutter RW, Murphy TV. Poliomyelitis prevention in the United States. Updated recommendations of the Advisory Committee on Immunization Practices (ACIP). MMWR Recomm Rep. 2000 May 9;49(RR-5):1–22.

7. Sutter RW, Kew OM, Cochi SL, Aylward RB. Poliovirus vaccine—live. In: Plotkin SA, Orenstein WA, Offit PA, editors. Vaccines. 6th ed. Philadelphia: Saunders Elsevier; 2012. p. 598–645.

8. Vidor E, Plotkin SA. Poliovirus vaccine—inactivated. In: Plotkin SA, Orenstein WA, Offit PA, editors. Vaccines. 6th ed. Philadelphia: Saunders Elsevier; 2012. pp. 573–97.

9. World Health Organization. Polio vaccines: WHO position paper—March, 2016. Wkly Epidemiol Rec. 2016 Mar 25;91(12):145–68.

10. World Health Organization. Wild poliovirus weekly update. World Health Organization; 2014 [cited 2016 Sep. 25]. Available from: http://www.polioeradication.org/Dataandmonitoring/Poliothisweek.aspx.

A HISTORY OF POLIO ERADICATION EFFORTS

Eric E. Mast, Stephen L. Cochi

Before licensing of the inactivated (1955) and live attenuated (1961) polio vaccines, poliomyelitis was ubiquitous and distributed globally. Poliovirus infected most people in childhood, causing paralysis in approximately 1 in 200. Where vaccine was introduced, it had a rapid effect on the disease. In the United States, reported paralytic cases fell from approximately 20,000 per year in the early 1950s to 2,525 in 1960 and 61 in 1965. The last cases of naturally occurring paralytic polio in the United States were in 1979, when an outbreak occurred among the Amish in several Midwestern states.

By the early 1980s, the feasibility of globally eradicating polio was already being discussed. Several characteristics of poliovirus made it an ideal candidate for eradication, including the lack of an animal reservoir and the availability of an effective, inexpensive, easily administered oral polio vaccine (OPV). Furthermore, experience in Cuba and Brazil had demonstrated the ability of mass vaccination

campaigns to interrupt poliovirus transmission. In 1988, the World Health Assembly formally resolved to eradicate poliomyelitis by 2000, giving birth to the Global Polio Eradication Initiative (GPEI).

The strategy of wild poliovirus (WPV) eradication was organized around 4 "pillars":

- Strengthening routine immunization service delivery to achieve high infant vaccination coverage with OPV.

- Conducting supplementary immunization activities (SIAs) in the form of mass vaccination campaigns for children, either at the national or subnational level. In polio-endemic countries and other countries with active WPV transmission, SIAs are typically conducted every 4–8 weeks until transmission has been stopped.

- Surveillance for acute flaccid paralysis (AFP) and confirmation of polio by laboratory testing of stool samples. AFP surveillance is a critical component in

countries both with and without polio, where the surveillance system is expected to detect nonpolio cases of AFP at a rate of at least 1 per 100,000 per year in industrialized countries and 2 per 100,000 per year in developing countries. Environmental surveillance—the testing of sewage for polioviruses—is also a sensitive tool for poliovirus detection and plays an important role in poliovirus surveillance.

- Conducting targeted "mop-up" vaccination campaigns in a focal geographic area around any confirmed polio cases.

The GPEI made rapid early progress, with a reduction in the number of polio-endemic countries from 125 countries in 1988 to 10 in 2001, polio-free certification in the Americas Region (1994), Western Pacific Region (2000), and European Region (2002) and eradication of WPV type 2 in 1999. However, the goal of eradication by 2000 was not achieved, and progress stagnated during the next decade due to major programmatic challenges including conflict, political instability, hard-to-reach populations, and poor infrastructure. Determined programmatic innovation was needed to overcome these challenges. In India, for example, a series of operational innovations were developed and implemented to improve vaccination service delivery and reach chronically undervaccinated groups—groups that were often outside the reach of the formal health care delivery system. In addition, vaccine innovations were brought to fruition, most importantly the division of OPV into monovalent components (mOPV1 and mOPV3) for the first time since they had been combined into the trivalent vaccine in the 1960s. These monovalent vaccines and, later on, the bivalent (types 1 and 3) vaccine greatly increased immunogenicity, because interference by the more robust type 2 component was removed.

By 2011, the GPEI was at a crossroads. The last WPV case in India was reported in early 2011. This success answered the question of feasibility—if polio could be eradicated in India, it

could be eradicated any- where. However, in the 3 remaining countries where endemic wild polio- virus transmission had never been interrupted— Nigeria, Pakistan, and Afghanistan—case counts were increasing, and polio- virus importations from the polio-endemic coun- tries caused multiple out- breaks in many countries that had previously been polio free. In October 2011, GPEI's independent moni- toring board issued a crit- ical report, stating bluntly that the program was "not on track to interrupt poliovirus transmission" and that "polio eradication needs to be treated as a global health emergency" if the ultimate goal of the program was ever to be achieved. This report led to the World Health Assembly declaring global polio eradication "a pro- grammatic emergency for global public health" in 2012. In addition, the World Health Organization declared the international spread of WPV to previ- ously polio-free countries to be "a public health emergency of international concern" in 2014, trigger- ing oversight by an emer- gency committee under the International Health Regulations.

The World Health Assembly declaration of polio eradication as a public health emergency in 2012 initiated a new era in which emergency oper- ations were established in GPEI partner agencies and at national and subnational levels in the last remaining polio-endemic countries of Nigeria, Pakistan, and Afghanistan to complete eradication. Substantial progress has been achieved with the renewed efforts. WPV type 3 was last detected in 2012, and polio-free certification in the Southeast Asia Region was announced in 2014. Four WPV cases were reported in Nigeria in August 2016; these are the first cases reported in the country since July 2014. No WPV cases have been detected elsewhere in Africa since August 2014. As of September 14, 2016, Afghanistan, Pakistan, and Nigeria were the last three countries with endemic WPV type 1 transmis- sion, and 26 cases had been reported worldwide in 2016.

In May 2013, the 66th World Health Assembly endorsed the Polio Eradication and Endgame Strategic Plan 2013–2018. This plan provides a time- line for completion of polio eradication by eliminating all paralytic polio due to both WPV and vaccine-derived polioviruses (VDPVs). VDPVs are very rare strains of poliovirus, genetically changed by mutations from the original strain contained in OPV, which can emerge in locations where childhood vaccination coverage is low. To prevent type 2 VDPV emergence, which accounted for 79% of the circulating VDPVs in 2014–2015, a coordinated global switch in all countries from use of trivalent (types 1, 2 and 3) OPV to bivalent OPV (types 1 and 3) was implemented in April 2016. To mitigate risks by increasing population immunity to poliovirus type 2, inactivated poliovirus vaccine (IPV) is being introduced in all countries where it has not been in use. The plan also has an objective to contain poliovirus and certify interruption of poliovirus transmission. In order to contain poliovirus, laboratories with samples containing poliovirus will need to destroy or consolidate and safely store those samples. Requirements for certifying a WHO region as free of WPV include the absence of any WPV

for a minimum of 3 years in all countries of the region and the presence of certification-standard surveillance in all countries during that 3-year period. Planning is also underway to prepare for the period after polio eradication is certified, so that polio eradication assets in high priority countries can be leveraged and transitioned to improve global health as part of polio eradication's legacy.

BIBLIOGRAPHY

1. Dowdle WR, Cochi SL. Global eradication of poliovirus: history and rationale. In: Selmer BL, Wimmer E, editors. Molecular Biology of Picornaviruses. Washington, DC: ASM Press; 2002. pp. 473–80.

2. el-Sayed N, el-Gamal Y, Abbassy AA, Seoud I, Salama M, Kandeel A, et al. Monovalent type 1 oral poliovirus vaccine in newborns. N Engl J Med. 2008 Oct 16;359(16):1655–65.

3. Global Polio Eradication Initiative. Polio eradication and endgame strategic plan, 2013–2018. Geneva: World Health Organization; 2013 [cited 2016 Sep. 25]. Available from: http://www.polioeradication.org/resourcelibrary/strategyandwork.aspx.

4. Hagan JE, Wassilak SG, Craig AS, Tangermann RH, Diop OM, Burns CC,

et al. Progress toward polio eradication—worldwide, 2014–2015. MMWR Morb Mortal Wkly Rep. 2015 May 22;64(19):527–31.

5. Independent Monitoring Board of the Global Polio Eradication Initiative. Report October 2011. Geneva2011 [cited 2016 Sep. 25]. Available from: http://www.polioeradication.org/Portals/0/Document/Aboutus/Governance/IMB/4IMBMeeting/IMBReportOctober2011.pdf.

6. Jenkins HE, Aylward RB, Gasasira A, Donnelly CA, Abanida EA, Koleosho-Adelekan T, et al. Effectiveness of immunization against paralytic poliomyelitis in Nigeria. N Engl J Med. 2008 Oct 16;359(16):1666–74.

7. Snider CJ, Diop OM, Burns CC, Tangermann RH, Wassilak SG. Surveillance systems to track progress toward polio eradication—worldwide, 2014–2015. MMWR Morb Mortal Wkly Rep. 2016 Apr 8;65(13):346–51.

8. Sutter RW, John TJ, Jain H, Agarkhedkar S, Ramanan PV, Verma H, et al. Immunogenicity of bivalent types 1 and 3 oral poliovirus vaccine: a randomised, double-blind, controlled trial. Lancet. 2010 Nov 13;376(9753):1682–8.

9. World Health Organization. List of innovations in the India Polio Eradication Program. 2013 [cited 2016 Sep. 25]. Available from: http://www.polioeradication.org/Portals/0/Document/Resources/StrategyWork/EAP/EAP_annex1.pdf.

Q FEVER

Gilbert J. Kersh

INFECTIOUS AGENT

The gram-negative intracellular bacterium *Coxiella burnetii*.

TRANSMISSION

Most commonly through inhalation of aerosols or dust contaminated with dried birth fluids or excreta from infected animals (usually cattle, sheep, or goats). *C. burnetii* is highly infectious and persists in the environment. Infections via ingestion of contaminated, unpasteurized dairy products and human-to-human transmission via sexual contact have been rarely reported.

EPIDEMIOLOGY

Distributed worldwide; the prevalence is highest in African and Middle Eastern countries. Reported rates of human infection are higher in France and Australia than in the United States. The largest known Q fever outbreak reported to date involved approximately 4,000 human cases and occurred during 2007–2010 in the Netherlands. Travelers who visit rural areas or farms with cattle, sheep, goats, or other livestock may be exposed to Q fever. Occupational exposure to infected animals (such as in farmers, veterinarians, butchers, meat packers, and seasonal or migrant farm workers), particularly during parturition, poses a high risk for disease transmission.

CLINICAL PRESENTATION

It is estimated that more than half of acute infections are mild or asymptomatic. Incubation period is typically 2–3 weeks but may be shorter after exposure to large numbers of organisms. The most common presentation of acute infection is a self-limiting influenzalike illness, with pneumonia or hepatitis in more severe acute infections. Chronic infections occur primarily in patients with preexisting cardiac valvulopathies, vascular abnormalities, or immunosuppression. Women infected during pregnancy are at risk for adverse pregnancy outcomes unless treated. The most common manifestations of chronic disease are endocarditis and endovascular infections.

DIAGNOSIS

Serologic evidence of a 4-fold rise in phase II IgG by indirect fluorescent antibody test between paired sera taken 3–4 weeks apart is the gold standard for diagnosis of acute infection. A single high serum phase II IgG titer (>1:128) in conjunction with clinical evidence of infection may be considered evidence of probable Q fever. PCR assays may be used on whole blood or serum samples in the early stages of illness and before initiation of antibiotic therapy. *C. burnetii* may be detected in infected tissues by using immunohistochemical staining or DNA detection methods or by direct isolation of the agent via culture. Q fever is a nationally notifiable disease.

TREATMENT

Doxycycline is the treatment of choice for acute Q fever. Pregnant women, children aged <8 years with mild illness, and patients allergic to doxycycline may be treated with alternative antibiotics such as trimethoprim-sulfamethoxazole. Treatment for acute Q fever is not recommended for asymptomatic people or for those whose symptoms have resolved. Chronic *C. burnetii* infections require long-term combination therapy with agents such as doxycycline, hydroxychloroquine, trimethoprim-sulfamethoxazole, fluoroquinolones, and rifampin.

PREVENTION

Avoid areas where potentially infected animals are kept, and avoid consumption of unpasteurized dairy products. A human vaccine for Q fever has been developed and used in Australia, but it is not available in the United States.

CDC website: www.cdc.gov/qfever

BIBLIOGRAPHY

1. Anderson A, Bijlmer H, Fournier PE, Graves S, Hartzell J, Kersh GJ, et al. Diagnosis and management of Q fever— United States, 2013: recommendations from CDC and the Q Fever Working Group. MMWR Recomm Rep. 2013 Mar 29;62(RR-03):1–30.

2. Cohen NJ, Papernik M, Singleton J, Segreti J, Eremeeva ME. Q fever in an American tourist returned from Australia. Travel Med Infect Dis. 2007 May;5(3):194–5.

3. Delord M, Socolovschi C, Parola P. Rickettsioses and Q fever in travelers (2004–2013). Travel Med Infect Dis. 2014 Sep-Oct;12(5):443–58.

4. Jensenius M, Davis X, von Sonnenburg F, Schwartz E, Keystone JS, Leder K, et al. Multicenter GeoSentinel analysis of rickettsial diseases in international travelers, 1996–2008. Emerg Infect Dis. 2009 Nov;15(11):1791–8.

5. Kobbe R, Kramme S, Gocht A, Werner M, Lippert U, May J, et al. Travel-associated *Coxiella burnetii* infections: three cases of Q fever with different clinical manifestation. Travel Med Infect Dis. 2007 Nov;5(6):374–9.

6. Million M, Thuny F, Richet H, Raoult D. Long-term outcome of Q fever endocarditis: a 26-year personal survey. Lancet Infect Dis. 2010 Aug;10(8):527–35.

7. Roest HI, Tilburg JJ, van der Hoek W, Vellema P, van Zijderveld FG, Klaassen CH, et al. The Q fever epidemic in The Netherlands: history, onset, response and reflection. Epidemiol Infect. 2011 Jan;139(1):1–12.

8. Ta TH, Jimenez B, Navarro M, Meije Y, Gonzalez FJ, Lopez-Velez R. Q Fever in returned febrile travelers. J Travel Med. 2008 Mar-Apr;15(2):126–9.

RABIES

Brett W. Petersen, Ryan M. Wallace, David R. Shlim

INFECTIOUS AGENTS

Rabies is a fatal, acute, progressive encephalomyelitis caused by neurotropic viruses in the family Rhabdoviridae, genus *Lyssavirus*. Numerous and diverse variants of lyssaviruses are found in a wide variety of animal species throughout the world, all of which may cause fatal human rabies. Rabies virus is by far the most common lyssavirus infection of humans. Tens of millions of potential human exposures and tens of thousands of deaths from rabies virus occur each year.

TRANSMISSION

The normal and most successful mode of transmission is inoculation of saliva from the bite of a rabid animal. Clinical signs of rabies in an animal are not always obvious because of the broad spectrum of disease manifestations. Rabies virus is neurotropic and gains access to the peripheral nervous system by being taken up at a nerve synapse at the site of the bite. The virus travels through peripheral nerves to the central nervous system before traveling back out through the peripheral nervous system. After reaching the salivary glands, virus can be secreted allowing the transmission cycle to repeat. Exposure of rabies virus to highly innervated tissue may increase the risk of successful infection. In addition to saliva, rabies virus may also be found in nervous tissues (central and peripheral) and tears. Infection from nonbite exposures, such as organ transplantation from infected humans, does occur.

All mammals are believed to be susceptible to infection, but major rabies reservoirs are terrestrial carnivores and bats. Although dogs are the main reservoir in developing countries, the epidemiology of the disease differs from one region or country to another. All patients with mammal bites should be medically evaluated. **Bat bites anywhere in the world are a cause of concern and an indication to consider prophylaxis.**

EPIDEMIOLOGY

Lyssaviruses, the causative agent for the disease rabies, have been found on all continents except Antarctica. Rabies virus is classified into 2 major genetic lineages: canine and New World bat. These 2 lineages can be further classified into rabies virus variants based on the reservoir species in which they circulate. Regionally, different viral variants are adapted to various mammalian hosts and perpetuate in dogs and wildlife, such as bats, foxes, jackals, mongooses, raccoons, and skunks. Canine rabies remains enzootic in many areas of the world, including Africa, Asia, and parts of Central and South America.

Timely and specific information about the global occurrence of rabies is often difficult to find. Surveillance levels vary, and reporting status can change suddenly as a result of disease reintroduction or emergence. The rate of rabies exposures in travelers is at best an estimate and may range from 16 to 200 per 100,000 travelers.

CLINICAL PRESENTATION

Clinical illness in humans begins following invasion of the peripheral and then central nervous system and culminates in acute fatal encephalitis. After infection the asymptomatic incubation period is variable, but signs and symptoms most commonly develop within several weeks to several months after exposure. Pain and paresthesia at the site of exposure are often the first symptoms of disease. The disease then progresses rapidly from a nonspecific, prodromal phase with fever and vague symptoms to an acute, progressive encephalitis. The neurologic phase may be characterized by anxiety, paresis, paralysis, and other signs of encephalitis; spasms of swallowing muscles can be stimulated by the sight, sound, or perception of water (hydrophobia); and delirium and convulsions can develop, followed rapidly by coma and

death. Once clinical signs manifest, patients die quickly in the absence of intensive supportive care.

DIAGNOSIS

The diagnosis may be relatively simple in a patient with a compatible history and a classic clinical presentation (Box 3-4). However, clinical suspicion and prioritization of differential diagnoses may be complicated by variations in clinical presentation and a lack of exposure history. The exposure history is difficult to elicit if the risk of exposure to rabies was not recognized, the exposure was not discussed with friends and family, and several weeks to months have elapsed since the exposure.

Definitive antemortem diagnosis requires high-complexity experimental test methods on multiple samples (such as serum, cerebrospinal fluid [CSF], saliva, and skin biopsy from the nape of the neck), which can be collected sequentially if initial testing is negative and clinical suspicion is high. Additional detailed information on diagnostic testing may be obtained from CDC (www.cdc.gov/rabies/specific_groups/doctors/ante_mortem.html). Rising levels of rabies virus–neutralizing antibodies, particularly in the CSF, is diagnostic in an unvaccinated, encephalitic patient. Rabies is a nationally notifiable disease.

TREATMENT

There is not yet an evidence-based "best practices" medical approach to treating patients with rabies; most patients are managed with symptomatic and palliative supportive care. An

---

BOX 3-4. **World Health Organization, human rabies case definition**

Clinical case definition: a person presenting with an acute neurologic syndrome (encephalitis) dominated by forms of hyperactivity (furious rabies) or paralytic syndromes (dumb rabies) progressing towards coma and death, usually by respiratory failure, within 7–10 days after the first symptom if no intensive care is instituted.

Human rabies:
  Suspected: A case that is compatible with the clinical case definition.

  Probable: A suspected case plus history of contact with a suspected rabid animal.

  Confirmed: A suspected case that is laboratory-confirmed.

experimental approach, known as the Milwaukee protocol, involves inducing coma and treating with antiviral drugs, but it remains controversial. Rabies is still considered universally fatal for practical purposes, and preventive measures are the only way to optimize survival after a bite from a rabid animal.

PREVENTION

Rabies in travelers is best prevented by having a comprehensive strategy. This consists of (1) education about risks and the need to avoid bites from mammals, especially high-risk rabies reservoir species; (2) consultation with travel health professionals to determine if preexposure vaccination is recommended; (3) knowing how to prevent rabies after a bite; and (4) knowing how to obtain postexposure prophylaxis (PEP). The last may involve urgent importation of rabies biologics or international travel to where PEP is available. Travelers who have died of rabies either did not seek PEP or received inadequate care when they did.

Avoiding Animal Bites

Travelers to rabies-enzootic countries should be warned about the risk of rabies exposure and educated as to how to avoid animal bites. Travelers should avoid free-roaming mammals, avoid provoking domestic animals, and avoid contact with bats and other wildlife. Although nonhuman primates are rarely rabid, they are a common source of bites, mainly on the Indian subcontinent. In most instances these nonhuman primates cannot be followed up for rabies assessments, and the bite victims are recommended to receive PEP. Awareness of this risk and simple prevention is particularly effective. Travelers should be advised to not approach or otherwise interact with monkeys or carry food while monkeys are near, especially around monkeys that are habituated to tourists. Travelers should be educated to not handle bats or other wildlife and consider the need for personal protective equipment before entering caves where bats may be found, given the risk for exposures to rabies virus, histoplasmosis, Marburg virus (see Ebola Virus Disease and Marburg Virus Disease section this chapter), or other bat-associated pathogens. Many bats have tiny teeth, and wounds may not be readily apparent. Any suspected or documented bite or wound from a bat should be grounds for seeking PEP.

Children are at higher risk for rabies exposure and subsequent illness because of their inquisitive nature and inability to read behavioral cues from dogs and other animals. The smaller stature of children makes them more likely to experience severe bites to high-risk areas, such as the face and head. Also contributing to the higher risk is their attraction to animals and the possibility that they may not report an exposure.

Preexposure Vaccination

Preexposure rabies vaccination may be recommended for certain international travelers based on the occurrence of animal rabies in the country of destination; the availability of antirabies biologics; the intended activities of the traveler, especially in remote areas; and the traveler's duration of stay. A decision to receive preexposure rabies immunization may also be based on the likelihood of repeat travel to at-risk destinations or long-term travel to a high-risk destination. Preexposure vaccination may be recommended for veterinarians, animal handlers, field biologists, cavers, missionaries, and certain laboratory workers. Table 3-15 provides criteria for preexposure vaccination. Regardless of whether preexposure vaccine is administered, travelers going to areas where the risk of rabies is high should be encouraged to purchase medical evacuation insurance (see Chapter 2, Travel Insurance, Travel Health Insurance, & Medical Evacuation Insurance).

In the United States, preexposure vaccination consists of a series of 3 intramuscular injections given on days 0, 7, and 21 or 28 in the deltoid with human diploid cell rabies vaccine (HDCV) or purified chick embryo cell (PCEC) vaccine (Table 3-16). Travelers should receive all 3 preexposure immunizations before travel. If 3 doses of rabies vaccine cannot be completed before travel, the traveler should not start the series, as few data exist to guide PEP after a partial immunization series.

Preexposure vaccination does not eliminate the need for additional medical attention after a rabies exposure, but it simplifies PEP. Preexposure vaccination may also provide some protection when an exposure to rabies virus is unrecognized

Table 3-15. Criteria for preexposure immunization for rabies

RISK CATEGORY	NATURE OF RISK	TYPICAL POPULATIONS	PREEXPOSURE REGIMEN
Continuous	Virus present continuously, often in high concentrations Specific exposures likely to go unrecognized Bite, nonbite, or aerosol exposure	Rabies research laboratory workers,[1] rabies biologics production workers	Primary course; serologic testing every 6 months; booster vaccination if antibody titer is below acceptable level[2]
Frequent	Exposure usually episodic with source recognized, but exposure might also be unrecognized Bite, nonbite, or aerosol exposure possible	Rabies diagnostic laboratory workers,[1] cavers, veterinarians and staff, and animal-control and wildlife workers in areas where rabies is enzootic. All people who frequently handle bats.	Primary course; serologic testing every 2 years; booster vaccination if antibody titer is below acceptable level[2]
Infrequent (greater than general population)	Exposure nearly always episodic with source recognized Bite or nonbite exposure	Veterinarians and animal control staff working with terrestrial carnivores in areas where rabies is uncommon to rare; veterinary students; and travelers visiting areas where rabies is enzootic and immediate access to medical care, including biologics, is limited	Primary course; no serologic testing or booster vaccination
Rare (general population)	Exposure always episodic, with source recognized Bite or nonbite exposure	US population at large, including people in rabies-epizootic areas	No preexposure immunization necessary

[1] Judgment of relative risk and extra monitoring of vaccination status of laboratory workers are the responsibility of the laboratory supervisor (see www.cdc.gov/biosafety/publications/bmbl5 for more information).
[2] Preexposure booster immunization consists of 1 dose of human diploid cell (rabies) vaccine or purified chick embryo cell vaccine, 1.0-mL dose, intramuscular (deltoid area). Per Advisory Committee on Immunization Practices recommendations, minimum acceptable antibody level is complete virus neutralization at a 1:5 serum dilution by the rapid fluorescent focus inhibition test, which is equivalent to approximately 0.1 IU/mL. A booster dose should be administered if titer falls below this level in populations that remain at risk.

or PEP might be delayed. Travelers who have completed a 3-dose preexposure rabies immunization series or have received full PEP are considered previously vaccinated and do not require routine boosters. Routine testing for rabies virus–neutralizing antibody is not recommended for international travelers who are not otherwise in the frequent or continuous risk categories (Table 3-15).

Wound Management

Any animal bite or scratch should be thoroughly cleaned with copious amounts of soap and water, povidone iodine, or other substances with virucidal activity. All travelers should be informed that immediately cleaning bite wounds as soon as possible substantially reduces the risk of rabies virus infection, especially when followed by timely administration of PEP. For unvaccinated patients,

Table 3-16. Preexposure immunization for rabies[1]

VACCINE	DOSE (ML)	NUMBER OF DOSES	SCHEDULE (DAYS)[2]	ROUTE
HDCV, Imovax (Sanofi)	1.0	3	0, 7, and 21 or 28	IM
PCEC, RabAvert (Novartis)	1.0	3	0, 7, and 21 or 28	IM

Abbreviations: HDCV, human diploid cell vaccine; IM, intramuscular; PCEC, purified chick embryo cell.
[1] Patients who are immunosuppressed by disease or medications should postpone preexposure vaccinations and consider avoiding activities for which rabies preexposure prophylaxis is indicated during the period of expected immunosuppression. If this is not possible, immunosuppressed people who are at risk for rabies should have their antibody titers checked after vaccination.
[2] Every attempt should be made to adhere to recommended schedules; however, for most minor deviations (delays of a few days for individual doses), vaccination can be resumed as though the traveler were on schedule. If 3 doses of rabies vaccine cannot be completed before travel, the traveler should not start the series, as few data exist to guide PEP after a partial immunization series.

wounds that might require suturing should have the suturing delayed for a few days. If suturing is necessary to control bleeding or for functional or cosmetic reasons, rabies immune globulin (RIG) should be injected into all wounded tissues before suturing. The use of local anesthetic is not contraindicated in wound management.

Postexposure Prophylaxis

IN TRAVELERS WHO RECEIVED PREEXPOSURE VACCINATION

PEP for someone previously vaccinated consists of 2 doses of modern cell culture vaccine given on days 0 and 3 after the exposure. The booster doses do not have to be the same brand as the one in the original preexposure immunization series.

IN TRAVELERS WHO DID NOT RECEIVE PREEXPOSURE VACCINATION

PEP for an unvaccinated patient consists of administration of RIG (20 IU/kg for human RIG and 40 IU/kg for equine RIG) and a series of 4 injections of rabies vaccine over 14 days, or 5 doses over a 1-month period in immunosuppressed patients (Table 3-17). After wound cleansing, as much of the dose-appropriate volume of RIG (Table 3-17) as is anatomically feasible should be injected at the wound site. The intent is to put the RIG in the areas where saliva may have contaminated wounded tissue. If the wound is small and on a distal extremity such as a finger or toe, the health care provider must use clinical judgment to decide how much RIG to inject to avoid local tissue compression and complications. Any

remaining dose should be administered intramuscularly at a site distant from the site of vaccine administration. If the wounds are extensive, the dose-appropriate volume of RIG must not be exceeded. If the volume is inadequate to inject all the wounds, the RIG may be diluted with normal saline to ensure sufficient volume to inject in all of the wounds. This is a particular issue in children whose body weight may be small in relation to the size and number of wounds.

RIG is difficult to access in many countries. If modern cell culture vaccine is available but access to RIG is delayed, the vaccine series should be started as soon as possible, and RIG may be added to the regimen up to and including day 7. After day 7, RIG is unlikely to provide benefit, as antibodies would be expected to be present from the patient's own vaccine-derived immune response.

Because rabies virus can persist in tissue for a long time before invading a peripheral nerve, a traveler who has sustained a bite that is suspicious for rabies should receive full PEP, including RIG, even if a considerable length of time has passed since the initial exposure. If there is a scar, or the patient remembers where the bite occurred, an appropriate amount of RIG should be injected in that area.

Human RIG is manufactured by plasmapheresis of blood from hyperimmunized volunteers. The total quantity of commercially produced human RIG falls short of worldwide demand, and it is not available in many developing countries. Equine RIG or purified fractions of equine RIG may be available in some developing countries

Table 3-17. Postexposure immunization for rabies[1]

IMMUNIZATION STATUS	VACCINE/ PRODUCT	DOSE	NUMBER OF DOSES	SCHEDULE (DAYS)[2]	ROUTE
Not previously vaccinated	RIG plus	20 IU/kg body weight	1	0	Infiltrated at bite site (if possible); remainder IM
Not previously vaccinated	HDCV or PCEC	1.0 mL	4[3]	0, 3, 7, 14 (28 if immunocompromised[4])	IM
Previously vaccinated[5,6]	HDCV or PCEC	1.0 mL	2	0, 3	IM

Abbreviations: RIG, rabies immune globulin; IM, intramuscular; HDCV, human diploid cell vaccine; PCEC, purified chick embryo cell.
[1] All postexposure prophylaxis should begin with immediate, thorough cleansing of all wounds with soap and water, povidone iodine, or other substances with virucidal activity.
[2] Every attempt should be made to adhere to recommended schedules; however, for most minor deviations (delays of a few days for individual doses), vaccination can be resumed as though the traveler were on schedule. When substantial deviations occur, immune status should be assessed by serologic testing 7–14 days after the final dose is administered.
[3] Five vaccine doses for the immunosuppressed patient. The first 4 vaccine doses are given on the same schedule as for an immunocompetent patient, and the fifth dose is given on day 28; patient follow-up should include monitoring antibody response. See www.cdc.gov/mmwr/preview/mmwrhtml/rr5902a1.htm for more information.
[4] CDC recommends 4 postexposure vaccine doses, on days 0, 3, 7, and 14, unless the patient is immunocompromised in some way, in which case a fifth dose is given at day 28.
[5] Preexposure immunization with HDCV or PCEC, prior postexposure prophylaxis with HDCV or PCEC, or people previously vaccinated with any other type of rabies vaccine and a documented history of positive rabies virus neutralizing antibody response to the prior vaccination.
[6] RIG is not recommended.

where human RIG might not be available. Such products are preferable to no RIG.

The incidence of adverse events after the use of modern equine-derived RIG is low (0.8%–6.0%), and most reactions are minor. However, such products are not regulated by the Food and Drug Administration, and their use cannot be recommended unequivocally. In addition, unpurified antirabies serum of equine origin might still be used in some countries where neither human nor equine RIG is available. The use of this antirabies serum is associated with higher rates of serious adverse reactions, including anaphylaxis and serum sickness.

Different PEP schedules, alternative routes of administration, and other rabies vaccines besides HDCV and PCEC may be used abroad. For example, commercially available purified Vero cell rabies vaccine and purified duck embryo cell vaccine are acceptable alternatives if available. However, other rabies vaccines or PEP regimens might require additional prophylaxis or confirmation of adequate rabies virus neutralizing antibody titers. Assistance in managing complicated PEP scenarios can be obtained from experienced travel medicine professionals, health departments, and CDC.

Rabies vaccine was once manufactured from viruses grown in animal brains, and some of these vaccines are still in use in developing countries. Typically, the brain-derived vaccines, also known as nerve tissue vaccines, can be identified if the traveler is offered a large-volume injection (5 mL) daily for approximately 14–21 days. Because of variability of potency in these preparations, which may limit effectiveness, and the risk of adverse reactions, the traveler should not accept these vaccines but travel to a location where acceptable vaccines and RIG are available.

Rabies Vaccine

VACCINE SAFETY AND ADVERSE REACTIONS

Travelers should be advised that they may experience local reactions after vaccination such as pain, erythema, swelling, or itching at the injection site, or mild systemic reactions such as headache, nausea, abdominal pain, muscle aches, and dizziness. Approximately 6% of people receiving booster vaccinations with HDCV may experience systemic hypersensitivity reactions characterized by urticaria, pruritus, and malaise. The likelihood of these reactions may be less with PCEC. Once initiated, rabies PEP should not be interrupted or discontinued because of local or mild systemic reactions to rabies vaccine. If an adverse event occurs with one of the vaccine types, consider switching to the alternative vaccine for the remainder of the series.

PRECAUTIONS AND CONTRAINDICATIONS

Pregnancy is not a contraindication to PEP. In infants and children, the dose of HDCV or PCEC for preexposure or PEP is the same as that recommended for adults. The dose of RIG for PEP is based on body weight (Table 3-17).

CDC website: www.cdc.gov/rabies

BIBLIOGRAPHY

1. Gautret P, Parola P. Rabies vaccination for international travelers. Vaccine. 2012 Jan 5;30(2):126–33.

2. Gautret P, Tantawichien T, Vu Hai V, Piyaphanee W. Determinants of pre-exposure rabies vaccination among foreign backpackers in Bangkok, Thailand. Vaccine. 2011 May 23;29(23):3931–4.

3. Malerczyk C, Detora L, Gniel D. Imported human rabies cases in Europe, the United States, and Japan, 1990 to 2010. J Travel Med. 2011 Nov-Dec;18(6):402–7.

4. Mills DJ, Lau CL, Weinstein P. Animal bites and rabies exposure in Australian travellers. Med J Aust. 2011 Dec 19;195(11-12):673–5.

5. Rupprecht CE, Briggs D, Brown CM, Franka R, Katz SL, Kerr HD, et al. Use of a reduced (4-dose) vaccine schedule for postexposure prophylaxis to prevent human rabies: recommendations of the Advisory Committee on Immunization Practices. MMWR Recomm Rep. 2010 Mar 19;59(RR-2):1–9.

6. Rupprecht CE, Gibbons RV. Clinical practice. Prophylaxis against rabies. N Engl J Med. 2004 Dec 16;351(25):2626–35.

7. Smith A, Petrovic M, Solomon T, Fooks A. Death from rabies in a UK traveller returning from India. Euro Surveill. 2005 Jul;10(30):E050728 5.

8. van Thiel PP, de Bie RM, Eftimov F, Tepaske R, Zaaijer HL, van Doornum GJ, et al. Fatal human rabies due to Duvenhage virus from a bat in Kenya: failure of treatment with coma-induction, ketamine, and antiviral drugs. PLoS Negl Trop Dis. 2009;3(7):e428.

9. Warrell MJ, Warrell DA. Rabies and other lyssavirus diseases. Lancet. 2004 Mar 20;363(9413):959–69.

10. World Health Organization. WHO expert consultation on rabies. World Health Organ Tech Rep Ser. 2005;931:1–88.

INTRADERMAL RABIES PREEXPOSURE IMMUNIZATION

David R. Shlim

3

Few topics in travel medicine prompt more concern and persistent questions than the prevention of rabies in travelers. Although we understand the basics of rabies prevention for travelers, the logistics of providing this care in a timely fashion remain a challenge. Unimmunized travelers who are exposed to rabies and other lyssaviruses require proper wound care, infiltration of human rabies immune globulin (RIG), and a series of 4 or 5 doses of rabies vaccine intramuscularly over a 2- to 4-week period. Travelers who receive 3 doses of rabies vaccine before travel need to receive 2 more doses of rabies vaccine, 3 days apart, after a viral exposure. Notably, human RIG and equine RIG are often unavailable in developing countries, although modern cell culture rabies vaccines are increasingly available. Thus, preexposure rabies immunization can facilitate the traveler's access to adequate postexposure rabies prophylaxis.

One limiting factor in the use of preexposure rabies immunization is the cost of the vaccine in most developed countries. In the United States, rabies vaccine may cost more than $300 per dose, resulting in a cost to the patient in excess of $900 for three 1.0-mL intramuscular injections. As a way of decreasing the cost of preexposure immunization, some practitioners have used a 0.1-mL dose of rabies vaccine administered intradermally.

At approximately $45 per dose in the early 1980s, many people already considered the vaccine too expensive. Thus, intradermal rabies immunization began almost as soon as the intramuscular human diploid cell vaccine (HDCV) was manufactured. By reconstituting the 1.0 mL of vaccine in the vial, practitioners could draw up approximately eight 0.1-mL doses. One problem was that the entire vial had to be used within a few hours of reconstituting, meaning that a provider

had to either be in a busy clinic or line up groups of people, such as families, for rabies immunization at the same time.

Early studies of the immune response to intradermal rabies vaccine, using HDCV and later other rabies vaccines, were uniformly encouraging. Virtually 100% of vaccinees seroconverted. A 1982 statement by the US Advisory Committee on Immunization Practices (ACIP) reviewed data on >1,500 vaccinees and declared, "It appears that, with this vaccine, the 0.1-mL intradermal (ID) regimen is an acceptable alternative to the currently approved 1.0-mL intramuscular (IM) regimen for preexposure prophylaxis." They called upon manufacturers to produce a product with appropriate packaging and labeling.

In 1986, the Mérieux Institute (now Sanofi Pasteur) received approval to market a 0.1-mL dose in an individual syringe. Sharing reconstituted vials of 1.0 mL between patients remained off-label.

Although the new product solved the logistical problem of providing individual travelers with an ID dose, the cost of the prepackaged ID dose was 75% of the full 1.0-mL IM dose.

As ID rabies immunization was being implemented, a death from rabies in an American Peace Corps volunteer in Kenya brought the enthusiasm for ID immunization to a temporary halt. The 23-year-old female volunteer died of rabies after a bite from a stray puppy that she had adopted. She had received 3 doses of ID rabies vaccine in Kenya, finishing 6 months before the bite. She did not suspect that the dog had rabies, even though it died shortly after biting her. As a result, she did not seek postexposure boosters. Serum drawn at the onset of her symptoms revealed she did not have an adequate antibody response. The Peace Corps medical personnel wondered why the recent ID immunization had not been effective. Concerned that she may have had an atypical response to immunization, they tested serum specimens from 11 other Peace Corps volunteers in Kenya who had been immunized at the same time. To their surprise, 9 of 11 also had an inadequate immunologic response. As a control group, Peace Corps volunteers who had received rabies ID preexposure immunization in Nepal and Morocco were also tested, and 31 of 79 had an inadequate antibody response.

Studies were undertaken to confirm the potency of the vaccine lot, maintenance of the cold chain, the method of administration, and the effect of concomitant medication. None of these factors proved to be an entirely adequate explanation. For example, chloroquine taken as an antimalarial medication during ID rabies immunization reduced the levels of antibody induced. However, the seroconversion rate among those taking chloroquine was still adequate, and the volunteers in Morocco and Nepal were not taking chloroquine. After the investigation, it was recommended that people using ID preexposure immunization should complete the course before starting chloroquine and traveling abroad or else use the IM regimen.

ACIP continued to endorse the concept of ID preexposure rabies immunization in a 1999 statement on rabies prevention. However, 3 lots of a prepackaged rabies ID vaccine were recalled in 2000 for having a potency that fell below the specification level before the expiration date. In 2001, the ID rabies vaccine was withdrawn from the market. Since then, authorities in the United States have not recommended sharing 1.0-mL vials for ID rabies immunization, as the manufacturer has not applied for the appropriate packaging and labeling to the Food and Drug Administration (FDA). This lack of endorsement of ID preexposure immunization has frustrated some travel medicine professionals.

Based on recent data, the World Health Organization has recommended the use of ID preexposure rabies immunization as an alternative to IM immunization. A recent study of 420 Australian travelers given a modified ID rabies preexposure immunization (2 doses on day 0, 2 doses on day 7, and 1 dose on day 21–28) documented a seroconversion rate of 98.3%. Although using only 0.5 mL of vaccine total might save money, this

(continued)

INTRADERMAL RABIES PREEXPOSURE IMMUNIZATION (CONTINUED)

regimen does not alleviate the challenge of needing to identify several travelers in a few hours or use multiple doses from a single-use vial.

Neither ACIP nor FDA are likely to endorse the use of 1.0-mL vials of rabies vaccine for multiple-dose ID use unless the manufacturer requests that indication. Until then, the use of ID rabies vaccine will remain off-label in the United States. The current status of ID rabies immunization in the United States reflects a regulatory situation and ACIP opinion, and is not a comment on the effectiveness of ID rabies preexposure immunization for travelers elsewhere.

BIBLIOGRAPHY

1. Bernard KW, Fishbein DB, Miller KD, Parker RA, Waterman S, Sumner JW, et al. Pre-exposure rabies immunization with human diploid cell vaccine: decreased antibody responses in persons immunized in developing countries. Am J Trop Med Hyg. 1985 May;34(3):633–47.

2. CDC. Recommendation of the Immunization Practices Advisory Committee (ACIP). Supplementary statement on pre-exposure rabies prophylaxis by the intradermal route. MMWR Morb Mortal Wkly Rep. 1982 Jun 4;31(21):279–80, 85.

3. Mills DJ, Lau CL, Fearnley EJ, Weinstein P. The immunogenicity of a modified intradermal pre-exposure rabies vaccination schedule--a case series of 420 travelers. J Travel Med. 2011 Sep-Oct;18(5):327–32.

*Perspectives sections are written as editorial discussions aiming to add depth and clinical perspective to the official recommendations contained in the book. The views and opinions expressed in this section are those of the author and do not necessarily represent the official position of CDC.

RICKETTSIAL (SPOTTED & TYPHUS FEVERS) & RELATED INFECTIONS, INCLUDING ANAPLASMOSIS & EHRLICHIOSIS

William L. Nicholson, Christopher D. Paddock

INFECTIOUS AGENTS

Rickettsial infections are caused by various bacterial species from the genera *Rickettsia*, *Orientia*, *Ehrlichia*, *Neorickettsia*, *Neoehrlichia*, and *Anaplasma* (Table 3-18). *Rickettsia* spp. are classically divided into the typhus group and spotted fever group (SFG). *Orientia* spp. make up the scrub typhus group. The rickettsial pathogens most likely to be encountered during travel outside the United States include *R. africae* (African tick-bite fever), *R. conorii* (Mediterranean spotted fever), *R. rickettsii* (known as both Rocky Mountain spotted fever and Brazilian spotted fever), *O. tsutsugamushi* (scrub typhus), and *R. typhi* (murine or fleaborne typhus).

TRANSMISSION

Most rickettsial pathogens are transmitted by ectoparasites such as fleas, lice, mites, and ticks. Organisms can be transmitted by bites from these ectoparasites or by inoculating infectious fluids or feces from the ectoparasites into the skin. Inhaling or inoculating conjunctiva with infectious material may also cause infection for some of these organisms. The specific vectors that transmit each rickettsial pathogen are listed in Table 3-18. Transmission of some rickettsial diseases after transfusion or organ transplantation is rare but has been reported.

EPIDEMIOLOGY

All age groups are at risk for rickettsial infections during travel to endemic areas. Both short and long-term travelers are at risk for infection. Transmission is increased during outdoor activities in the spring and summer months when ticks and fleas are most active; however, infection can occur throughout the year. Because of the 5- to 14-day incubation period for most rickettsial diseases, tourists often do not experience symptoms during their trip, and disease onset may coincide with their return home or develop within a week after returning. Although the most commonly diagnosed rickettsial diseases in travelers are usually in the spotted fever or typhus groups, travelers may acquire a wide range of rickettsioses, including emerging and newly recognized species (Table 3-18).

Tickborne spotted fever rickettsioses are the most frequently reported travel-associated rickettsial infections. Those who go on safari—especially those walking in the bush, game hunters, and ecotourists in southern Africa—are at risk for African tick-bite fever, which consistently remains the most commonly reported rickettsial infection acquired during travel. Mediterranean spotted fever is less commonly reported but occurs over an even larger region, including much of Europe, Africa, India, and the Middle East. Rocky Mountain spotted fever (also known as Brazilian spotted fever and other local names) is reported throughout much of the Western Hemisphere, including Canada, the United States, Mexico, and several countries in Central and South America including Argentina, Brazil, Colombia, Costa Rica, and Panama. Clusters of illness may be reported in families or in geographic areas. Contact with dogs in rural and urban settings and outdoor activities such as hiking, hunting, fishing, and camping increase the risk of infection.

Scrub typhus, which is transmitted by trombiculid mites encountered in high grass and brush, is endemic in northern Japan, Southeast Asia, the western Pacific Islands, northern Australia, China,

Table 3-18. Classification, primary vector, and reservoir occurrence of rickettsiae known to cause disease in humans

ANTIGENIC GROUP	DISEASE	SPECIES	VECTOR	ANIMAL RESERVOIR(S)	GEOGRAPHIC DISTRIBUTION
Anaplasma	Human anaplasmosis	Anaplasma phagocytophilum A. platys A. ovis "A. capra"	Tick	Small mammals, rodents, deer Dogs Sheep Goats	Primarily United States, worldwide Venezuela Cyprus, Iran China
Ehrlichia	Human ehrlichiosis	Ehrlichia chaffeensis E. muris E. ewingii E. canis	Tick	Deer, wild and domestic dogs, domestic ruminants, rodents Dogs	Common in United States, possibly worldwide Venezuela
Neoehrlichia	Neoehrlichiosis	Neoehrlichia mikurensis	Tick	Rodents	Europe, Asia
Neorickettsia	Sennetsu fever, neorickettsiosis	Neorickettsia sennetsu	Trematode (ingestion)	Fish	Japan, Malaysia, possibly other parts of Asia
Scrub typhus	Scrub typhus	Orientia tsutsugamushi	Larval mite (chigger)	Rodents	Asia-Pacific region from maritime Russia and China to Indonesia and North Australia to Afghanistan
Spotted fever	Rickettsiosis	Rickettsia aeschlimannii	Tick	Unknown	South Africa, Morocco, Mediterranean littoral
	African tick-bite fever	R. africae	Tick	Ruminants	Sub-Saharan Africa, West Indies
	Rickettsialpox	R. akari	Mite	House mice, wild rodents	Countries of the former Soviet Union, South Africa, Korea, Turkey, Balkan countries, United States

Disease	Organism	Vector	Reservoir	Distribution
Queensland tick typhus	*R. australis*	Tick	Rodents	Australia, Tasmania
Mediterranean spotted fever or Boutonneuse fever	*R. conorii*	Tick	Dogs, rodents	Southern Europe, southern and western Asia, Africa, India
Cat flea rickettsiosis	*R. felis*	Flea	Domestic cats, rodents, opossums	Europe, North and South America, Africa, Asia
Far Eastern spotted fever	*R. heilongjiangensis*	Tick	Rodents	Far East of Russia, Northern China, eastern Asia
Aneruptive fever	*R. helvetica*	Tick	Rodents	Central and northern Europe, Asia
Flinders Island spotted fever, Thai tick typhus	*R. honei*, including strain "marmionii"	Tick	Rodents, reptiles	Australia, Thailand
Japanese spotted fever	*R. japonica*	Tick	Rodents	Japan
Mediterranean spotted fever–like disease	*R. massiliae*	Tick	Unknown	France, Greece, Spain, Portugal, Switzerland, Sicily, central Africa, Mali, and Argentina
Mediterranean spotted fever–like illness	*R. monacensis*	Tick	Lizards, possibly birds	Europe, North Africa
Maculatum infection; Tidewater spotted fever; American boutonneuse fever	*R. parkeri*	Tick	Rodents	North and South America
Tickborne lymphadenopathy, *Dermacentor*-borne necrosis and lymphadenopathy	*R. raoultii*	Tick	Unknown	Europe, Asia
Rocky Mountain spotted fever Brazilian spotted fever	*R. rickettsia*	Tick	Rodents	North, Central, and South America
North Asian tick typhus, Siberian tick typhus	*R. sibirica*	Tick	Rodents	Russia, China, Mongolia
Lymphangitis-associated rickettsiosis	*R. sibirica mongolotimonae*	Tick	Rodents	Southern France, Portugal, China, Africa

(continued)

3

Table 3-18. Classification, primary vector, and reservoir occurrence of rickettsiae known to cause disease in humans (continued)

ANTIGENIC GROUP	DISEASE	SPECIES	VECTOR	ANIMAL RESERVOIR(S)	GEOGRAPHIC DISTRIBUTION
	Tickborne lymphadenopathy (TIBOLA), *Dermacentor*-borne necrosis and lymphadenopathy (DEBONEL)	*R. slovaca*	Tick	Lagomorphs, rodents	Southern and eastern Europe, Asia
Typhus fever	Epidemic typhus, sylvatic typhus	*R. prowazekii*	Human body louse, flying squirrel ectoparasites, possibly some ticks	Humans, flying squirrels	Central Africa; Asia; Central, North, and South America
	Murine typhus, fleaborne typhus	*R. typhi*	Flea	Rodents	Tropical and subtropical areas worldwide

maritime areas, and several parts of south-central Russia, India, and Sri Lanka. More than 1 million cases occur annually. Most travel-acquired cases of scrub typhus occur during visits to rural areas in endemic countries for activities such as camping, hiking, or rafting, but urban cases have also been described.

R. typhi and R. felis, which are transmitted by fleas, are widely distributed, especially throughout the tropics and subtropics and in port cities and coastal regions with rodents. Humans exposed to flea-infested cats, dogs, and peridomestic animals while traveling in endemic regions, or who enter or sleep in areas infested with rodents, are at most risk for fleaborne rickettsioses. Murine typhus has been reported among travelers returning from southeastern Asia, Africa, and the Mediterranean Basin. In the United States, most cases are reported from Hawaii, California, and Texas.

R. akari, the causative agent of rickettsialpox, is transmitted by house-mouse mites, and circulates in mainly urban centers in Ukraine, South Africa, Korea, the Balkan states, and the United States. Outbreaks of rickettsialpox most often occur after contact with infected rodents and their mites, especially during natural die-offs or exterminations of infected rodents that cause the mites to seek out new hosts, including humans. The agent may spill over and occasionally be found in other wild rodent populations.

Epidemic typhus caused by R. prowazekii infection is rarely reported among tourists but can occur in impoverished communities and refugee populations where body lice are prevalent. Outbreaks often occur during colder months.

Travelers at most risk for epidemic typhus include those who may visit areas with large homeless populations, impoverished areas, refugee camps, and regions that have recently experienced war or natural disasters. Active foci of epidemic typhus are known in the Andes regions of South America and some parts of Africa (including but not limited to Burundi, Ethiopia, and Rwanda). Louseborne epidemic typhus does not regularly occur in the United States, but a zoonotic reservoir occurs in the southern flying squirrel, and sporadic sylvatic typhus cases are reported. Tick-associated reservoirs of R. prowazekii have been described in Ethiopia, Mexico, and Brazil, but the role of ticks in the natural transmission of R. prowazekii has not been characterized.

Ehrlichiosis and anaplasmosis are tickborne infections most commonly reported in the United States. A variety of species are implicated in infection, but E. chaffeensis and A. phagocytophilum are most common. Infections with various Ehrlichia and Anaplasma spp. have also been reported in Europe, Asia, and South America. Neoehrlichia mikurensis is a tickborne pathogen that occurs in Europe and Asia and perhaps in Africa. Sennetsu fever, caused by Neorickettsia sennetsu, occurs in Japan, Malaysia, and possibly other parts of Asia. This disease can be contracted from eating raw infected fish.

CLINICAL PRESENTATION

Rickettsioses are difficult to diagnose, even by health care providers experienced with these diseases. Most symptomatic rickettsial diseases cause a moderately severe illness, but some, such as Rocky Mountain spotted fever, Mediterranean spotted fever, scrub typhus, and epidemic typhus, may be life threatening and can be fatal in 20%–60% of untreated cases, so prompt treatment is essential.

Clinical presentations vary with the causative agent and patient; however, common symptoms that typically develop within 1–2 weeks of infection include fever, headache, malaise, rash, nausea, and vomiting. Many rickettsioses are accompanied by a maculopapular, vesicular, or petechial rash or sometimes an eschar at the site of the tick bite. African tick-bite fever is typically milder than some other rickettsioses, but recovery is improved with treatment. It should be suspected in a patient who presents with fever, headache, myalgia, and an eschar (tache noir) after recent travel to southern Africa. Mediterranean spotted fever is a potentially life-threatening rickettsial infection and should be suspected in patients with rash, fever, and eschar after recent travel to northern Africa or the Mediterranean. Rocky Mountain spotted fever is frequently characterized by fever, headache, nausea, and abdominal pain; a rash is commonly reported, but eschars are not. Scrub typhus should be suspected in patients with a fever, headache, and myalgia after recent travel to Asia; eschar, lymphadenopathy, cough, and

3

encephalitis may be present. Patients with murine or epidemic typhus usually present with a severe but nonspecific febrile illness, and approximately half will also present with a rash. Ehrlichiosis and anaplasmosis should be suspected in febrile patients with leukopenia and thrombocytopenia and mild to moderately elevated levels of hepatic transaminases.

DIAGNOSIS

Diagnosis is usually based on clinical recognition and serology. Serologic testing provides stronger evidence when acute- and convalescent-phase serum samples are compared; a ≥4-fold rise in titer is diagnostic. PCR assays and immunohisto-chemical analyses may also be helpful, but useful results are highly dependent upon the specimen submitted. If an eschar is present, a swab or biopsy sample of the lesion can be evaluated by PCR and provides a species-specific diagnosis. If ehrlichio-sis or anaplasmosis is suspected, PCR of a whole-blood specimen provides the best diagnostic test. A buffy coat may provide presumptive evidence of infection if examined to identify characteris-tic intraleukocytic morulae. Contact the CDC Rickettsial Zoonoses Branch at 404-639-1075 for further information. Ehrlichiosis, anaplasmosis, and spotted fever rickettsiosis are nationally noti-fiable diseases.

TREATMENT

Treatment of patients with possible rickettsioses should be started when disease is suspected and should never await confirmatory testing, as certain infections can be rapidly progressive.

Immediate empiric treatment with a tetracycline, most commonly doxycycline, is recommended for all ages. Almost all other broad-spectrum antibi-otics are not helpful. Chloramphenicol may be an alternative in some cases, but its use is associated with more deaths, particularly for *R. rickettsii*. In some areas, tetracycline-resistant scrub typhus has been reported. Azithromycin may be an effec-tive alternative. *Anaplasma phagocytophilum* infections may respond to rifampin, which may be an alternate drug for pregnant patients. Expert advice should be sought if alternative agents are being considered.

PREVENTION

No vaccine is available for preventing rickettsial infections. Antibiotics are not recommended for prophylaxis of rickettsial diseases and should not be given to asymptomatic people.

Travelers should be instructed to minimize exposure to biting arthropods during travel (including lice, fleas, ticks, mites) and to animal reservoirs (particularly dogs) when traveling in endemic areas. The proper use of insect or tick repellents on skin or clothing, self-examination after visits to vector-infested areas, and wearing protective clothing are ways to reduce risk. These precautions are especially important for people with underlying conditions that may compro-mise their immune systems, as these people may be more susceptible to severe disease. For more detailed information, see Chapter 2, Protection against Mosquitoes, Ticks, & Other Arthropods.

CDC website: www.cdc.gov/ticks

BIBLIOGRAPHY

1. Biggs HM, Behravesh CB, Bradley KK, Dahlgren FS, Drexler NA, Dumler JS, et al. Diagnosis and manage-ment of tickborne rickettsial diseases: Rocky Mountain spotted fever and other spotted fever group rickett-sioses, ehrlichioses, and anaplasmosisUnited States. MMWR Recomm Rep. 2016;65(2):1–44.

2. Demeester R, Claus M, Hildebrand M, Vlieghe E, Bottieau E. Diversity of life-threatening complications due to Mediterranean spotted fever in returning travel-ers. J Travel Med. 2010 Mar-Apr;17(2):100–4.

3. Hendershot EF, Sexton DJ. Scrub typhus and rickettsial diseases in international travelers: a review. Curr Infect Dis Rep. 2009 Jan;11(1):66–72.

4. Jensenius M, Davis X, von Sonnenburg F, Schwartz E, Keystone JS, Leder K, et al. Multicenter GeoSentinel analysis of rickettsial diseases in international travelers, 1996–2008. Emerg Infect Dis. 2009 Nov;15(11):1791–8.

5. Li H, Zheng YC, Ma L, Jia N, Jiang BG, Jiang RR, et al. Human infection with a novel tick-borne *Anaplasma* species in China: a surveillance study. Lancet Infect Dis. 2015 Jun;15(6):663–70.

6. Nachega JB, Bottieau E, Zech F, Van Gompel A. Travel-acquired scrub typhus: emphasis on the differential diagnosis, treatment, and prevention strategies. J Travel Med. 2007 Sep-Oct;14(5):352–5.

7. Paddock CD, Fernandez S, Echenique GA, Sumner JW, Reeves WK, Zaki SR, et al. Rocky Mountain spotted fever in Argentina. Am J Trop Med Hyg. 2008 Apr;78(4):687–92.

8. Raoult D, Parola P, editors. Rickettsial Diseases. New York: Informa Healthcare USA, Inc; 2007.

9. Roch N, Epaulard O, Pelloux I, Pavese P, Brion JP, Raoult D, et al. African tick bite fever in elderly patients: 8 cases in French tourists returning from South Africa. Clin Infect Dis. 2008 Aug 1;47(3):e28–35.

10. Silaghi C, Beck R, Oteo JA, Pfeffer M, Sprong H. Neoehrlichiosis: an emerging tick-borne zoonosis caused by *Candidatus* Neoehrlichia mikurensis. Exp Appl Acarol. 2016 Mar;68(3):279–97.

RUBELLA

Emmaculate J. Lebo, Cristina V. Cardemil, Susan E. Reef

INFECTIOUS AGENT

Rubella virus (family Togaviridae, genus *Rubivirus).*

TRANSMISSION

Person-to-person contact or droplets shed from the respiratory secretions of infected people. People may shed virus from 7 days before the onset of the rash to approximately 5–7 days after rash onset. Transmission from mother to fetus can also occur, with the highest risk of congenital rubella syndrome (CRS) if infection occurs in the first trimester. Infants with CRS can transmit virus for up to 1 year after birth.

EPIDEMIOLOGY

Even though endemic rubella virus transmission was declared eliminated in the Americas in 2015, rubella virus continues to circulate widely, especially in Africa, the Middle East, and South and Southeast Asia. Globally, >100,000 infants are born each year with CRS, and >80% of those are born in Africa and some countries in South and Southeast Asia. In the United States, endemic rubella virus transmission was interrupted in 2001 and elimination was verified in 2004, but imported cases continue to occur. From 2004 through 2015, a median of 9 (range, 3–18) imported cases were reported annually in the United States, and 9 CRS cases were reported during the same period.

CLINICAL PRESENTATION

Average incubation period is 14 days (range, 12–23 days). Usually presents as a nonspecific, maculopapular, generalized rash that lasts ≤3 days with generalized lymphadenopathy. Rash may be preceded by low-grade fever, malaise, anorexia, mild conjunctivitis, runny nose, and sore throat. Adolescents and adults, especially women, can also present with transient arthritis. Asymptomatic rubella virus infections are common. Infection during early pregnancy can lead to miscarriage, fetal death, or CRS with severe birth defects.

DIAGNOSIS

Demonstration of specific rubella IgM or significant increase in rubella IgG in acute- and convalescent-phase specimens. RT-PCR can be used to detect virus infection; viral culture is also acceptable but is time-consuming and expensive. Rubella is a nationally notifiable disease.

TREATMENT

Supportive care.

PREVENTION

All travelers aged ≥12 months who do not have acceptable evidence of immunity to rubella (documented by ≥1 dose of rubella-containing vaccine on or after the first birthday, laboratory evidence of immunity, or birth before 1957) should be vaccinated with measles-mumps-rubella (MMR) vaccine. Before departure from the United States, infants aged 6–11 months should receive 1 dose of MMR vaccine (for measles protection), and children aged ≥12 months and adults should receive 2 doses of MMR vaccine ≥28 days apart on or after the first birthday. MMR vaccine is contraindicated during pregnancy. Pregnant women who do not have acceptable evidence of rubella immunity should not travel to countries where rubella is endemic or areas with known rubella outbreaks, especially during the first 20 weeks of pregnancy, and should be vaccinated immediately postpartum. Health care providers should also ensure that all women of childbearing age and recent immigrants are up-to-date on their immunization against rubella or have evidence of immunity to rubella, because these groups are at the highest risk for maternal-fetal transmission of rubella virus.

CDC website: www.cdc.gov/rubella

BIBLIOGRAPHY

1. CDC. Rubella. In: Hamborsky J, Kroger A, Wolfe S, editors. Epidemiology and Prevention of Vaccine-Preventable Diseases. 13th ed. Washington, DC: Public Health Foundation; 2015. pp. 275–89.

2. CDC. Summary of notifiable infectious diseases and conditions—United States, 2013. MMWR Morb Mortal Wkly Rep. 2015 Oct 23;62(53):1–122.

3. Papania MJ, Wallace GS, Rota PA, Icenogle JP, Fiebelkorn AP, Armstrong GL, et al. Elimination of endemic measles, rubella, and congenital rubella syndrome from the Western hemisphere: the US experience. JAMA Pediatr. 2014 Feb;168(2):148–55.

4. Reef SE, Plotkin SA. Rubella vaccine. In: Plotkin SA, Orenstein WA, Offit PA, editors. Vaccines. 6th ed. Philadelphia: Saunders Elsevier; 2012. pp. 688–717.

5. Reef SE, Redd SB, Abernathy E, Kutty P, Icenogle JP. Evidence used to support the achievement and maintenance of elimination of rubella and congenital rubella syndrome in the United States. J Infect Dis. 2011 Sep 1;204 Suppl 2:S593–7.

6. Vynnycky E, Adams EJ, Cutts FT, Reef SE, Navar AM, Simons E, et al. Using seroprevalence and immunisation coverage data to estimate the global burden of congenital rubella syndrome, 1996–2010: a systematic review. PLoS One. 2016;11(3):e0149160.

7. World Health Organization. Rubella vaccines: WHO position paper. Wkly Epidemiol Rec. 2011 July 15, 2011;86(29):301–16.

SALMONELLOSIS (NONTYPHOIDAL)

Jennifer C. Hunter, Louise K. Francois Watkins

INFECTIOUS AGENT

Salmonella enterica subspecies *enterica* is a gram-negative, rod-shaped bacillus. More than 2,500 *Salmonella* serotypes have been identified. Nontyphoidal salmonellosis refers to illnesses caused by all serotypes of *Salmonella* except for Typhi, Paratyphi A, Paratyphi B (tartrate negative), and Paratyphi C.

TRANSMISSION

Usually through the consumption of food or water contaminated with animal feces. Transmission can also occur through direct contact with infected animals or their environment and directly between humans.

EPIDEMIOLOGY

Nontyphoidal salmonellae are a leading cause of bacterial diarrhea worldwide; they are estimated to cause approximately 153 million cases of gastroenteritis and 57,000 deaths globally each year. The risk of *Salmonella* infection among travelers returning to the United States varies by region of the world visited. The incidence of laboratory-confirmed infections from 2004 through 2009 was 7.1 cases per 100,000 among travelers to

Latin America and the Caribbean, 5.8 cases per 100,000 among travelers to Asia, and 25.8 cases per 100,000 among travelers to Africa. The true number of illnesses is much higher, because most ill people do not have a stool specimen tested. US travelers with salmonellosis were most likely to report visiting the following countries: Mexico (38% of travel-associated salmonellosis), India (9%), Jamaica (7%), the Dominican Republic (4%), China (3%), and the Bahamas (2%); these findings are influenced by the number of travelers to different destinations. A systematic review of travelers' diarrhea etiology studies published from 2002 through 2011 found that *Salmonella* was detected in <5% of patients who had traveled to Latin America, the Caribbean, and South Asia and in 5%–15% of patients who had traveled to Africa or Southeast Asia. *Salmonella* infection and carriage have been reported among internationally adopted children.

CLINICAL PRESENTATION

Gastroenteritis is the most common clinical presentation of nontyphoidal *Salmonella* infection. The incubation period is typically 6–72 hours; while atypical, illness has been documented even 14 days after exposure. Illness is commonly manifested as acute diarrhea, abdominal pain, fever, and sometimes vomiting. The illness usually lasts 4–7 days, and most people recover without treatment. Approximately 5% of people develop bacteremia or focal infection (such as meningitis or osteomyelitis). Salmonellosis outcomes differ by serotype. Infections with some serotypes, including Dublin and Choleraesuis, are more likely to result in invasive infections. Rates of invasive infections and death are generally higher among infants, older adults, and people with immunosuppressive conditions (including HIV), hemoglobinopathies, and malignant neoplasms. Infection with antibiotic-resistant organisms has been associated with a higher risk of bloodstream infection and hospitalization.

DIAGNOSIS

Culturing organisms continues to be the mainstay of clinical diagnostic testing for nontyphoidal *Salmonella* infection. Approximately 90% of isolates are obtained from routine stool culture, but isolates are also obtained from blood, urine, abscesses, cerebrospinal fluid, and other sites of infection. Although culture-independent diagnostic tests are increasingly used by clinical laboratories to diagnose *Salmonella* infection, isolates are needed for serotyping and antimicrobial susceptibility testing. *Salmonella* isolate submission requirements vary by state, but most states mandate that *Salmonella* isolates or clinical material be submitted to the local or state public health laboratory. To understand submission requirements in a particular state, clinical laboratories are advised to review the disease reporting and mandatory isolate submission regulations of that state. Salmonellosis is a nationally notifiable disease.

TREATMENT

Current recommendations are to treat most patients with uncomplicated *Salmonella* infection with oral rehydration therapy but not with antimicrobial agents. Antimicrobial therapy should be considered for patients who are severely ill (for example, those with severe diarrhea, high fever, or manifestations of extraintestinal infection) and for people at increased risk of invasive disease (infants, older adults, and the debilitated or immunosuppressed). When antimicrobial therapy is indicated, empiric treatment is usually required until susceptibility data are available. Resistance to antimicrobial agents varies by serotype and geographic region. Fluoroquinolones are considered first-line treatment in adult travelers. However, resistance to fluoroquinolones among *Salmonella* strains is rising globally. In a study of international travelers diagnosed with *S. enterica* serotype Enteritidis infection in the United States, 24% of isolates showed decreased susceptibility to fluoroquinolones compared with only 3% of isolates from patients with no history of international travel. Azithromycin can be used for children and is an alternative agent for adults returning from Latin America or Asia, where resistance in this organism to fluoroquinolones may exceed 10%. Azithromycin resistance has been documented in multiple settings globally but is not commonly reported. Resistance to older antimicrobial agents (chloramphenicol, ampicillin, and trimethoprim-sulfamethoxazole) has been present for many years; these should not be considered first-line empiric agents in returning travelers (see Chapter 2, Travelers' Diarrhea).

PREVENTION

No vaccine is available against nontyphoidal *Salmonella* infection. Preventive measures are aimed at avoiding foods and drinks at high risk for contamination; frequent handwashing, especially after contacting animals or their environment; and taking food and water precautions (see Chapter 2, Food & Water Precautions).

CDC website: www.cdc.gov/salmonella

BIBLIOGRAPHY

1. American Public Health Association. Salmonellosis. In: Heymann DL, editor. Control of Communicable Diseases Manual. 19th ed. Washington, DC: American Public Health Association; 2008. pp. 534–40.
2. Association of Public Health Laboratories. State legal requirements for submission of isolates and other clinical materials by clinical laboratories: a review of state approaches 2015 [cited 2016 Sep. 26]. Available from: https://www.aphl.org/aboutAPHL/publications/Documents/StateRequirements_Appendix_v6.pdf.
3. Brooks JT, Matyas BT, Fontana J, DeGroot MA, Beuchat LR, Hoekstra M, et al. An outbreak of *Salmonella* serotype Typhimurium infections with an unusually long incubation period. Foodborne Pathog Dis. 2012 Mar;9(3):245–8.
4. Iwamoto M, Huang JY, Cronquist AB, Medus C, Hurd S, Zansky S, et al. Bacterial enteric infections detected by culture-independent diagnostic tests—FoodNet, United States, 2012–2014. MMWR Morb Mortal Wkly Rep. 2015 Mar 13;64(9):252–7.
5. Johnson LR, Gould LH, Dunn JR, Berkelman R, Mahon BE, FoodNet Travel Working Group. *Salmonella* infections associated with international travel: a Foodborne Diseases Active Surveillance Network (FoodNet) study. Foodborne Pathog Dis. 2011 Sep;8(9):1031–7.
6. Jones TF, Ingram LA, Cieslak PR, Vugia DJ, Tobin-D'Angelo M, Hurd S, et al. Salmonellosis outcomes differ substantially by serotype. J Infect Dis. 2008 Jul 1; 198(1):109–14.
7. Kendall ME, Crim S, Fullerton K, Han PV, Cronquist AB, Shiferaw B, et al. Travel-associated enteric infections diagnosed after return to the United States, Foodborne Diseases Active Surveillance Network (FoodNet), 2004–2009. Clin Infect Dis. 2012 Jun;54 Suppl 5:S480–7.
8. Kirk MD, Pires SM, Black RE, Caipo M, Crump JA, Devleesschauwer B, et al. World Health Organization estimates of the global and regional disease burden of 22 foodborne bacterial, protozoal, and viral diseases, 2010: a data synthesis. PLoS Med. 2015 Dec;12(12):e1001921.
9. O'Donnell AT, Vieira AR, Huang JY, Whichard J, Cole D, Karp BE. Quinolone-resistant *Salmonella enterica* serotype Enteritidis infections associated with international travel. Clin Infect Dis. 2014 Nov 1;59(9):e139–41.
10. Steffen R, Hill DR, DuPont HL. Traveler's diarrhea: a clinical review. JAMA. 2015 Jan 6;313(1):71–80.

SARCOCYSTOSIS

Douglas H. Esposito

INFECTIOUS AGENT

Intracellular coccidian protozoan parasites in the genus *Sarcocystis*.

TRANSMISSION

Humans are the natural definitive host for *Sarcocystis hominis* and *S. suihominis*, acquired by eating undercooked sarcocyst-containing beef or pork. Aberrant, dead-end intermediate-host infection can occur in humans with *S. nesbitti* and possibly other species when food, water, or soil contaminated with the feces from a sporocyst-shedding definitive host (likely a reptile) are ingested.

EPIDEMIOLOGY

Human intestinal sarcocystosis occurs worldwide, but the prevalence is poorly defined and may vary regionally. Outbreaks of symptomatic muscular sarcocystosis among tourists in Malaysia suggest that intermediate-host infection may be of public health significance. Most reported cases have been acquired in the tropics and subtropics, particularly in Southeast Asia.

CLINICAL PRESENTATION

Most people with intestinal sarcocystosis are asymptomatic or experience mild gastroenteritis, though severe illness has been described. Differences in symptoms and illness severity and duration may reflect the number and species of the sarcocysts ingested. The disease is thought to be self-limited in immunocompetent hosts.

Intermediate-host infection may range from asymptomatic to severe and debilitating. In those with symptoms, onset occurs in the first 2 weeks after infection, and symptoms typically resolve in weeks to months. However, some patients may remain symptomatic for years. The most common symptoms are fever, fatigue, myalgia, headache, cough, and arthralgia. Less frequent are wheezing, nausea, vomiting, diarrhea, rash, lymphadenopathy, and symptoms reflecting cardiac involvement such as palpitations. Fever and muscle pain may be relapsing and can occur in 2 distinct phases: early (beginning during the second week after infection) and late (beginning during the sixth week after infection). Early-phase disease may reflect a generalized vasculitis, and late-phase disease may coincide with the onset of a diffuse focal myositis.

DIAGNOSIS

Intestinal sarcocystosis should be considered in patients with gastroenteritis and a history of eating raw or undercooked meat. Oocysts or sporocysts can be confirmed in stool by light or fluorescence microscopy; PCR is not widely available, and no serologic assays have been validated for use in humans.

Muscular sarcocystosis should be considered in people presenting with myalgia, with or without fever, and a history of travel to a tropical or subtropical region, especially Malaysia. However, diagnosis during the early phase of infection is difficult because of the lack of specificity of symptoms and clinical and laboratory findings. In the absence of an alternate diagnosis, serial investigations for evidence of myositis and eosinophilia should be considered. In those with myositis, trichinellosis should be excluded. Confirmation of muscular sarcocystosis requires biopsy and histologic observation of sarcocysts in muscle. Diagnostic assistance is available through CDC (www.cdc.gov/dpdx; dpdx@cdc.gov).

TREATMENT

There are no proven medical treatments for sarcocystosis. Trimethoprim-sulfamethoxazole may have activity against schizonts in the early phase of muscular sarcocystosis, but data are scant. Glucocorticoids and nonsteroidal antiinflammatories may improve the symptoms associated with myositis.

PREVENTION

Intestinal sarcocystosis can be prevented by thoroughly cooking or freezing meat, which kills the infective bradyzoites. Muscular sarcocystosis can be prevented with standard food and water precautions (see Chapter 2: Food & Water Precautions).

CDC website: www.cdc.gov/parasites/ sarcocystosis/index.html

BIBLIOGRAPHY

1. Arness MK, Brown JD, Dubey JP, Neafie RC, Granstrom DE. An outbreak of acute eosinophilic myositis attributed to human *Sarcocystis* parasitism. Am J Trop Med Hyg. 1999 Oct;61(4):548–53.

2. Esposito DH, Stich A, Epelboin L, Malvy D, Han PV, Bottieau E, et al. Acute muscular sarcocystosis: an international investigation among ill travelers returning from Tioman Island, Malaysia, 2011–2012. Clin Infect Dis. 2014 Nov 15;59(10):1401–10.

3. Fayer R, Esposito DH, Dubey JP. Human infections with *Sarcocystis* species. Clin Microbiol Rev. 2015 Apr;28(2):295–311.

4. Italiano CM, Wong KT, AbuBakar S, Lau YL, Ramli N, Syed Omar SF, et al. *Sarcocystis nesbitti* causes

acute, relapsing febrile myositis with a high attack rate: description of a large outbreak of muscular sarcocystosis in Pangkor Island, Malaysia, 2012. PLoS Negl Trop Dis. 2014 May;8(5):e2876.

5. Slesak G, Schafer J, Langeheinecke A, Tappe D. Prolonged clinical course of muscular sarcocystosis and effectiveness of cotrimoxazole among travelers to Tioman Island, Malaysia, 2011–2014. Clin Infect Dis. 2015 Jan 15;60(2):329.

6. Tappe D, Stich A, Langeheinecke A, von Sonnenburg F, Muntau B, Schafer J, et al. Suspected new wave of muscular sarcocystosis in travellers returning from Tioman Island, Malaysia, May 2014. Euro Surveill. 2014;19(21).

SCABIES

Diana Martin

INFECTIOUS AGENT

The human itch mite, *Sarcoptes scabiei* var. *hominis*.

TRANSMISSION

Transmission of scabies occurs through prolonged skin-to-skin contact with a person with conventional scabies. Crusted scabies (formerly called Norwegian scabies) is a more severe form of scabies in which a person is infested with a large number of mites and is more highly contagious. Indirect transmission may occur through contact with objects contaminated by a person with crusted scabies but is rare if the person has conventional scabies.

EPIDEMIOLOGY

Scabies occurs worldwide and is transmitted most easily in settings where skin contact is common. Crusted scabies most commonly occurs among elderly, disabled, debilitated, or immunosuppressed people, often in institutional settings. Skin conditions are the most common complaint among European travelers to tropical countries, and scabies is a more common skin infection among travelers with longer travel (>8 weeks).

CLINICAL PRESENTATION

Symptoms occur 2–6 weeks after a person is first infested. However, if someone has had scabies before, symptoms appear much sooner (1–4 days after exposure). Conventional scabies is characterized by intense itching, particularly at night, and by a papular or papulovesicular erythematous rash. Crusted scabies is characterized by widespread crusts and scales that contain large numbers of mites, although itching may be less than in conventional scabies.

DIAGNOSIS

Scabies is generally diagnosed by identifying burrows in a patient with itching and by observing the characteristic rash. Diagnosis can be confirmed by microscopically identifying mites, mite eggs, or scybala (mite feces); however, microscopic identification of mites is far less sensitive than clinical diagnosis. Crusted scabies is often misdiagnosed as psoriasis but can be accurately diagnosed using skin scrapings due to the high number of mites in the sores.

TREATMENT

Permethrin (5%) cream is considered by many to be the drug of choice. Ivermectin is reported to be safe and effective to treat scabies. Ivermectin is not currently FDA-approved for scabies but can be considered for off-label use in patients in whom treatment has failed or who cannot tolerate other approved medications. Crusted scabies must be treated more aggressively; a combination of permethrin and ivermectin is recommended.

PREVENTION

Avoid prolonged skin-to-skin contact with people who have conventional scabies and even brief skin-to-skin contact with people who have crusted scabies. Contact with items such as clothing and bed linens that have been used by an infested person should be avoided, especially if the person has crusted scabies.

BIBLIOGRAPHY

1. Ansart S, Perez L, Jaureguiberry S, Danis M, Bricaire F, Caumes E. Spectrum of dermatoses in 165 travelers returning from the tropics with skin diseases. Am J Trop Med Hyg. 2007 Jan;76(1):184–6.

2. Bouvresse S, Chosidow O. Scabies in healthcare settings. Curr Opin Infect Dis. 2010 Apr;23(2):111–8.

3. Chosidow O. Clinical practices. Scabies. N Engl J Med. 2006 Apr 20;354(16):1718–27.

4. Currie BJ, McCarthy JS. Permethrin and ivermectin for scabies. N Engl J Med. 2010 Feb 25;362(8):717–25.

5. Davis JS, McGloughlin S, Tong SY, Walton SF, Currie BJ. A novel clinical grading scale to guide the management of crusted scabies. PLoS Negl Trop Dis. 2013;7(9):e2387.

6. Davis RF, Johnston GA, Sladden MJ. Recognition and management of common ectoparasitic diseases in travelers. Am J Clin Dermatol. 2009;10(1):1–8.

7. Hengge UR, Currie BJ, Jager G, Lupi O, Schwartz RA. Scabies: a ubiquitous neglected skin disease. Lancet Infect Dis. 2006 Dec;6(12):769–79.

8. Heukelbach J, Feldmeier H. Scabies. Lancet. 2006 May 27;367(9524):1767–74.

9. O'Brien BM. A practical approach to common skin problems in returning travellers. Travel Med Infect Dis. 2009 May;7(3):125–46.

CDC website: www.cdc.gov/parasites/scabies

SCHISTOSOMIASIS

Susan Montgomery

INFECTIOUS AGENT

Schistosomiasis is caused by helminth parasites of the genus *Schistosoma*. Other helminth infections are discussed in the Helminths, Soil-Transmitted section earlier in this chapter.

TRANSMISSION

Waterborne transmission occurs when larval cercariae, found in contaminated bodies of freshwater, penetrate the skin.

EPIDEMIOLOGY

An estimated 85% of the world's cases of schistosomiasis are in Africa, where prevalence rates can exceed 50% in local populations. *Schistosoma mansoni* and *S. haematobium* are distributed throughout Africa; only *S. haematobium* is found in areas of the Middle East, and *S. japonicum* is found in Indonesia and parts of China and Southeast Asia (Map 3-12). Although schistosomiasis had been eliminated in Europe for decades, transmission of *S. haematobium* was reported in Corsica in 2014, when cases were identified among travelers who had bathed in the Cavu River. Two other species can infect humans: *S. mekongi*, found in Cambodia and Laos, and *S. intercalatum*, found in parts of Central and West Africa. These 2 species are rarely reported causes of human infection. Many countries endemic for schistosomiasis have established control programs, but others have not. Countries where development has led to widespread improvements in sanitation and water safety, as well as successful schistosomiasis control programs, may have eliminated this disease. However, there are currently no international guidelines for certification of elimination.

All ages are at risk for infection from freshwater exposure in endemic areas. Swimming, bathing, and wading in contaminated freshwater can result in infection. Human schistosomiasis is not acquired by contact with saltwater (oceans or seas). The distribution of schistosomiasis is very focal and determined by the presence of competent snail vectors, inadequate sanitation, and

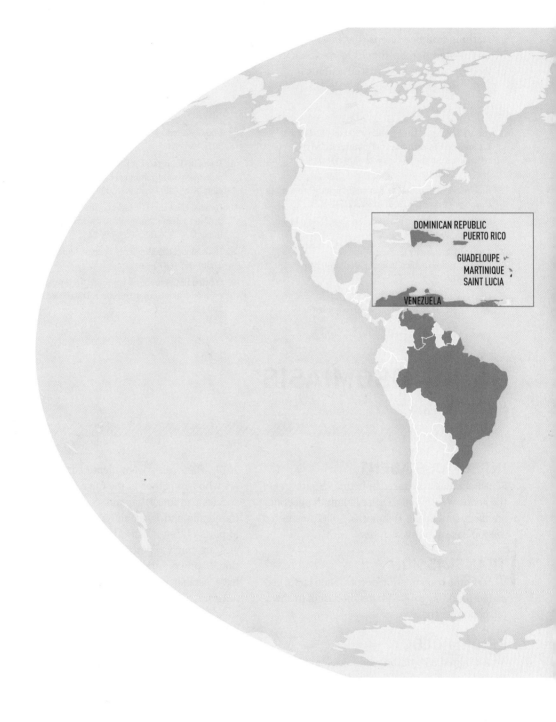

MAP 3-12. **Distribution of schistosomiasis**[1]

[1] The distribution of schistosomiasis is very focal; however, surveillance for schistosomiasis is limited in most countries. Therefore, this map shades entire countries where schistosomiasis transmission has been reported. The exception to this is France, where schistosomiasis has been reported on several islands, such as Guadeloupe, Martinique, and Corsica.

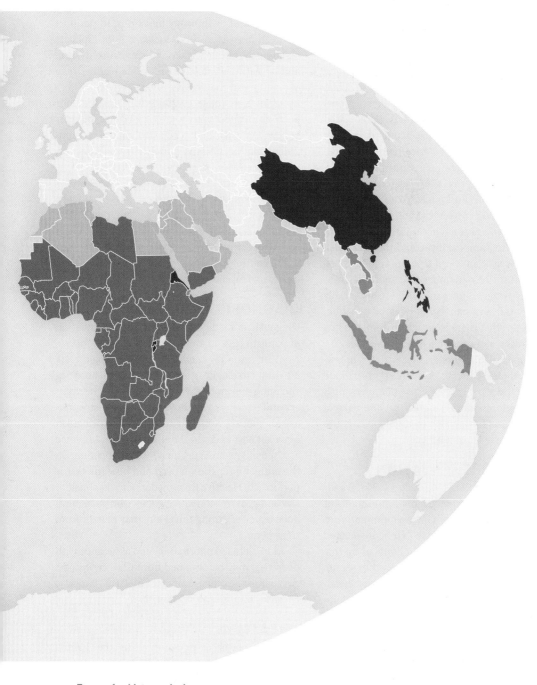

3

Types of schistosomiasis

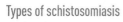 Low Risk for Hepatic-Intestinal

Low Risk for both Hepatic-Intestinal and Urinary

Low Risk for Urinary

Hepatic-Intestinal

Both Hepatic-Intestinal and Urinary

Not Endemic

infected humans. The specific snail vectors can be difficult to identify, and whether snails are infected with human schistosome species can only be determined in the laboratory.

The geographic distribution of cases of schistosomiasis acquired by travelers reflects travel and immigration patterns. Most travel-associated cases of schistosomiasis are acquired in sub-Saharan Africa. Sites in Africa frequently visited by travelers are common sites of infection. These sites include rivers and water sources in the Banfora region (Burkina Faso) and areas populated by the Dogon people (Mali), Lake Malawi, Lake Tanganyika, Lake Victoria, the Omo River (Ethiopia), the Zambezi River, and the Nile River. However, as visitors travel to more remote sites, it is important to remember that most freshwater surface water sources in Africa are potentially contaminated and can be sources of infection. A local claim that there is no schistosomiasis in a body of freshwater is not necessarily reliable.

The types of travelers and expatriates potentially at increased risk for infection include adventure travelers, Peace Corps volunteers, missionaries, soldiers, and ecotourists. Outbreaks of schistosomiasis have occurred among adventure travelers on river trips in Africa.

CLINICAL PRESENTATION

The incubation period is typically 14–84 days for acute schistosomiasis (Katayama syndrome), but chronic infection can remain asymptomatic for years. Penetration of cercariae can be associated with a rash that develops within hours or up to a week after contaminated water exposures. Acute schistosomiasis is characterized by fever, headache, myalgia, diarrhea, and respiratory symptoms. Eosinophilia is often present, as well as painful hepatomegaly or splenomegaly.

The clinical manifestations of chronic schistosomiasis are the result of host immune responses to schistosome eggs. Eggs, secreted by adult worm pairs living in the bloodstream, become lodged in the capillaries of organs and cause granulomatous reactions. *S. mansoni* and *S. japonicum* eggs most commonly lodge in the blood vessels of the liver or intestine and can cause diarrhea, constipation, and blood in the stool. Chronic inflammation can lead to bowel wall ulceration, hyperplasia, and

polyposis and, with heavy infections, to periportal liver fibrosis. *S. haematobium* eggs typically lodge in the urinary tract and can cause dysuria and hematuria. Calcifications in the bladder may appear late in the disease. *S. haematobium* infection can also cause genital symptoms and has been associated with increased risk of bladder cancer. As with acute schistosomiasis, eosinophilia may be present during chronic infection with any species.

Rarely, central nervous system manifestations of schistosomiasis may develop; this is thought to result from aberrant migration of adult worms or eggs depositing in the spinal cord or brain. Signs and symptoms are related to ectopic granulomas in the central nervous system and can present as transverse myelitis.

DIAGNOSIS

Diagnosis is made by microscopic identification of parasite eggs in stool (*S. mansoni* or *S. japonicum*) or urine (*S. haematobium*). Serologic tests are useful to diagnose light infections because egg shedding may not be consistent such as in travelers and in others who have not had schistosomiasis previously. Antibody tests do not distinguish between past and current infection. Immunologic test sensitivity and specificity vary, depending on the antigen preparation used and how the test is performed. Health care providers should consider screening asymptomatic people who may have been exposed during travel and may benefit from treatment.

More detailed information and assistance with diagnosis may be obtained from CDC (www.cdc.gov/parasites/schistosomiasis or CDC Parasitic Diseases Inquiries, 404-718-4745).

TREATMENT

Schistosomiasis is uncommon in the United States, and clinicians unfamiliar with management of schistosomiasis should consult an infectious disease or tropical medicine specialist for diagnosis and treatment. Praziquantel is used to treat schistosomiasis. Praziquantel is most effective against adult forms of the parasite and requires an immune response to the adult worm to be fully effective. Host immune response differences may affect individual response to treatment with praziquantel. Although a single course of treatment is usually curative, the immune response in lightly infected patients may be less robust, and repeat treatment may be needed after 2–4 weeks to increase effectiveness.

PREVENTION

No vaccine is available. No drugs for preventing infection are available. Preventive measures are primarily avoiding wading, swimming, or other contact with freshwater in disease-endemic countries. Untreated piped water coming directly from freshwater sources may contain cercariae, but filtering with fine-mesh filters, heating bathing water to 122°F (50°C) for 5 minutes, or allowing water to stand for ≥24 hours before exposure can prevent infection.

Swimming in adequately chlorinated swimming pools is safe, even in disease-endemic countries, although confirming adequate levels of chlorination is difficult. Vigorous towel-drying after accidental exposure to water has been suggested as a way to remove cercariae before they can penetrate, but this may only prevent some infections and should not be recommended as a preventive measure. Topical applications of insect repellents such as DEET can block penetrating cercariae, but the effect depends on the repellent formulation, may be short-lived, and cannot reliably prevent infection.

CDC website: www.cdc.gov/parasites/ schistosomiasis

BIBLIOGRAPHY

1. Berry A, Mone H, Iriart X, Mouahid G, Aboo O, Boissier J, et al. Schistosomiasis haematobium, Corsica, France. Emerg Infect Dis. 2014 Sep;20(9):1595–7.

2. Bierman WF, Wetsteyn JC, van Gool T. Presentation and diagnosis of imported schistosomiasis: relevance of eosinophilia, microscopy for ova, and serology. J Travel Med. 2005 Jan-Feb;12(1):9–13.

3. Clerinx J, Van Gompel A. Schistosomiasis in travellers and migrants. Travel Med Infect Dis. 2011 Jan;9(1):6–24.

4. Corachan M. Schistosomiasis and international travel. Clin Infect Dis. 2002 Aug 15;35(4):446–50.

5. Grobusch MP, Muhlberger N, Jelinek T, Bisoffi Z, Corachan M, Harms G, et al. Imported schistosomiasis in Europe: sentinel surveillance data from TropNetEurop. J Travel Med. 2003 May-Jun;10(3):164–9.

6. Meltzer E, Artom G, Marva E, Assous MV, Rahav G, Schwartzt E. Schistosomiasis among travelers: new aspects of an old disease. Emerg Infect Dis. 2006 Nov;12(11):1696–700.

7. Nicolls DJ, Weld LH, Schwartz E, Reed C, von Sonnenburg F, Freedman DO, et al. Characteristics of schistosomiasis in travelers reported to the GeoSentinel Surveillance Network 1997–2008. Am J Trop Med Hyg. 2008 Nov;79(5):729–34.

8. Ross AG, Bartley PB, Sleigh AC, Olds GR, Li Y, Williams GM, et al. Schistosomiasis. N Engl J Med. 2002 Apr 18;346(16):1212–20.

9. Ross AG, Vickers D, Olds GR, Shah SM, McManus DP. Katayama syndrome. Lancet Infect Dis. 2007 Mar;7(3):218–24.

10. World Health Organization Expert Committee. Prevention and control of schistosomiasis and soil-transmitted helminthiasis. World Health Organ Tech Rep Ser. 2002;912:1–57.

3

SEXUALLY TRANSMITTED DISEASES

Emily J. Weston, Kimberly Workowski

INFECTIOUS AGENT

Sexually transmitted diseases (STDs) are the infections and resulting clinical syndromes caused by approximately 30 infectious organisms.

TRANSMISSION

Sexual activity is the predominant mode of transmission, through genital, anal, or oral mucosal contact.

EPIDEMIOLOGY

STDs are among the most common infectious diseases and can be caused by bacterial, viral, and parasitic pathogens. Annually, an estimated 19.7 million sexually transmitted infections occur in the United States alone. Worldwide, an estimated 498 million cases of chlamydia, gonorrhea, syphilis, and trichomoniasis occur each year. Some STDs are more prevalent in developing countries (chancroid, lymphogranuloma venereum [LGV], granuloma inguinale [donovanosis]) or in specific regions (gonorrhea with treatment failure and decreased susceptibility to cephalosporins in Asia) and may be imported into other countries by travelers returning from such locales. Infection with multiple STDs is common. Additionally, infection with an STD can facilitate the sexual transmission of HIV. Casual sexual relationships occur frequently during travel to foreign countries. In a systematic review published in 2010, the pooled prevalence of travel-associated casual sex among foreign travelers was 20.4%. In addition, commercial sex in various destinations, such as Southeast Asia, attracts many foreign travelers. Commercial sex workers in some regions have high rates of STDs, including HIV, and travelers who have sex with them risk acquiring these infections.

Knowledge of the clinical presentation, frequency of infection, and antimicrobial resistance patterns is needed to manage STDs that occur in travelers. Assessing risk for men who have sex with men is important because of the recent increased rates of infectious syphilis, gonorrhea with treatment failure and decreased susceptibility to cephalosporins, and LGV in various geographic locations.

CLINICAL PRESENTATION

Many infections, such as chlamydia and gonorrhea, may be asymptomatic, so screening for these infections and serologic testing for syphilis should be encouraged among travelers who report high-risk behaviors. Any traveler with sexual exposure who develops vaginal, urethral, or rectal discharge, an unexplained rash or genital lesion, or genital or pelvic pain should be advised to cease sexual activity and promptly seek medical evaluation.

Some systemic infections are acquired through sexual transmission (such as hepatitis A, hepatitis B, hepatitis C, HIV, syphilis, Zika infection). Human papillomavirus (HPV) infection is usually subclinical and asymptomatic and most often clears spontaneously within 2 years. However, persistent HPV infection can lead to genital warts, cervical and other anogenital cancers, and oropharyngeal cancer. Because many travelers do not volunteer a history of sexual contact during travel, clinicians should inquire about sexual exposures when caring for returned travelers.

DIAGNOSIS

Genital ulcer evaluation should include a serologic test for syphilis and a culture or PCR test for genital herpes. If exposure occurred in areas where chancroid is more common (Africa, Asia, and Latin America), a test for *Haemophilus ducreyi* should also be performed. Lymphadenopathy can accompany genital ulceration with chancroid infections, as well as with LGV and donovanosis. If painful perianal ulcers are present or mucosal ulcers are detected on anoscopy, presumptive therapy should include a regimen for anogenital herpes. LGV should be suspected in a traveler with tender unilateral inguinal or femoral lymphadenopathy or proctocolitis. Presumptive treatment for LGV should be considered for men who have sex with men and who have proctitis and perianal or mucosal ulcers, after obtaining specific testing for *Chlamydia trachomatis* (culture, direct immunofluorescence, or nucleic acid testing) from relevant specimens (genital lesions, rectal, or lymph node). Of note, for patients presenting with proctitis, *C. trachomatis* nucleic acid amplification testing of a rectal specimen is recommended. While a positive result is not a definitive diagnosis of LGV, the results might aid in the presumptive clinical diagnosis of LGV proctitis. Donovanosis is endemic in India, Papua New Guinea, central Australia, and southern Africa and is diagnosed with a crush tissue preparation from the lesion.

Testing specimens from the anatomic site of exposure with nucleic acid amplification tests can detect *C. trachomatis* and *Neisseria gonorrhoeae*. Culture and antibiotic susceptibility testing should be considered when gonorrhea is suspected, because of geographic differences in antimicrobial susceptibility. Various diagnostic methods are available to identify the cause of an abnormal vaginal discharge, including microscopic evaluation and pH testing of vaginal secretions, DNA probe-based testing, nucleic acid amplification testing, and culture.

Diagnosis of anogenital warts is made by visual inspection, with confirmation by biopsy if clinically indicated.

Anyone who seeks evaluation for STDs, or is diagnosed with an STD, should be screened for HIV infection. People seeking STD care known to be HIV-infected should be provided linkage to HIV care and treatment services.

TREATMENT

Evaluation, management, and follow-up of STDs should be based on standard guidelines (CDC and the World Health Organization). The prevalence of antimicrobial resistance in different areas should be considered when selecting treatment regimens. Early detection and treatment are important, as many STDs are asymptomatic.

STDs can often result in serious and long-term complications, including pelvic inflammatory disease, infertility, stillbirths and neonatal infections, anogenital and other cancers, and an increased risk for HIV acquisition and transmission.

PREVENTION

The prevention and control of STDs are based on accurate risk assessment, education, counseling, early identification of asymptomatic infection, and effective treatment of patients and their sex partners. Pretravel advice should include specific messages with strategies to avoid acquiring or transmitting STDs. Abstinence or mutual monogamy with an uninfected partner is the most reliable way to avoid acquiring and transmitting STDs.

For people whose sexual behaviors place them at risk for STDs, correct and consistent use of the male latex condom can reduce the risk of HIV infection and other STDs, including chlamydia, gonorrhea, and trichomoniasis. Preventing lower genital tract infections might reduce the risk of pelvic inflammatory disease in women. Correct and consistent use of male latex condoms also reduces the risk of HPV infection, genital herpes, syphilis, and chancroid, although data are limited. Only water-based lubricants (such as K-Y Jelly or glycerin) should be used with latex condoms because oil-based lubricants (such as petroleum jelly, shortening, mineral oil, or massage oil) can weaken latex condoms. Spermicides containing nonoxynol-9 are not recommended for STD/HIV prevention, as nonoxynol-9 may disrupt genital or rectal epithelium and has been associated with an increased risk of HIV transmission. Contraceptive methods that are not mechanical barriers do not protect against HIV or other STDs.

Prompt evaluation of sexual partners is necessary to prevent reinfection and disrupt transmission of many STDs. Preexposure vaccination is among the most effective methods for preventing some STDs. Two HPV vaccines are available and licensed for girls and women aged 9–26 years to prevent cervical precancers and cancers: the quadrivalent HPV and the bivalent HPV vaccine. The quadrivalent vaccine also prevents genital warts and is recommended for boys and men aged 9–26 years as well as girls and women. All travelers should be considered candidates for both hepatitis A and hepatitis B vaccines, as these infections can be sexually transmitted. Hepatitis B vaccine is recommended for all people being evaluated or treated for an STD. In addition, hepatitis A and hepatitis B vaccines are recommended for men who have sex with men and injection drug users. Travelers, particularly those at high risk for acquiring HIV infection, may consider discussing preexposure prophylaxis with their health care providers (see www.cdc.gov/hiv/prep and HIV section in this chapter).

CDC website: www.cdc.gov/std

BIBLIOGRAPHY

1. CDC. Human papillomavirus vaccination: recommendations of the Advisory Committee on Immunization Practices (ACIP). MMWR Recomm Rep. 2014 Aug 29;63(RR-05):1–30.

2. CDC. Recommendations for the laboratory-based detection of *Chlamydia trachomatis* and *Neisseria gonorrhoeae*—2014. MMWR Recomm Rep. 2014 Mar 14;63(RR-02):1–19.

3. CDC. Sexually transmitted diseases treatment guidelines, 2015. MMWR Recomm Rep. 2015 Jun 5;64(RR-03):1–137.

4. CDC. Supplemental information and guidance for vaccination providers regarding use of 9-valent HPV vaccine. 2015 [cited 2016 Sep. 26]. Available from: http://www.cdc.gov/hpv/downloads/9vhpv-guidance.pdf.

5. Korzeniewski K, Juszczak D. Travel-related sexually transmitted infections. Int Marit Health. 2015;66(4):238–46.

6. Lahra MM, Lo YR, Whiley DM. Gonococcal antimicrobial resistance in the Western Pacific Region. Sex Transm Infect. 2013 Dec;89 Suppl 4:iv19–23.

7. Stoner BP, Cohen SE. Lymphogranuloma Venereum 2015: clinical presentation, diagnosis, and treatment. Clin Infect Dis. 2015 Dec 15;61 Suppl 8: S865–73.

8. Unemo M, Nicholas RA. Emergence of multidrug-resistant, extensively drug-resistant and untreatable gonorrhea. Future Microbiol. 2012 Dec;7(12):1401–22.

9. Vivancos R, Abubakar I, Hunter PR. Foreign travel, casual sex, and sexually transmitted infections: systematic review and meta-analysis. Int J Infect Dis. 2010 Oct;14(10):e842–51.

10. World Health Organization. Baseline report on global sexually transmitted infection surveillance 2012. 2013 [cited 2016 Sep. 26]. Available from: http://www.who.int/reproductivehealth/publications/rtis/9789241505895/en/.

11. World Health Organization. Global incidence and prevalence of selected curable sexually transmitted infections–2008. Geneva 2012 [cited 2016 Sep. 26]. Available from: http://www.who.int/reproductive-health/publications/rtis/stisestimates/en/.

12. World Health Organization. Report on global sexually transmitted infection surveillance 2013. 2014 [cited 2016 Sep. 26]. Available from: www.who.int/reproductivehealth/publications/rtis/stis-surveillance-2013/en/.

SEX & TOURISM

Kimberly A. Workowski, Elissa Meites

TRAVEL AND SEXUAL HEALTH

Whether or not sex is the purpose of a trip, sex with a new partner is common during travel of any length. An estimated 5%–50% of international travelers have sex with a new partner while abroad, increasing their chances of developing a sexually transmitted disease (STD). Travelers may be unaware of the high prevalence of HIV and STDs in certain countries, particularly among commercial sex workers. For example, antibiotic-resistant gonorrhea has been considered a public health threat since it was first identified internationally.

The mainstays of sexually transmitted infection prevention (condoms, and vaccinations against hepatitis A, hepatitis B, and human papillomavirus), contraception, and other prescription medications may not be subject to US quality control standards in manufacturing, storage, or distribution when obtained in other countries. Condoms that are low quality, stored improperly, or past their expiration date are more likely to break. Clinicians seeing travelers at high risk for acquiring HIV infection should consider discussing preexposure prophylaxis with them (see www.cdc.gov/hiv/prep and HIV section in this chapter).

Any sexually active adult may benefit from consulting a clinician about partners, practices, prevention of STDs and unintended pregnancy, and recommended screening tests to check for HIV and treatable STDs. Travelers should also be alert to attempts at coercion or fraud from previously unknown partners professing romantic interest, especially in relationships beginning exclusively online. People who have experienced a high-risk sexual encounter should consider taking medications for postexposure prophylaxis of HIV or unintended pregnancy within 72 hours. These and other prescription medications can be costly or difficult to obtain overseas, but US consular officers may be able to assist in locating needed medical services. See Box 3-5 for a summary of sexual health recommendations for travelers.

SEX TOURISM

"Sex tourism" has been defined as travel planned specifically to procure sex. Sex tourism most commonly involves male tourists traveling to economically disadvantaged countries to pay for sex with female sex workers. In certain regions, commercial sex work is legal and culturally acceptable. However, travelers should be aware that HIV and STD infections are common among commercial sex workers. Also, sex tourism helps to support sex trafficking, among the largest criminal industries in the world, in which victims are forced to perform sex work. Travelers should be familiar with applicable US and local laws and should report known or suspected violations promptly to the authorities. The regional security officer at the local US embassy or foreign law enforcement officials can assist.

(continued)

3

BOX 3-5. # Summary of sexual health recommendations for travelers

BEFORE TRAVEL

1. Obtain recommended vaccinations, including those that protect against sexually transmitted infections.
2. Get recommended tests for HIV and treatable STDs. Be aware of STD symptoms in case any develop.
3. Pack sufficient quantities of needed prescription medications and supplies. Check condom packaging and expiration dates.
4. Review local laws and contact information for medical and law enforcement services.

DURING TRAVEL

5. Use good judgment in choosing consensual adult sex partners.
6. Condoms, used consistently and correctly, can decrease the risk of HIV and STDs.
7. If indicated, be prepared to start taking medications for HIV postexposure prophylaxis or unintended pregnancy within 72 hours after a high-risk sexual encounter.
8. Never engage in sex with a minor (<18 years old), child pornography, or trafficking activities in any country.
9. Report suspicious activity to US and local authorities as soon as it occurs.

AFTER TRAVEL

10. To avoid exposing sex partners at home, see a clinician to get recommended tests for HIV and treatable STDs.

SEXUAL ABUSE AND THE LAW

Although commercial sex work may be legal in some countries, sex trafficking, sex with a minor, and child pornography are always criminal activities according to US law and can be prosecuted in the United States even if the behavior occurred abroad. The Trafficking Victims Protection Act makes it illegal to recruit, entice, or obtain a person of any age to engage in commercial sex acts or to benefit from such activities. Federal law also bars US residents from engaging in sexual or pornographic activities with a child aged <18 years anywhere in the world, regardless of local age of consent, or to travel abroad for the purpose of having sex with a minor. In addition, child pornography, including sexual photographs or videos of minors in foreign countries, is illegal in the United States. These crimes are subject to prosecution with penalties of up to 30 years in prison.

Nearly 2 million children around the world are victims of commercial sexual exploitation, and roughly 1 million children are victims of trafficking. Children abused by sex tourists suffer not only sexual abuse but also poverty, homelessness, and physical, emotional, and psychological abuse, as well as health problems including illnesses, addictions, malnourishment, infections, physical injuries, and STDs.

If you suspect child sexual exploitation occurring overseas, you can report tips anonymously by using the Operation Predator smartphone app (https://itunes.apple.com/us/app/operation-predator/id695130859), calling the Homeland Security Investigations Tip Line toll-free at 866-347-2423, or submitting the information online at www.ice.gov/tips. In the United States, the National Center for Missing & Exploited Children's Cybertipline collects reports of child prostitution and other crimes against children (toll-free at 800-843-5678, www.cybertipline.com). At least 8,000 Americans have been arrested for child sex exploitation and 99 Americans have been convicted for child sex tourism since 2003, when the federal PROTECT Act was passed to strengthen the US government's prosecution of crimes related to sex tourism.

Americans and US permanent residents account for an estimated 25% of child sex tourists worldwide and up to 80% in Latin America. These are typically Caucasian men aged ≥40 and have been traced visiting Mexico, Central and South America (Brazil, Colombia, Costa Rica, Dominican Republic), Southeast Asia (Cambodia, India, Laos, Philippines, Thailand), Eastern Europe (Estonia, Latvia, Lithuania, Russia), and other regions.

To combat child sexual abuse, some international hotels and other tourism services have voluntarily adopted a code of conduct that includes training and reporting suspicious activities. Tourist establishments supporting this initiative to protect children from sex tourism are listed online (www.thecode.org). For more ways you can help, see the Department of State list of 15 ways to fight human trafficking (www.state.gov/j/tip/id/help).

BIBLIOGRAPHY

1. Abdullah AS, Ebrahim SH, Fielding R, Morisky DE. Sexually transmitted infections in travelers: implications for prevention and control. Clin Infect Dis. 2004 Aug 15;39(4):533–8.

2. CDC. Sexually transmitted diseases treatment guidelines, 2015. MMWR Recomm Rep. 2015 Jun 5;64(RR-03):1–137.

3. Marrazzo JM. Sexual tourism: implications for travelers and the destination culture. Infect Dis Clin North Am. 2005 Mar;19(1):103–20.

4. Newman WJ, Holt BW, Rabun JS, Phillips G, Scott CL. Child sex tourism: extending the borders of sexual offender legislation. Int J Law Psychiatry. 2011 Mar-Apr;34(2):116–21.

5. Vivancos R, Abubakar I, Hunter PR. Foreign travel, casual sex, and sexually transmitted infections: systematic review and meta-analysis. Int J Infect Dis. 2010 Oct;14(10):e842–51.

Perspectives sections are written as editorial discussions aiming to add depth and clinical perspective to the official recommendations contained in the book. The views and opinions expressed in this section are those of the authors and do not necessarily represent the official position of CDC.

SHIGELLOSIS

Anna Bowen

INFECTIOUS AGENT

Shigellosis is an acute infection of the intestine caused by bacteria in the genus *Shigella*. There are 4 species of *Shigella*: *Shigella dysenteriae, S. flexneri, S. boydii,* and *S. sonnei* (also referred to as group A, B, C, and D, respectively). Several distinct serotypes are recognized within the first 3 species.

TRANSMISSION

Because only humans and higher primates carry *Shigella*, transmission occurs via the fecal-oral route, including through direct person-to-person or sexual contact or indirectly through contaminated food, water, or fomites. Since as few as 10 organisms can cause infection, shigellosis is easily transmitted. It can be acquired even during short-term travel to settings with Western-style amenities. In the United States, *S. sonnei* infection is usually transmitted through interpersonal contact, particularly among young children and their caregivers; however, an estimated 30% of US shigellosis is foodborne. Foodborne outbreaks have been linked to contaminated foods commonly consumed raw and to infected food handlers. Outbreaks have also been traced to contaminated drinking water, swimming in contaminated water, and sexual contact between men.

EPIDEMIOLOGY

Worldwide, *Shigella* is estimated to cause 80–165 million cases of disease and 600,000 deaths annually. *Shigella* spp. are endemic in temperate and tropical climates. Transmission of *Shigella* spp. is most likely when hygiene and sanitation are insufficient. Shigellosis is predominantly caused by *S. sonnei* in industrialized countries, whereas *S. flexneri* prevails in the developing world. Infections caused by *S. boydii* and *S. dysenteriae* are less common globally but can make up a substantial proportion of *Shigella* spp. isolated in sub-Saharan Africa and South Asia. *Shigella* spp. are detected in the stools of 5%–18% of patients with travelers' diarrhea, and recent studies in Australia and Canada found that 40%–50% of locally diagnosed shigellosis cases were associated with international travel. In a study of travel-associated enteric infections diagnosed after return to the United States, *Shigella* was the third most common bacterial pathogen isolated by clinical laboratories (of note, these laboratories did not test for enterotoxigenic *Escherichia coli*, a common cause of travelers' diarrhea). Many infections caused by *S. dysenteriae* (56%) and *S. boydii* (44%) were travel-associated, but infections caused by *S. flexneri* and *S. sonnei* were less often associated with travel (24% and 12%, respectively). In this study, the risk of infection caused by *Shigella* spp. was highest for people traveling to Africa, followed by Central America, South America, and Asia. In 2014–2015, a large outbreak of ciprofloxacin-resistant *S. sonnei* infections occurred in the United States after travelers to India, Haiti, the Dominican Republic, and other countries returned with shigellosis. Outbreaks of infections caused by multidrug-resistant *Shigella*, including isolates resistant to azithromycin or ciprofloxacin, have been reported in Australia, Europe, Taiwan, Canada, and the United States among men who have sex with men. Infections caused by Shiga toxin–producing *S. flexneri* and *S. dysenteriae* have been reported repeatedly among travelers to Haiti and the Dominican Republic.

CLINICAL PRESENTATION

Illness typically begins 0.5–4 days after exposure. The symptoms of shigellosis typically last 4–7 days. Disease severity varies according to species; serotype *S. dysenteriae* serotype 1 (Sd1) is the agent of epidemic dysentery, while *S. sonnei* commonly causes milder, nondysenteric diarrheal illness. However, *Shigella* of any species can cause severe illness among people with compromised immune systems. Shigellosis is characterized by watery, bloody, or mucoid diarrhea; fever; stomach cramps; and nausea. Occasionally, patients experience vomiting, seizures (young children), or postinfectious arthritis. Hemolytic uremic syndrome can occur after infection with Shiga toxin–producing strains.

DIAGNOSIS

Rapid diagnostic tests for shigellosis are used in some US laboratories; however, shigellosis should be confirmed through culture of a stool specimen or rectal swab. *Shigella* isolates may then be speciated and serotyped and their antimicrobial susceptibilities determined to help guide treatment. Fecal specimens should be processed rapidly because *Shigella* often does not survive for long outside the body. Shigellosis is a nationally notifiable disease.

TREATMENT

Although antimicrobial treatment, when given early in the course of illness, can slightly shorten the duration of symptoms and of carriage, shigellosis can be mild and typically resolves within 4–7 days without treatment. When treatment is required for shigellosis associated with travel outside the United States, a fluoroquinolone or ceftriaxone may be used empirically until antimicrobial susceptibility data are available. However, clinicians should be aware that rates of multidrug resistance among *Shigella* spp., including resistance to fluoroquinolones, azithromycin, and third- and fourth-generation cephalosporins, are high outside the United States, particularly in South and East Asia.

PREVENTION

No vaccines are available for *Shigella*. The best defense against shigellosis is thorough, frequent

3

handwashing, strict adherence to standard food and water safety precautions (see Chapter 2, Food & Water Precautions), and minimizing fecal-oral exposures during sexual contact. Alcohol-based hand sanitizers may be a useful adjunct to washing hands with soap and water or when soap and water are not available.

CDC website: www.cdc.gov/shigella

BIBLIOGRAPHY

1. American Academy of Pediatrics. *Shigella* infections. In: Kimberlin DW, Brady MT, Jackson MA, Long SS, editors. Red Book: 2015 Report of the Committee on Infectious Diseases. 30th ed. Elk Grove Village, IL: American Academy of Pediatrics; 2015. pp. 706–9.

2. Baker KS, Dallman TJ, Ashton PM, Day M, Hughes G, Crook PD, et al. Intercontinental dissemination of azithromycin-resistant shigellosis through sexual transmission: a cross-sectional study. Lancet Infect Dis. 2015 Aug;15(8):913–21.

3. Bardhan P, Faruque AS, Naheed A, Sack DA. Decrease in shigellosis-related deaths without *Shigella* spp.-specific interventions, Asia. Emerg Infect Dis. 2010 Nov;16(11):1718–23.

4. CDC. Importation and domestic transmission of Shigella sonnei resistant to ciprofloxacin—United States, May 2014–February 2015. MMWR Morb Mortal Wkly Rep. 2015 Apr 3;64(12):318–20.

5. Gray MD, Lacher DW, Leonard SR, Abbott J, Zhao S, Lampel KA, et al. Prevalence of Shiga toxin-producing Shigella species isolated from French travellers returning from the Caribbean: an emerging pathogen with international implications. Clin Microbiol Infect. 2015 Aug;21(8):765.e9–.e14.

6. Hoffmann C, Sahly H, Jessen A, Ingiliz P, Stellbrink HJ, Neifer S, et al. High rates of quinolone-resistant strains of *Shigella sonnei* in HIV-infected MSM. Infection. 2013 Oct;41(5):999–1003.

7. Kendall ME, Crim S, Fullerton K, Han PV, Cronquist AB, Shiferaw B, et al. Travel-associated enteric infections diagnosed after return to the United States, Foodborne Diseases Active Surveillance Network (FoodNet), 2004–2009. Clin Infect Dis. 2012 Jun;54 Suppl 5:S480–7.

8. Lane CR, Sutton B, Valcanis M, Kirk M, Walker C, Lalor K, et al. Travel destinations and sexual behavior as indicators of antibiotic resistant shigella strains—Victoria, Australia. Clin Infect Dis. 2016 Mar 15;62(6):722–9.

9. Nygren BL, Schilling KA, Blanton EM, Silk BJ, Cole DJ, Mintz ED. Foodborne outbreaks of shigellosis in the USA, 1998–2008. Epidemiol Infect. 2013 Feb;141(2):233–41.

10. Wong MR, Reddy V, Hanson H, Johnson KM, Tsoi B, Cokes C, et al. Antimicrobial resistance trends of *Shigella* serotypes in New York City, 2006–2009. Microb Drug Resist. 2010 Jun;16(2):155–61.

3

SMALLPOX & OTHER ORTHOPOXVIRUS-ASSOCIATED INFECTIONS

Andrea M. McCollum

INFECTIOUS AGENT

Smallpox is caused by variola virus, genus *Orthopoxvirus*. Other members of this genus that cause infection in humans are vaccinia virus, monkeypox virus, and cowpox virus. In 1980, the World Health Organization officially declared smallpox to be eradicated.

TRANSMISSION

Smallpox

Person to person, principally respiratory; less commonly through contact with infectious skin lesions or scabs.

Monkeypox

Zoonotic transmission followed by person-to-person, principally respiratory; less commonly through contact with infectious skin lesions or scabs. African rodents and primates may harbor the virus and could infect humans, but the reservoir host is unknown.

Vaccinia

Vaccinia virus is the live-virus component of contemporary smallpox vaccines. Rarely, social contacts of people recently vaccinated for smallpox develop infections with vaccinia virus when their skin comes into contact with fluid from the inoculation lesion. Zoonotic infections via contact with infected animals with vaccinialike viruses have been reported in Colombia, Brazil, and India.

Cowpox

Contact with infected animals; transmission between humans has not been observed.

EPIDEMIOLOGY

Smallpox

Eradicated globally. A single confirmed case of smallpox would almost certainly be the result of an intentional act (bioterrorism) and would be considered an emergency.

Monkeypox

Endemic in tropical forested regions of West and Central Africa, notably the Congo Basin. Rodents imported from West Africa were the source of a 2003 outbreak of human monkeypox in the United States. Monkeypox is endemic in the Democratic Republic of the Congo (DRC) and occurs sporadically in neighboring countries (Republic of the Congo, Central African Republic, Sudan). Refugees and immigrants who have recently left DRC may harbor monkeypox virus infection, but reports of this are rare. Short-term travelers to monkeypox-endemic areas would not generally be at risk.

Vaccinia

Infections with wild vaccinialike viruses have been reported among cattle and buffalo herders in India and among dairy workers in southern Brazil and Colombia. Travelers who have direct (hands-on) contact with affected bovines may be at risk for acquiring cutaneous infection.

Cowpox

Human infections with cowpox and cowpox-like viruses have been reported in Europe and the Caucasus (cowpox and Akhmeta virus in Georgia). Travelers who have direct (hands-on) contact with affected bovines, felines, rodents, or captive exotics (zoo animals) may be at risk for cutaneous infection.

CLINICAL PRESENTATION

Smallpox

Infections present with acute onset of fever >101°F (38.3°C), malaise, head and body aches, and sometimes vomiting. This phase is followed by a rash characterized by firm, deep-seated vesicles or pustules in the same stage of development. Clinically, the most common rash illness likely to be confused with smallpox is varicella (chickenpox).

Monkeypox

Clinically similar to smallpox, with a febrile prodrome followed by a widespread vesiculopustular rash involving the palms and soles. One feature distinctive to monkeypox is marked lymphadenopathy.

Vaccinia and Cowpox

Human infections with vaccinia, wild vaccinialike viruses, cowpox, and cowpoxlike viruses are most often self-limited, characterized by localized pustular (and in cowpox, occasionally ulcerative) lesions. Fever and other constitutional symptoms may occur briefly after lesions first appear. Lesions can be painful and can persist for weeks. People who are immunocompromised or who have exfoliative skin conditions (such as eczema or atopic dermatitis) are at higher risk of severe illness or death.

DIAGNOSIS

Orthopoxvirus infection is confirmed by PCR or virus isolation. Health care providers can refer to the CDC smallpox website (https://emergency.cdc.gov/agent/smallpox) for guidance in the application of a clinical algorithm designed to aid in distinguishing orthopoxvirus infections from other disseminated rash illnesses, namely chickenpox.

TREATMENT

Mainly supportive, to include hydration, nutritional supplementation, and prevention of secondary infections. Vaccinia and cowpox lesions should remain covered until the scab detaches to diminish chances of spreading virus to other parts of the body or to another person. Health care providers managing orthopoxvirus infection in a patient who is at high risk for severe outcome (such as a patient who is immunocompromised or has an underlying skin condition) or ocular infections should consult with CDC to explore treatment options (770-488-7100). Investigational use of antivirals could be considered.

BIBLIOGRAPHY

1. Baxby D, Bennett M, Getty B. Human cowpox 1969-93: a review based on 54 cases. Br J Dermatol. 1994 Nov;131(5):598–607.

2. Levine RS, Peterson AT, Yorita KL, Carroll D, Damon IK, Reynolds MG. Ecological niche and geographic distribution of human monkeypox in Africa. PLoS One. 2007;2(1):e176.

3. Nakazawa Y, Emerson GL, Carroll DS, Zhao H, Li Y, Reynolds MG, et al. Phylogenetic and ecologic perspectives of a monkeypox outbreak, southern Sudan, 2005. Emerg Infect Dis. 2013 Feb;19(2):237–45.

4. Reynolds MG, Emerson GL, Pukuta E, Karhemere S, Muyembe JJ, Bikindou A, et al. Detection of human monkeypox in the Republic of the Congo following intensive community education. Am J Trop Med Hyg. 2013 May;88(5):982–5.

5. Trindade GS, Guedes MI, Drumond BP, Mota BE, Abrahao JS, Lobato ZI, et al. Zoonotic vaccinia virus: clinical and immunological characteristics in a naturally infected patient. Clin Infect Dis. 2009 Feb 1;48(3):e37–40.

PREVENTION

Smallpox vaccine is not recommended for international travelers. Smallpox vaccination is recommended only for laboratory workers who handle variola virus (the agent of smallpox) or closely related orthopoxviruses and health care and public health officials who would be designated first responders in the event of an intentional release of variola virus. In addition, members of the US military may be required to receive the vaccine.

For other orthopoxvirus infections, avoid contact with rodents and sick or dead animals, including pets and domestic ruminants (cattle, buffalo), and direct contact with ill humans. For more information about monkeypox and other orthopoxviruses, contact the CDC Poxvirus Inquiry Line (404-639-4129).

CDC websites: http://emergency.cdc.gov/agent/smallpox and www.cdc.gov/poxvirus/monkeypox/index.html

STRONGYLOIDIASIS

Francisca Abanyie

INFECTIOUS AGENT

An intestinal nematode, *Strongyloides stercoralis*.

TRANSMISSION

Filariform larvae found in contaminated soil penetrate human skin. Person-to-person transmission is rare but documented.

EPIDEMIOLOGY

Endemic in the tropics and subtropics and in limited foci elsewhere, including in Appalachia and the southeastern United States. Estimates of global prevalence exceed 100 million. Most documented infections in the United States occur in immigrants, refugees, and military veterans who have lived in endemic areas for long periods of time. Risk for short-term travelers is low, but infections can occur.

CLINICAL PRESENTATION

Most infections are asymptomatic. With acute infections, a localized, pruritic, erythematous papular rash can develop at the site of skin penetration, followed by pulmonary symptoms (a Löffler-like pneumonitis), diarrhea, abdominal pain, and eosinophilia. Migrating larvae in the skin cause larva currens, a serpiginous urticarial rash.

Immunocompromised people, especially those receiving systemic corticosteroids, those with human T cell lymphotropic virus type 1 infection, those with hematologic malignancies, or who have had organ transplants, are at risk for hyperinfection or disseminated disease, characterized by abdominal pain, diffuse pulmonary infiltrates, and septicemia or meningitis from enteric bacteria. The death rate from untreated hyperinfection and disseminated strongyloidiasis is high.

DIAGNOSIS

Peripheral blood eosinophilia is common in intestinal strongyloidiasis but often absent in disseminated strongyloidiasis. Rhabditiform larvae can be visualized on microscopic examination of stool, either directly or by culture on agar plates. Repeated stool examinations or examination of duodenal contents may be necessary. Hyperinfection and disseminated strongyloidiasis are diagnosed by examining stool, sputum, cerebrospinal fluid, and other body fluids and tissues,

which typically contain high numbers of filariform larvae. Serologic testing is available through commercial laboratories and through the National Institutes of Health and CDC (www.cdc.gov/dpdx; 404-718-4745; parasites@cdc.gov).

TREATMENT

Treatment of choice for acute, chronic, and disseminated disease or hyperinfection is ivermectin. The alternative is albendazole, although it is associated with lower cure rates. Prolonged or repeated treatment may be necessary in patients with hyperinfection, disseminated disease, or coinfection with human T cell lymphotropic virus 1, as relapse can occur.

PREVENTION

No vaccine or preventative drugs are available. Protective measures include wearing shoes when walking in areas where humans may have defecated. It may be reasonable to perform serologic testing on patients who have been at high risk for *Strongyloides* infection and who will either be placed on glucocorticosteroids, other immunosuppressive drug regimens, or who will undergo procedures such as transplantation that involve immunosuppression. If indicated, these patients should be treated before immunosuppression. Empiric treatment may be considered in people deemed at high risk of strongyloidiasis in whom immediate immunosuppression is required.

CDC website: www.cdc.gov/parasites/strongyloides

BIBLIOGRAPHY

1. Keiser PB, Nutman TB. *Strongyloides stercoralis* in the immunocompromised population. Clin Microbiol Rev. 2004 Jan;17(1):208–17.

2. Olsen A, van Lieshout L, Marti H, Polderman T, Polman K, Steinmann P, et al. Strongyloidiasis—the most neglected of the neglected tropical diseases? Trans R Soc Trop Med Hyg. 2009 Oct;103(10):967–72.

3. Puthiyakunnon S, Boddu S, Li Y, Zhou X, Wang C, Li J, et al. Strongyloidiasis—an insight into its global prevalence and management. PLoS Negl Trop Dis. 2014 Aug;8(8):e3018.

4. Seybolt LM, Christiansen D, Barnett ED. Diagnostic evaluation of newly arrived asymptomatic refugees with eosinophilia. Clin Infect Dis. 2006 Feb 1;42(3):363–7.

5. Siddiqui AA, Berk SL. Diagnosis of *Strongyloides stercoralis* infection. Clin Infect Dis. 2001 Oct 1;33(7):1040–7.

TAENIASIS

Paul T. Cantey, Jeffrey L. Jones

INFECTIOUS AGENT

Taenia solium (pork tapeworm) and *T. saginata* or *T. asiatica* (beef tapeworm).

TRANSMISSION

Eating raw or undercooked contaminated pork or beef.

EPIDEMIOLOGY

The highest prevalences are in Latin America, Africa, and South and Southeast Asia. Taeniasis has been reported at lower rates in Eastern Europe, Spain, and Portugal. Tapeworm infections are unusual in travelers.

CLINICAL PRESENTATION

The incubation period is 8–10 weeks for *T. solium* and 10–14 weeks for *T. saginata*. Symptoms may include abdominal discomfort, weight loss, anorexia, nausea, insomnia, weakness, perianal pruritus, and nervousness. Symptoms are less likely for *T. solium* infection than for *T. saginata* infection.

DIAGNOSIS

Presence of eggs, proglottids (segments), or tapeworm antigens in the feces or on anal swabs. Differentiation of *T. solium* from *T. saginata* and *T. asiatica* is based on morphology of the scolex and gravid proglottids.

TREATMENT

Praziquantel is the drug of choice, except in the setting of symptomatic neurocysticercosis (see Cysticercosis in this chapter). Niclosamide is an alternative but is not as widely available.

PREVENTION

Avoid undercooked meat.

CDC website: www.cdc.gov/parasites/taeniasis

BIBLIOGRAPHY

1. Cantey PT, Coyle CM, Sorvillo FJ, Wilkins PP, Starr MC, Nash TE. Neglected parasitic infections in the United States: cysticercosis. Am J Trop Med Hyg. 2014 May;90(5):805–9.
2. Garcia HH, Gonzalez AE, Evans CA, Gilman RH, Cysticercosis Working Group in Peru. *Taenia solium* cysticercosis. Lancet. 2003 Aug 16;362(9383):547–56.
3. Wittner M, White ACJ, Tanowitz HB. *Taenia* and other tapeworm infections. In: Guerrant R.L., Walker D.H., Weller P.F., editors. Tropical Infectious Diseases: Principles, Pathogens and Practice. 3rd ed. Philadelphia: Saunders Elsevier; 2011. pp. 839–47.

TETANUS

Tejpratap S. P. Tiwari

INFECTIOUS AGENT

Clostridium tetani, a spore-forming, anaerobic, gram-positive bacterium. Bacteria are ubiquitous in the environment.

TRANSMISSION

Contact with nonintact skin, usually via injuries from contaminated objects. "Tetanus-prone" wounds include those contaminated with dirt, human or animal excreta, or saliva; punctures; burns; crush injuries; or injuries with necrotic tissue.

EPIDEMIOLOGY

Distributed worldwide; more common in rural and agricultural regions, areas where contact with soil or animal excreta is likely, and areas where immunization is inadequate. Tetanus can affect any age group.

CLINICAL PRESENTATION

Incubation period is 10 days (range, 3–21 days). Acute symptoms typically include muscle rigidity and spasms, often in the jaw and neck. Symptoms of less common forms of tetanus (localized or cephalic) can include muscle spasms confined to the injury site, head or face lesions, and flaccid cranial nerve palsies. Progression from these forms to generalized tetanus may occur. Severe tetanus can lead to respiratory failure and death. Case-fatality ratios are high even where modern intensive care is available.

DIAGNOSIS

Diagnosis is made clinically; no confirmatory laboratory tests are available. Tetanus is a nationally notifiable disease.

TREATMENT

Tetanus requires hospitalization, treatment with human tetanus immune globulin (TIG), a tetanus toxoid booster, agents to control muscle spasm, aggressive wound care, and antibiotics. Metronidazole is the most appropriate antibiotic. The wound should be debrided widely and excised if possible.

PREVENTION

Ensure adequate immunity to tetanus by completing the childhood primary vaccine series with tetanus toxoid, a booster dose during adolescence, and at 10-year intervals thereafter during adulthood. For heavily contaminated wounds, a booster dose may be given if more than 5 years have elapsed since the last dose. For detailed information regarding the tetanus vaccine, visit www.cdc.gov/vaccines/vpd-vac/tetanus. Additional tetanus prophylaxis with TIG may be required in wounded patients.

CDC website: www.cdc.gov/tetanus

BIBLIOGRAPHY

1. CDC. Updated recommendations for use of tetanus toxoid, reduced diphtheria toxoid and acellular pertussis (Tdap) vaccine from the Advisory Committee on Immunization Practices, 2010. MMWR Morb Mortal Wkly Rep. 2011 Jan 14;60(1):13–5.

2. Farrar JJ, Yen LM, Cook T, Fairweather N, Binh N, Parry J, et al. Tetanus. J Neurol Neurosurg Psychiatry. 2000 Sep;69(3):292–301.

3. World Health Organization. Tetanus vaccine. Wkly Epidemiol Rec. 2006 May 19;81(20):198–208.

TICKBORNE ENCEPHALITIS

Marc Fischer, Ingrid B. Rabe, Pierre E. Rollin

INFECTIOUS AGENT

Tickborne encephalitis (TBE) virus is a single-stranded RNA virus that belongs to the genus *Flavivirus*. TBE virus has 3 subtypes: European, Siberian, and Far Eastern.

TRANSMISSION

TBE virus is transmitted to humans through the bite of an infected tick of the *Ixodes* species,

primarily *I. ricinus* (European subtype) or *I. persulcatus* (Siberian and Far Eastern subtypes). The virus is maintained in discrete areas of deciduous forests. Ticks act as both vector and virus reservoir, and small rodents are the primary amplifying host. TBE can also be acquired by ingesting unpasteurized dairy products (such as milk and cheese) from infected goats, sheep, or cows. TBE virus transmission has infrequently been reported through laboratory exposure and slaughtering viremic animals. Direct person-to-person spread of TBE virus occurs only rarely, through blood transfusion or breastfeeding.

EPIDEMIOLOGY

TBE is endemic in focal areas of Europe and Asia, extending from eastern France to northern Japan and from northern Russia to Albania. Approximately 5,000–13,000 TBE cases are reported each year, with large annual fluctuations. Russia has the largest number of reported cases. The highest disease incidence has been reported from western Siberia, Slovenia, and the Baltic States (Estonia, Latvia, Lithuania). Other European countries with reported cases or known endemic areas include Albania, Austria, Belarus, Bosnia, Croatia, Czech Republic, Denmark, Finland, France, Germany, Hungary, Italy, Norway, Poland, Romania, Serbia, Slovakia, Sweden, Switzerland, and Ukraine. Asian countries with reported TBE cases or virus activity include China, Japan, Kazakhstan, Kyrgyzstan, Mongolia, and South Korea.

Most cases occur from April through November, with peaks in early and late summer when ticks are active. The incidence and severity of disease are highest in people aged ≥50 years. Most cases occur in areas <2,500 ft (750 m). In the last 30 years, the geographic range of TBE virus appears to have expanded to new areas, and the virus has been found at altitudes up to and above 5,000 ft (1,500 m). These trends are likely due to a complex combination of changes in diagnosis and surveillance, human activities and socioeconomic factors, and ecology and climate.

The overall risk of acquiring TBE for an unvaccinated visitor to a highly endemic area during the TBE virus transmission season has been estimated at 1 case per 10,000 person-months of exposure. Most TBE virus infections result from tick bites acquired in forested areas through activities such as camping; hiking; fishing; bicycling; collecting mushrooms, berries, or flowers; and outdoor occupations such as forestry or military training. The risk is negligible for people who remain in urban or unforested areas and who do not consume unpasteurized dairy products.

Vector tick population density and infection rates in TBE virus-endemic foci are highly variable. For example, TBE virus infection rates in *I. ricinus* in central Europe vary from <0.1% to approximately 5%, depending on geographic location and time of year, while rates of up to 40% have been reported in *I. persulcatus* in Siberia. The number of TBE cases reported from a country depends on the ecology and geographic distribution of TBE virus, the intensity of diagnosis and surveillance, and the vaccine coverage in the population. Therefore, the number of human TBE cases reported from an area may not be a reliable predictor of a traveler's risk for infection. The same ticks that transmit TBE virus can also transmit other pathogens, including *Borrelia burgdorferi* (the agent for Lyme disease), *Anaplasma phagocytophilum* (anaplasmosis), and *Babesia* spp. (babesiosis), and simultaneous infection with multiple organisms has been described.

From 2000 through 2015, 7 cases of TBE among US travelers to Europe and China were reported. TBE is not a nationally notifiable disease in the United States, and additional cases may have occurred.

CLINICAL PRESENTATION

Approximately two-thirds of infections are asymptomatic. The median incubation period for TBE is 8 days (range, 4–28 days). The incubation period for milkborne exposure is usually shorter (3–4 days). Acute neuroinvasive disease is the most commonly recognized clinical manifestation of TBE virus infection. However, TBE disease often presents with milder forms of the disease or a biphasic course:

- First phase: nonspecific febrile illness with headache, myalgia, and fatigue. Usually lasts for several days and may be followed by an afebrile and relatively asymptomatic period. Up to two-thirds of patients recover without any further illness.

3

- Second phase: central nervous system involvement resulting in aseptic meningitis, encephalitis, or myelitis. Findings include meningeal signs, altered mental status, cognitive dysfunction, ataxia, rigidity, seizures, tremors, cranial nerve palsies, and limb paresis.

Disease severity increases with age. Although TBE tends to be less severe in children, residual symptoms and neurologic deficits have been described. Clinical course and long-term outcome also vary by TBE virus subtype:

- The European subtype is associated with milder disease, a case-fatality ratio of <2%, and neurologic sequelae in up to 30% of patients.

- The Far Eastern subtype is often associated with a more severe disease course, including a case-fatality ratio of 20%–40% and higher rates of severe neurologic sequelae.

- The Siberian subtype is more frequently associated with chronic or progressive disease and has a case-fatality ratio of 2%–3%.

DIAGNOSIS

TBE should be suspected in travelers who develop a nonspecific febrile illness that progresses to neuroinvasive disease within 4 weeks of arriving from an endemic area. A history of tick bite may be a clue to this diagnosis; however, approximately 30% of TBE patients do not recall a tick bite.

Serology is typically used for laboratory diagnosis. IgM-capture ELISA performed on serum or cerebrospinal fluid is virtually always positive during the neuroinvasive phase of the illness. Vaccination history, date of onset of symptoms, and information regarding other flaviviruses known to circulate in the geographic area that may cross-react in serologic assays need to be considered when interpreting results. During the first phase of the illness, TBE virus or viral RNA can sometimes be detected in serum samples by virus isolation or RT-PCR. However, by the time neurologic symptoms are recognized, the virus or viral RNA is usually undetectable. Therefore, virus

isolation and RT-PCR should not be used to rule out a diagnosis of TBE. Clinicians should contact their state or local health department, the CDC Viral Special Pathogens Branch (404-639-1115), or CDC Division of Vector-Borne Diseases (970-221-6400) for assistance with diagnostic testing.

TREATMENT

There is no specific antiviral treatment for TBE; therapy consists of supportive care and management of complications.

PREVENTION

Personal Protection Measures

Travelers should avoid consuming unpasteurized dairy products and use all measures to avoid tick bites (see Chapter 2, Protection against Mosquitoes, Ticks, & Other Arthropods).

Vaccine

No TBE vaccines are licensed or available in the United States. Two inactivated cell culture-derived TBE vaccines are available in Europe, in adult and pediatric formulations: FSME-IMMUN (Baxter, Austria) and Encepur (Novartis, Germany). Two other inactivated TBE vaccines are available in Russia: TBE-Moscow (Chumakov Institute, Russia) and EnceVir (Microgen, Russia). Immunogenicity studies suggest that the European and Russian vaccines should provide cross-protection against all 3 TBE virus subtypes. At least 1 other TBE vaccine is produced in China, but information regarding this vaccine is not available in the English literature.

For both FSME-IMMUN and Encepur, the primary vaccination series consists of 3 doses. The specific recommended intervals between doses vary by country and vaccine (Table 3-19). Although no formal efficacy trials of these vaccines have been conducted, indirect evidence suggests that their efficacy is >95%. Vaccine failures have been reported, particularly in people aged ≥50 years.

Because the routine primary vaccination series requires ≥6 months for completion, most travelers to TBE-endemic areas will find avoiding tick bites to be more practical than vaccination. However, an accelerated vaccination schedule has

Table 3-19. Tickborne encephalitis (TBE) vaccines licensed in Europe and Russia[1]

TRADE NAME (MANUFACTURER, LOCATION)	AGE (Y)	DOSE	ROUTE	PRIMARY SERIES	FIRST BOOSTER (Y)	SUBSEQUENT BOOSTERS (Y)
FSME-IMMUN (Baxter, Austria)	≥16	0.5 mL	IM	3 doses (0, 1–3 mo, 6–15 mo)[2]	3	5[3]
FSME-IMMUN Junior (Baxter, Austria)	1–15	0.25 mL	IM	3 doses (0, 1–3 mo, 6–15 mo)[2]	3	5
Encepur-Adults (Novartis, Germany)	≥17	0.5 mL	IM	3 doses (0, 1–3 mo, 9–12 mo)[4]	3	5[3]
Encepur-Children (Novartis, Germany)	1–11	0.25 mL	IM	3 doses (0, 1–3 mo, 9–12 mo)[4]	3	5
EnceVir (Microgen, Russia)	≥3	0.5 mL	IM	2 doses (0, 5–7 mo)[5]	1	3
TBE-Moscow (Chumakov Institute, Russia)	≥3	0.5 mL	IM	2 doses (0, 1–7 mo)	1	3

Abbreviation: IM, intramuscular.
[1] No TBE vaccines are licensed or available in the United States. FSME-IMMUN, FSME-IMMUN Junior, Encepur-Adults, and Encepur-Children are licensed in Europe and EnceVir and TBE-Moscow are licensed in Russia.
[2] If a rapid immune response is required, the second dose can be administered 2 weeks after the first dose.
[3] Booster doses recommended every 3 years for people aged ≥50 years.
[4] An accelerated schedule has been used with 3 doses given on days 0, 7, and 21. After the primary series, the first booster dose is administered at 12–18 months.
[5] For emergency situations, there is a rapid primary series schedule of 0 and 1–2 months.

been evaluated for both European vaccines, and results in seroconversion rates are similar to those observed with the standard vaccination schedule. Travelers anticipating high-risk exposures, such as working or camping in forested areas or farmland, adventure travel, or living in TBE-endemic countries for an extended period of time, may wish to be vaccinated in Europe.

CDC website: www.cdc.gov/vhf/tbe

BIBLIOGRAPHY

1. Amicizia D, Domnich A, Panatto D, Lai PL, Cristina ML, Avio U, et al. Epidemiology of tick-borne encephalitis (TBE) in Europe and its prevention by available vaccines. Hum Vaccin Immunother. 2013 May;9(5):1163–71.

2. CDC. Tick-borne encephalitis among US travelers to Europe and Asia—2000-2009. MMWR Morb Mortal Wkly Rep. 2010 Mar 26;59(11):335–8.

3. Committee to Advise on Tropical Medicine and Travel (CATMAT). Statement on tick-borne encephalitis. An Advisory Committee Statement (ACS). Can Commun Dis Rep. 2006 Apr 1;32(ACS-3):1–18.

4. Donoso Mantke O, Escadafal C, Niedrig M, Pfeffer M, Working Group for Tick-Borne Encephalitis Virus. Tick-borne encephalitis in Europe, 2007 to 2009. Euro Surveill. 2011;16(39).

5. Kollaritsch H, Paulke-Korinek M, Holzmann H, Hombach J, Bjorvatn B, Barrett A. Vaccines and vaccination against tick-borne encephalitis. Expert Rev Vaccines. 2012 Sep;11(9):1103–19.

6. Kunze U. The International Scientific Working Group on Tick-Borne Encephalitis (ISW TBE): Review of 17 years of activity and commitment. Ticks Tick Borne Dis. 2016 Apr;7(3):399–404.

7. Ruzek D, Dobler G, Donoso Mantke O. Tick-borne encephalitis: pathogenesis and clinical implications. Travel Med Infect Dis. 2010 Jul;8(4):223–32.

8. Steffen R. Epidemiology of tick-borne encephalitis (TBE) in international travellers to Western/Central Europe and conclusions on vaccination recommendations. J Travel Med. 2016 Apr;23(4).

9. Suss J. Tick-borne encephalitis 2010: epidemiology, risk areas, and virus strains in Europe and Asia—an overview. Ticks Tick Borne Dis. 2011 Mar;2(1):2–15.

10. World Health Organization. Vaccines against tick-borne encephalitis: WHO position paper. Wkly Epidemiol Rec. 2011 Jun 10;86(24):241–56.

TOXOPLASMOSIS

Jeffrey L. Jones

INFECTIOUS AGENT

Toxoplasma gondii, an intracellular coccidian protozoan parasite.

TRANSMISSION

Ingestion of soil, water, or food contaminated with cat feces, ingestion of undercooked meat, congenital transmission when a woman becomes infected during pregnancy, and contaminated blood transfusion and organ transplantation.

EPIDEMIOLOGY

T. gondii is endemic throughout most of the world. Risk is higher in developing and tropical countries, especially when people eat undercooked meat, drink untreated water, or are extensively exposed to soil.

CLINICAL PRESENTATION

Incubation period is 5–23 days. Symptoms may include influenzalike symptoms or a mononucleosis syndrome with prolonged fever, lymphadenopathy, elevated liver enzymes, lymphocytosis, and weakness. Rarely, chorioretinitis or disseminated disease can occur in immunocompetent people. In severely immunocompromised people, severe and even fatal toxoplasmic encephalitis, pneumonitis, and other systemic illnesses can occur, most often from reactivation of a previous infection. Infants with congenital toxoplasmosis are often asymptomatic, but eye disease, neurologic disease, or other systemic symptoms can occur, and learning disabilities, cognitive deficits, or visual impairments may develop later in life.

DIAGNOSIS

Serologic testing for *T. gondii* antibodies. Eye disease is diagnosed by ocular examination. Diagnosis of toxoplasmic encephalitis in immunocompromised people (most often seen in people with AIDS) can be based on typical clinical course and identification of ≥1 mass lesion by CT, MRI, or other radiographic testing. Biopsy may be needed to make a definitive diagnosis.

TREATMENT

Treatment is reserved for those with severe disease or who are immunocompromised. A number of regimens are available, including pyrimethamine, sulfadiazine, and leukovorin. Alternative treatment regimens include clindamycin, atovaquone, and azithromycin.

PREVENTION

Food and water precautions (see Chapter 2, Food & Water Precautions). Avoid direct contact with soil or sand that may be contaminated with cat feces. If caring for a cat, change the litter box daily. If pregnant or immunocompromised, avoid changing cat litter if possible, and do not adopt or handle stray cats.

CDC website: www.cdc.gov/parasites/ toxoplasmosis

BIBLIOGRAPHY

1. Anand R, Jones CW, Ricks JH, Sofarelli TA, Hale DC. Acute primary toxoplasmosis in travelers returning from endemic countries. J Travel Med. 2012 Jan-Feb;19(1):57–60.

2. Bottieau E, Clerinx J, Van den Enden E, Van Esbroeck M, Colebunders R, Van Gompel A, et al. Infectious mononucleosis-like syndromes in febrile

travelers returning from the tropics. J Travel Med. 2006 Jul-Aug;13(4):191–7.

3. Montoya JG, Liesenfeld O. Toxoplasmosis. Lancet. 2004 Jun 12;363(9425):1965–76.

4. Montoya JG, Remington JS. Management of *Toxoplasma gondii* infection during pregnancy. Clin Infect Dis. 2008 Aug 15;47(4):554–66.

5. Panel on Opportunistic Infections in HIV-Infected Adults and Adolescents. Guidelines for the prevention and treatment of opportunistic infections in HIV-infected adults and adolescents: recommendations from the Centers for Disease Control and Prevention, the National Institutes of Health, and the HIV Medicine Association of the Infectious Diseases Society of America. [updated Aug 17 2016; cited 2016 Sep. 26]. Available from: https://aidsinfo.nih.gov/contentfiles/lvguidelines/adult_oi.pdf.

6. Sepulveda-Arias JC, Gomez-Marin JE, Bobic B, Naranjo-Galvis CA, Djurkovic-Djakovic O. Toxoplasmosis as a travel risk. Travel Med Infect Dis. 2014 Nov-Dec;12(6 Pt A):592–601.

TRYPANOSOMIASIS, AFRICAN (SLEEPING SICKNESS)

Francisca Abanyie

INFECTIOUS AGENT

Two subspecies of the protozoan parasite *Trypanosoma brucei* (*T. b. rhodesiense* and *T. b. gambiense*).

TRANSMISSION

The bite of an infected tsetse fly (*Glossina* spp.). Bloodborne and congenital transmission are rare.

EPIDEMIOLOGY

Endemic in rural sub-Saharan Africa. *T. b. rhodesiense* is found in eastern and southeastern Africa, mainly Tanzania, Uganda, Malawi, Zambia, and Zimbabwe. *T. b. gambiense* is found in central Africa and in limited areas of West Africa, primarily in Democratic Republic of the Congo, Central African Republic, Angola, South Sudan, Guinea, Cameroon, Gabon, Côte d'Ivoire, Congo, Chad, and northern Uganda. World Health Organization (WHO) maps of African trypanosomiasis cases, by country, are available at www.who.int/trypanosomiasis_african/country/foci_AFRO/en.

In 2014, 3,796 sleeping sickness cases were reported to the World Health Organization; *T. b. gambiense* accounted for >98% of cases. Many cases, however, are probably not recognized nor reported. Tsetse flies inhabit rural, densely vegetated areas; people who only travel to urban areas are not at risk. Flies bite during the day, and <1% are infected. Risk of infection increases with the number of fly bites, which is not always directly correlated with duration of travel. Cases imported into the United States are rare.

CLINICAL PRESENTATION

T. b. rhodesiense

Clinical manifestations generally appear within 1–3 weeks of the infective bite and may include high fever, a chancre at the bite site, skin rash, headache, myalgia, thrombocytopenia, and less commonly, splenomegaly, renal failure, or cardiac dysfunction. Central nervous system involvement can occur within a month of infection and results in sleep cycle disturbance, mental deterioration, and eventually death.

T. b. gambiense

Clinical manifestations generally appear months to years after infection and are nonspecific. Signs and symptoms may include intermittent fever, headache, malaise, myalgia, arthralgia, facial edema, pruritus, lymphadenopathy, and weight loss. Central nervous system involvement occurs after several months to years of infection and is characterized by daytime somnolence and nighttime sleep disturbance, severe headache, and a range of neurologic manifestations including mood disorders, behavior change, focal deficits, and endocrine disorders. The clinical course of disease caused by *T. b. gambiense* is generally less severe than that caused by *T. b. rhodesiense*, but both are fatal if not treated.

DIAGNOSIS

Bites are characteristically painful, and a chancre may develop at the bite location. Diagnosis is made by identifying parasites in specimens of blood, chancre fluid or tissue, lymph node aspirate, or cerebrospinal fluid. Buffy-coat preparations concentrate the parasite, enabling easier visualization for diagnosis. Diagnostic assistance is available through CDC (www.cdc.gov/dpdx; 404-718-4745; parasites@cdc.gov).

TREATMENT

Infection can usually be cured by a course of antitrypanosomal therapy, although long-term sequelae, including permanent damage to the central nervous system, may remain. Treatment drugs (suramin, melarsoprol, eflornithine) are provided by CDC under investigational protocols. Choice of treatment drug depends on species causing infection (*T. b. rhodesiense* or *T. b. gambiense*) and stage of disease. Clinicians can consult with CDC for assistance with treatment.

PREVENTION

Avoid tsetse fly bites. Travelers should wear clothing of wrist and ankle length made of medium-weight fabric in neutral colors, as tsetse flies are attracted to bright or dark colors and can bite through lightweight clothing. Permethrin-impregnated clothing and use of DEET repellent may reduce the number of fly bites.

CDC website: www.cdc.gov/parasites/sleepingsickness

BIBLIOGRAPHY

1. Brun R, Blum J, Chappuis F, Burri C. Human African trypanosomiasis. Lancet. 2010 Jan 9;375(9709):148–59.
2. Franco JR, Simarro PP, Diarra A, Jannin JG. Epidemiology of human African trypanosomiasis. Clinical epidemiology. 2014;6:257–75.
3. Simarro PP, Franco JR, Cecchi G, Paone M, Diarra A, Ruiz Postigo JA, et al. Human African trypanosomiasis in non-endemic countries (2000–2010). J Travel Med. 2012 Jan-Feb;19(1):44–53.

TRYPANOSOMIASIS, AMERICAN (CHAGAS DISEASE)

Susan Montgomery

INFECTIOUS AGENT

The protozoan parasite *Trypanosoma cruzi*.

TRANSMISSION

Typically through feces of an infected triatomine insect (reduviid bug), may occur when a bug bite is scratched or by consuming food or beverages contaminated with infected bug feces; may also be transmitted through blood transfusion or organ transplantation and from mother to infant.

EPIDEMIOLOGY

Endemic in many parts of Mexico and Central and South America. In the United States, Chagas disease is primarily a disease of immigrants from endemic areas of Latin America. The risk to travelers is extremely low, but they could be at risk if staying in poor-quality housing or from consuming contaminated food or beverages in endemic areas.

CLINICAL PRESENTATION

Acute illness typically develops ≥1 week after exposure and lasts up to 60 days. A chagoma may develop at the site of infection; for example, the Romaña sign (edema of the eyelid and ocular tissues). Most infected people never develop symptoms but remain infected throughout their lives. Approximately 20%–30% of patients will develop chronic manifestations of Chagas disease after a prolonged period without any clinical disease. Chronic Chagas disease usually affects the heart; clinical signs include conduction system abnormalities, ventricular arrhythmias, and in late-stage disease, congestive cardiomyopathy. Less common chronic gastrointestinal problems (such as megaesophagus or megacolon) may develop with or without cardiac manifestations. Reactivation disease can occur in immunocompromised patients.

DIAGNOSIS

During the acute phase, parasites may be detectable in fresh preparations of buffy coat or stained peripheral blood specimens; PCR testing may also help detect acute infection. After the acute phase, diagnosis requires 2 or more serologic tests (most commonly, ELISA, immunoblot, and immunofluorescent antibody test) to detect *T. cruzi*–specific antibodies. PCR is not a useful diagnostic test for chronic-phase infections since parasites are not detectable in the peripheral blood during this phase.

TREATMENT

Antitrypanosomal drug treatment is always recommended for acute, early congenital, and reactivated *T. cruzi* infection and for chronic *T. cruzi* infection in children aged <18 years old. In adults, treatment is usually recommended. In the United States, treatment drugs (benznidazole and nifurtimox) are provided by CDC under investigational protocols. Contact CDC (chagas@cdc.gov; 404-718-4745) for assistance with clinical management.

PREVENTION

Insect precautions (see Chapter 2, Protection against Mosquitoes, Ticks, & Other Arthropods) and food and water precautions (see Chapter 2, Food & Water Precautions). Avoid sleeping in thatch, mud, and adobe housing in endemic areas; using insecticides in and around such homes is also protective. Impregnated bed nets are helpful. Screening blood and organs for Chagas disease prevents transmission via transfusion or transplantation.

CDC website: www.cdc.gov/parasites/chagas

BIBLIOGRAPHY

1. Bern C. Antitrypanosomal therapy for chronic Chagas' disease. N Engl J Med. 2011 Jun 30;364(26):2527–34.

2. Bern C, Montgomery SP, Herwaldt BL, Rassi A Jr, Marin-Neto JA, Dantas RO, et al. Evaluation and treatment of Chagas disease in the United States: a systematic review. JAMA. 2007 Nov 14;298(18):2171–81.

3. Carter YL, Juliano JJ, Montgomery SP, Qvarnstrom Y. Acute Chagas disease in a returning traveler. Am J Trop Med Hyg. 2012 Dec;87(6):1038–40.

4. Rassi A Jr, Rassi A, Marin-Neto JA. Chagas disease. Lancet. 2010 Apr 17;375(9723):1388–402.

TUBERCULOSIS

Philip LoBue

INFECTIOUS AGENT

Mycobacterium tuberculosis is a rod-shaped, non-motile, slow-growing, acid-fast bacterium.

TRANSMISSION

Tuberculosis (TB) transmission occurs when a contagious patient coughs, spreading bacilli through the air. Bovine TB (caused by the closely related *M. bovis*) can be transmitted by consuming unpasteurized dairy products from infected cattle.

EPIDEMIOLOGY

Globally, 9.6 million new TB cases and 1.5 million TB-related deaths are estimated to occur each year. TB occurs throughout the world, but the incidence varies (see Map 3-13). In the United States, the annual incidence is 3 per 100,000 population, but in some countries in sub-Saharan Africa and Asia, the annual incidence is several hundred per 100,000.

Drug-resistant TB is of increasing concern. Multidrug-resistant (MDR) TB is resistant to the 2 most effective drugs, isoniazid and rifampin. Extensively drug-resistant (XDR) TB is resistant to isoniazid and rifampin, any fluoroquinolone, and ≥1 of 3 injectable second-line drugs (amikacin, kanamycin, or capreomycin). MDR TB is less common than drug-susceptible TB, but approximately 480,000 new cases of MDR TB are diagnosed each year, and some countries have proportions of MDR TB in excess of 25% (see Table 3-20). MDR and XDR TB are of particular concern among HIV-infected or other immunocompromised people. As of 2014, XDR TB had been reported in 105 countries.

Before leaving the United States, travelers who anticipate possible prolonged exposure to TB (such as those who would spend time in health care facilities, correctional facilities, or homeless shelters) or those who plan to stay for years in an endemic country should have a 2-step tuberculin skin test (TST) or a single interferon-γ release assay (IGRA), either the QuantiFERON TB test (Gold In-Tube version) or T-SPOT.TB test (see *Perspectives*: Tuberculin Skin Testing of Travelers, later in this chapter). If the predeparture test result is negative, a single TST or IGRA should be repeated 8–10 weeks after returning from travel. Because people with HIV infection or other immunocompromising conditions are more likely to have an impaired response to either a skin or blood test, travelers should inform their clinicians about such conditions.

The risk of TB transmission on an airplane does not appear to be higher than in any other enclosed space. To prevent TB transmission, people who have infectious TB (TB that can be transmitted to other people) should not travel by commercial airplanes or other commercial conveyances. Only TB of the lung is infectious, and health department authorities determine whether a person is infectious based on the person's chest radiograph, sputum tests, symptoms, and treatment received. The World Health Organization (WHO) has issued guidelines for notifying passengers who might have been exposed to TB aboard airplanes. Passengers concerned about possible exposure to TB should see their primary health care provider or visit their local health department clinic for evaluation.

Bovine TB (*M. bovis*) is a risk in travelers who consume unpasteurized dairy products in countries where *M. bovis* in cattle is common. Mexico is a common place of infection for US travelers.

CLINICAL PRESENTATION

TB disease can affect any organ but most commonly occurs in the lungs (70%–80%). Common TB symptoms include prolonged cough, fever, decreased appetite, weight loss, night sweats, and coughing up blood (hemoptysis). The most common sites for TB outside the lungs are the lymph nodes, pleura, bones and joints, brain and spinal cord lining (meningitis), kidneys, bladder, and genitalia.

Infection is manifested by a positive TST or IGRA result 8–10 weeks after exposure. Overall, only 5%–10% of otherwise healthy people have an infection that progresses to disease during their lifetime. Progression to disease can occur weeks to decades after initial infection. People with TB disease have symptoms or other manifestations of illness such as an abnormal chest radiograph. In the remainder, the infection remains in a latent state (latent TB infection or LTBI) in which the infected person has no symptoms and cannot spread TB to others. The risk of progression is much higher in immunosuppressed people (8%–10% per year in HIV-infected people not receiving antiretroviral therapy). People who are receiving tumor necrosis factor inhibitors to treat rheumatoid arthritis and other chronic inflammatory conditions are also at increased risk for disease progression.

DIAGNOSIS

Diagnosis of TB disease is confirmed by culturing *M. tuberculosis* from sputum or other respiratory specimens for pulmonary TB and from other affected body tissues or fluids for extrapulmonary TB. On average, it takes about 2 weeks to culture and identify *M. tuberculosis*, even with rapid culture techniques. A preliminary diagnosis of TB can be made when acid-fast bacilli are seen by microscope on sputum smear or in other body tissues or fluids. However, microscopy cannot distinguish between *M. tuberculosis* and nontuberculous mycobacteria. This is particularly problematic in countries such as the United States where TB incidence is low. Nucleic acid amplification tests are more rapid than culture and specific for *M. tuberculosis*. They are also more sensitive than the acid-fast bacillus smear but less sensitive than culture. A diagnosis of TB disease can be made by using clinical criteria in the absence of microbiologic confirmation. However, laboratory testing should be performed when feasible to confirm the diagnosis. Molecular tests for drug resistance can be performed directly on specimens and can guide initial treatment while culture results

are pending. Culture-based susceptibility testing is recommended for all patients with a positive culture, regardless of the availability of molecular testing, to make a final determination on the appropriate drug regimen. LTBI is diagnosed by a positive TST or IGRA after further examinations (such as chest radiograph, symptom review) have excluded TB disease. Tuberculosis is a nationally notifiable disease.

TREATMENT

People with LTBI can be treated to prevent progression to TB disease. American Thoracic Society (ATS)/CDC guidelines for treatment of LTBI recommend 9 months of isoniazid as the preferred treatment. The combination regimen of isoniazid and rifapentine given as 12 weekly doses using directly observed therapy is recommended as equivalent to 9 months of isoniazid for treating LTBI in otherwise healthy patients aged ≥12 years who are at higher risk of developing active TB, for example after recent exposure to contagious TB. For people who have been exposed to isoniazid-resistant, rifampin-susceptible TB or who cannot tolerate isoniazid, 4 months of rifampin is a reasonable alternative. Travelers who suspect that they have been exposed to TB should inform their health care provider of the possible exposure and receive medical evaluation. CDC and ATS have published guidelines for targeted testing and treatment of LTBI. Because drug resistance is relatively common in some parts of the world, travelers who have TST or IGRA conversion associated with international travel should consult experts in infectious diseases or pulmonary medicine.

TB disease is treated with a multiple-drug regimen administered by directly observed therapy for 6–9 months (usually isoniazid, rifampin, ethambutol, and pyrazinamide for 2 months, followed by isoniazid and rifampin for an additional 4 months) if the TB is not MDR TB. MDR TB treatment is more difficult, requiring 4–6 drugs for 18–24 months; it should be managed by an expert in MDR TB. ATS/CDC/Infectious Diseases Society of America have published guidelines on TB treatment (www.cdc.gov/mmwr/preview/mmwrhtml/rr5211a1.htm).

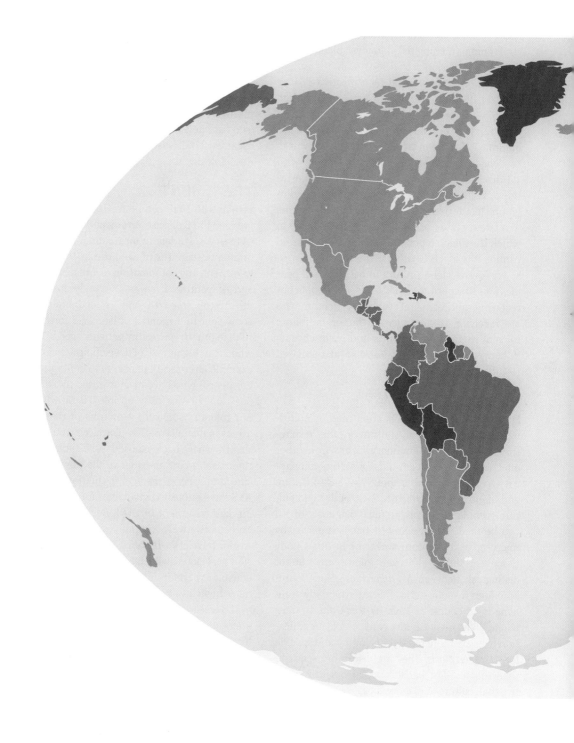

MAP 3-13. **Estimated tuberculosis incidence rates**[1]

[1] Disease data source: World Health Organization. Global Tuberculosis Report 2015 (WHO/HTM/TB/2015.22). 2015 (accessed June 23, 2016). Available from: http://apps.who.int/iris/bitstream/10665/191102/1/9789241565059_eng.pdf.

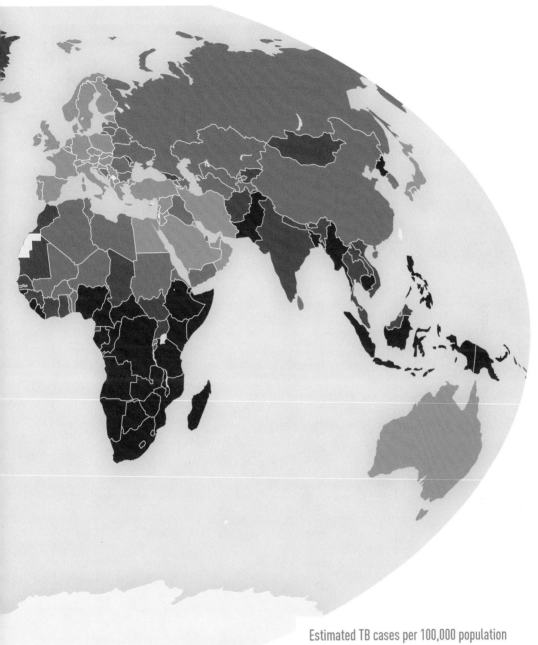

3

Estimated TB cases per 100,000 population

- 201–582
- 101–200
- 26–100
- 1–25
- No estimate

Table 3-20. Estimated proportion of MDR TB cases in high-burden countries

COUNTRY	% OF NEW TB CASES THAT ARE MDR	% OF RETREATMENT TB CASES THAT ARE MDR
Armenia	9.4	43
Azerbaijan	13	28
Bangladesh	1.4	29
Belarus	34	69
Bulgaria	2.3	23
Burma	5.0	27
China	5.7	26
Democratic Republic of Congo	2.2	11
Estonia	19	62
Ethiopia	1.6	12
Georgia	12	39
India	2.2	15
Indonesia	1.9	12
Kazakhstan	26	58
Kyrgyzstan	26	55
Latvia	8.2	30
Lithuania	14	49
Moldova	24	62
Nigeria	2.9	14
Pakistan	3.7	18
Philippines	2.0	21
Russia	19	49
South Africa	1.8	6.7
Tajikistan	8.1	52
Ukraine	22	56
Uzbekistan	23	62
Vietnam	4.0	23

PREVENTION

Travelers should avoid exposure to TB patients in crowded and enclosed environments (such as health care facilities, correctional facilities, or homeless shelters). Travelers who will be working in hospitals or health care settings where TB patients are likely to be encountered should be advised to consult infection control or occupational health experts about procedures for obtaining personal respiratory protective devices (such as N-95 respirators), along with respirator selection and training.

Based on WHO recommendations, bacillus Calmette-Guérin (BCG) vaccine is used once at birth in most developing countries to reduce the severe consequences of TB in infants and children. However, BCG vaccine has variable efficacy in preventing the adult forms of TB and interferes with testing for LTBI with the TST. Therefore, BCG is not routinely recommended for use in the United States. Recently, some experts have advocated BCG vaccination for health care providers who are likely to be exposed to MDR or XDR TB patients in settings where the TB infection control measures recommended in the United States are not fully implemented. BCG may offer some protection in this circumstance; however, people who receive BCG vaccination must follow all recommended TB infection control precautions to the extent possible. Additionally, IGRA is preferred over the TST for pre- and post-travel testing in people vaccinated with BCG.

To prevent infections due to *M. bovis*, travelers should also avoid eating or drinking unpasteurized dairy products.

CDC website: www.cdc.gov/tb

BIBLIOGRAPHY

1. American Thoracic Society and CDC. Diagnostic standards and classification of tuberculosis in adults and children. Am J Respir Crit Care Med. 2000 Apr;161(4 Pt 1):1376–95.

2. American Thoracic Society and CDC. Targeted tuberculin testing and treatment of latent tuberculosis infection. Am J Respir Crit Care Med. 2000 Apr;161(4 Pt 2):S221–47.

3. CDC. Availability of an assay for detecting *Mycobacterium tuberculosis*, including rifampin-resistant strains, and considerations for its use—United States, 2013. MMWR Morb Mortal Wkly Rep. 2013 Oct 18;62(41):821–7.

4. CDC. Recommendations for use of an isoniazid-rifapentine regimen with direct observation to treat latent *Mycobacterium tuberculosis* infection. MMWR Morb Mortal Wkly Rep. 2011 Dec 9;60(48):1650–3.

5. CDC. Treatment of tuberculosis. MMWR Recomm Rep. 2003 Jun 20;52(RR-11):1–77.

6. CDC. Updated guidelines for using interferon gamma release assays to detect *Mycobacterium tuberculosis* infection, United States. MMWR Recomm Rep. 2010.

7. Jensen PA, Lambert LA, Iademarco MF, Ridzon R. Guidelines for preventing the transmission of *Mycobacterium tuberculosis* in health-care settings, 2005. MMWR Recomm Rep. 2005 Dec 30;54(RR-17):1–141.

8. Seaworth BJ, Armitige LY, Aronson NE, Hoft DF, Fleenor ME, Gardner AF, et al. Multidrug-resistant tuberculosis. Recommendations for reducing risk during travel for healthcare and humanitarian work. Ann Am Thorac Soc. 2014 Mar;11(3):286–95.

9. World Health Organization. Global tuberculosis report 2015. 20th ed. Geneva: World Health Organization; 2015 [cited 2016 Sep. 26]. Available from: http://www.who.int/tb/publications/global_report/en/.

10. World Health Organization. Tuberculosis and air travel: guidelines for prevention and control. 3rd ed. Geneva: World Health Organization; 2008 [cited 2016 Sep. 26]. Available from: http://www.who.int/tb/publications/tb-airtravel-guidance/en/.

TUBERCULIN SKIN TESTING OF TRAVELERS

Philip LoBue

3

Screening for asymptomatic tuberculosis (TB) infections should only be carried out among travelers who will be at risk of acquiring TB if they are exposed at their destinations (see the preceding section on Tuberculosis). Screening with a tuberculin skin test (TST) in very low-risk travelers may result in false-positive test results, leading to unnecessary additional screening or unnecessary treatment. Using screening tests in very low-prevalence populations will likely produce more false positives than true positives.

Therefore, the TST should be considered only for travelers who are spending years in a country with a high risk of TB or for those travelers who will spend any length of time in routine contact with health care facilities, prisons, or homeless shelter populations. The general recommendation is that people at low risk for exposure to TB, which includes most travelers, do not need to be screened before or after travel.

For travelers who anticipate a long stay or contact with a high-risk population, careful pretravel screening should be carried out with use of 2-step pretravel TST screening. For 2-step TSTs, people whose baseline TSTs yield a negative result are retested 1–3 weeks after the initial test; if the second test result is negative, they are considered not infected. If the second test result is positive, they are classified as having had previous TB infection. The 2-step TST is recommended in this population for the following reasons:

- The use of 2-step testing can reduce the number of positive TSTs that would otherwise be misclassified as recent skin test conversions during future periodic screenings.
- Certain people who were infected with *Mycobacterium tuberculosis* years earlier exhibit waning delayed-type hypersensitivity to tuberculin. When they are skin tested years after infection, they might have a false-negative TST result (even though they are truly infected). However, the first TST might stimulate the ability to react to subsequent tests, resulting in a "booster" reaction. When the test is repeated, the reaction might be misinterpreted as a new infection (recent conversion) rather than a boosted reaction.

Two-step testing is important for travelers who will have potential prolonged or substantial TB exposure. Two-step testing before travel will detect boosting and potentially prevent "false conversions"—positive TST results that appear to indicate infection acquired during travel, but which are really the result of previous TB infection. This distinction is particularly important if the traveler is going to a country where multidrug-resistant (MDR) and extensively drug-resistant XDR TB are present: it would be critical to know whether the person's skin test had been positive before travel.

If the 2-step pretravel TST result is negative, the traveler should have a repeat TST 8–10 weeks after returning from the trip. During extended (>6 months) stays in or repeated travel to high-risk settings, a TST should be performed every 6–12 months, depending on the risk of exposure while traveling outside the United States, and 8–10 weeks after final return. Two-step testing should be considered for the baseline testing of people who report no history of a recent TST and who will receive repeated TSTs as part of ongoing monitoring.

People who have repeat TSTs must be tested with the same commercial antigen, since switching antigens can also lead to false TST conversions. Two commercial tuberculin skin test antigens are approved by the Food and Drug Administration (FDA) and are commercially available in the United States: Aplisol (JHP Pharmaceuticals) and Tubersol (Sanofi Pasteur).

An alternative to the 2-step TST is a single FDA-approved interferon-γ release assay (IGRA), either the QuantiFERON TB test (Gold In-Tube versions) or T-SPOT.TB test. IGRAs, which require a blood draw, are approximately as specific as TST in people who have not been vaccinated with bacillus Calmette-Guérin (BCG) and are much more specific in BCG-vaccinated populations. For a traveler whose time before departure is short, a single-step TST would be an acceptable alternative if time is insufficient for the 2-step TST and the IGRAs are not available.

In general, it is best not to mix tests. There is up to 15% discordance between TST and IGRA, usually with the TST positive and the IGRA negative. There are multiple reasons for the discordance, and in any single person, it is often difficult to be confident about the reason for discordance. However, if the clinician decides to mix tests,

it is better to go from TST to IGRA than the other way around, because the likelihood of having a discordant result with the TST negative and the IGRA positive is much lower. Such discordant results may become unavoidable as more medical establishments switch from TSTs to IGRAs.

The use of TSTs among travelers who are visiting friends and relatives in TB-endemic areas should take into account that the rate of TST positivity in people visiting their country of birth is often high. In a study among 53,000 adults in Tennessee, the prevalence of a positive TST among the foreign born was 11 times that among the US born (34% vs 3%). Confirming TST status before travel would prevent the conclusion that a positive TST after travel was due to recent infection.

BIBLIOGRAPHY

1. Al-Jahdali H, Memish ZA, Menzies D. Tuberculosis in association with travel. Int J Antimicrob Agents. 2003 Feb;21(2):125–30.

2. Brown ML, Henderson SJ, Ferguson RW, Jung P. Revisiting tuberculosis risk in Peace Corps Volunteers, 2006-13. J Travel Med. 2016 Jan;23(1).

3. Cobelens FG, van Deutekom H, Draayer-Jansen IW, Schepp-Beelen AC, van Gerven PJ, van Kessel RP, et al. Risk of infection with *Mycobacterium tuberculosis* in travellers to areas of high tuberculosis endemicity. Lancet. 2000 Aug 5;356(9228):461–5.

4. Haley CA, Cain KP, Yu C, Garman KF, Wells CD, Laserson KF. Risk-based screening for latent tuberculosis infection. South Med J. 2008 Feb;101(2):142–9.

5. Johnston VJ, Grant AD. Tuberculosis in travellers. Travel Med Infect Dis. 2003 Nov;1(4):205–12.

6. Leder K, Tong S, Weld L, Kain KC, Wilder-Smith A, von Sonnenburg F, et al. Illness in travelers visiting friends and relatives: a review of the GeoSentinel Surveillance Network. Clin Infect Dis. 2006 Nov 1;43(9):1185–93.

7. Mancuso JD, Tobler SK, Keep LW. Pseudoepidemics of tuberculin skin test conversions in the US Army after recent deployments. Am J Respir Crit Care Med. 2008 Jun 1;177(11):1285–9.

8. Mazurek M, Jereb J, Vernon A, LoBue P, Goldberg S, Castro K. Updated guidelines for using interferon gamma release assays to detect *Mycobacterium tuberculosis* infection—United States, 2010. MMWR Recomm Rep. 2010 Jun 25;59(RR-5):1–25.

9. Seaworth BJ, Armitige LY, Aronson NE, Hoft DF, Fleenor ME, Gardner AF, et al. Multidrug-resistant tuberculosis. Recommendations for reducing risk during travel for healthcare and humanitarian work. Ann Am Thorac Soc. 2014 Mar;11(3):286–95.

10. Villarino ME, Burman W, Wang YC, Lundergan L, Catanzaro A, Bock N, et al. Comparable specificity of 2 commercial tuberculin reagents in persons at low risk for tuberculous infection. JAMA. 1999 Jan 13;281(2):169–71.

Perspectives sections are written as editorial discussions aiming to add depth and clinical perspective to the official recommendations contained in the book. The views and opinions expressed in this section are those of the author and do not necessarily represent the official position of CDC.

TYPHOID & PARATYPHOID FEVER

Michael C. Judd, Eric D. Mintz

INFECTIOUS AGENT

Salmonella enterica serotypes Typhi and Paratyphi A, Paratyphi B (tartrate negative), and Paratyphi C cause a potentially severe and occasionally life-threatening bacteremic illness referred to respectively as typhoid and paratyphoid fever, and collectively as enteric fever.

TRANSMISSION

Humans are the only source of these bacteria; no animal or environmental reservoirs have been identified. Typhoid and paratyphoid fever are most often acquired through consumption of water or food that has been contaminated by feces of an acutely infected or convalescent person or a chronic, asymptomatic carrier. Transmission through sexual contact, especially among men who have sex with men, has been documented rarely.

EPIDEMIOLOGY

An estimated 26 million cases of typhoid fever and 5 million cases of paratyphoid fever occur worldwide each year, causing 215,000 deaths. In the United States, approximately 300 culture-confirmed cases of typhoid fever and 80 cases of paratyphoid fever caused by *S. enterica* serotype Paratyphi A are reported each year. Cases of paratyphoid fever caused by serotypes Paratyphi B (tartrate negative) and Paratyphi C are rarely reported. Approximately 85% of typhoid fever and 90% of paratyphoid fever cases in the United States are among international travelers; of those, 75% of typhoid and 90% of paratyphoid fever cases are caused by serotype Paratyphi A acquired by travelers to southern Asia (such as India, Pakistan, or Bangladesh). Other high-risk regions for typhoid and paratyphoid fever include Africa and Southeast Asia; lower-risk regions include East Asia, South America, and the Caribbean.

Travelers who are visiting friends and relatives are at increased risk (see Chapter 8, Immigrants Returning Home to Visit Friends and Relatives [VFRs]). Although the risk of acquiring typhoid or paratyphoid fever increases with the duration of stay, travelers have acquired typhoid fever even during visits of <1 week to countries where the disease is highly endemic (such as India, Pakistan, or Bangladesh).

CLINICAL PRESENTATION

The incubation period of typhoid and paratyphoid infections is 6–30 days. The onset of illness is insidious, with gradually increasing fatigue and a fever that increases daily from low-grade to as high as 102°F–104°F (38°C–40°C) by the third to fourth day of illness. Headache, malaise, and anorexia are nearly universal, and abdominal pain, diarrhea, or constipation are common. Hepatosplenomegaly can often be detected. A transient, macular rash of rose-colored spots can occasionally be seen on the trunk. Fever is commonly lowest in the morning, reaching a peak in late afternoon or evening. This clinical presentation is often confused with malaria, and typhoid fever should be suspected in a person with a history of travel to an endemic area who is not responding to antimalarial medication. Untreated, the disease can last for a month. The serious complications of typhoid fever generally occur after 2–3 weeks of illness and may include life-threatening intestinal hemorrhage or perforation.

DIAGNOSIS

Infection with typhoid or paratyphoid fever results in a low-grade septicemia. Although blood culture is the mainstay of diagnosis in typhoid and paratyphoid fever, a single culture is positive in only approximately 50% of cases. Multiple cultures increase the sensitivity and may be required to make the diagnosis. Bone marrow culture increases the diagnostic yield to approximately 80% of cases and is relatively unaffected by prior or concurrent antibiotic use. Stool culture is not usually positive during the first week of illness, so blood culture is preferred. Urine culture has no higher diagnostic yield than stool culture for acute cases.

The Widal test is unreliable but is widely used in developing countries because of its low cost. It is a serologic assay that may react in patients with typhoid or paratyphoid fever, but is not specific and false positives may occur. Serologic assays are not an adequate substitute for blood, stool, or bone marrow culture.

Because there is no definitive serologic test for typhoid or paratyphoid fever, the initial diagnosis often has to be made clinically. The combination of a history of risk for infection and a gradual onset of fever that increases in severity over several days should raise suspicion of typhoid or paratyphoid fever. Typhoid fever is a nationally notifiable disease.

TREATMENT

Specific antimicrobial therapy shortens the clinical course of enteric fever and reduces the risk for death. Fluoroquinolones are recommended for empiric treatment of enteric fever in adults, but quinolone resistance is >80% for Typhi and Paratyphi A infections in travelers to South and Southeast Asia, which suggests that treatment failures will occur. Injectable third-generation cephalosporins are often the empiric drug of choice when the possibility of fluoroquinolone resistance is high. Azithromycin and ceftriaxone are increasingly used to treat typhoid fever or paratyphoid fever because of the emergence of multidrug-resistant strains, although increasing resistance to azithromycin in Typhi strains has been documented outside the United States. In contrast, no cases of ceftriaxone resistance have been reported among Typhi and Paratyphi A isolates tested by the CDC National Antimicrobial Monitoring System through 2013. Additional data on antimicrobial resistance among enteric fever cases in the United States can be found at www.cdc.gov/narmsnow.

Patients treated with an antibiotic may continue to have fever for 3–5 days, although the height of the fever generally decreases each day. Patients may actually feel worse during the several days it takes for the fever to end. If fever in a person with culture-confirmed typhoid or paratyphoid fever does not subside within 5 days, alternative antimicrobial agents or other foci of infection such as abscesses, bone or joint infections, and other extraintestinal sites should be considered.

PREVENTION

Food and Water

Safe food and water precautions and frequent handwashing (especially before meals) are important in preventing typhoid and paratyphoid fever (see Chapter 2, Food & Water Precautions). Although vaccines are recommended to prevent typhoid fever, they are not 100% effective; therefore, even vaccinated travelers should follow recommended food and water precautions. For paratyphoid fever, food and water precautions are the only prevention method, as no vaccines are available.

Vaccine

INDICATIONS FOR USE

CDC recommends typhoid vaccine for travelers to areas where there is an increased risk of exposure to *S. enterica* serotype Typhi. Destination-specific vaccine recommendations are available at the CDC Travelers' Health website (www.cdc.gov/travel).

Two typhoid vaccines are available in the United States:

- Vi capsular polysaccharide vaccine (ViCPS) (Typhim Vi, manufactured by Sanofi Pasteur) for intramuscular use

- Oral live attenuated vaccine (Vivotif, manufactured from the Ty21a strain of serotypeTyphi by PaxVax)

Both typhoid vaccines protect 50%–80% of recipients; travelers should be reminded that typhoid immunization is not 100% effective, and typhoid fever could still occur. Available typhoid vaccines offer no protection against paratyphoid fever.

VACCINE ADMINISTRATION

Table 3-21 provides information on vaccine dosage, administration, and revaccination. The time required for primary vaccination differs for the 2 vaccines, as do the lower age limits.

Primary vaccination with ViCPS consists of one 0.5 mL (25 mg) dose administered intramuscularly. One dose should be given ≥2 weeks before travel. The manufacturer does not recommend the vaccine for infants and for children <2 years old. A booster dose is recommended every 2 years for people who remain at risk.

Primary vaccination with oral Ty21a vaccine consists of 4 capsules, 1 taken every other day. The capsules should be kept refrigerated (not frozen), and all 4 doses must be taken to achieve maximum efficacy. Each capsule should be taken with cool liquid no warmer than 98.6°F (37°C), approximately 1 hour before a meal and ≥2 hours after a previous meal. This regimen should be completed ≥1 week before potential exposure. What to do when a dose of the oral vaccine is missed or taken late is unclear. Some suggest that minor deviations in the dosing schedule, such as taking a dose one day late, may not have a large effect on how well the vaccine works. However, we are unaware of any studies showing the effect of such deviations; thus, if 4 doses are not completed as directed, optimal immune response may not be achieved. The vaccine manufacturer recommends that Ty21a not be administered to infants or to children aged <6 years. A booster dose is recommended every 5 years for people who remain at risk.

VACCINE SAFETY AND ADVERSE REACTIONS

Adverse reactions to Ty21a vaccine are rare and mainly consist of abdominal discomfort, nausea, vomiting, and rash. ViCPS vaccine is most often associated with headache (16%–20%) and injection-site reactions (7%). Adverse reactions should be reported to the Vaccine Adverse Event Reporting System by visiting https://vaers.hhs.gov/index or calling 1-800-822-7967.

PRECAUTIONS AND CONTRAINDICATIONS

No information is available on the safety of these vaccines in pregnancy; it is prudent on theoretical grounds to avoid vaccinating pregnant women. However, the benefits of vaccinating pregnant women may outweigh potential risks when the likelihood of typhoid exposure is high;

Table 3-21. Vaccines to prevent typhoid fever

VACCINATION	AGE (Y)	DOSE, MODE OF ADMINISTRATION	NUMBER OF DOSES	DOSING INTERVAL	BOOSTING INTERVAL
Oral, Live Attenuated Ty21a Vaccine (Vivotif)[1]					
Primary series	≥6	1 capsule,[2] oral	4	48 hours	Not applicable
Booster	≥6	1 capsule,[2] oral	4	48 hours	Every 5 years
Vi Capsular Polysaccharide Vaccine (Typhim Vi)					
Primary series	≥2	0.5 mL, intramuscular	1	Not applicable	Not applicable
Booster	≥2	0.5 mL, intramuscular	1	Not applicable	Every 2 years

[1] The vaccine must be kept refrigerated (35.6°F–46.4°F, 2°C–8°C).
[2] Administer with cool liquid no warmer than 98.6°F (37°C).

the inactivated vaccine (ViCPS) may be considered in these situations. Live attenuated Ty21a vaccine should not be given to pregnant women or immunocompromised travelers, including those infected with HIV. The intramuscular vaccine presents a theoretically safer alternative for immunocompromised travelers. (The Advisory Committee on Immunization Practices does not recommend against vaccinating household contacts of immunocompromised people with Ty21a; although vaccine organisms can be shed transiently in the stool of vaccine recipients, secondary transmission of vaccine organisms has not been documented.) The only contraindication to vaccination with ViCPS vaccine is a history of severe local or systemic reactions after a previous dose. Neither vaccine should be given to people with an acute febrile illness.

Theoretical concerns have been raised about the immunogenicity of live, attenuated Ty21a vaccine in people concurrently receiving antimicrobial agents (including antimalarial chemoprophylaxis), viral vaccines, or immune globulin. The growth of the live Ty21a strain is inhibited in vitro by various antibacterial agents, and vaccination with Ty21a should be delayed for >72 hours after the administration of any antibacterial agent. Available data do not suggest that simultaneous administration of oral polio or yellow fever vaccine decreases the immunogenicity of Ty21a. If typhoid vaccination is warranted, it should not be delayed because of administration of viral vaccines. Simultaneous administration of Ty21a and immune globulin does not appear to pose a problem.

CDC website: www.cdc.gov/typhoid-fever

BIBLIOGRAPHY

1. Beeching NJ, Clarke PD, Kitchin NR, Pirmohamed J, Veitch K, Weber F. Comparison of two combined vaccines against typhoid fever and hepatitis A in healthy adults. Vaccine. 2004 Nov 15;23(1):29–35.

2. Buckle GC, Walker CL, Black RE. Typhoid fever and paratyphoid fever: systematic review to estimate global morbidity and mortality for 2010. J Glob Health. 2012 Jun;2(1):010401.

3. Crump JA, Mintz ED. Global trends in typhoid and paratyphoid fever. Clin Infect Dis. 2010 Jan 15;50(2):241–6.

4. Date KA, Newton AE, Medalla F, Blackstock A, Richardson L, McCullough A, et al. Changing patterns in enteric fever incidence and increasing antibiotic resistance of enteric fever isolates in the United States, 2008–2012. Clin Infect Dis. 2016 Aug 1;63(3):322–9.

5. Effa EE, Bukirwa H. Azithromycin for treating uncomplicated typhoid and paratyphoid fever (enteric fever). Cochrane Database Syst Rev. 2008(4):CD006083.

6. Gupta SK, Medalla F, Omondi MW, Whichard JM, Fields PI, Gerner-Smidt P, et al. Laboratory-based surveillance of paratyphoid fever in the United States: travel and antimicrobial resistance. Clin Infect Dis. 2008 Jun 1;46(11):1656–63.

7. Lynch MF, Blanton EM, Bulens S, Polyak C, Vojdani J, Stevenson J, et al. Typhoid fever in the United States, 1999–2006. JAMA. 2009 Aug 26;302(8):859–65.

8. Parry CM, Hien TT, Dougan G, White NJ, Farrar JJ. Typhoid fever. N Engl J Med. 2002 Nov 28;347(22):1770–82.

9. Steinberg EB, Bishop R, Haber P, Dempsey AF, Hoekstra RM, Nelson JM, et al. Typhoid fever in travelers: who should be targeted for prevention? Clin Infect Dis. 2004 Jul 15;39(2):186–91.

10. Wain J, Pham VB, Ha V, Nguyen NM, To SD, Walsh AL, et al. Quantitation of bacteria in bone marrow from patients with typhoid fever: relationship between counts and clinical features. J Clin Microbiol. 2001 Apr;39(4):1571–6.

VARICELLA (CHICKENPOX)

Mona Marin, Adriana S. Lopez

INFECTIOUS AGENT

Varicella-zoster virus, a member of the herpesvirus family. Humans are the only reservoir of the virus, and disease occurs only in humans. After primary infection as varicella (chickenpox), the virus remains dormant in the sensory-nerve ganglia and can reactivate at a later time, causing herpes zoster (shingles).

TRANSMISSION

Varicella-zoster virus is transmitted from person to person, primarily via the respiratory route by inhalation of aerosols from vesicular fluid of skin lesions of varicella or herpes zoster; it can also spread by direct contact with the vesicular fluid of skin lesions and possibly infected respiratory tract secretions. The varicella zoster virus enters the host through the upper respiratory tract or the conjunctiva. Varicella is a highly contagious viral disease with secondary attack ratios of approximately 85% (range, 61%–100%) in susceptible household contacts; contagiousness after community exposure is lower. Herpes zoster is approximately 20% as infectious as varicella; in susceptible people, contact with herpes zoster rash causes varicella, not herpes zoster. The period of communicability of patients with varicella is estimated to begin 1–2 days before the onset of rash and ends when all lesions are crusted, typically 4–7 days after onset of rash in immunocompetent people, but this period may be longer in immunocompromised people. Patients with herpes zoster are contagious while they have active, vesicular lesions (usually 7–10 days).

In utero infection can also occur as a result of transplacental passage of the virus during maternal varicella infection.

EPIDEMIOLOGY

Varicella occurs worldwide. In temperate climates, varicella tends to be a childhood disease, with peak incidence among preschool and school-aged children and during late winter and early spring. In these countries, <5% of adults are susceptible to varicella. In tropical climates, the highest incidence was described in the driest, coolest months; overall, infection tends to be acquired later in childhood, resulting in higher susceptibility among adults than in temperate climates, especially in less densely populated areas.

With the implementation of the childhood varicella vaccination program in the United States in 1996, substantial declines have occurred in disease incidence, and, although varicella is still endemic, the risk of exposure to varicella zoster virus is higher in most other parts of the world than it is in the United States.

Because varicella is endemic worldwide, all susceptible travelers are at risk of contracting varicella during travel. Additionally, exposure to herpes zoster poses a risk for varicella in susceptible travelers, although localized herpes zoster is much less contagious than varicella. Travelers at highest risk for severe varicella are infants, adults, and immunocompromised people without evidence of immunity (see criteria for evidence of immunity in "Prevention," below).

CLINICAL PRESENTATION

Varicella is generally a mild disease in children, and most people recover without serious complications. The average incubation period is 14–16 days (range, 10–21 days). Infection is often characterized by a short (1- or 2-day) prodromal period (fever, malaise), although this may be absent in children, and a pruritic rash consisting of crops of macules, papules, and vesicles (typically 250–500 lesions), which appear in ≥3 successive waves and resolve by crusting. Characteristic for varicella is the presence of lesions in different stages of development at the same time. Serious complications can occur, most commonly in infants, adults, and immunocompromised people. Complications include secondary bacterial infections of skin lesions sometimes resulting in bacteremia/sepsis, pneumonia, cerebellar ataxia, encephalitis, and hemorrhagic conditions; rarely (about 1 case in 40,000), these complications may result in death.

Modified varicella, also known as breakthrough varicella, can occur in vaccinated people. Breakthrough varicella is usually mild, with <50 lesions, low or no fever, and shorter duration of rash. The rash may be atypical in appearance with fewer vesicles and predominance of maculopapular lesions. Breakthrough varicella is contagious, although less so than varicella in unvaccinated people.

DIAGNOSIS

Varicella is often diagnosed clinically on the basis of a generalized maculopapulovesicular rash. The clinical diagnosis of varicella in the United States has become increasingly challenging as a growing proportion of cases occur in vaccinated people in whom disease is mild and rash is atypical. Although not routinely recommended, laboratory diagnosis is likely to become increasingly useful. Varicella is a nationally notifiable disease.

For laboratory confirmation, skin lesions are the preferred specimen. Vesicular swabs or scrapings and scabs from crusted lesions can be used to identify varicella-zoster virus DNA by PCR (preferred method as it is the most sensitive and specific) or direct fluorescent antibody. In the absence of vesicles or scabs, scrapings of maculopapular lesions can be collected for testing. Serologic tests may also be used to confirm disease but are less reliable than PCR or direct fluorescent antibody methods for virus identification.

- A significant rise in serum varicella IgG titers from acute- and convalescent-phase samples by any standard serologic assay can confirm a diagnosis retrospectively; these antibody tests may not be reliable in immunocompromised people.

- Of note, testing for varicella-zoster IgM by using commercial kits is not recommended, because available methods lack sensitivity and specificity; false-positive IgM results are common in the presence of high IgG levels.

TREATMENT

Treatment with antivirals is not routinely recommended for otherwise healthy children with varicella. Treatment with oral acyclovir should be considered for people at increased risk for moderate to severe disease, such as people aged >12 years, people with chronic cutaneous or pulmonary disorders, people who are receiving long-term salicylate therapy, and people who are receiving short, intermittent, or aerosolized courses of corticosteroids. Intravenous acyclovir is recommended for immunocompromised people, including patients being treated with high-dose corticosteroids for ≥2 weeks, and people with serious, virally mediated complications (such as pneumonia). Therapy initiated within 24 hours of onset maximizes efficacy.

PREVENTION

Vaccine

All people, including those traveling or living abroad, should be assessed for varicella immunity, and those who do not have evidence of immunity or contraindications to vaccination should receive age-appropriate vaccination. Vaccination against varicella is not a requirement for entry into any country (including the United States), but people who do not have evidence of immunity should be considered at risk for varicella during international travel. Evidence of immunity to varicella includes any of the following:

- Documentation of age-appropriate vaccination:
  - Preschool-aged children (≥12 months through 3 years of age): 1 dose
  - School-aged children (≥4 years of age), adolescents, and adults: 2 doses

- Laboratory evidence of immunity or laboratory confirmation of disease

- Birth in the United States before 1980 (not a criterion for health care personnel, pregnant women, and immunocompromised people)

- A health care provider's diagnosis of varicella or verification of a history of varicella

- A health care provider's diagnosis of herpes zoster or verification of a history of herpes zoster

Varicella vaccine contains live, attenuated varicella-zoster virus. Single-antigen varicella vaccine is licensed for people aged ≥12 months, and the combination measles-mumps-rubella-varicella (MMRV) vaccine is licensed only for children 1–12 years. CDC recommends varicella vaccination for all people aged ≥12 months without evidence of immunity to varicella who do not have contraindications to the vaccine: 1 dose for children aged 1–3 years and 2 doses for people aged ≥4 years. The minimum interval between doses is 3 months for children aged <13 years and 4 weeks for people aged ≥13 years. Contraindications for vaccination include allergy to vaccine components, immune-compromising conditions or treatments, and pregnancy. When evidence of immunity is uncertain, a possible history of varicella is not a contraindication to varicella vaccination. Vaccine effectiveness is approximately 80% after 1 dose and 95% after 2 doses.

VACCINE SAFETY AND ADVERSE REACTIONS

The varicella vaccine is generally well tolerated. The most common adverse events after vaccination are self-limited injection-site reactions (pain, soreness, redness, and swelling). Fever or a varicellalike rash, usually consisting of a few lesions at the injection site or generalized rash with a small number of lesions, are reported less frequently.

Compared with use of MMR and varicella vaccines at the same visit, use of MMRV vaccine is associated with a higher risk for fever and febrile seizures 5–12 days after the first dose among children aged 12–23 months and approximately 1 additional febrile seizure for every 2,300–2,600 MMRV vaccine doses administered. Use of separate MMR and varicella vaccines avoids this increased risk for fever and febrile seizures in this age group. For detailed information regarding the varicella vaccine, visit www.cdc.gov/vaccines/vpd-vac/varicella/default.htm.

POSTEXPOSURE PROPHYLAXIS

Vaccine

Varicella vaccine is recommended for postexposure administration for unvaccinated healthy people aged ≥12 months and without other evidence of immunity, to prevent or modify the disease. The vaccine should be administered as soon as possible within 5 days after exposure to rash, if there are no contraindications to use. Among children, protective efficacy was reported as ≥90% when vaccination occurred within 3 days of exposure. No data are available regarding a potential benefit of administering a second dose to 1-dose vaccine recipients after exposure. However, administration of the second dose is recommended for exposed people to bring them up-to-date on vaccination and for best protection against future exposures.

Varicella Zoster Immune Globulin

People without evidence of immunity who have contraindications for vaccination and who are at risk for severe varicella and complications are recommended to receive postexposure prophylaxis with varicella zoster immune globulin. The varicella zoster immune globulin product licensed in the United States is VariZIG.

People who should receive VariZIG after exposure include immunocompromised people, pregnant women without evidence of immunity, and some infants. VariZIG provides maximum benefit when administered as soon as possible after exposure but may be effective if administered as late as 10 days after exposure. In the United States, VariZIG can be obtained from FFF Enterprises, Temecula, California, by calling 800-843-7477 or visiting www.fffenterprises.com or from ASD Healthcare, Frisco, Texas, by calling 800-746-6273 or visiting www.asdhealthcare.com.

If VariZIG is not available, intravenous immune globulin (IVIG) can be considered (also within 10 days of exposure). Additionally, in the absence of both VariZIG and IVIG, some experts recommend prophylaxis with acyclovir (80 mg/kg/day in 4 divided doses for 7 days; maximum dose, 800 mg, 4 times per day), beginning 7–10 days after exposure for people without evidence of immunity and with contraindications for varicella vaccination. Published data on the benefit of acyclovir as postexposure prophylaxis among immunocompromised people are limited.

CDC website: www.cdc.gov/chickenpox

BIBLIOGRAPHY

1. American Academy of Pediatrics. Varicella-zoster infections. In: Kimberlin DW, Brady MT, Jackson MA, Long SS, editors. Red Book: 2015 Report of the Committee on Infectious Diseases. 30th ed. Elk Grove Village, IL: American Academy of Pediatrics; 2015. pp. 846–59.

2. Bialek SR, Perella D, Zhang J, Mascola L, Viner K, Jackson C, et al. Impact of a routine two-dose varicella vaccination program on varicella epidemiology. Pediatrics. 2013 Nov;132(5):e1134–40.

3. CDC. Updated recommendations for use of VariZIG—United States, 2013. MMWR Morb Mortal Wkly Rep. 2013 Jul 19;62(28):574–6.

4. Gershon AA, Takahasi M, Seward JF. Varicella vaccine. In: Plotkin SA, Orenstein WA, Offit PA, editors. Vaccines. 6th ed. Philadelphia: Saunders Elsevier; 2012. pp. 837–69.

5. Harpaz R, Ortega-Sanchez IR, Seward JF. Prevention of herpes zoster: recommendations of the Advisory Committee on Immunization Practices (ACIP). MMWR Recomm Rep. 2008 Jun 6;57(RR-5):1–30.

6. Marin M, Broder KR, Temte JL, Snider DE, Seward JF. Use of combination measles, mumps, rubella, and varicella vaccine: recommendations of the Advisory Committee on Immunization Practices (ACIP). MMWR Recomm Rep. 2010 May 7;59(RR-3):1–12.

7. Marin M, Guris D, Chaves SS, Schmid S, Seward JF. Prevention of varicella: recommendations of the Advisory Committee on Immunization Practices (ACIP). MMWR Recomm Rep. 2007 Jun 22;56(RR-4):1–40.

8. World Health Organization. WHO vaccine-preventable diseases: monitoring system. 2016 global summary 2016 [cited 2016 Sep. 26]. Available from: http://apps.who.int/immunization_monitoring/globalsummary/schedules?sc%5Bd%5D=&sc%5Bv%5D%5B%5D=VARICELLA&sc%5BOK%5D=OK.

VIRAL HEMORRHAGIC FEVERS

Barbara Knust, Mary Choi

INFECTIOUS AGENTS

Viral hemorrhagic fevers (VHFs) are caused by several families of enveloped RNA viruses: filoviruses (Ebola and Marburg hemorrhagic fever, also see the Ebola Virus Disease and Marburg Virus Disease section in this chapter), arenaviruses (Lassa fever, lymphocytic choriomeningitis virus [LCMV], Lujo, Guanarito, Machupo, Junin, Sabia, and Chapare viruses), bunyaviruses (Rift Valley fever [RVF], Crimean-Congo hemorrhagic fever [CCHF], and hantaviruses), and flaviviruses (dengue, yellow fever, Omsk hemorrhagic fever, Kyasanur Forest disease, and Alkhurma viruses) (also see the Dengue and Yellow Fever sections in this chapter).

TRANSMISSION

Some VHFs are spread person-to-person through direct contact with symptomatic patients, body fluids, or cadavers, or through inadequate infection control in a hospital setting (filoviruses, arenaviruses, CCHF virus). Zoonotic spread may occur from contact with the following:

- Livestock via slaughter or consumption of raw meat from infected animals or unpasteurized milk (CCHF, RVF, Alkhurma viruses)

- Rodents or insectivores (arenaviruses, hantaviruses) via direct contact with the animal, or inhalation of or contact with materials contaminated with rodent excreta

- Vectorborne transmission via mosquito (RVF virus) or tick (CCHF, Omsk, Kyasanur Forest disease, Alkhurma viruses) bites or by crushing infected ticks

EPIDEMIOLOGY

The viruses that cause VHF are distributed over much of the globe. Each virus is associated with 1 or more nonhuman host or vector species, restricting the virus and the initial contamination to the areas inhabited by these species. The diseases caused by these viruses are seen in people living in or having visited these areas. Humans are incidental hosts for these enzootic diseases; however, person-to-person transmission of some viruses can occur. Specific viruses are addressed below.

Lassa Fever and Other Arenaviral Diseases

Arenaviruses are transmitted from rodents to humans, except Tacaribe virus, which was found in bats but has not been reported to cause disease in humans. Most infections are mild, but some result in hemorrhagic fever with high death rates. Old World (eastern hemisphere) and New World (western hemisphere) viruses cause the following diseases:

- Old World arenaviruses: Lassa virus (Lassa fever), Lujo virus, and LCMV (meningitis, encephalitis, and congenital fetal infection in normal hosts, severe disease with multiple organ failure in organ transplant recipients). Lassa fever occurs across rural West Africa, with hyperendemic areas in Sierra Leone, Guinea, Liberia, and Nigeria. Lujo virus has been recently described in Zambia and the Republic of South Africa during a health care–associated outbreak.

- New World arenaviruses: Junin (Argentine hemorrhagic fever), Machupo (Bolivian hemorrhagic fever), Guanarito (Venezuelan hemorrhagic fever), Sabia (Brazilian hemorrhagic fever), and the recently discovered Chapare virus (single case in Bolivia).

Reservoir host species are Old World rats and mice (family Muridae, subfamily Murinae) and New World rats and mice (family Muridae, subfamily Sigmodontinae). These rodent types are found worldwide, including Europe, Asia, Africa, and the Americas. Virus is transmitted through inhalation of aerosols from rodent urine, ingestion of rodent-contaminated food, or direct contact of broken skin or mucosa with rodent excreta. Risk of Lassa virus infection is associated with peridomestic rodent exposure, where inappropriate food storage increases the risk for exposure. Several cases of Lassa fever have been confirmed in international travelers staying in traditional dwellings in the countryside. Health

care–associated transmission of Lassa, Lujo, and Machupo viruses has occurred through droplet and direct contact exposures.

Rift Valley Fever and Other Bunyaviral Diseases

RVF primarily affects livestock, causing stillbirths and high mortality in neonatal cattle, sheep, and goats. In humans, RVF virus infection causes fever, hemorrhage, encephalitis, and retinitis. RVF virus is endemic in sub-Saharan Africa. Sporadic outbreaks have occurred in humans in Egypt, Madagascar, and Mauritania. Large epidemics occurred in Kenya, Somalia, and Tanzania in 1997–1998 and 2006–2007; Saudi Arabia and Yemen in 2000; Madagascar in 1990 and 2008; and South Africa, Botswana, Namibia, and Mauritania in 2010. RVF virus is transmitted to livestock by mosquitoes, while people become infected more frequently through direct contact with clinically affected animals or their body fluids, including slaughter or consumption of infected animals.

CCHF is endemic where ticks of the genus *Hyalomma* are found in Africa and Eurasia, including South Africa, the Balkans, the Middle East, Russia, and western China, and is highly endemic in Turkey, Afghanistan, Iran, and Pakistan. The first human cases were reported in Spain in 2016. The *Hyalomma* ticks are primarily associated with livestock but will also bite humans. Livestock and other tick hosts may develop CCHF viremia from tick bites but do not develop clinical disease. CCHF virus is transmitted to humans by infected ticks or direct handling and preparation of fresh carcasses of infected animals, usually domestic livestock. Nosocomial human-to-human transmission can occur through droplet or direct contact.

Hantaviruses cause hantavirus pulmonary syndrome (HPS) and hemorrhagic fever with renal syndrome (HFRS). The viruses that cause HPS are present in the New World; those that cause HFRS occur worldwide. The viruses that cause both HPS and HFRS are transmitted to humans through contact with urine, feces, or saliva of infected rodents. Travelers staying in rodent-infested dwellings are at risk for HPS and

3

HFRS. Human-to-human transmission of hantavirus has been reported only with Andes virus in Chile and Argentina.

CLINICAL PRESENTATION

Signs and symptoms vary by disease, but in general, patients with VHF present with abrupt onset of fever, myalgias, and prostration, followed in severe forms by coagulopathy with a petechial rash or ecchymoses and sometimes overt bleeding. Gastrointestinal symptoms (diarrhea, vomiting, abdominal pain) are commonly observed. Vascular endothelial damage leads to shock and pulmonary edema, and liver injury is common. Signs seen with specific viruses include renal failure (HFRS), ecchymoses and bruises (CCHF), pharyngitis, retrosternal pain, hearing loss in adults and anasarca in newborns (Lassa fever), and spontaneous abortion and birth defects (Lassa virus and LCMV). Laboratory abnormalities include elevations in liver enzymes, initial drop in leukocyte count, and thrombocytopenia. Because the incubation period may be as long as 21 days, patients may not develop illness until returning from travel; therefore, a thorough travel and exposure history is critical.

DIAGNOSIS

US-based clinicians should notify local health authorities immediately of any suspected cases of VHF occurring in patients residing in the United States, or notify the CDC directly regarding any patients requiring evacuation to the United States (contact the CDC Emergency Operations Center at 770-488-7100). Appropriate personal protective equipment is indicated for any patients where Lassa, Lujo, South American arenaviruses, or CCHFV infection is suspected and includes droplet and contact precautions. Whole blood or serum may be tested for virologic (RT-PCR, antigen detection, virus isolation) and immunologic (IgM, IgG) evidence of infection. Tissue may be tested by immunohistochemistry, RT-PCR, and virus isolation. Blood collected within a few hours after death by cardiac puncture can be used for diagnosis.

TREATMENT

Ribavirin is effective if given early in course of disease for treating Lassa fever and other Old World arenaviruses, New World arenaviruses, and potentially CCHF, but it is not approved by the Food and Drug Administration (FDA) for these indications. Convalescent-phase plasma is effective in treating Argentine hemorrhagic fever. Intravenous ribavirin can be obtained for compassionate use through FDA from Valeant Pharmaceuticals (Aliso Viejo, California). Requests should be initiated by the provider through FDA (301-796-1500 or after hours 866-300-4374), with simultaneous notification to Valeant Pharmaceuticals: 800-548-5100, extension 5 (domestic telephone). The process is explained on FDA's website (www. fda.gov/Drugs/DevelopmentApprovalProcess/ HowDrugsareDevelopedandApproved/Approval Applications/InvestigationalNewDrugIND Application/ucm090039.htm).

PREVENTION

The risk of acquiring VHF is very low for international travelers. Travelers at increased risk for exposure include those engaging in animal research, health care workers, and others providing care for patients in the community without adequate personal protection, particularly where outbreaks of VHF are occurring.

Prevention should focus on avoiding unprotected contact with people suspected of having VHF or host or vector species in endemic countries. Travelers should not visit locations where an outbreak is occurring, avoid contact with rodents, and avoid blood or body fluids of livestock in RVF- and CCHF-endemic areas. To prevent vectorborne disease, travelers should use insecticide-treated bed nets and wear insect repellent.

Standard precautions and contact and droplet precautions for suspected VHF patients are recommended to avoid transmission. Direct contact should be avoided with corpses of patients suspected of having died of CCHF or arenavirus infection. Investigational vaccines exist for Argentine hemorrhagic fever and RVF; however, neither is approved by FDA, nor are they commonly available in the United States.

BIBLIOGRAPHY

1. Ergonul O, Holbrook MR. Crimean-Congo hemorrhagic fever. In: Guerrant RL, Walker DH, Weller PF, editors. Tropical Infectious Diseases: Principles, Pathogens and Practice. 3rd ed. Philadelphia: Elsevier; 2011. pp. 466–9.

2. Gunther S, Lenz O. Lassa virus. Crit Rev Clin Lab Sci. 2004;41(4):339–90.

3. Heyman P, Vaheri A, Lundkvist A, Avsic-Zupanc T. Hantavirus infections in Europe: from virus carriers to a major public-health problem. Expert Rev Anti Infect Ther. 2009 Mar;7(2):205–17.

4. Marty AM, Jahrling PB, Geisbert TW. Viral hemorrhagic fevers. Clin Lab Med. 2006 Jun;26(2):345–86, viii.

5. Ozkurt Z, Kiki I, Erol S, Erdem F, Yilmaz N, Parlak M, et al. Crimean-Congo hemorrhagic fever in eastern Turkey: clinical features, risk factors and efficacy of ribavirin therapy. J Infect. 2006 Mar;52(3):207–15.

6. Paweska JT, Sewlall NH, Ksiazek TG, Blumberg LH, Hale MJ, Lipkin WI, et al. Nosocomial outbreak of novel arenavirus infection, southern Africa. Emerg Infect Dis. 2009 Oct;15(10):1598–602.

7. Peters CJ, Makino S, Morrill JC. Rift valley fever. In: Guerrant RL, Walker DH, Weller PF, editors. Tropical Infectious Diseases: Principles, Pathogens and Practice. 3rd ed. Philadelphia: Saunders Elsevier; 2011. pp. 462–5.

8. Peters CJ, Zaki SR. Overview of viral hemorrhagic fevers. In: Guerrant RL, Walker DH, Weller PF, editors. Tropical Infectious Diseases: Principles, Pathogens and Practice. 3rd ed. Philadelphia: Elsevier; 2011. pp. 441–8.

9. Rollin PE, Nichol ST, Zaki S, Ksiazek TG. Arenaviruses and filoviruses. In: Jorgensen JH, Pfaller MA, Carroll KC, Funke G, Landry ML, Richter SS, et al., editors. Manual of Clinical Microbiology. 11th ed. Washington, DC: ASM Press; 2015. pp. 1669–86.

10. Wahl-Jensen V, Peters CJ, Jahrling PB, Feldman H, Kuhn JH. Filovirus infections. In: Guerrant RL, Walker DH, Weller PF, editors. Tropical Infectious Diseases: Principles, Pathogens and Practice. 3rd ed. Philadelphia: Elsevier; 2011. pp. 483–91.

YELLOW FEVER

Mark D. Gershman, J. Erin Staples

INFECTIOUS AGENT

Yellow fever virus (YFV) is a single-stranded RNA virus that belongs to the genus *Flavivirus*.

TRANSMISSION

Vectorborne transmission occurs via the bite of an infected mosquito, primarily *Aedes* or *Haemagogus* spp. Nonhuman and human primates are the main reservoirs of the virus, with anthroponotic (human-to-vector-to-human) transmission occurring. There are 3 transmission cycles for yellow fever: sylvatic (jungle), intermediate (savannah), and urban.

- The sylvatic (jungle) cycle involves transmission of the virus between nonhuman primates and mosquito species found in the forest canopy. The virus is transmitted via mosquitoes from monkeys to humans when the humans encroach into the jungle during occupational or recreational activities.

- In Africa, an intermediate (savannah) cycle involves transmission of YFV from tree hole-breeding *Aedes* spp. to humans living or working in jungle border areas. In this cycle, the virus may be transmitted from monkeys to humans or from human to human via these mosquitoes.

- The urban cycle involves transmission of the virus between humans and peridomestic mosquitoes, primarily *Ae. aegypti*.

Humans infected with YFV experience the highest levels of viremia and can transmit the virus to mosquitoes shortly before onset of fever and for the first 3–5 days of illness. Given the high level of viremia, bloodborne transmission theoretically can occur via transfusion or needlesticks. One case of perinatal transmission of wild-type YFV has been documented from a woman who developed symptoms of yellow fever 3 days before giving birth. The infant tested positive for YFV RNA and died of fulminant yellow fever on the 12th day of life.

EPIDEMIOLOGY

Yellow fever occurs in sub-Saharan Africa and tropical South America, where it is endemic and intermittently epidemic (see Tables 3-22 and 3-23 for a list of countries with risk of YFV transmission). Most yellow fever disease in humans is due to sylvatic or intermediate transmission cycles. However, urban yellow fever occurs periodically in Africa and sporadically in the Americas. In areas of Africa with persistent circulation of YFV, natural immunity accumulates with age, and thus, infants and children are at highest risk for disease. In South America, yellow fever occurs most frequently in unimmunized young men who are exposed to mosquito vectors through their work in forested areas.

RISK FOR TRAVELERS

A traveler's risk for acquiring yellow fever is determined by various factors, including immunization status, location of travel, season, duration of exposure, occupational and recreational activities while traveling, and local rate of virus transmission at the time of travel. Although reported cases of human disease are the principal indicator of disease risk, case reports may be absent because of a low level of transmission, a high level of immunity in the population (because of vaccination, for example), or failure of local surveillance systems to detect cases. This "epidemiologic silence" does not equate to absence of risk and should not lead to travel without taking protective measures.

YFV transmission in rural West Africa is seasonal, with an elevated risk during the end of the rainy season and the beginning of the dry season (usually July–October). However, YFV may be episodically transmitted by *Ae. aegypti* even during the dry season in both rural and densely settled urban areas.

The risk for infection in South America is highest during the rainy season (January–May, with a peak incidence in February and March). Given the high level of viremia that may occur in infected humans and the widespread distribution of *Ae. aegypti* in many towns and cities, South America is at risk for a large-scale urban epidemic.

From 1970 through 2015, a total of 10 cases of yellow fever were reported in unvaccinated travelers from the United States and Europe who traveled to West Africa (5 cases) or South America (5 cases). Eight (80%) of these 10 travelers died. There has been only 1 documented case of yellow fever in

3

Table 3-22. Countries with risk of yellow fever virus (YFV) transmission[1]

AFRICA			CENTRAL AND SOUTH AMERICA
Angola	Ethiopia[2]	Nigeria	Argentina[2]
Benin	Gabon	Senegal	Bolivia[2]
Burkina Faso	The Gambia	Sierra Leone	Brazil[2]
Burundi	Ghana	South Sudan	Colombia[2]
Cameroon	Guinea	Sudan[2]	Ecuador[2]
Central African Republic	Guinea-Bissau	Togo	French Guiana
Chad[2]	Kenya[2]	Uganda	Guyana
Congo, Republic of the	Liberia		Panama[2]
Côte d'Ivoire	Mali[2]		Paraguay
Democratic Republic of the Congo[2]	Mauritania[2]		Peru[2]
Equatorial Guinea	Niger[2]		Suriname
			Trinidad and Tobago[2]
			Venezuela[2]

[1] Countries or areas where "a risk of YFV transmission is present," as defined by the World Health Organization, are countries or areas where "yellow fever has been reported currently or in the past, plus vectors and animal reservoirs currently exist" (see the current country list within the *International Travel and Health* publication (Annex 1) at www.who.int/ith/en/index.html).

[2] These countries are not holoendemic (only a portion of the country has risk of yellow fever transmission). See Maps 3-14 and 3-15 and yellow fever vaccine recommendations (Yellow Fever & Malaria Information, by Country) for details.

Table 3-23. Countries with low potential for exposure to yellow fever virus (YFV)[1]

AFRICA
Eritrea[2]
Rwanda[3]
São Tomé and Príncipe[3]
Somalia[2]
Tanzania[3]
Zambia[2]

[1] Countries listed in this table are not contained on the official World Health Organization list of countries with risk of YFV transmission (Table 3-22). Therefore, proof of yellow fever vaccination should not be required if traveling from any of these countries to another country with a vaccination entry requirement (unless that country requires proof of yellow fever vaccination from all arriving travelers; see Table 3-26). An exception is Bolivia, which requires yellow fever vaccination for people traveling from or transiting through any of the 6 countries with low potential for exposure, in addition to those with risk of YFV transmission.

[2] These countries are classified as "low potential for exposure to YFV" in only some areas; the remaining areas of these countries are classified as having no risk of exposure to YFV.

[3] The entire area of these countries is classified as "low potential for exposure to YFV."

a vaccinated traveler. This nonfatal case occurred in a traveler from Spain who visited several West African countries in 1988. In early 2016, >15 long-term travelers from Africa and Asia developed yellow fever disease after visiting Angola, where one of the largest urban outbreaks was occurring. Reportedly, none of the ill travelers was vaccinated.

The risk of acquiring yellow fever is difficult to predict because of variations in ecologic determinants of virus transmission. For a 2-week stay, the estimated risks for illness and death due to yellow fever for an unvaccinated traveler visiting an endemic area in:

- West Africa are 50 per 100,000 and 10 per 100,000, respectively

- South America are 5 per 100,000 and 1 per 100,000, respectively

The risk of illness during outbreaks of the disease is likely higher. These estimates are a rough guideline based on the risk to indigenous populations, often during peak transmission season. Thus, these risk estimates may not accurately reflect the risk to travelers, who may have a different immunity profile, take precautions against getting bitten by mosquitoes, and have less outdoor exposure.

The risk of acquiring yellow fever in South America is lower than that in Africa, because the mosquitoes that transmit the virus between monkeys in the forest canopy in South America do not often come in contact with humans. Additionally, there is a relatively high level of immunity in local residents because of vaccine use, which might reduce the risk of transmission.

CLINICAL PRESENTATION

Asymptomatic or clinically inapparent infection is believed to occur in most people infected with YFV. For people who develop symptomatic illness, the incubation period is typically 3–6 days. The initial illness presents as a nonspecific influenzalike syndrome with sudden onset of fever, chills, headache, backache, myalgia, prostration, nausea, and vomiting. Most patients improve after the initial presentation. After a brief remission of hours to a day, approximately 15% of patients progress to a more serious or toxic form of the disease, characterized by jaundice, hemorrhagic symptoms, and eventually shock and multisystem organ failure. The case-fatality ratio for severe cases with hepatorenal dysfunction is 20%–50%.

DIAGNOSIS

The preliminary diagnosis is based on the patient's clinical features, places and dates of travel, and activities. Laboratory diagnosis is best performed by:

- Virus isolation or nucleic acid amplification tests performed early in the illness for YFV or yellow fever viral RNA. However, by the time more overt symptoms are recognized, the virus or viral RNA might be undetectable. Therefore, virus isolation and nucleic acid amplification should not be used to rule out a diagnosis of yellow fever.

- Serologic assays to detect virus-specific IgM and IgG antibodies. Because of cross-reactivity between antibodies raised against other flaviviruses, more specific antibody testing, such as a plaque reduction neutralization test, should be done to confirm the infection.

Clinicians should contact their state or local health department or call the CDC Arboviral Diseases Branch at 970-221-6400 for assistance with diagnostic testing for yellow fever infections and for questions about antibody response to vaccination. Yellow fever is a nationally notifiable disease.

TREATMENT

There are no specific medications to treat YFV infections; treatment is directed at symptomatic relief or life-saving interventions. Rest, fluids, and use of analgesics and antipyretics may relieve symptoms of fever and aching. Care should be taken to avoid medications, such as aspirin or nonsteroidal anti-inflammatory drugs, which may increase the risk for bleeding. Infected people should be protected from further mosquito exposure (staying indoors or under a mosquito net) during the first few days of illness, so they do not contribute to the transmission cycle.

PREVENTION

Personal Protection Measures

The best way to prevent mosquitoborne diseases, including yellow fever, is to avoid mosquito bites (see Chapter 2, Protection against Mosquitoes, Ticks, & Other Arthropods).

Vaccine

Yellow fever is preventable by a relatively safe, effective vaccine. All yellow fever vaccines currently manufactured are live-attenuated viral vaccines. Only one yellow fever vaccine is licensed for use in the United States (Table 3-24). Studies comparing the reactogenicity and immunogenicity of various yellow fever vaccines, including those manufactured outside the United States, suggest that there is no substantial difference in the reactogenicity or immune response generated by the various vaccines. Thus, people who receive yellow fever vaccines in other countries should be considered protected against yellow fever.

INDICATIONS FOR USE

Yellow fever vaccine is recommended for people aged ≥9 months who are traveling to or living in areas with risk for YFV transmission in South America and Africa. In addition, some countries require proof of yellow fever vaccination for entry. See the Yellow Fever & Malaria Information, by Country section at the end of this chapter for more detailed information on the requirements and recommendations for yellow fever vaccination for specific countries.

Because of the risk of serious adverse events after yellow fever vaccination, clinicians should only vaccinate people who (1) are at risk of exposure to YFV or (2) require proof of vaccination to enter a country. To further minimize the risk of serious adverse events, clinicians should carefully observe the contraindications and consider the precautions to vaccination before administering

Table 3-24. Vaccine to prevent yellow fever

VACCINE	TRADE NAME (MANUFACTURER)	AGE	DOSE	ROUTE	SCHEDULE	BOOSTER
17D yellow fever vaccine	YF-Vax (Sanofi Pasteur)	≥9 months[1]	0.5 mL[2]	SC	1 dose	Not recommended for most[3]

Abbreviation: SC, subcutaneous.
[1] Ages 6–8 months and ≥60 years are precautions and age <6 months is a contraindication to the use of yellow fever vaccine.
[2] YF-Vax is available in single-dose and multiple-dose (5-dose) vials.
[3] For further details regarding revaccination, see "Vaccine Administration" in this section.

Table 3-25. Contraindications and precautions to yellow fever vaccine administration

CONTRAINDICATIONS	PRECAUTIONS
• Allergy to vaccine component[1] • Age <6 months • Symptomatic HIV infection or CD4 T lymphocytes <200/mm³ (or <15% of total lymphocytes in children aged <6 years)[2] • Thymus disorder associated with abnormal immune-cell function • Primary immunodeficiencies • Malignant neoplasms • Transplantation • Immunosuppressive and immunomodulatory therapies	• Age 6–8 months • Age ≥60 years • Asymptomatic HIV infection and CD4 T lymphocytes 200–499/mm³ (or 15%–24% of total lymphocytes in children aged <6 years)[2] • Pregnancy • Breastfeeding

[1] If vaccination is considered essential because of a high risk for acquiring yellow fever, desensitization can be performed under direct supervision of a physician experienced in the management of anaphylaxis
[2] Symptoms of HIV are classified in 1) Adults and Adolescents, Table 1. CDC. 1993 Revised classification system for HIV infection and expanded surveillance case definition for AIDS among adolescents and adults. MMWR Recomm Rep 1992;41(RR-17). Available from: www.cdc.gov/mmwr/preview/mmwrhtml/00018871.htm and 2) Panel on Antiretroviral Therapy and Medical Management of HIV-Infected Children. Guidelines for the use of antiretroviral agents in pediatric HIV infection. 2010. Available from http://aidsinfo.nih.gov/ContentFiles/PediatricGuidelines.pdf. pp. 20–2.

yellow fever vaccine (Table 3-25). For additional information, refer to the yellow fever vaccine recommendations of the Advisory Committee on Immunization Practices (ACIP) at www.cdc.gov/vaccines/hcp/acip-recs/vacc-specific/yf.html.

VACCINE ADMINISTRATION

For all eligible people, a single injection of reconstituted vaccine should be administered subcutaneously. Until recently, revaccination has been required by certain countries at 10-year intervals to comply with International Health Regulations (IHR) of the World Health Organization (WHO). However, in 2014, the WHO Strategic Advisory Group of Experts on Immunization concluded that a single primary dose of yellow fever vaccine provides sustained immunity and lifelong protection against yellow fever disease and that a booster dose is not needed. That year the World Health Organization adopted the recommendation to remove the 10-year booster dose requirement from the IHR after a 2-year transition period. As of July 11, 2016, a completed International Certificate of Vaccination or Prophylaxis is valid for the lifetime of the vaccinee and countries cannot require proof of revaccination (booster) against yellow fever as a condition of entry, even if the last vaccination was more than 10 years prior.

The Advisory Committee on Immunization Practices (ACIP) also stated that a single dose of yellow fever vaccine provides long-lasting protection and is adequate for most travelers. However, these guidelines specify that additional doses of yellow fever vaccine are recommended for the following groups of travelers:

- Women who were pregnant when they received their initial dose of vaccine: they should receive 1 additional dose of yellow fever vaccine before their next travel that puts them at risk for yellow fever.

- People who received a hematopoietic stem cell transplant after receiving a dose of yellow fever vaccine: they should be revaccinated before their next travel that puts them at risk for yellow fever as long as they are sufficiently immunocompetent to be safely vaccinated.

- People who were infected with HIV when they received their last dose of yellow fever vaccine: they should receive a dose every 10 years if they continue to be at risk for yellow fever virus infection.

The updated recommendations also note that a booster dose may be considered for travelers who received their last dose of yellow fever vaccine

≥10 years previously and who will be in a higher-risk setting based on season, location, activities, and duration of their travel. This would include travelers who plan to spend a prolonged period in endemic areas, or those traveling to highly endemic areas such as rural West Africa during peak transmission season or an area with an ongoing outbreak. All current ACIP yellow fever vaccine recommendations can be found on the ACIP website at www.cdc.gov/vaccines/hcp/acip-recs/vacc-specific/yf.html.

Although booster doses of yellow fever vaccine are not recommended for most travelers, and despite the recent changes to the IHR, clinicians and travelers should review the entry requirements for destination countries. At the time this edition goes to press it is uncertain when and if all countries with yellow fever vaccination requirements will adopt and fully implement this change that is stipulated by the IHR. See the yellow fever vaccination requirements on the CDC Travelers' Health website (wwwnc.cdc.gov/travel/destinations/list) for more information on country-specific recommendations and requirements.

VACCINE SAFETY AND ADVERSE REACTIONS

COMMON ADVERSE REACTIONS

Reactions to yellow fever vaccine are generally mild; 10%–30% of vaccinees report mild systemic adverse events. Reported events typically include low-grade fever, headache, and myalgia that begin within days after vaccination and last 5–10 days. Approximately 1% of vaccinees temporarily curtail their regular activities because of these reactions.

SEVERE ADVERSE REACTIONS

Hypersensitivity—Immediate hypersensitivity reactions, characterized by rash, urticaria, or bronchospasm are uncommon. Anaphylaxis after yellow fever vaccine is reported to occur at a rate of 1.3 cases per 100,000 doses administered.

Yellow Fever Vaccine–Associated Neurologic Disease (YEL-AND)—YEL-AND represents a conglomerate of clinical syndromes, including meningoencephalitis, Guillain-Barré syndrome, acute disseminated encephalomyelitis, and rarely, cranial nerve palsies. Historically, YEL-AND was seen primarily among infants as encephalitis, but more recent reports have been among people of all ages. YEL-AND is rarely fatal.

Among all cases of YEL-AND reported globally, almost all occurred in first-time vaccine recipients. The onset of illness for documented cases in the United States is 2–56 days after vaccination. The incidence of YEL-AND in the United States is 0.8 per 100,000 doses administered. The rate is higher in people aged ≥60 years, with a rate of 2.2 per 100,000 doses.

Yellow Fever Vaccine–Associated Viscerotropic Disease (YEL-AVD)—YEL-AVD is a severe illness similar to wild-type disease, with vaccine virus proliferating in multiple organs and often leading to multiple organ dysfunction syndrome or multiorgan failure and death. Since the initial cases of YEL-AVD were published in 2001, >100 confirmed and suspected cases have been reported throughout the world.

YEL-AVD has been reported to occur only after the first dose of yellow fever vaccine; worldwide, there have been no laboratory-confirmed reports of YEL-AVD following booster doses. For YEL-AVD cases reported in the United States, the median time from yellow fever vaccination until symptom onset is 4 days (range, 1–18 days). The case-fatality ratio for all reported YEL-AVD cases in the United States is approximately 46%. The incidence of YEL-AVD in the United States is 0.3 cases per 100,000 doses of vaccine administered. The rate is higher for people aged ≥60 years, with a rate of 1.2 per 100,000 doses. The rate is even higher for people aged ≥70 years.

CONTRAINDICATIONS

INFANTS YOUNGER THAN 6 MONTHS

Yellow fever vaccine is contraindicated for infants aged <6 months. This contraindication was instituted in the late 1960s in response to a high rate of YEL-AND documented in vaccinated young infants (50–400 per 100,000). The mechanism of increased neurovirulence in infants is unknown but may be due to the immaturity of the blood-brain barrier, higher or more prolonged viremia, or immune system immaturity.

HYPERSENSITIVITY

Yellow fever vaccine is contraindicated for people with a history of acute hypersensitivity reaction to a previous dose of the vaccine, as well as those who have a history of an allergic reaction to any of the vaccine components, including eggs, egg products, chicken proteins, or gelatin. The stopper used in vials of vaccine also contains dry natural latex rubber, which may cause an allergic reaction.

If vaccination of a person with a questionable history of hypersensitivity to any of the vaccine components is considered essential because of a high risk for acquiring yellow fever, skin testing, as described in the vaccine package insert, should be performed under close medical supervision. If a person has a positive skin test to the vaccine or has severe egg sensitivity and the vaccination is recommended, desensitization, as described in the package insert, can be performed under direct supervision of a physician experienced in the management of anaphylaxis.

ALTERED IMMUNE STATUS

Thymus Disorder—Yellow fever vaccine is contraindicated for people with a thymus disorder that is associated with abnormal immune cell function, such as thymoma or myasthenia gravis. If travel to a yellow fever–endemic area cannot be avoided in a person with such a thymus disorder, a medical waiver should be provided and counseling on protective measures against mosquito bites should be emphasized. Because there is no evidence of immune dysfunction or increased risk of yellow fever vaccine–associated serious adverse events in people who have undergone incidental surgical removal of their thymus or have had indirect radiation therapy in the distant past, these people can be given yellow fever vaccine if recommended or required.

HIV Infection—Yellow fever vaccine is contraindicated for people with AIDS or other clinical manifestations of HIV, including people with CD4 T lymphocyte values <200/mm³ or <15% of total lymphocytes for children aged <6 years. This recommendation is based on a potential increased risk of encephalitis in this population.

If travel to a yellow fever–endemic area cannot be avoided by a person with severe immune suppression based on CD4 counts (<200/mm³ or <15% total lymphocytes for children aged <6 years) or symptomatic HIV, a medical waiver should be provided, and counseling on protective measures against mosquito bites should be emphasized. See the following section, Precautions, for other HIV-infected people not meeting the above criteria.

Immunodeficiencies (other than thymus disorder or HIV infection)—Yellow fever vaccine is contraindicated for people with primary immunodeficiencies, as well as those with malignant neoplasms or transplantation that might be associated with immunosuppression caused either by treatment or the underlying condition. While there are no data on the use of yellow fever vaccine in these people, they presumably are at increased risk for yellow fever vaccine–associated serious adverse events (see Chapter 8, Immunocompromised Travelers). If someone with an immunodeficiency cannot avoid travel to a yellow fever–endemic area, a medical waiver should be provided, and counseling on protective measures against mosquito bites should be emphasized.

Immunosuppressive and Immunomodulatory Therapies—Yellow fever vaccine is contraindicated for people whose immunologic response is either suppressed or modulated by current or recent radiation therapies or drugs. Drugs with known immunosuppressive or immunomodulatory properties include, but are not limited to, high-dose systemic corticosteroids, alkylating drugs, antimetabolites, tumor necrosis factor-α inhibitors (such as etanercept), interleukin-1 and interleukin-6 blocking agents (such as anakinra and tocilizumab), or other monoclonal antibodies targeting immune cells (such as rituximab or alemtuzumab). There are no specific data on the use of yellow fever vaccine in people receiving these therapies. However, these people are presumed to be at increased risk for yellow fever vaccine–associated serious adverse events, and the use of live attenuated vaccines is contraindicated in the package insert for most of these therapies (see Chapter 8, Immunocompromised Travelers).

Live viral vaccines should be deferred in people who have discontinued these therapies until immune function has improved. If travel to a yellow fever–endemic area cannot be avoided for someone receiving immunosuppressive or immunomodulatory therapies, a medical waiver should be provided and counseling on protective measures against mosquito bites should be emphasized.

Family members of people with altered immune status, who themselves have no contraindications, can receive yellow fever vaccine.

PRECAUTIONS

INFANTS AGED 6–8 MONTHS

Age 6–8 months is a precaution for yellow fever vaccination. Two cases of YEL-AND have been reported among infants aged 6–8 months. In infants <6 months of age, the rates of YEL-AND are elevated (50–400 per 100,000). By 9 months of age, risk for YEL-AND is believed to be substantially lower. ACIP generally recommends that, whenever possible, travel to yellow fever–endemic countries should be postponed or avoided for children aged 6–8 months. If travel is unavoidable, the decision of whether to vaccinate these infants needs to balance the risks of YFV exposure with the risk for adverse events after vaccination.

ADULTS 60 YEARS OF AGE OR OLDER

Age ≥60 years is a precaution for yellow fever vaccination, particularly if this is the first dose of the yellow fever vaccine given. From adverse events passively reported to the Vaccine Adverse Events Reporting System (VAERS), the rate of serious adverse events in people aged ≥60 years was 7.7 per 100,000 doses distributed, compared with 3.8 per 100,000 for all vaccine recipients. The risk of YEL-AND and YEL-AVD is also increased in this age group, at 2.2 and 1.2 per 100,000 doses, respectively, compared with 0.8 and 0.3 per 100,000 for all vaccine recipients. Given that YEL-AVD has been reported exclusively, and YEL-AND almost exclusively, in primary vaccine recipients, caution should be exercised with older travelers who may be receiving yellow fever vaccine for the first time. If travel is unavoidable, the decision to vaccinate travelers aged ≥60 years needs to weigh the risks and benefits of the vaccination in the context of their destination-specific risk for exposure to YFV.

HIV INFECTION

Asymptomatic HIV infection with CD4 T lymphocyte values 200–499/mm³ or 15%–24% of total lymphocytes for children aged <6 years is a precaution for yellow fever vaccination (see also the discussion

of HIV infection in the Contraindications section above). Large prospective, randomized trials have not been performed to adequately address the safety and efficacy of yellow fever vaccine among this group. Retrospective and prospective studies that combined included >500 HIV-infected people reported no serious adverse events among patients considered moderately immunosuppressed based on their CD4 counts. However, HIV infection has been associated with a reduced immunologic response to a number of inactivated and live attenuated vaccines, including yellow fever vaccine. The mechanisms for the diminished immune response in HIV-infected people are uncertain but appear to be correlated with HIV RNA levels and CD4 T cell counts.

If an asymptomatic HIV-infected person with moderate immune suppression (CD4 T lymphocyte values 200–499/mm³ or 15%–24% of total lymphocytes for children aged <6 years) is traveling to a yellow fever–endemic area, vaccination may be considered. Vaccinated people should be monitored closely after vaccination; if an adverse event occurs, the state health department or CDC should be notified and a report made to VAERS. However, if international travel requirements—not risk of yellow fever—are the only reason to vaccinate an HIV-infected person, the person should be excused from immunization and issued a medical waiver to fulfill health regulations.

If an asymptomatic HIV-infected person has no evidence of immune suppression based on CD4 counts (CD4 T lymphocyte values ≥500/mm³ or ≥25% of total lymphocytes for children aged <6 years), yellow fever vaccine can be administered if recommended.

Because vaccinating asymptomatic HIV-infected people might be less effective than vaccinating people not infected with HIV, measuring their neutralizing antibody response to vaccination should be considered before travel. Contact the state health department or the CDC Arboviral Diseases Branch (970-221-6400) to discuss serologic testing.

PREGNANCY

Pregnancy is a precaution for yellow fever vaccine administration. The safety of yellow fever

3

vaccination during pregnancy has not been studied in a large prospective trial. However, a study of women who were vaccinated with yellow fever vaccine early in their pregnancies found no major malformations in their infants. A slight increased risk was noted for minor, mostly skin, malformations in infants. A higher rate of spontaneous abortions in pregnant women receiving the vaccine was reported but not substantiated in a subsequent study. The proportion of women vaccinated during pregnancy who develop YFV-specific IgG antibodies is variable depending on the study (39% or 98%) and may be correlated with the trimester in which they received the vaccine. Because pregnancy may affect immunologic function, serologic testing can be considered to document a protective immune response to the vaccine.

If travel is unavoidable and the vaccination risks are felt to outweigh the risks of YFV exposure, pregnant women should be excused from immunization and issued a medical waiver to fulfill health regulations. Pregnant women who must travel to areas where YFV exposure is likely should be vaccinated. Although there are no specific data, ACIP recommends that a woman wait 4 weeks after receiving the yellow fever vaccine before conceiving.

BREASTFEEDING

Breastfeeding is a precaution for yellow fever vaccine administration. Three YEL-AND cases have been reported in exclusively breastfed infants whose mothers were vaccinated with yellow fever vaccine. All 3 infants were diagnosed with encephalitis and aged <1 month at the time of exposure. Further research is needed to document the risk of potential vaccine exposure through breastfeeding. Until more information is available, yellow fever vaccine should be avoided in breastfeeding women. However, when travel of nursing mothers to a yellow fever–endemic area cannot be avoided or postponed, these women should be vaccinated.

OTHER CONSIDERATIONS

There are no data regarding possible increased adverse events or decreased vaccine efficacy after administration of yellow fever vaccine to patients with other chronic medical conditions (such as renal disease, hepatitis C virus infection, other liver disease, or diabetes mellitus). Caution should be used if considering vaccination of such patients. Factors to consider in assessing patients' general level of immune competence include disease severity, duration, clinical stability, complications, and comorbidities.

SIMULTANEOUS ADMINISTRATION OF OTHER VACCINES AND DRUGS

No evidence exists that inactivated vaccines interfere with the immune response to yellow fever vaccine. Therefore, inactivated vaccines can be administered either simultaneously or at any time before or after yellow fever vaccination. ACIP recommends that yellow fever vaccine be given at the same time as other live viral vaccines. Otherwise, the clinician should wait 30 days between vaccinations, as the immune response to a live viral vaccine might be impaired if administered within 30 days of another live viral vaccine. One study involving the simultaneous administration of yellow fever and measles-mumps-rubella (MMR) vaccines in children found a decrease in the immune response against yellow fever, mumps, and rubella when the vaccines were given on the same day versus 30 days apart. Additional studies are needed to confirm these findings, but they suggest that if possible, yellow fever and MMR should be given 30 days apart. Limited data suggest oral Ty21a typhoid vaccine, a live bacterial vaccine, can be administered simultaneously or at any interval before or after yellow fever vaccine. There are no data on the immune response to live attenuated influenza and yellow fever vaccines administered simultaneously. However, data from live attenuated influenza and MMR found no evidence of interference.

INTERNATIONAL CERTIFICATE OF VACCINATION OR PROPHYLAXIS (ICVP)

The IHR allow countries to require proof of yellow fever vaccination documented on an ICVP as a condition of entry for travelers arriving from certain countries, even if only in transit, to prevent importation and indigenous transmission of YFV. Some countries require evidence of vaccination from all entering travelers, which includes

Table 3-26. Countries that require proof of yellow fever vaccination from all arriving travelers[1]

Angola	Ghana
Burundi	Guinea-Bissau
Cameroon	Liberia
Central African Republic	Mali
Congo, Republic of the	Niger
Côte d'Ivoire	Sierra Leone
Democratic Republic of the Congo	Togo
French Guiana	Uganda
Gabon	

[1] Country requirements for yellow fever vaccination are subject to change at any time; therefore, CDC encourages travelers to check with the destination country's embassy or consulate before departure.

direct travel from the United States (Table 3-26). Some countries do not require an ICVP for infants younger than a certain age (see Yellow Fever & Malaria Information, by Country section at the end of this chapter for specific age requirements). A traveler who has a specific contraindication to yellow fever vaccine and who cannot avoid travel to a country requiring vaccination should request a waiver from a physician before embarking on travel (see the Medical Waivers [Exemptions] section below). Travelers who arrive in a country that has a yellow fever vaccination entry requirement without proof of yellow fever vaccination or a medical waiver may be quarantined for up to 6 days, refused entry, or vaccinated on site.

AUTHORIZATION TO PROVIDE VACCINATIONS AND TO VALIDATE THE ICVP

People who received a yellow fever vaccination after December 15, 2007, must provide proof of vaccination on the new ICVP. If the person received the vaccine before December 15, 2007, their original International Certificate of Vaccination against Yellow Fever (ICV) card is still valid as proof of vaccination. Vaccinees should receive a completed ICVP (Figure 3-2), validated (stamped and signed) with the stamp of the center where the vaccine was given (see below). An incomplete or inaccurate ICVP is not valid. Failure to secure validations can cause a traveler to be quarantined, denied entry, or possibly revaccinated at the point of entry to a country. Revaccination at the point of entry is not a recommended option for the traveler.

Clinics may purchase ICVPs, CDC 731 (formerly PHS 731), from the US Government Printing Office (http://bookstore.gpo.gov, 866-512-1800). This certificate of vaccination (ICVP) is valid beginning 10 days after the date of primary vaccination. As of July 2016, the yellow fever vaccine booster requirement was eliminated in the IHR and a completed ICVP is considered valid for the lifetime of the vaccinee.

PEOPLE AUTHORIZED TO SIGN THE ICVP AND DESIGNATED YELLOW FEVER VACCINATION CENTERS

The ICVP must be signed by a medical provider, who may be a licensed physician or a health care worker designated by the physician, supervising the administration of the vaccine (Figure 3-2). A signature stamp is not acceptable. Yellow fever vaccination must be given at a certified center in possession of an official "uniform stamp," which can be used to validate the ICVP.

State health departments are responsible for designating nonfederal yellow fever vaccination centers and issuing uniform stamps to clinicians. Information about the location and hours of yellow fever vaccination centers may be obtained by visiting CDC's website at wwwnc.cdc.gov/travel/yellow-fever-vaccination-clinics-search.aspx.

INTERNATIONAL CERTIFICATE OF VACCINATION OR PROPHYLAXIS
Certificat international de vaccination ou de prophylaxie

This is to certify that / Nous certifions que (1) Jane Mary Doe [name – nom] (2) 22 March 1960 [date of birth – né(e) le] F [sex – de sexe] United States [nationality – et de nationalité]

[passport number] (national identification document, if applicable – document d'identification nationale, le cas échéant) whose signature follows / dont la signature suit (3) Jane Mary Doe

has on the date indicated been vaccinated or received prophylaxis against / a été vacciné(e) ou a reçu une prophylaxie à la date indiquée (4) Yellow Fever [name of disease or condition – nom de la maladie ou de l'affection] in accordance with the International Health Regulations. / conformément au Règlement sanitaire international.

Vaccine or prophylaxis Vaccin ou agent prophylactique	Date	Signature and professional status of supervising clinician Signature et titre du professionel de santé responsable	Manufacturer and batch no. of vaccine or prophylaxis Fabricant du vaccin ou de l'agent prophylactique et numéro du lot	Certificate valid from: until: Certificat valable à partir du : jusqu'au :	Official stamp of the administering center Cachet officiel du centre habilité
(4) Yellow Fever	(5) 15 June 2018	(6) John M. Smith, MD	[Batch (or lot) #]	(7) 25 June 2018; life of person vaccinated	[(8)]

FIGURE 3-2. Example International Certificate of Vaccination or Prophylaxis (ICVP)

(1) Name should appear exactly as on the patient's passport.

(2, 5, 7) All dates should be entered with the day in numerals, followed by the month in letters, then the year. For example: in the above example, the patient's date of birth is 22 March 1960.

(3) This space is for the patient's signature.

(4) For a yellow fever vaccination, "Yellow Fever" should be written in both spaces. Should the ICVP be used for a required vaccination or prophylaxis against another disease or condition (following an amendment to the International Health Regulations or by recommendation of the World Health Organization), that disease or condition should be written in this space. Other vaccinations may be listed on the other side.

(5) The date on which the vaccination is given should be entered as shown above.

(6) A handwritten signature of the clinician—either the stamp holder or another health care provider authorized by the stamp holder—administering or supervising the administration of the vaccine (or prophylaxis) should appear in this box. A signature stamp is not acceptable.

(7) The certificate of yellow fever vaccination (ICVP) is valid beginning 10 days after the date of primary vaccination, which should be noted in the box for "certificate valid from." As of July 2016, the yellow fever vaccine booster requirement was eliminated in the IHR, and a completed ICVP is considered valid for the lifetime of the vaccinee. Suggested wording to write in the ICVP box for "certificate valid until" is "life of person vaccinated." However, it is uncertain when and if all countries with yellow fever vaccination entry requirements will adopt this change. For the most recent information on yellow fever vaccination entry requirements by country, consult the destination pages of the CDC Travelers' Health website.

(8) The Uniform Stamp of the vaccinating center should appear in this box.

Medical Waivers (Exemptions)

For medical contraindications, a clinician who has decided to issue a waiver should fill out and sign the Medical Contraindications to Vaccination section of the ICVP (Figure 3-3). The clinician should also do the following:

- Give the traveler a signed and dated exemption letter on letterhead stationery, clearly stating the contraindications to vaccination and bearing the stamp used by the yellow fever vaccination center to validate the ICVP.

MEDICAL CONTRAINDICATION TO VACCINATION
Contre-indication médicale à la vaccination

This is to certify that immunization against
Je soussigné(e) certifie que la vaccination contre

_____ for
(Name of disease – Nom de la maladie)   pour

_____ is medically
(Name of traveler – Nom du voyageur)   est médicalement

contraindicated because of the following conditions:
contre-indiquée pour les raisons suivantes:

_____

_____

_____

                                    _____
                                    (Signature and address of physician)
                                    (Signature et adresse du médecin)

FIGURE 3-3. Medical Contraindication to Vaccination section of the International Certificate of Vaccination or Prophylaxis (ICVP)

- Inform the traveler of any increased risk for yellow fever infection associated with lack of vaccination and how to minimize this risk by avoiding mosquito bites.

Reasons other than medical contraindications are not acceptable for exemption from vaccination. The traveler should be advised that issuance of a waiver does not guarantee its acceptance by the destination country. To improve the likelihood that the waiver will be accepted at the destination country, clinicians can suggest that the traveler take the following additional measures before beginning travel:

- Obtain specific and authoritative advice from the embassy or consulate of the destination country or countries.

- Request documentation of requirements for waivers from embassies or consulates and retain these, along with the completed Medical Contraindication to Vaccination section of the ICVP.

REQUIREMENTS VERSUS RECOMMENDATIONS

Country entry _requirements_ for proof of yellow fever vaccination under the IHR differ from CDC's _recommendations_. Yellow fever vaccine entry requirements are established by countries to prevent the importation and transmission of YFV and are allowed under the IHR. Travelers must comply with these to enter the country, unless they have been issued a medical waiver. Certain countries require vaccination from travelers arriving from all countries (Table 3-26), while some countries require vaccination only for travelers coming from a country with risk of YFV transmission (see Yellow Fever & Malaria Information, by Country at the end of this chapter). WHO defines those areas with risk of YFV transmission as countries or areas where yellow fever has been reported currently or in the past, plus where vectors and animal reservoirs exist. Country requirements are subject to change at any time; therefore, CDC encourages travelers to check with the relevant embassy or consulate before departure.

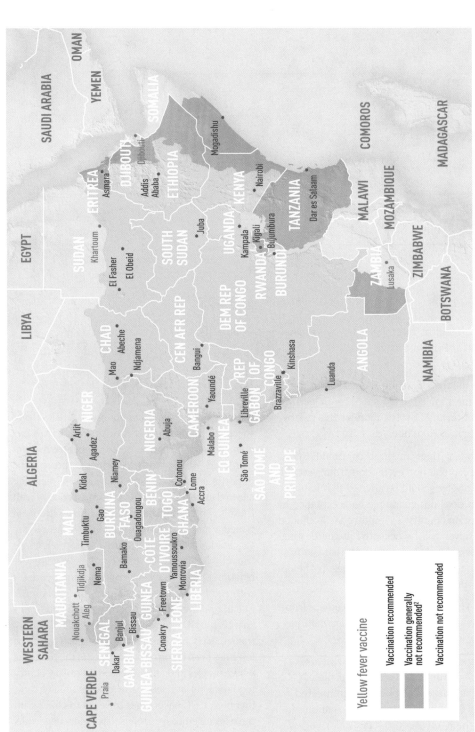

MAP 3-14. Yellow fever vaccine recommendations in Africa[1]

Yellow fever vaccine

Vaccination recommended

Vaccination generally not recommended[2]

Vaccination not recommended

[1] Current as of January 2017. This map is an updated version of the 2010 map created by the Informal WHO Working Group on the Geographic Risk of Yellow Fever.

[2] Yellow fever (YF) vaccination is generally not recommended in areas where there is low potential for YF virus exposure. However, vaccination might be considered for a small subset of travelers to these areas who are at increased risk for exposure to YF virus because of prolonged travel, heavy exposure to mosquitoes, or inability to avoid mosquito bites. Consideration for vaccination of any traveler must take into account the traveler's risk of being infected with YF virus, country entry requirements, and individual risk factors for serious vaccine-associated adverse events (such as age or immune status).

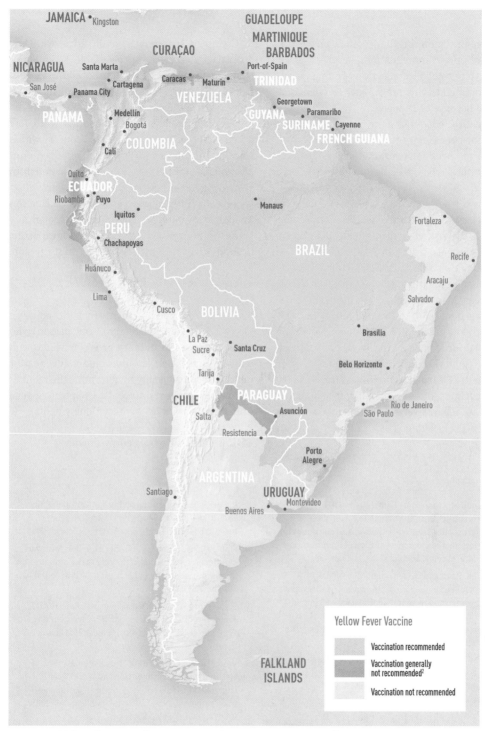

MAP 3-15. Yellow fever vaccine recommendations in the Americas¹

¹ Current as of January 2017. This map is an updated version of the 2010 map created by the Informal WHO Working Group on the Geographic Risk of Yellow Fever.

² Yellow fever (YF) vaccination is generally not recommended in areas where there is low potential for YF virus exposure. However, vaccination might be considered for a small subset of travelers to these areas who are at increased risk for exposure to YF virus because of prolonged travel, heavy exposure to mosquitoes, or inability to avoid mosquito bites. Consideration for vaccination of any traveler must take into account the traveler's risk of being infected with YF virus, country entry requirements, and individual risk factors for serious vaccine-associated adverse events (such as age or immune status).

The information in the section on yellow fever vaccine recommendations is advice given by CDC to prevent YFV infections among travelers. Recommendations are subject to change at any time because of changes in YFV circulation; therefore, CDC encourages travelers to check the destination pages for up-to-date vaccine information and to check for relevant travel notices on the CDC website before departure (www.cdc.gov/travel).

Yellow fever vaccine recommendations for travelers going to specific destinations are based on the risk classification for YFV transmission: endemic, transitional, low potential for exposure, and no risk. Yellow fever vaccination is recommended for travel to endemic and transitional areas (Maps 3-14 and 3-15). Although vaccination is generally not recommended for travel to areas with low potential for exposure, it might be considered for a small subset of travelers whose itinerary could place them at increased risk for exposure to YFV (such as prolonged travel, heavy exposure to mosquitoes, or inability to avoid mosquito bites). Yellow fever vaccination is not recommended in areas with no risk.

Countries that only contain areas with low potential for exposure to YFV (Table 3-23) are not included on the official WHO list of countries with risk of YFV transmission (Table 3-22). Therefore, proof of yellow fever vaccination should not be required if traveling from a country with low potential for exposure to YFV to a country with a vaccination entry requirement (unless that country requires proof of yellow fever vaccination from all arriving travelers; see Table 3-26). An exception is Bolivia, which requires yellow fever vaccination for people traveling from or transiting through any of the 6 countries with low potential for exposure, in addition to those with risk of YFV transmission.

VACCINATION FOR TRAVEL ON MILITARY ORDERS

Because military requirements may exceed those indicated in this publication, any person who plans to travel on military orders (civilians and military personnel) should contact the nearest military medical facility to determine the requirements for his or her trip (see also Chapter 8, Special Considerations for US Military Deployments).

CDC website: www.cdc.gov/yellowfever

BIBLIOGRAPHY

1. Gershman MD, Staples JE, Bentsi-Enchill AD, Breugelmans JG, Brito GS, Camacho LA, et al. Viscerotropic disease: case definition and guidelines for collection, analysis, and presentation of immunization safety data. Vaccine. 2012 Jul 13;30(33):5038–58.

2. Jentes ES, Poumerol G, Gershman MD, Hill DR, Lemarchand J, Lewis RF, et al. The revised global yellow fever risk map and recommendations for vaccination, 2010: consensus of the Informal WHO Working Group on Geographic Risk for Yellow Fever. Lancet Infect Dis. 2011 Aug;11(8):622–32.

3. Lindsey NP, Rabe IB, Miller ER, Fischer M, Staples JE. Adverse event reports following yellow fever vaccination, 2007-13. J Travel Med. 2016 May;23(5).

4. Monath TP, Cetron MS. Prevention of yellow fever in persons traveling to the tropics. Clin Infect Dis. 2002 May 15;34(10):1369–78.

5. Staples JE, Bocchini JA, Jr., Rubin L, Fischer M. Yellow fever vaccine booster doses: recommendations of the Advisory Committee on Immunization Practices, 2015. MMWR Morb Mortal Wkly Rep. 2015 Jun 19;64(23):647–50.

6. Staples JE, Gershman M, Fischer M. Yellow fever vaccine: recommendations of the Advisory Committee on Immunization Practices (ACIP). MMWR Recomm Rep. 2010 Jul 30;59(RR-7):1–27.

7. Staples JE, Monath TP, Gershman MD, Barrett ADT. Yellow fever vaccine. In: Plotkin SA, Orenstein WA, Offit PA, editors. Vaccines. 7th ed. Philadelphia: Elsevier; In press.

8. World Health Organization. International Health Regulations, 2005. Geneva: World Health Organization; 2008 [cited 2016 Sep. 27]. Available from: http://whqlibdoc.who.int/publications/2008/9789241580410_eng.pdf.

9. World Health Organization. Vaccines and vaccination against yellow fever. WHO position paper—June 2013. Wkly Epidemiol Rec. 2013 Jul 5;88(27):269–83.

A HISTORY OF YELLOW FEVER VACCINATION REQUIREMENTS

Mark D. Gershman

3

The history of yellow fever vaccination requirements is best understood in the larger context of the history of international measures to prevent the spread of infectious diseases. The first international disease control measures were instituted in Europe in the 14th century in an attempt to prevent the spread of bubonic plague. Subsequently, cholera became the next major target of international disease control efforts. The lack of agreement between countries on the most effective means of disease prevention and lack of consistency in quarantine regulations eventually led to a series of International Sanitary Conferences.

The first International Sanitary Conference was held in Paris in 1851, and others were held periodically until 1944. Several international health organizations, including the Health Organization of the League of Nations, were established to oversee the various international regulations on disease control. The onset of World War II in 1939 severely disrupted the international public health functions of these organizations. The United Nations Relief and Rehabilitation Administration (UNRRA) was created by the

Allies in 1943 to provide economic assistance to war-ravaged European nations, assist refugees, and conduct public health functions. (The UNRRA is unrelated to the more familiar United Nations organization, founded in 1945.) The public health responsibilities included the oversight of international quarantine activities, particularly those delineated in the updated International Sanitary Conventions of 1944, which contained yellow fever control measures. (The live attenuated 17D yellow fever vaccine had been developed and put into use by the late 1930s.) Specific provisions for national governments included quarantining a traveler from an endemic area who did not possess a valid vaccination certificate. This provision, which directed countries how to deal with unvaccinated travelers who may have been exposed to yellow fever virus, was the precursor to formal yellow fever vaccination requirements.

In order for the provisions of the Sanitary Conventions of 1944 to be carried out, areas where yellow fever was endemic had to be delineated. The conventions delegated this responsibility to the UNRRA, which appointed

the Expert Commission on Quarantine. This commission created the first official map of yellow fever–endemic areas in 1945. Soon after the end of World War II, the responsibilities of the UNRRA were assumed by the newly formed World Health Organization (WHO), which appointed the Yellow Fever Panel. In 1949, the Yellow Fever Panel modified the original UNRRA map and issued its first report, which recommended that "measures may be applied permanently against arrivals from endemic areas."

The International Sanitary Regulations (ISR), drafted by WHO to replace the previous International Sanitary Conventions, were adopted by the World Health Assembly in 1951. The ISR stipulated that "vaccination against yellow fever shall be required of any person leaving an infected local area on an international voyage and proceeding to a yellow fever receptive area." Although only alluded to in previous International Sanitary Conventions, this was the first regulatory language that overtly mandated yellow fever vaccination requirements for country entry. The ISR were modified and renamed

(continued)

A HISTORY OF YELLOW FEVER VACCINATION REQUIREMENTS (CONTINUED)

the International Health Regulations (IHR) in 1969; the IHR were completely revised in 2005, the most current iteration. The text regarding yellow fever vaccination requirements has been gradually modified. The IHR (2005) stipulate, "Vaccination against yellow fever may be required of any traveler leaving an area where the Organization has determined that a risk of yellow fever transmission is present."

In 1960, WHO started to publish annually a listing of all the national yellow fever vaccination requirements in the booklet *Vaccination Certificate Requirements for International Travel*. This booklet gradually evolved into the WHO's *International Travel and Health*. The book is no longer published, but the material remains online and lists country-specific yellow fever vaccination requirements, which are updated regularly. To keep its list current, WHO sends a questionnaire to all member countries yearly requesting any updates to their vaccination requirements. CDC publishes these same country requirements.

BIBLIOGRAPHY

1. Strode GK, editor. Yellow Fever. 1st ed. New York: McGraw Hill; 1951.
2. Wilder-Smith A, Martinez L, Rietveld A, Duclos P, Hardiman M, Gollogly L. World Health Organization and International Travel and Health. Travel Med Infect Dis. 2007 May;5(3):147–9.
3. World Health Organization. International Health Regulations (1969): 1st annotated edition. Geneva: World Health Organization; 1971.
4. World Health Organization. International Health Regulations, 2005. Geneva: World Health Organization; 2008 [cited 2016 Sep. 27]. Available from: http://whqlibdoc. who.int/publications/2008/ 9789241580410_eng.pdf.
5. World Health Organization. International Sanitary Regulations: 2nd annotated edition. Geneva: World Health Organization; 1961.

YERSINIOSIS

L. Hannah Gould, Cindy R Friedman

INFECTIOUS AGENT

Facultative anaerobic gram-negative coccobacilli in the genus *Yersinia* (most commonly *Yersinia enterocolitica* serogroups O:3; O:5,27; O:8; and O:9).

TRANSMISSION

Consuming or handling contaminated food, most commonly raw or undercooked pork products; milk that was not pasteurized, inadequately pasteurized, or contaminated after pasteurization; or untreated water. Also transmitted by direct or indirect contact with animals.

EPIDEMIOLOGY

Most common in northern Europe (particularly Scandinavia), Japan, and Canada. In temperate climates, risk is higher in cooler months. The incidence among travelers to developing countries is generally low. A US study found that approximately 6% of *Y. enterocolitica* infections were travel associated. People with high iron levels are at higher risk of infection and severe disease.

CLINICAL PRESENTATION

Incubation period is 4–6 days (range, 1–14 days). Symptoms include fever, abdominal pain (may mimic appendicitis), and diarrhea (may be bloody and can persist for several weeks). Necrotizing enterocolitis has been described in young infants. Reactive arthritis affecting the wrists, knees, and ankles can occur, usually 1 month after the initial diarrhea episode, resolving after 1–6 months.

Erythema nodosum can also occur, manifesting as painful, raised red or purple lesions along the trunk and legs, usually resolving spontaneously within 1 month.

DIAGNOSIS

Isolation of the organism from stool, blood, bile, wound, throat swab, mesenteric lymph node, cerebrospinal fluid, or peritoneal fluid. If yersiniosis is suspected, the clinical laboratory should be notified and instructed to culture on CIN agar.

TREATMENT

Most infections are self-limited. Antibiotics should be given for moderate to severe cases. *Y. enterocolitica* isolates are usually susceptible to trimethoprim-sulfamethoxazole, aminoglycosides, third-generation cephalosporins, fluoroquinolones, and tetracyclines; they are typically resistant to first-generation cephalosporins and most penicillins. Antimicrobial therapy has no effect on postinfectious sequelae.

PREVENTION

Avoid eating raw or undercooked pork products, unpasteurized milk products, and untreated water (see Chapter 2, Food & Water Precautions). Wash hands with soap and water before eating and preparing food, after contact with animals, and after handling raw meat.

CDC website: www.cdc.gov/yersinia

BIBLIOGRAPHY

1. Cover TL, Aber RC. *Yersinia enterocolitica*. N Engl J Med. 1989 Jul 6;321(1):16–24.
2. Kendall ME, Crim S, Fullerton K, Han PV, Cronquist AB, Shiferaw B, et al. Travel-associated enteric infections diagnosed after return to the United States, Foodborne Diseases Active Surveillance Network (FoodNet), 2004–2009. Clin Infect Dis. 2012 Jun;54 Suppl 5:S480–7.
3. Mead PS. *Yersinia* species, including plague. In: Bennett JE, Dolin R, Blaser MJ, editors. Mandell, Douglas, and Bennett's Principles and Practice of Infectious Diseases. 8th ed. Philadelphia: Saunders Elsevier; 2015. pp. 2615–7.
4. Perdikogianni C, Galanakis E, Michalakis M, Giannoussi E, Maraki S, Tselentis Y, et al. *Yersinia enterocolitica* infection mimicking surgical conditions. Pediatr Surg Int. 2006 Jul;22(7):589–92.

ZIKA

Tai-Ho Chen, J. Erin Staples, Marc Fischer

INFECTIOUS AGENT

Zika virus is a single-stranded RNA virus of the Flaviviridae family, genus *Flavivirus*.

TRANSMISSION

Transmission occurs through the bite of an infected *Aedes* species mosquito. Intrauterine, perinatal, sexual, laboratory, and possible transfusion-associated transmission also have been reported. Although Zika viral particles were found in the breast milk of 1 woman, and virus RNA has been detected in breast milk of 2 additional women, transmission of Zika virus through breastfeeding has not been documented.

EPIDEMIOLOGY

Zika virus was first identified in Uganda in 1947. Before 2007, only sporadic human cases were reported from countries in Africa and Asia. In 2007, the first documented Zika virus disease outbreak was reported in the Federated States of Micronesia. In subsequent years, outbreaks of Zika virus disease were identified in countries in Southeast Asia and the Western Pacific. Zika virus was identified for the first time in the Western hemisphere in 2015, when large outbreaks were reported in Brazil. Since then, the virus spread throughout much of the Americas. (See www.cdc.gov/travel for current CDC travel notices for Zika virus.)

CLINICAL PRESENTATION

Most Zika virus infections are asymptomatic. Symptomatic infections are generally mild. Commonly reported signs and symptoms include fever, maculopapular rash, arthralgia, and conjunctivitis. Other symptoms include myalgia and headache. During the outbreak in Brazil in 2015, the Ministry of Health of Brazil reported a marked increase in the number of infants born with microcephaly, although it is not known how many of these cases were associated with Zika virus infection. Zika virus RNA was subsequently identified in tissues from several infants with microcephaly and from fetal losses in women who were infected during pregnancy. (See Box 3-6 for more information about Zika and pregnancy.) Guillain-Barré syndrome also has been reported in some patients after Zika virus infection.

DIAGNOSIS

Zika virus infection should be considered in patients with acute onset of fever, maculopapular rash, arthralgia, or conjunctivitis who live in or have traveled to an area with ongoing transmission in the 2 weeks preceding illness onset. Because dengue and chikungunya virus infections share a similar geographic distribution and symptoms with Zika, patients with suspected Zika virus infection should also be evaluated and managed for possible dengue or chikungunya

virus infection. Other considerations in the differential diagnosis include malaria, rubella, measles, parvovirus, adenovirus, enterovirus, leptospirosis, rickettsiosis, and group A streptococcal infections.

For people with suspected Zika virus disease, Zika virus rRT-PCR should be performed on urine specimens collected <14 days after onset of symptoms or serum specimens collected <7 days after onset of symptoms. A positive rRT-PCR result confirms Zika virus infection, and no antibody testing is indicated. Serum IgM antibody testing should be performed if rRT-PCR is negative or for samples collected ≥7 days after illness onset. However, these serologic assays can be positive because of cross-reacting antibodies against related flaviviruses, such as dengue or yellow fever viruses. Virus-specific neutralization testing can be used to discriminate between cross-reacting antibodies in primary flavivirus infections, although neutralizing antibodies might still yield cross-reactive results in people who were previously infected or vaccinated against a related flavivirus (secondary flavivirus infection).

Health care providers are encouraged to report suspected Zika virus disease cases to their state or local health departments to facilitate diagnosis and mitigate the risk of local transmission in areas where *Aedes* species mosquitoes are active. Zika virus disease is a nationally

---

BOX 3-6. Zika in pregnancy

Zika virus infection in a pregnant woman can cause microcephaly and other congenital brain abnormalities in the fetus. CDC recommends that pregnant women not travel to any area with ongoing local transmission of Zika virus. Pregnant women who travel to these areas should talk to their health care provider first and strictly follow steps to prevent mosquito bites. Women who are trying to become pregnant should consult with their health care provider before traveling to an area with ongoing local transmission and strictly follow steps to avoid mosquito bites during the trip.

People who have traveled to an area with Zika and have a pregnant partner should use condoms or not have sex (vaginal, anal, or oral) during the pregnancy.

Travelers who have returned from areas with Zika virus transmission should consider preconception counseling with their health care provider and wait to attempt conception until the risk for sexual transmission is believed to be minimal. For more information, visit www.cdc.gov/zika.

Health care providers can contact the CDC Zika Pregnancy Hotline (770-488-7100, ZikaMCH@cdc.gov or ZikaPregnancy@cdc.gov, or fax 404-718-2200) for clinical consultation on Zika virus infection in pregnancy.

notifiable condition. State health departments should report laboratory-confirmed cases to CDC according to the Council of States and Territorial Epidemiologists case definitions. Pregnant women with laboratory evidence of Zika virus infection should be reported to the US Zika Pregnancy Registry or the Puerto Rico Zika Active Pregnancy Surveillance System for clinical follow-up.

TREATMENT

No specific antiviral treatment is available for Zika virus disease. Treatment is generally supportive and can include rest, fluids, and use of analgesics and antipyretics. Aspirin and other nonsteroidal antiinflammatory drugs (NSAIDs) should be avoided until dengue can be ruled out to reduce the risk of hemorrhage. People infected with Zika, dengue, or chikungunya virus should be protected from further mosquito exposure during the first week of illness to reduce the risk of local transmission. Pregnant women with laboratory evidence of Zika virus infection should be evaluated and managed for possible adverse pregnancy outcomes.

PREVENTION

Avoiding mosquito bites can protect against Zika virus infection (see Chapter 2, Protection against Mosquitoes, Ticks, & Other Arthropods). Using condoms during sexual contact with people with possible Zika virus infection also may reduce transmission risk. For more information on sexual transmission of Zika, see Zika and Sexual Transmission on the CDC website (www.cdc.gov/zika/transmission/sexual-transmission.html). Zika virus likely can be spread through blood transfusions. Blood donors returning from areas with active transmission of Zika virus should defer donation for 4 weeks after return (or 4 weeks after resolution of symptoms, if they become ill with symptoms consistent with Zika virus). Mothers are encouraged to breastfeed infants even in areas where Zika virus is circulating, as available evidence indicates the benefits of breastfeeding outweigh any theoretical risks associated with Zika virus infection transmission through breast milk.

CDC website: http://www.cdc.gov/zika

BIBLIOGRAPHY

1. Besnard M, Lastere S, Teissier A, Cao-Lormeau V, Musso D. Evidence of perinatal transmission of Zika virus, French Polynesia, December 2013 and February 2014. Euro Surveill. 2014;19(13).

2. Duffy MR, Chen TH, Hancock WT, Powers AM, Kool JL, Lanciotti RS, et al. Zika virus outbreak on Yap Island, Federated States of Micronesia. N Engl J Med. 2009 Jun 11;360(24):2536–43.

3. Food and Drug Administration. Recommendations for donor screening, deferral, and product management to reduce the risk of transfusion—transmission of Zika virus. 2016 [cited 2016 Sep. 27]. Available from: http://www.fda.gov/downloads/BiologicsBloodVaccines/GuidanceComplianceRegulatoryInformation/Guidances/Blood/UCM486360.pdf.

4. Foy BD, Kobylinski KC, Chilson Foy JL, Blitvich BJ, Travassos da Rosa A, Haddow AD, et al. Probable non-vector-borne transmission of Zika virus, Colorado, USA. Emerg Infect Dis. 2011 May;17(5):880–2.

5. Hayes EB. Zika virus outside Africa. Emerg Infect Dis. 2009 Sep;15(9):1347–50.

6. Petersen EE, Polen KN, Meaney-Delman D, Ellington SR, Oduyebo T, Cohn A, et al. Update: interim guidance for health care providers caring for women of reproductive age with possible Zika virus exposure—United States, 2016. MMWR Morb Mortal Wkly Rep. 2016;65(12):315–22.

7. Petersen LR, Jamieson DJ, Powers AM, Honein MA. Zika Virus. N Engl J Med. 2016 Apr 21;374(16):1552–63.

8. Staples JE, Dziuban EJ, Fischer M, Cragan JD, Rasmussen SA, Cannon MJ, et al. Interim guidelines for the evaluation and testing of infants with possible congenital Zika virus infection – United States, 2016. MMWR Morb Mortal Wkly Rep. 2016;65(3):63–7.

YELLOW FEVER & MALARIA INFORMATION, BY COUNTRY

Mark D. Gershman, Emily S. Jentes, Rhett J. Stoney (Yellow Fever)
Kathrine R. Tan, Paul M. Arguin, Stefanie F. Steele (Malaria)

The following pages present country-specific information on yellow fever vaccine requirements and recommendations (see Table 3-27) and malaria transmission information and prophylaxis recommendations. Fourteen country-specific maps of malaria transmission areas, 11 country-specific maps depicting yellow fever vaccine recommendations, and a reference map of China are included to aid in interpreting the information. The information was accurate at the time of publication; however, this information is subject to change at any time as a result of changes in disease transmission or, in the case of yellow fever, changing country entry requirements. Updated information reflecting changes since publication can be found in the online version of this book (www.cdc.gov/yellowbook) and on the CDC Travelers' Health website (www.cdc.gov/travel). General recommendations for other vaccines to consider during the pretravel consultation can be found on the CDC Travelers' Health website (www.cdc.gov/travel).

YELLOW FEVER

Since publication of the 2016 edition of *CDC Health Information for International Travel*, additional country-specific data has been made available on the geographic risk of yellow fever virus (YFV) transmission. Based on a review of these data by the WHO Scientific and Technical Advisory Group on Geographical Yellow Fever Risk Mapping (in which CDC participates), an updated yellow fever vaccination recommendation was made for Rwanda.

Revaccination against yellow fever was previously required by certain countries at 10-year intervals to comply with International Health Regulations (IHR). In 2014, the World Health Assembly (of WHO) adopted the recommendation to amend the IHR by removing the 10-year booster dose requirement, and stipulated a 2-year transition period for this change. Consequently, as of July 11, 2016, a completed International Certificate of Vaccination or Prophylaxis (ICVP) is valid for the lifetime of the vaccinee. Moreover, countries cannot require proof of revaccination (booster) against yellow fever as a condition of entry, even if the last vaccination was more than 10 years prior.

In the United States, the Advisory Committee on Immunization Practices (ACIP) published a new recommendation in 2015 that one dose of yellow fever vaccine provides long-lasting protection and is adequate for most travelers. The recommendation also identifies specific groups of travelers who should receive additional doses and others for whom additional doses may be considered. For details, see the Yellow Fever section earlier in this chapter. For the most up-to-date information about yellow fever vaccine boosters, consult the CDC Travelers' Health website or the specific publication posted on the ACIP website (www.cdc.gov/mmwr/pdf/wk/mm6423.pdf).

Ultimately, the clinician's decision whether or not to vaccinate any traveler must take into account the traveler's risk of being infected with YFV, country entry requirements, and individual risk factors for serious adverse events after yellow fever vaccination (such as age and immune status). For a thorough discussion of yellow fever and guidance for vaccination, see the Yellow Fever section earlier in this chapter.

NOTE: Despite the recent changes to the IHR regarding yellow fever vaccine boosters, it is uncertain when and if all countries with current yellow fever vaccination entry

requirements will adopt this change. Even if countries do modify their official policies to extend the validity period of the ICVP from 10 years to the lifetime of the vaccinee, there is no guarantee that all national border officials will be aware of such policy change or be able to enforce it appropriately. CDC obtains information yearly from WHO about official country entry requirements. WHO likely will not be asking countries about yellow fever vaccine booster entry requirements in the yearly questionnaires, because it will be assumed that countries are complying with the amended IHR. This could leave a gap in the foreseeable future in accurate published information about entry requirements for yellow fever vaccine boosters for certain countries. Past experience has demonstrated that information given by consulates and embassies about vaccination requirements is often not accurate. Therefore, providers and travelers should not rely solely on such information when determining current yellow fever vaccination entry requirements for specific destinations. With the caveats described above, readers should refer to the online version of this book (www.cdc.gov/yellowbook) and the CDC Travelers'

Health website (www.cdc.gov/travel) for any reported updates to country entry requirements since publication of this edition.

MALARIA

The following recommendations to protect travelers from malaria were developed using the best available data from multiple sources. Countries are not required to submit malaria surveillance data to CDC. On an ongoing basis, CDC actively solicits data from multiple sources, including World Health Organization (main and regional offices); national malaria control programs; international organizations, such as the International Society of Travel Medicine; CDC overseas staff; US military; academic, research, and aid organizations; and published records from the medical literature. The reliability and accuracy of those data are also assessed. If the information is available, trends in malaria incidence and other data are considered in the context of malaria control activities within a given country, or other mitigating factors such as natural disasters, wars, and other events that may affect the ability to control malaria or accurately count and report it. Factors such as the volume of travel to that country and the number of acquired cases reported in the US

Table 3-27. Categories of recommendations for yellow fever vaccination

YELLOW FEVER VACCINATION CATEGORY	RATIONALE FOR RECOMMENDATION
Recommended	Vaccination recommended for all travelers ≥9 months of age to areas with endemic or transitional yellow fever risk, as determined by persistent or periodic YFV transmission.
Generally not recommended	Vaccination generally not recommended in areas where the potential for YFV exposure is low, as determined by absence of reports of human yellow fever and past evidence suggestive of only low levels of YFV transmission. However, vaccination might be considered for a small subset of travelers who are at increased risk for exposure to YFV because of prolonged travel, heavy exposure to mosquitoes, or inability to avoid mosquito bites.
Not recommended	Vaccination not recommended in areas where there is no risk of YFV transmission, as determined by absence of past or present evidence of YFV circulation in the area or environmental conditions not conducive to YFV transmission.

Abbreviation: YFV, yellow fever virus.

surveillance system are also examined. Based on all those considerations, recommendations are developed to try to accurately describe areas of the country where transmission occurs, substantial occurrences of antimalarial drug resistance, the proportions of species present, and the recommended chemoprophylaxis options.

The recommendations for malaria prevention include estimates of relative risk for US travelers. This means that compared to a hypothetical average country with malaria transmission, US travelers to some countries can be at higher than average or lower than average risk for malaria infection. The designations high, moderate, low, and very low have been used to describe the estimated relative risk for a traveler to that country.

These recommendations should be used in conjunction with an individual risk assessment, taking into account not only the destination country but also the detailed itinerary including specific cities, types of accommodation, season, and style of travel, as well as special health conditions such as pregnancy.

Several medications are available for malaria chemoprophylaxis. When deciding on which drug to use, clinicians should consider the specific itinerary, length of trip, cost of the drugs, previous adverse reactions to antimalarials, drug allergies, and medical history.

For a thorough discussion of malaria and guidance for prophylaxis, see the Malaria section earlier in this chapter.

COUNTRY-SPECIFIC INFORMATION

AFGHANISTAN

YELLOW FEVER

Requirements: Required if traveling from a country with risk of YFV transmission.[1]
Recommendations: None.

MALARIA

Areas with malaria: April–December in all areas <2,500 m (8,202 ft).
Estimated relative risk of malaria for US travelers: Moderate.[3]
Drug resistance[4]: Chloroquine.
Malaria species: *P. vivax* 80%–90%, *P. falciparum* 10%–20%.
Recommended chemoprophylaxis: Atovaquone-proguanil, doxycycline, or mefloquine.

ALBANIA

YELLOW FEVER

Requirements: Required if traveling from a country with risk of YFV transmission and ≥1 year of age.[1]
Recommendations: None.

MALARIA

No malaria transmission.

ALGERIA

YELLOW FEVER

Requirements: Required if traveling from a country with risk of YFV transmission and ≥1 year of age, including transit >12 hours in an airport located in a country with risk of YFV transmission.[1]
Recommendations: None.

MALARIA

No malaria transmission.

AMERICAN SAMOA (US)

YELLOW FEVER

No requirements or recommendations.

MALARIA

No malaria transmission.

ANDORRA

YELLOW FEVER

No requirements or recommendations.

MALARIA

No malaria transmission.

ANGOLA

YELLOW FEVER

Requirements: Required for arriving travelers from all countries if traveler is ≥9 months of age.

*All footnotes are located on page 424.

Recommendations: *Recommended* for all travelers ≥9 months of age.

MALARIA

Areas with malaria: All.
Estimated relative risk of malaria for US travelers: High.
Drug resistance[4]: Chloroquine.
Malaria species: *P. falciparum* 90%, *P. ovale* 5%, *P. vivax* 5%.
Recommended chemoprophylaxis: Atovaquone-proguanil, doxycycline, or mefloquine.

ANGUILLA (UK)

YELLOW FEVER

No requirements or recommendations.

MALARIA

No malaria transmission.

ANTARCTICA

YELLOW FEVER

No requirements or recommendations.

MALARIA

No malaria transmission.

ANTIGUA AND BARBUDA

YELLOW FEVER

Requirements: Required if traveling from a country with risk of YFV transmission and ≥1 year of age.[1]
Recommendations: None.

MALARIA

No malaria transmission.

ARGENTINA *(see Map 3-16.)*

YELLOW FEVER

Requirements: None.
Recommendations:
Recommended for travelers ≥9 months of age going to Corrientes and Misiones Provinces.
Generally not recommended for travelers going to Formosa Province and designated areas of Chaco, Jujuy, and Salta Provinces (see Map 3-16).
Not recommended for all travelers whose itineraries are limited to areas and provinces not listed above.

MALARIA

No malaria transmission.

ARMENIA

YELLOW FEVER

No requirements or recommendations.

MALARIA

No malaria transmission.

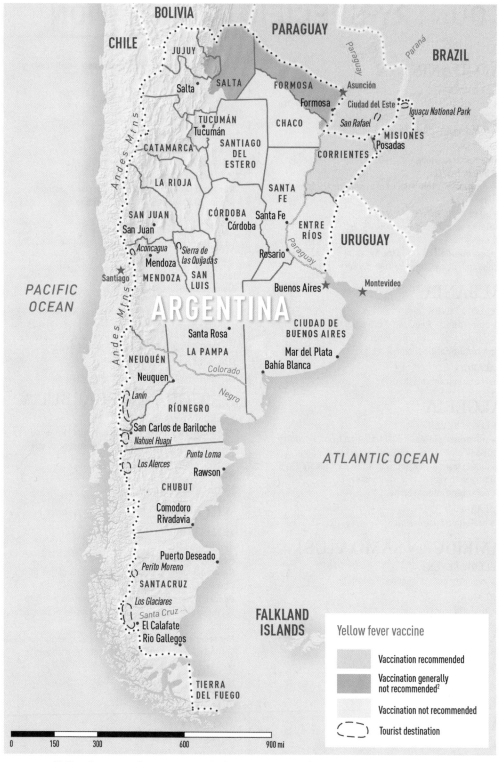

MAP 3-16. **Yellow fever vaccine recommendations in Argentina**[1]

[1,2] See footnotes on page 424.

ARUBA

YELLOW FEVER
No requirements or recommendations.

MALARIA
No malaria transmission.

AUSTRALIA

YELLOW FEVER
Requirements: Required if traveling from a country with risk of YFV transmission and ≥1 year of age, including transit >12 hours in an airport located in a country with risk of YFV transmission.[1] This requirement excludes Galápagos Islands in Ecuador and the island of Tobago and is limited to Misiones Province in Argentina.
Recommendations: None.

MALARIA
No malaria transmission.

AUSTRIA

YELLOW FEVER
No requirements or recommendations.

MALARIA
No malaria transmission.

AZERBAIJAN

YELLOW FEVER
No requirements or recommendations.

MALARIA
No malaria transmission.

AZORES (PORTUGAL)

YELLOW FEVER
No requirements or recommendations.

MALARIA
No malaria transmission.

BAHAMAS, THE

YELLOW FEVER
Requirements: Required if traveling from a country with risk of YFV transmission and ≥1 year of age, including transit >12 hours in an airport located in a country with risk of YFV transmission.[1] This requirement excludes Guyana, Suriname, and Trinidad and Tobago.
Recommendations: None.

MALARIA
No malaria transmission.

BAHRAIN

YELLOW FEVER
Requirements: Required if traveling from a country with risk of YFV transmission and ≥9 months of age, including transit >12 hours in an airport located in a country with risk of YFV transmission.[1]

Recommendations: None.

MALARIA
No malaria transmission.

BANGLADESH

YELLOW FEVER
Requirements: Required if traveling from a country with risk of YFV transmission and ≥1 year of age.[1]
Recommendations: None.

MALARIA
Areas with malaria: All areas, except in the city of Dhaka.
Estimated relative risk of malaria for US travelers: Low.
Drug resistance[4]: Chloroquine.
Malaria species: *P. falciparum* 90%, *P. vivax* 10%, *P. malariae* rare.
Recommended chemoprophylaxis: Atovaquone-proguanil, doxycycline, or mefloquine.

BARBADOS

YELLOW FEVER
Requirements: Required if traveling from a country with risk of YFV transmission and ≥1 year of age, including transit >12 hours in an airport located in a country with risk of YFV transmission.[1] This requirement excludes Guyana and Trinidad and Tobago.
Recommendations: None.

MALARIA
No malaria transmission.

BELARUS

YELLOW FEVER
No requirements or recommendations.

MALARIA
No malaria transmission.

BELGIUM

YELLOW FEVER
No requirements or recommendations.

MALARIA
No malaria transmission.

BELIZE

YELLOW FEVER
Requirements: Required if traveling from a country with risk of YFV transmission and ≥1 year of age, including transit in an airport located in a country with risk of YFV transmission.[1]
Recommendations: None.

MALARIA
Areas with malaria: Rare locally transmitted cases. None in Belize City and islands frequented by tourists, such as Ambergris Caye.

*All footnotes are located on page 424.

Estimated relative risk of malaria for US travelers: Very low.
Drug resistance[4]: None.
Malaria species: *P. vivax* 100%.
Recommended chemoprophylaxis: Mosquito avoidance only.

BENIN

YELLOW FEVER

Requirements: Required if traveling from a country with risk of YFV transmission and ≥1 year of age, including transit in an airport located in a country with risk of YFV transmission.[1]
Recommendations: *Recommended* for all travelers ≥9 months of age.

MALARIA

Areas with malaria: All.
Estimated relative risk of malaria for US travelers: High.
Drug resistance[4]: Chloroquine.
Malaria species: *P. falciparum* >85%, *P. ovale* 5%–10%, *P. vivax* rare.
Recommended chemoprophylaxis: Atovaquone-proguanil, doxycycline, or mefloquine.

BERMUDA (UK)

YELLOW FEVER

No requirements or recommendations.

MALARIA

No malaria transmission.

BHUTAN

YELLOW FEVER

Requirements: Required if traveling from a country with risk of YFV transmission, including transit in an airport located in a country with risk of YFV transmission.[1]
Recommendations: None.

MALARIA

Areas with malaria: Rare cases in rural areas <1,700 m (5,577 ft) in districts along the southern border shared with India. Rare seasonal cases May–September in Lhuentse, Monggar, Punakha, Trashigang, Trongsa, Tsirang, Yangtse, and Wangdue. None in districts of Bumthang, Gaza, Haa, Paro, and Thimphu.
Estimated relative risk of malaria for US travelers: Very low.
Drug resistance[4]: Chloroquine.
Malaria species: *P. falciparum* 70%, *P. vivax* 30%.
Recommended chemoprophylaxis: Mosquito avoidance only.

BOLIVIA *(see Maps 3-17 and 3-18.)*

YELLOW FEVER

Requirements: Required if traveling from a country with risk of YFV transmission and ≥1 year of age, including transit >12 hours in an airport located in a country with risk of YFV transmission. This includes

*All footnotes are located on page 424.

São Tomé and Príncipe, Rwanda, Somalia, Tanzania, Zambia, and designated areas of Eritrea.[1]
Recommendations:
Recommended for all travelers ≥9 months of age traveling to the following areas <2,300 m in elevation[2] and east of the Andes Mountains: the entire departments of Beni, Pando, Santa Cruz, and designated areas (see Map 3-17) of Chuquisaca, Cochabamba, La Paz, and Tarija departments.
Not recommended for travelers whose itineraries are limited to areas >2,300 m in elevation[2] and all areas not listed above, including the cities of La Paz and Sucre.

MALARIA

Areas with malaria: All areas <2,500 m (8,202 ft). None in the city of La Paz (see Map 3-18).
Estimated relative risk of malaria for US travelers: Low.
Drug resistance[4]: Chloroquine.
Malaria species: *P. vivax* 93%, *P. falciparum* 7%.
Recommended chemoprophylaxis: Atovaquone-proguanil, doxycycline, mefloquine, or primaquine[5].

BONAIRE

YELLOW FEVER

Requirements: Required if traveling from a country with risk of YFV transmission and ≥6 months of age.[1] This requirement applies only to travelers going to Bonaire, Saba, or Sint Eustatius.
Recommendations: None.

MALARIA

No malaria transmission.

BOSNIA AND HERZEGOVINA

YELLOW FEVER

No requirements or recommendations.

MALARIA

No malaria transmission.

BOTSWANA *(see Map 3-19.)*

YELLOW FEVER

Requirements: Required if traveling from or having passed through a country with risk of YFV transmission and ≥1 year of age, including transit in an airport located in a country with risk of YFV transmission.[1]
Recommendations: None.

MALARIA

Areas with malaria: Present in the following districts: Central and North West (including Chobe National Park). None in the cities of Francistown and Gaborone (see Map 3-19).
Estimated relative risk of malaria for US travelers: Low.
Drug resistance[4]: Chloroquine.
Malaria species: *P. falciparum* 90%, *P. vivax* 5%, *P. ovale* 5%.
Recommended chemoprophylaxis: Atovaquone-proguanil, doxycycline, or mefloquine.

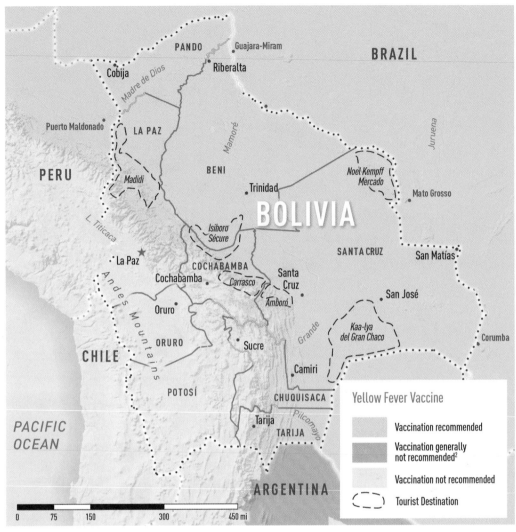

MAP 3-17. Yellow fever vaccine recommendations in Bolivia[1]

[1,2] See footnotes on page 424.

BRAZIL *(see Maps 3-20 and 3-21.)*

YELLOW FEVER

Requirements: None.

Recommendations:

Recommended for all travelers ≥9 months of age going to the following areas: the entire states of Acre, Amapá, Amazonas, Distrito Federal (including the capital city of Brasília), Goiás, Maranhão, Mato Grosso, Mato Grosso do Sul, Minas Gerais, Pará, Rondônia, Roraima, Tocantins, and designated areas (see Map 3-20) of the following states: Bahia, Paraná, Piauí, Rio Grande do Sul, Santa Catarina, and São Paulo (state). Vaccination is also recommended for travelers visiting Iguaçu Falls.

*All footnotes are located on page 424.

Not recommended for travelers whose itineraries are limited to areas not listed above, including the cities of Fortaleza, Recife, Rio de Janeiro, Salvador, and São Paulo (see Map 3-20).

MALARIA

Areas with malaria: All areas of the states of Acre, Amapá, Amazonas, Rondonia, and Roraima. Also present in the states of Maranhão, Mato Grosso, and Para, but rare cases in their capital cities. Rare cases in the rural areas of the states of Espirito Santo, Goias, Mato Grasso do Sul, Piaui, and Tocantins. Rare cases in the rural forested areas of the states of Rio de Janeiro and São Paulo. No malaria in the cities of Brasilia, Rio de Janeiro, São Paulo, and none at Iguaçu Falls (see Map 3-21).

Estimated relative risk of malaria for US travelers: Low.

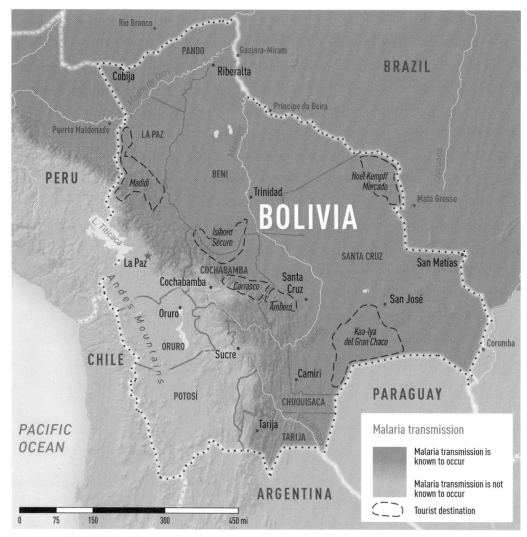

MAP 3-18. Malaria in Bolivia

Drug resistance[4]: Chloroquine.
Malaria species: *P. vivax* 85%, *P. falciparum* 15%.
Recommended chemoprophylaxis: States of Acre, Amapá, Amazonas, Rondonia, and Roraima. States of Maranão, Mato Grosso, and Para (but not their capital cities): Atovaquone-proguanil, doxycycline, or mefloquine. Areas with rare cases: Mosquito avoidance only.

BRITISH INDIAN OCEAN TERRITORY, INCLUDES DIEGO GARCIA (UK)

YELLOW FEVER
Requirements: This territory has not stated its yellow fever vaccination certificate requirements.
Recommendations: None.

*All footnotes are located on page 424.

MALARIA
No malaria transmission.

BRUNEI

YELLOW FEVER
Requirements: Required if traveling from a country with risk of YFV transmission and ≥1 year of age, including transit >12 hours in an airport located in a country with risk of YFV transmission.[1]
Recommendations: None.

MALARIA
No malaria transmission.

BULGARIA

YELLOW FEVER
No requirements or recommendations.

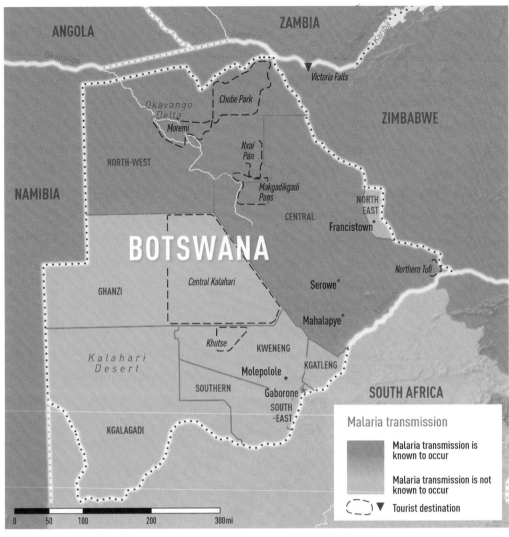

MAP 3-19. Malaria in Botswana

Malaria transmission

Malaria transmission is known to occur

Malaria transmission is not known to occur

Tourist destination

MALARIA
No malaria transmission.

BURKINA FASO

YELLOW FEVER

Requirements: Required if traveling from a country with risk of YFV transmission and ≥9 months of age, including transit in an airport located in a country with risk of YFV transmission.[1]

Recommendations: *Recommended* for all travelers ≥9 months of age.

MALARIA

Areas with malaria: All.

Estimated relative risk of malaria for US travelers: High.

*All footnotes are located on page 424.

Drug resistance[4]: Chloroquine.

Malaria species: *P. falciparum* >80%, *P. ovale* 5%–10%, *P. vivax* rare.

Recommended chemoprophylaxis: Atovaquone-proguanil, doxycycline, or mefloquine.

BURMA (MYANMAR)

YELLOW FEVER

Requirements: Required if traveling from a country with risk of YFV transmission and ≥1 year of age, including transit >12 hours in an airport located in a country with risk of YFV transmission.[1] Required also for nationals and residents of Burma (Myanmar) departing for a country with risk of YFV transmission.

Recommendations: None.

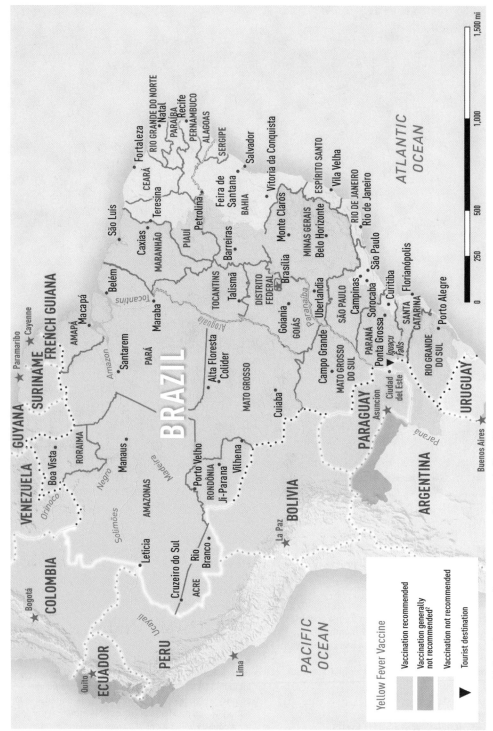

MAP 3-20. Yellow fever vaccine recommendations in Brazil[1]

[1,2] See footnotes on page 424.

Yellow Fever Vaccine

- Vaccination recommended
- Vaccination generally not recommended[2]
- Vaccination not recommended
- ► Tourist destination

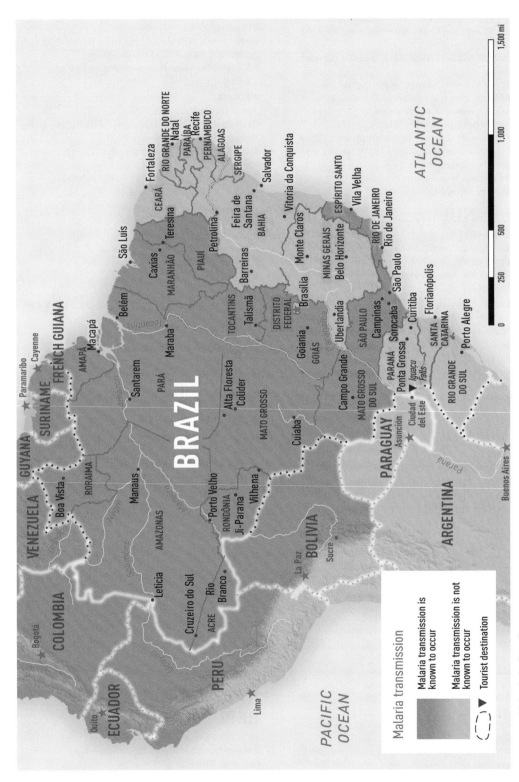

MAP 3-21. Malaria in Brazil

Malaria transmission

- Malaria transmission is known to occur
- Malaria transmission is not known to occur
- ▶ Tourist destination

MALARIA

Areas with malaria: Present at altitudes <1,000 m (3,281 ft), including Bagan. Rare transmission above 1,000 m.

Estimated relative risk of malaria for US travelers: Moderate.

Drug resistance[4]: Chloroquine and mefloquine.

Malaria species: *P. falciparum* 60%, *P. vivax* 35%; *P. malariae, P. ovale, P. knowlesi* rare.

Recommended chemoprophylaxis:
In the provinces of Bago, Kachin, Kayah, Kayin, Shan, and Tanintharyi below 1,000m (3,281 ft): Atovaquone-proguanil or doxycycline.

All other areas with malaria: Atovaquone-proguanil, doxycycline, or mefloquine.

BURUNDI

YELLOW FEVER

Requirements: Required for arriving travelers from all countries if traveler is ≥1 year of age.

Recommendations: *Recommended* for all travelers ≥9 months of age.

MALARIA

Areas with malaria: All.

Estimated relative risk of malaria for US travelers: Moderate.

Drug resistance[4]: Chloroquine.

Malaria species: *P. falciparum* 86%; *P. malariae, P. ovale, P. vivax* 14% combined.

Recommended chemoprophylaxis: Atovaquone-proguanil, doxycycline, or mefloquine.

CAMBODIA

YELLOW FEVER

Requirements: Required if traveling from a country with risk of YFV transmission and ≥1 year of age, including transit >12 hours in an airport located in a country with risk of YFV transmission.[1]

Recommendations: None.

MALARIA

Areas with malaria: Present throughout the country, including Siem Reap city. None in the city of Phnom Penh or at the temple complex at Angkor Wat.

Estimated relative risk of malaria for US travelers: Low.

Drug resistance[4]: Chloroquine and mefloquine.

Malaria species: *P. falciparum* 86%, *P. vivax* 12%, *P. malariae* 2%, *P. knowlesi* rare.

Recommended chemoprophylaxis:
In the provinces of Banteay Meanchey, Battambang, Kampot, Koh Kong, Odder Meanchey, Pailin, Preah Vihear, Pursat, and Siem Reap bordering Thailand: Atovaquone-proguanil or doxycycline.

All other areas with malaria: Atovaquone-proguanil, doxycycline, or mefloquine.

*All footnotes are located on page 424.

CAMEROON

YELLOW FEVER

Requirements: Required for arriving travelers from all countries if traveler is ≥9 months of age.

Recommendations: *Recommended* for all travelers ≥9 months of age.

MALARIA

Areas with malaria: All.

Estimated relative risk of malaria for US travelers: High.

Drug resistance[4]: Chloroquine.

Malaria species: *P. falciparum* >85%, *P. ovale* 5%–10%, *P. vivax* rare.

Recommended chemoprophylaxis: Atovaquone-proguanil, doxycycline, or mefloquine.

CANADA

YELLOW FEVER

No requirements or recommendations.

MALARIA

No malaria transmission.

CANARY ISLANDS (SPAIN)

YELLOW FEVER

No requirements or recommendations.

MALARIA

No malaria transmission.

CAPE VERDE

YELLOW FEVER

Requirements: Required if traveling from a country with risk of YFV transmission and ≥1 year of age, including transit >12 hours in an airport located in a country with risk of YFV transmission.[1]

Recommendations: None.

MALARIA

Areas with malaria: Limited cases in São Tiago Island.

Estimated relative risk of malaria for US travelers: Very low.

Drug resistance[4]: Chloroquine.

Malaria species: Primarily *P. falciparum*.

Recommended chemoprophylaxis: Mosquito avoidance only.

CAYMAN ISLANDS (UK)

YELLOW FEVER

No requirements or recommendations.

MALARIA

No malaria transmission.

CENTRAL AFRICAN REPUBLIC

YELLOW FEVER

Requirements: Required for arriving travelers from all countries if traveler is ≥9 months of age.

Recommendations: *Recommended* for all travelers ≥9 months of age.

MALARIA

Areas with malaria: All.
Estimated relative risk of malaria for US travelers: High.
Drug resistance[4]: Chloroquine.
Malaria species: *P. falciparum* 85%; *P. malariae, P. ovale, P. vivax* 15% combined.
Recommended chemoprophylaxis: Atovaquone-proguanil, doxycycline, or mefloquine.

CHAD

YELLOW FEVER

Requirements: Required if traveling from a country with risk of YFV transmission.[1]
Recommendations:
Recommended for all travelers ≥9 months of age traveling to areas south of the Sahara Desert (see Map 3-14).
Not recommended for travelers whose itineraries are limited to areas in the Sahara Desert (see Map 3-14).

MALARIA

Areas with malaria: All.
Estimated relative risk of malaria for US travelers: High.
Drug resistance[4]: Chloroquine.
Malaria species: *P. falciparum* 85%; *P. malariae, P. ovale, P. vivax* 15% combined.
Recommended chemoprophylaxis: Atovaquone-proguanil, doxycycline, or mefloquine.

CHILE

YELLOW FEVER

No requirements or recommendations.

MALARIA

No malaria transmission.

CHINA *(see Map 3-22.)*

YELLOW FEVER

Requirements: Required if traveling from a country with risk of YFV transmission and ≥1 year of age, including transit in an airport located in a country with risk of YFV transmission.[1] This requirement does not apply to travelers whose itineraries are limited to Hong Kong Special Administrative Region (SAR) and Macao SAR.
Recommendations: None.

MALARIA

Areas with malaria: Present in the counties along the China-Burma (Myanmar) border in Yunnan Province. Limited transmission in Motuo County in Tibet. No malaria in areas where most major river cruises pass.
Estimated relative risk of malaria for US travelers: Very low.
Drug resistance[4]: Chloroquine and mefloquine.
Malaria species: Primarily *P. vivax; P. falciparum* in Yunnan Province.

*All footnotes are located on page 424.

Recommended chemoprophylaxis:
Along China-Burma (Myanmar) border in the western part of Yunnan Province: Atovaquone-proguanil or doxycycline.
Motuo County in Tibet: Mosquito avoidance only.

CHRISTMAS ISLAND (AUSTRALIA)

YELLOW FEVER

Requirements: Required if traveling from a country with risk of YFV transmission and ≥1 year of age, including transit >12 hours in an airport located in a country with risk of YFV transmission.[1] This requirement excludes Galápagos Islands in Ecuador and the island of Tobago and is limited to Misiones Province in Argentina.
Recommendations: None.

MALARIA

No malaria transmission.

COCOS (KEELING) ISLANDS (AUSTRALIA)

YELLOW FEVER

Requirements: Required if traveling from a country with risk of YFV transmission and ≥1 year of age, including transit >12 hours in an airport located in a country with risk of YFV transmission.[1] This requirement excludes Galápagos Islands in Ecuador and the island of Tobago and is limited to Misiones Province in Argentina.
Recommendations: None.

MALARIA

No malaria transmission.

COLOMBIA *(see Maps 3-23 and 3-24.)*

YELLOW FEVER

Requirements: None.
Recommendations:
Recommended for all travelers ≥9 months of age except as mentioned below.
Generally not recommended for travelers to the cities of Barranquilla, Cali, Cartagena, and Medellín (see Map 3-23).
Not recommended for travelers whose itineraries are limited to all areas >2,300 m in elevation,[2] the department of San Andrès y Providencia, and the capital city of Bogotá.

MALARIA

Areas with malaria: All areas <1,700 m (5,577 ft). None in Bogotá, Cartagena, and Medellín (see Map 3-24).
Estimated relative risk of malaria for US travelers: Low.
Drug resistance[4]: Chloroquine.
Malaria species: *P. falciparum* 50%, *P. vivax* 50%.
Recommended chemoprophylaxis: Atovaquone-proguanil, doxycycline, or mefloquine.

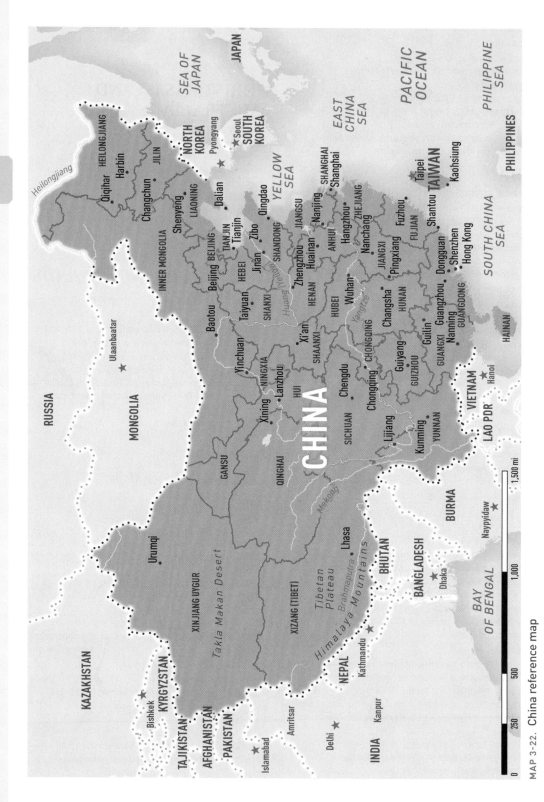

MAP 3-22. China reference map

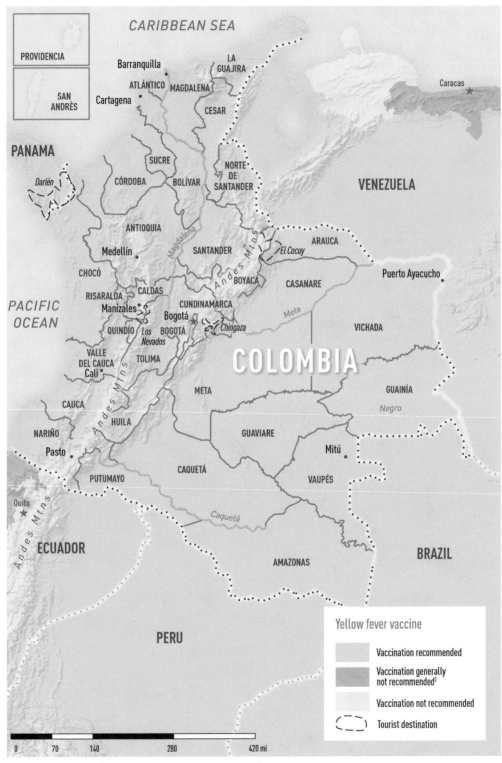

MAP 3-23. Yellow fever vaccine recommendations in Colombia[1]

[1,2] See footnotes on page 424.

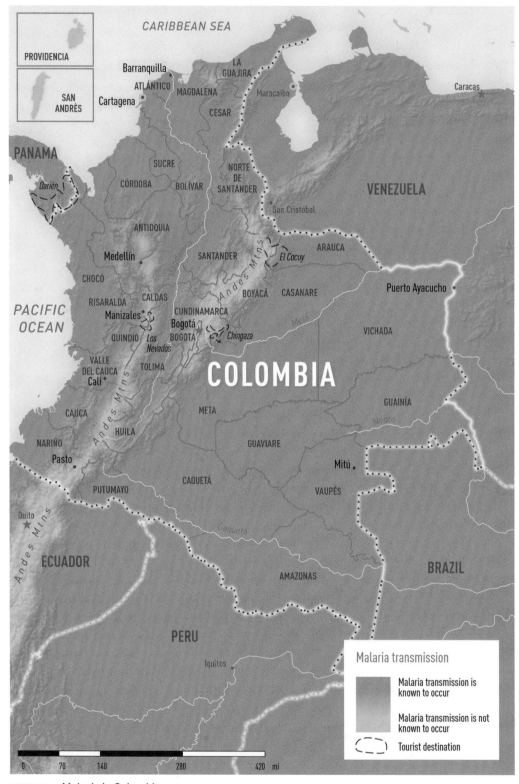

MAP 3-24. **Malaria in Colombia**

COMOROS

YELLOW FEVER

No requirements or recommendations.

MALARIA

Areas with malaria: All.
Estimated relative risk of malaria for US travelers: No data.
Drug resistance[4]: Chloroquine.
Malaria species: Primarily *P. falciparum*.
Recommended chemoprophylaxis: Atovaquone-proguanil, doxycycline, or mefloquine.

CONGO, REPUBLIC OF THE (CONGO-BRAZZAVILLE)

YELLOW FEVER

Requirements: Required for arriving travelers from all countries if traveler is ≥9 months of age.
Recommendations: *Recommended* for all travelers ≥9 months of age.

MALARIA

Areas with malaria: All.
Estimated relative risk of malaria for US travelers: High.
Drug resistance[4]: Chloroquine.
Malaria species: *P. falciparum* 90%, *P. ovale* 5%–10%, *P. vivax* rare.
Recommended chemoprophylaxis: Atovaquone-proguanil, doxycycline, or mefloquine.

COOK ISLANDS (NEW ZEALAND)

YELLOW FEVER

No requirements or recommendations.

MALARIA

No malaria transmission.

COSTA RICA

YELLOW FEVER

Requirements: Required if traveling from a country with risk of YFV transmission and ≥9 months of age, including transit >12 hours in an airport located in a country with risk of YFV transmission.[1] This requirement excludes Argentina, Burundi, Central African Republic, Chad, Congo, Côte d'Ivoire, Equatorial Guinea, Ethiopia, Guinea-Bissau, Guyana, Kenya, Mali, Mauritania, Niger, Panama, Paraguay, Rwanda, Senegal, South Sudan, Suriname, Togo, Trinidad and Tobago, and Uganda.
Recommendations: None.

MALARIA

No malaria transmission.

CÔTE D'IVOIRE (IVORY COAST)

YELLOW FEVER

Requirements: Required for arriving travelers from all countries if traveler is ≥9 months of age.

*All footnotes are located on page 424.

Recommendations: *Recommended* for all travelers ≥9 months of age.

MALARIA

Areas with malaria: All.
Estimated relative risk of malaria for US travelers: High.
Drug resistance[4]: Chloroquine.
Malaria species: *P. falciparum* 85%, *P. ovale* 5%–10%, *P. vivax* rare.
Recommended chemoprophylaxis: Atovaquone-proguanil, doxycycline, or mefloquine.

CROATIA

YELLOW FEVER

No requirements or recommendations.

MALARIA

No malaria transmission.

CUBA

YELLOW FEVER

No requirements or recommendations.

MALARIA

No malaria transmission.

CURAÇAO

YELLOW FEVER

Requirements: Required if traveling from a country with risk of YFV transmission and ≥6 months of age.[1]
Recommendations: None.

MALARIA

No malaria transmission.

CYPRUS

YELLOW FEVER

No requirements or recommendations.

MALARIA

No malaria transmission.

CZECH REPUBLIC

YELLOW FEVER

No requirements or recommendations.

MALARIA

No malaria transmission.

DEMOCRATIC REPUBLIC OF THE CONGO (CONGO-KINSHASA)

YELLOW FEVER

Requirements: Required for arriving travelers from all countries if traveler is ≥9 months of age.
Recommendations: *Recommended* for all travelers ≥9 months of age.

MALARIA

Areas with malaria: All.

Estimated relative risk of malaria for US travelers: High.
Drug resistance[4]: Chloroquine.
Malaria species: *P. falciparum* >90%, *P. ovale* 5%, *P. vivax* rare.
Recommended chemoprophylaxis: Atovaquone-proguanil, doxycycline, or mefloquine.

DENMARK

YELLOW FEVER
No requirements or recommendations.

MALARIA
No malaria transmission.

DJIBOUTI

YELLOW FEVER
Requirements: Required if traveling from a country with risk of YFV transmission and ≥1 year of age, including transit in an airport located in a country with risk of YFV transmission.[1]
Recommendations: None.

MALARIA
Areas with malaria: All.
Estimated relative risk of malaria for US travelers: No data.
Drug resistance[4]: Chloroquine.
Malaria species: *P. falciparum* 90%, *P. vivax* 5%–10%.
Recommended chemoprophylaxis: Atovaquone-proguanil, doxycycline, or mefloquine.

DOMINICA

YELLOW FEVER
Requirements: Required if traveling from a country with risk of YFV transmission and ≥1 year of age, including transit >12 hours in an airport located in a country with risk of YFV transmission.[1]
Recommendations: None.

MALARIA
No malaria transmission.

DOMINICAN REPUBLIC

YELLOW FEVER
No requirements or recommendations.

MALARIA
Areas with malaria: All areas (including resort areas), except none in the cities of Santiago and Santo Domingo.
Estimated relative risk of malaria for US travelers: Low.
Drug resistance[4]: None.
Malaria species: *P. falciparum* 100%.
Recommended chemoprophylaxis: Atovaquone-proguanil, chloroquine, doxycycline, or mefloquine.

EASTER ISLAND (CHILE)

YELLOW FEVER
Requirements: This country has not stated its yellow fever vaccination certificate requirements.

All footnotes are located on page 424.

Recommendations: None.
MALARIA
No malaria transmission.

ECUADOR, INCLUDING THE GALÁPAGOS ISLANDS
(see Maps 3-25 and 3-26.)

YELLOW FEVER
Requirements: Required if traveling from a country with risk of YFV transmission and ≥1 year of age, including transit >12 hours in an airport located in a country with risk of YFV transmission.[1]
Recommendations:
Recommended for all travelers ≥9 months of age traveling to areas <2,300 m in elevation[2] in the following provinces east of the Andes Mountains: Morona-Santiago, Napo, Orellana, Pastaza, Sucumbios, and Zamora-Chinchipe (see Map 3-25).
Generally not recommended for travelers whose itinerary is limited to areas <2,300 m in elevation[2] in the following provinces west of the Andes mountains: Esmeraldas, Guayas, Los Rios, Santa Elena, Santo Domingo de los Tsachilas, and designated areas of Azuay, Bolivar, Canar, Carchi, Chimborazo, Cotopaxi, El Oro, Imbabura, Loja, Pichincha, and Tungurahua (see Map 3-25).
Not recommended for travelers whose itineraries are limited to all areas >2,300 m in elevation,[2] the cities of Guayaquil and Quito, or the Galápagos Islands (see Map 3-25).

MALARIA
Areas with malaria: Areas at altitudes <1,500 m (4,921 ft) in the provinces of Carchi, Esmeraldas, Morona Santiago, Orellana, and Pastaza. Rare cases in other provinces in areas <1,500m (4,921 ft). Not present in the cities of Guayaquil and Quito or the Galápagos Islands (see Map 3-26).
Estimated relative risk of malaria for US travelers: Very low.
Drug resistance[4]: Chloroquine.
Malaria species: *P. vivax* 66%, *P. falciparum* 34%.
Recommended chemoprophylaxis: Areas with malaria in Carchi, Esmeraldas, Morona Santiago, Orellana, and Pastaza Provinces: Atovaquone-proguanil, doxycycline, or mefloquine.
Other areas with rare cases of malaria: Mosquito avoidance only.

EGYPT

YELLOW FEVER
Requirements: Required if traveling from a country with risk of YFV transmission and ≥9 months of age, including transit >12 hours in an airport located in a country with risk of YFV transmission. This includes Rwanda, Somalia, Tanzania, and Zambia and excludes Bolivia, Galapagos Islands, and Tobago.[1] In the absence of a vaccination certificate, the person will be

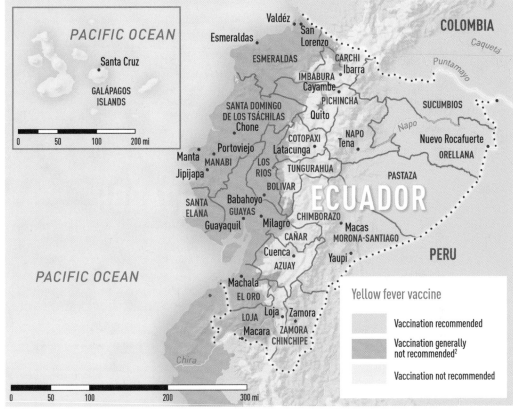

MAP 3-25. Yellow fever vaccine recommendations in Ecuador[1]

1,2 See footnotes on page 424.

Yellow fever vaccine

- Vaccination recommended
- Vaccination generally not recommended[2]
- Vaccination not recommended

detained in quarantine for up to 6 days after departure from an area at risk of yellow fever transmission.
Recommendations: None.

MALARIA
No malaria transmission.

EL SALVADOR

YELLOW FEVER
Requirements: Required if traveling from a country with risk of YFV transmission and ≥1 year of age, including transit >12 hours in an airport located in a country with risk of YFV transmission.[1]
Recommendations: None.

MALARIA
Areas with malaria: Rare cases along Guatemalan border.
Estimated relative risk of malaria for US travelers: Very low.
Drug resistance[4]: None.
Malaria species: *P. vivax* 99%, *P. falciparum* <1%.
Recommended chemoprophylaxis: Mosquito avoidance only.

*All footnotes are located on page 424.

EQUATORIAL GUINEA

YELLOW FEVER
Requirements: Required if traveling from a country with risk of YFV transmission and ≥6 months of age.[1]
Recommendations: *Recommended* for all travelers ≥9 months of age.

MALARIA
Areas with malaria: All.
Estimated relative risk of malaria for US travelers: High.
Drug resistance[4]: Chloroquine.
Malaria species: *P. falciparum* 85%; *P. malariae, P. ovale, P. vivax* 15% combined.
Recommended chemoprophylaxis: Atovaquone-proguanil, doxycycline, or mefloquine.

ERITREA

YELLOW FEVER
Requirements: Required if traveling from a country with risk of YFV transmission and ≥9 months of age, including transit >12 hours in an airport located in a country with risk of YFV transmission.[1]

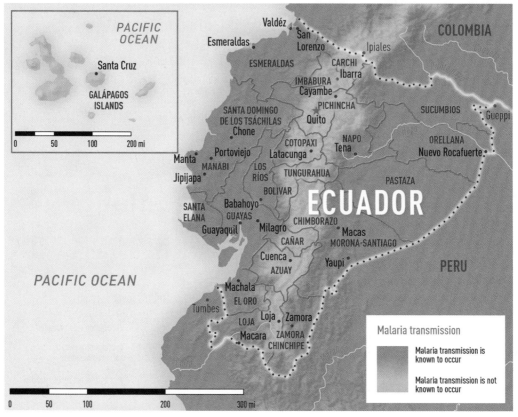

MAP 3-26. Malaria in Ecuador

Recommendations:
Generally not recommended for travelers going to the following states: Anseba, Debub, Gash Barka, Mae Kel, and Semenawi Keih Bahri.
Not recommended for all areas not listed above, including the Dahlak Archipelago (see Map 3-14).

MALARIA
Areas with malaria: All areas <2,200 m (7,218 ft). None in Asmara.
Estimated relative risk of malaria for US travelers: High.
Drug resistance[4]: Chloroquine.
Malaria species: *P. falciparum* 85%, *P. vivax* 10%–15%, *P. ovale* rare.
Recommended chemoprophylaxis: Atovaquone-proguanil, doxycycline, or mefloquine.

ESTONIA

YELLOW FEVER
No requirements or recommendations.

MALARIA
No malaria transmission.

ETHIOPIA *(see Maps 3-27 and 3-28.)*

YELLOW FEVER
Requirements: Required if traveling from a country with risk of YFV transmission and ≥9 months of age, including transit >12 hours in an airport located in a country with risk of YFV transmission.[1]
Recommendations:
Recommended for all travelers ≥9 months of age, except as mentioned below.
Generally not recommended for travelers whose itinerary is limited to the Afar and Somali Provinces (see Map 3-27).

MALARIA
Areas with malaria: All areas <2,500 m (8,202 ft), except none in the city of Addis Ababa (see Map 3-28).
Estimated relative risk of malaria for US travelers: Moderate.
Drug resistance[4]: Chloroquine.
Malaria species: *P. falciparum* 60%–70%, *P. vivax* 30%–40%, *P. malariae* and *P. ovale* rare.
Recommended chemoprophylaxis: Atovaquone-proguanil, doxycycline, or mefloquine.

*All footnotes are located on page 424.

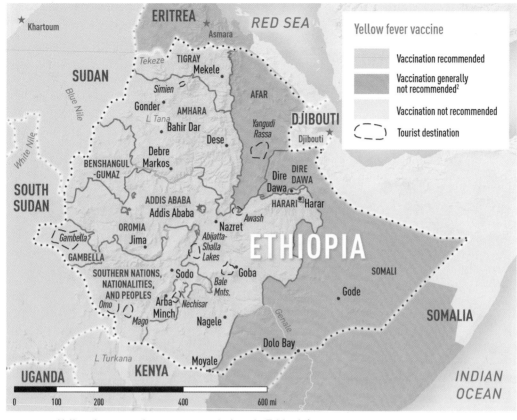

MAP 3-27. Yellow fever vaccine recommendations in Ethiopia[1]

[1,2] See footnotes on page 424.

FALKLAND ISLANDS (ISLAS MALVINAS)

YELLOW FEVER

No requirements or recommendations.

MALARIA

No malaria transmission.

FAROE ISLANDS (DENMARK)

YELLOW FEVER

No requirements or recommendations.

MALARIA

No malaria transmission.

FIJI

YELLOW FEVER

Requirements: Required if traveling from a country with risk of YFV transmission and ≥1 year of age, including transit >12 hours in an airport located in a country with risk of YFV transmission.[1]

Recommendations: None.

*All footnotes are located on page 424.

MALARIA

No malaria transmission.

FINLAND

YELLOW FEVER

No requirements or recommendations.

MALARIA

No malaria transmission.

FRANCE

YELLOW FEVER

No requirements or recommendations.

MALARIA

No malaria transmission.

FRENCH GUIANA

YELLOW FEVER

Requirements: Required for arriving travelers from all countries if traveler is ≥1 year of age.

Recommendations: *Recommended* for all travelers ≥9 months of age.

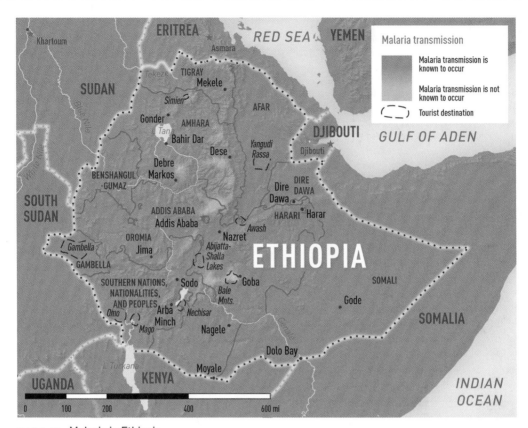

MAP 3-28. Malaria in Ethiopia

MALARIA

Areas with malaria: All areas, including Matoury, Macouria, and Kourou, except none in coastal areas west of Kourou and Cayenne City.

Estimated relative risk of malaria for US travelers: Low.

Drug resistance[4]**:** Chloroquine.

Malaria species: *P. vivax* >70%, *P. falciparum* 20%–30%, *P. malariae* rare

Recommended chemoprophylaxis: Atovaquone-proguanil, doxycycline, or mefloquine.

FRENCH POLYNESIA, INCLUDING THE ISLAND GROUPS OF SOCIETY ISLANDS (TAHITI, MOOREA, AND BORA-BORA), MARQUESAS ISLANDS (HIVA OA AND UA HUKA), AND AUSTRAL ISLANDS (TUBUAI AND RURUTU)

*All footnotes are located on page 424.

YELLOW FEVER

Requirements: Required if traveling from a country with risk of YFV transmission and ≥1 year of age, including transit >12 hours in an airport located in a country with risk of YFV transmission.[1]

Recommendations: None.

MALARIA

No malaria transmission.

GABON

YELLOW FEVER

Requirements: Required for arriving travelers from all countries if traveler is ≥1 year of age.

Recommendations: *Recommended* for all travelers ≥9 months of age.

MALARIA

Areas with malaria: All.

Estimated relative risk of malaria for US travelers: High.

Drug resistance[4]**:** Chloroquine.

Malaria species: *P. falciparum* 90%; *P. malariae, P. ovale, P. vivax* 10% combined.

Recommended chemoprophylaxis: Atovaquone-proguanil, doxycycline, or mefloquine.

GAMBIA, THE

YELLOW FEVER
Requirements: Required if traveling from a country with risk of YFV transmission and ≥9 months of age.[1]
Recommendations: *Recommended* for all travelers ≥9 months of age.

MALARIA
Areas with malaria: All.
Estimated relative risk of malaria for US travelers: High.
Drug resistance[4]**:** Chloroquine.
Malaria species: *P. falciparum* ≥85%, *P. ovale* 5%–10%, *P. malariae* and *P. vivax* rare.
Recommended chemoprophylaxis: Atovaquone-proguanil, doxycycline, or mefloquine.

GEORGIA

YELLOW FEVER
No requirements or recommendations.

MALARIA
No malaria transmission.

GERMANY

YELLOW FEVER
No requirements or recommendations.

MALARIA
No malaria transmission.

GHANA

YELLOW FEVER
Requirements: Required for arriving travelers from all countries if traveler is ≥9 months of age.
Recommendations: *Recommended* for all travelers ≥9 months of age.

MALARIA
Areas with malaria: All.
Estimated relative risk of malaria for US travelers: High.
Drug resistance[4]**:** Chloroquine.
Malaria species: *P. falciparum* 90%, *P. ovale* 5%–10%, *P. vivax* rare.
Recommended chemoprophylaxis: Atovaquone-proguanil, doxycycline, or mefloquine.

GIBRALTAR (UK)

YELLOW FEVER
No requirements or recommendations.

MALARIA
No malaria transmission.

GREECE

YELLOW FEVER
No requirements or recommendations.

MALARIA
Areas with malaria: Rare focal transmission May–Nov associated with imported malaria cases, limited to agricultural areas. None in tourist areas.
Estimated relative risk of malaria for US travelers: None.
Drug resistance: Not applicable.
Malaria species: *P. vivax* 100%.
Recommended chemoprophylaxis: None.

GREENLAND (DENMARK)

YELLOW FEVER
No requirements or recommendations.

MALARIA
No malaria transmission.

GRENADA

YELLOW FEVER
Requirements: Required if traveling from a country with risk of YFV transmission and ≥1 year of age, including transit >12 hours in an airport located in a country with risk of YFV transmission.[1]
Recommendations: None.

MALARIA
No malaria transmission.

GUADELOUPE (FRANCE)

YELLOW FEVER
Requirements: Required if traveling from a country with risk of YFV transmission and ≥1 year of age, including transit >12 hours in a country with risk of YFV transmission.[1]
Recommendations: None.

MALARIA
No malaria transmission.

GUAM (US)

YELLOW FEVER
No requirements or recommendations.

MALARIA
No malaria transmission.

GUATEMALA

YELLOW FEVER
Requirements: Required if traveling from a country with risk of YFV transmission and ≥1 year of age, including transit >12 hours in an airport located in a country with risk of YFV transmission.[1]
Recommendations: None.

*All footnotes are located on page 424.

MALARIA

Areas with malaria: Rural areas only at altitudes <1,500 m (4,921 ft). None in Antigua, Guatemala City, or Lake Atitlán.
Estimated relative risk of malaria for US travelers: Low.
Drug resistance[4]: None.
Malaria species: *P. vivax* 97%, *P. falciparum* 3%.
Recommended chemoprophylaxis: Escuintla Province: Atovaquone-proguanil, chloroquine, doxycycline, or mefloquine.
All other areas with malaria: Atovaquone-proguanil, chloroquine, doxycycline, mefloquine, or primaquine[5].

GUINEA

YELLOW FEVER

Requirements: Required if traveling from a country with risk of YFV transmission and ≥1 year of age.[1]
Recommendations: *Recommended* for all travelers ≥9 months of age.

MALARIA

Areas with malaria: All.
Estimated relative risk of malaria for US travelers: High.
Drug resistance[4]: Chloroquine.
Malaria species: *P. falciparum* >85%, *P. ovale* 5%–10%, *P. vivax* rare.
Recommended chemoprophylaxis: Atovaquone-proguanil, doxycycline, or mefloquine.

GUINEA-BISSAU

YELLOW FEVER

Requirements: Required for arriving travelers from all countries if traveler is ≥1 year of age.
Recommendations: *Recommended* for all travelers ≥9 months of age.

MALARIA

Areas with malaria: All.
Estimated relative risk of malaria for US travelers: Moderate.
Drug resistance[4]: Chloroquine.
Malaria species: *P. falciparum* >85%, *P. ovale* 5%–10%, *P. vivax* rare.
Recommended chemoprophylaxis: Atovaquone-proguanil, doxycycline, or mefloquine.

GUYANA

YELLOW FEVER

Requirements: Required if traveling from a country with risk of YFV transmission and ≥1 year of age, including transit in an airport located in a country with risk of YFV transmission.[1]
Recommendations: *Recommended* for all travelers ≥9 months of age.

MALARIA

Areas with malaria: All areas <900 m (2,953 ft). Rare cases in the cities of Amsterdam and Georgetown.

Estimated relative risk of malaria for US travelers: High.
Drug resistance[4]: Chloroquine.
Malaria species: *P. falciparum* 50%, *P. vivax* 50%.
Recommended chemoprophylaxis:
Areas with malaria except cities of Amsterdam and Georgetown: Atovaquone-proguanil, doxycycline, or mefloquine.
Cities of Georgetown and Amsterdam: Mosquito avoidance only.

HAITI

YELLOW FEVER

No requirements or recommendations.

MALARIA

Areas with malaria: All (including Port Labadee).
Estimated relative risk of malaria for US travelers: Moderate.
Drug resistance[4]: None.
Malaria species: *P. falciparum* 99%, *P. malariae* rare.
Recommended chemoprophylaxis: Atovaquone-proguanil, chloroquine, doxycycline, or mefloquine.

HONDURAS

YELLOW FEVER

Requirements: Required if traveling from a country with risk of YFV transmission and ≥1 year of age, including transit >12 hours in an airport located in a country with risk of YFV transmission.[1] This requirement excludes the Central African Republic, Panama, and South Sudan.
Recommendations: None.

MALARIA

Areas with malaria: Present throughout the country and in Roatán and other Bay Islands. None in San Pedro Sula and Tegucigalpa.
Estimated relative risk of malaria for US travelers: Moderate.
Drug resistance[4]: None.
Malaria species: *P. vivax* 93%, *P. falciparum* 7%.
Recommended chemoprophylaxis: Atovaquone-proguanil, chloroquine, doxycycline, mefloquine, or primaquine[5].

HONG KONG SAR (CHINA)

YELLOW FEVER

No requirements or recommendations.

MALARIA

No malaria transmission.

HUNGARY

YELLOW FEVER

No requirements or recommendations.

MALARIA

No malaria transmission.

*All footnotes are located on page 424.

3

ICELAND

YELLOW FEVER
No requirements or recommendations.

MALARIA
No malaria transmission.

INDIA *(see Map 3-29.)*

YELLOW FEVER
Requirements: Any traveler (except infants <6 months old) arriving by air or sea without a yellow fever vaccination certificate is detained in isolation for up to 6 days if that person—
1) arrives within 6 days of departure from an area with risk of YFV transmission,
2) has been in such an area in transit (except those passengers and members of flight crews who, while in transit through an airport in an area with risk of YFV transmission, remained in the airport during their entire stay and the health officer agrees to such an exemption),
3) arrives on a ship that started from or touched at any port in an area with risk of YFV transmission up to 30 days before its arrival in India, unless such a ship has been disinsected in accordance with the procedure recommended by WHO, or
4) arrives on an aircraft that has been in an area with risk of YFV transmission and has not been disinsected in accordance with the Indian Aircraft Public Health Rules, 1954, or as recommended by WHO.

The following are regarded as countries and areas with risk of YFV transmission:
Africa: Angola, Benin, Burkina Faso, Burundi, Cameroon, Central African Republic, Chad, Congo, Côte d'Ivoire, Democratic Republic of the Congo, Equatorial Guinea, Ethiopia, Gabon, The Gambia, Ghana, Guinea, Guinea-Bissau, Kenya, Liberia, Mali, Mauritania, Niger, Nigeria, Rwanda, Senegal, Sierra Leone, South Sudan, Sudan, Togo, and Uganda.
Americas: Argentina, Bolivia, Brazil, Colombia, Ecuador, French Guiana, Guyana, Panama, Paraguay, Peru, Suriname, Trinidad (Trinidad only), and Venezuela.
Note: When a case of yellow fever is reported from any country, that country is regarded by the government of India as a country with risk of YFV transmission and is added to the above list.
Recommendations: None.

MALARIA
Areas with malaria: All areas throughout the country, including cities of Bombay (Mumbai) and Delhi, except none in areas >2,000 m (6,562 ft) in Himachal Pradesh, Jammu and Kashmir, and Sikkim (see Map 3-29).
Estimated relative risk of malaria for US travelers: Moderate.
Drug resistance[4]: Chloroquine.

Malaria species: *P. vivax* 50%, *P. falciparum* >40%, *P. malariae* and *P. ovale* rare.
Recommended chemoprophylaxis: Atovaquone-proguanil, doxycycline, or mefloquine.

INDONESIA

YELLOW FEVER
Requirements: Required if traveling from a country with risk of YFV transmission and ≥9 months of age.[1]
Recommendations: None.

MALARIA
Areas with malaria: All areas of eastern Indonesia (provinces of Maluku, Maluku Utara, Nusa Tenggara Timur, Papua, and Papua Barat), including the town of Labuan Bajo and Komodo Islands in the Nusa Tenggara region. Rural areas of Kalimantan (Borneo), Nusa Tenggara Barat (includes the island of Lombok), Sulawesi, and Sumatra. Low transmission in rural areas of Java, including Pangandaran, Sukalumi, and Ujung Kulong. None in cities of Jakarta and Ubud, resort areas of Bali and Java, and Gili Islands and the Thousand Islands (Pulau Seribu).
Estimated relative risk of malaria for US travelers: Low.
Drug resistance[4]: Chloroquine (*P. falciparum* and *P. vivax*).
Malaria species: *P. falciparum* 57%, *P. vivax* 43%, *P. malariae*, *P. knowlesi*, *P. ovale* rare
Recommended chemoprophylaxis: Atovaquone-proguanil, doxycycline, or mefloquine.

IRAN

YELLOW FEVER
Requirements: Required if traveling from a country with risk of YFV transmission and ≥9 months of age, including transit >12 hours in an airport located in a country with risk of YFV transmission.
Recommendations: None.

MALARIA
Areas with malaria: Rural areas of Fars Province, Sistan-Baluchestan Province, and southern, tropical parts of Hormozgan and Kerman Provinces.
Estimated relative risk of malaria for US travelers: Very low.
Drug resistance[4]: Chloroquine.
Malaria species: *P. vivax* 93%, *P. falciparum* 7%.
Recommended chemoprophylaxis: Atovaquone-proguanil, doxycycline, or mefloquine.

IRAQ

YELLOW FEVER
Requirements: Required if traveling from a country with risk of YFV transmission and ≥9 months of age, including transit >12 hours in an airport located in a country with risk of YFV transmission.[1]
Recommendations: None.

*All footnotes are located on page 424.

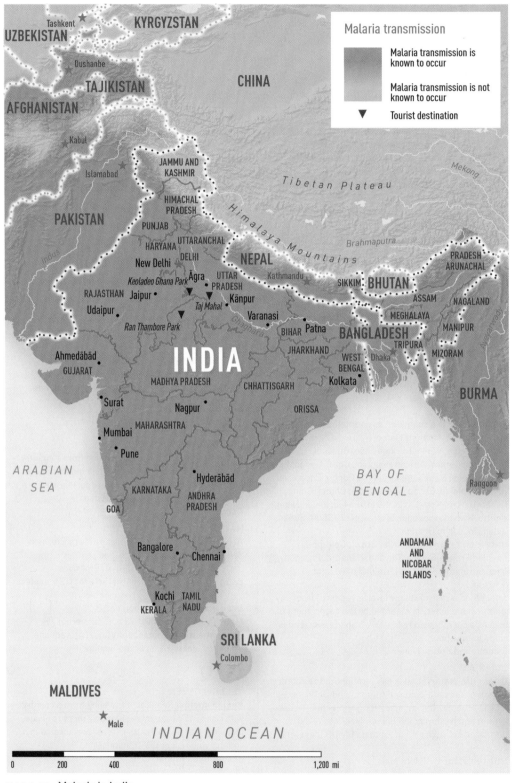

Malaria transmission

Malaria transmission is known to occur

Malaria transmission is not known to occur

▼ Tourist destination

MAP 3-29. Malaria in India

MALARIA
No malaria transmission.

IRELAND

YELLOW FEVER
No requirements or recommendations.

MALARIA
No malaria transmission.

ISRAEL

YELLOW FEVER
No requirements or recommendations.

MALARIA
No malaria transmission.

ITALY, INCLUDING HOLY SEE (VATICAN CITY)

YELLOW FEVER
No requirements or recommendations.

MALARIA
No malaria transmission.

JAMAICA

YELLOW FEVER
Requirements: Required if traveling from a country with risk of YFV transmission and ≥1 year of age, including transit in an airport located in a country with risk of YFV transmission.[1]
Recommendations: None.

MALARIA
No malaria transmission.

JAPAN

YELLOW FEVER
No requirements or recommendations.

MALARIA
No malaria transmission.

JORDAN

YELLOW FEVER
Requirements: Required if traveling from a country with risk of YFV transmission and ≥1 year of age, including transit >12 hours in an airport located in a country with risk of YFV transmission.[1]
Recommendations: None.

MALARIA
No malaria transmission.

KAZAKHSTAN

YELLOW FEVER
Requirements: Required if traveling from a country with risk of YFV transmission.[1]
Recommendations: None.

MALARIA
No malaria transmission.

*All footnotes are located on page 424.

KENYA *(see Maps 3-30 and 3-31.)*

YELLOW FEVER
Requirements: Required if traveling from a country with risk of YFV transmission and ≥1 year of age.[1]
Recommendations:
Recommended for all travelers ≥9 months of age, except as mentioned below.
Generally not recommended for travelers whose itinerary is limited to the following areas: the entire North Eastern Province; the states of Kilifi, Kwale, Lamu, Malindi, and Tanariver in the Coast Province; and the cities of Mombasa and Nairobi (see Map 3-30).

MALARIA
Areas with malaria: Present in all areas (including game parks) <2,500 m (8,202 ft) including the city of Nairobi (see Map 3-31).
Estimated relative risk of malaria for US travelers: Moderate.
Drug resistance[4]: Chloroquine.
Malaria species: *P. falciparum* >85%, *P. vivax* 5%–10%, *P. ovale* up to 5%.
Recommended chemoprophylaxis: Atovaquone-proguanil, doxycycline, or mefloquine.

KIRIBATI (FORMERLY GILBERT ISLANDS), INCLUDES TARAWA, TABUAERAN (FANNING ISLAND), AND BANABA (OCEAN ISLAND)

YELLOW FEVER
Requirements: Required if traveling from a country with risk of YFV transmission and ≥1 year of age.[1]
Recommendations: None.

MALARIA
No malaria transmission.

KOSOVO

YELLOW FEVER
Requirements: This country has not stated its yellow fever vaccination certificate requirements.
Recommendations: None.

MALARIA
No malaria transmission.

KUWAIT

YELLOW FEVER
No requirements or recommendations.

MALARIA
No malaria transmission.

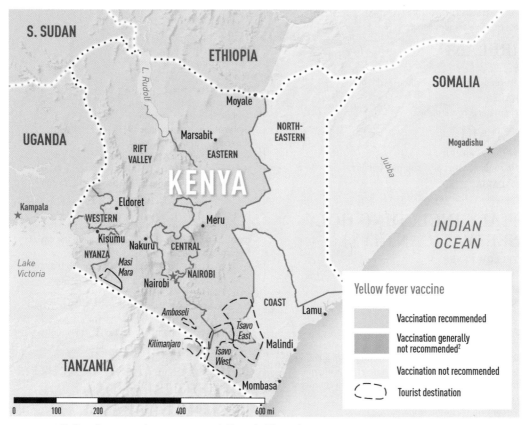

MAP 3-30. Yellow fever vaccine recommendations in Kenya[1]

[1,2] See footnotes on page 424.

KYRGYZSTAN

YELLOW FEVER

Requirements: Required if traveling from a country with risk of YFV transmission and ≥1 year of age, including transit >12 hours in an airport located in a country with risk of YFV transmission.[1]
Recommendations: None.

MALARIA
No malaria transmission.

LAOS

YELLOW FEVER

Requirements: Required if traveling from a country with risk of YFV transmission.[1]
Recommendations: None.

MALARIA

Areas with malaria: All, except none in the city of Vientiane.
Estimated relative risk of malaria for US travelers: Very low.
Drug resistance[4]: Chloroquine and mefloquine.

*All footnotes are located on page 424.

Malaria species: *P. falciparum* 65%, *P. vivax* 34%, *P. malariae* and *P. ovale* 1% combined.
Recommended chemoprophylaxis:
Along the Laos-Burma (Myanmar) border in the provinces of Bokeo and Louang Namtha, along the Laos-Thailand border in the province of Champasak and Saravan, along the Laos-Cambodia border, and along the Laos-Vietnam border: Atovaquone-proguanil or doxycycline.
All other areas with malaria: Atovaquone-proguanil, doxycycline, or mefloquine.

LATVIA

YELLOW FEVER
No requirements or recommendations.

MALARIA
No malaria transmission.

LEBANON

YELLOW FEVER
No requirements or recommendations.

MALARIA
No malaria transmission.

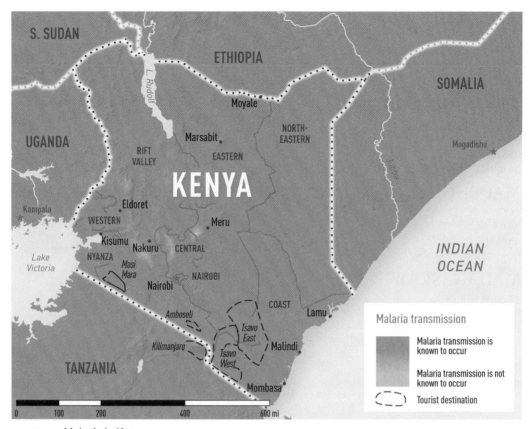

MAP 3-31. Malaria in Kenya

Malaria transmission

- Malaria transmission is known to occur
- Malaria transmission is not known to occur
- Tourist destination

LESOTHO

YELLOW FEVER

Requirements: Required if traveling from a country with risk of YFV transmission and ≥9 months of age, including transit >12 hours in an airport located in a country with risk of YFV transmission.[1]
Recommendations: None.

MALARIA

No malaria transmission.

LIBERIA

YELLOW FEVER

Requirements: Required for arriving travelers from all countries if traveler is ≥1 year of age.
Recommendations: *Recommended* for all travelers ≥9 months of age.

MALARIA

Areas with malaria: All.
Estimated relative risk of malaria for US travelers: High.
Drug resistance[4]: Chloroquine.
Malaria species: *P. falciparum* >85%, *P. ovale* 5%–10%, *P. vivax* rare.

*All footnotes are located on page 424.

Recommended chemoprophylaxis: Atovaquone-proguanil, doxycycline, or mefloquine.

LIBYA

YELLOW FEVER

Requirements: Required if traveling from a country with risk of YFV transmission and ≥1 year of age, including transit in an airport located in a country with risk of YFV transmission.
Recommendations: None.

MALARIA

No malaria transmission.

LIECHTENSTEIN

YELLOW FEVER

No requirements or recommendations.

MALARIA

No malaria transmission.

LITHUANIA

YELLOW FEVER

No requirements or recommendations.

MALARIA

No malaria transmission.

LUXEMBOURG

YELLOW FEVER

No requirements or recommendations.

MALARIA

No malaria transmission.

MACAU SAR (CHINA)

YELLOW FEVER

No requirements or recommendations.

MALARIA

No malaria transmission.

MACEDONIA

YELLOW FEVER

No requirements or recommendations.

MALARIA

No malaria transmission.

MADAGASCAR

YELLOW FEVER

Requirements: Required if traveling from a country with risk of YFV transmission and ≥9 months of age, including transit >12 hours in an airport located in a country with risk of YFV transmission.[1]

Recommendations: None.

MALARIA

Areas with malaria: All areas, except rare cases in the city of Antananarivo.

Estimated relative risk of malaria for US travelers: Moderate.

Drug resistance[4]: Chloroquine.

Malaria species: *P. falciparum* 85%, *P. vivax* 5%–10%, *P. ovale* 5%.

Recommended chemoprophylaxis: All areas except the city of Antananarivo: Atovaquone-proguanil, doxycycline, or mefloquine.
Antananarivo: Mosquito avoidance only.

MADEIRA ISLANDS (PORTUGAL)

YELLOW FEVER

No requirements or recommendations.

MALARIA

No malaria transmission.

MALAWI

YELLOW FEVER

Requirements: Required if traveling from a country with risk of YFV transmission and ≥1 year of age, including transit >12 hours in an airport located in a country with risk of YFV transmission.[1]

Recommendations: None.

MALARIA

Areas with malaria: All.

Estimated relative risk of malaria for US travelers: Moderate.

Drug resistance[4]: Chloroquine.

Malaria species: *P. falciparum* 90%; *P. malariae, P. ovale, P. vivax* 10% combined.

Recommended chemoprophylaxis: Atovaquone-proguanil, doxycycline, or mefloquine.

MALAYSIA

YELLOW FEVER

Requirements: Required if traveling from a country with risk of YFV transmission and ≥1 year of age, including transit >12 hours in an airport located in a country with risk of YFV transmission.[1]

Recommendations: None.

MALARIA

Areas with malaria: Present in rural areas. None in Georgetown, Kuala Lampur, and Penang State (includes Penang Island).

Estimated relative risk of malaria for US travelers: Low.

Drug resistance[4]: Chloroquine.

Malaria species: *P. falciparum, P. vivax, P. knowlesi, P. malariae, P. ovale.*

Recommended chemoprophylaxis: Rural areas: Atovaquone-proguanil, doxycycline, or mefloquine.

MALDIVES

YELLOW FEVER

Requirements: Required if traveling from a country with risk of YFV transmission and ≥1 year of age, including transit >12 hours in an airport located in a country with risk of YFV transmission.[1]

Recommendations: None.

MALARIA

No malaria transmission.

MALI

YELLOW FEVER

Requirements: Required for arriving travelers from all countries if traveler is ≥1 year of age.

Recommendations:

Recommended for all travelers ≥9 months of age going to areas south of the Sahara Desert (see Map 3-14).

Not recommended for travelers whose itineraries are limited to areas in the Sahara Desert (see Map 3-14).

MALARIA

Areas with malaria: All.

Estimated relative risk of malaria for US travelers: High.

Drug resistance[4]: Chloroquine.

Malaria species: *P. falciparum* >85%, *P. ovale* 5%–10%, *P. vivax* rare.

Recommended chemoprophylaxis: Atovaquone-proguanil, doxycycline, or mefloquine.

*All footnotes are located on page 424.

MALTA

YELLOW FEVER

Requirements: Required if traveling from a country with risk of YFV transmission and ≥9 months of age, including transit >12 hours in an airport located in a country with risk of YFV transmission.[1] If indicated on epidemiologic grounds, infants <9 months of age are subject to isolation or surveillance if coming from an area with risk of YFV transmission.

Recommendations: None.

MALARIA

No malaria transmission.

MARSHALL ISLANDS

YELLOW FEVER

No requirements or recommendations.

MALARIA

No malaria transmission.

MARTINIQUE (FRANCE)

YELLOW FEVER

Requirements: Required if traveling from a country with risk of YFV transmission and ≥1 year of age, including transit >12 hours in an airport located in a country with risk of YFV transmission.[1]

Recommendations: None.

MALARIA

No malaria transmission.

MAURITANIA

YELLOW FEVER

Requirements: Required if traveling from a country with risk of YFV transmission and ≥1 year of age.[1]

Recommendations:

Recommended for all travelers ≥9 months of age traveling to areas south of the Sahara Desert (see Map 3-14).

Not recommended for travelers whose itineraries are limited to areas in the Sahara Desert (see Map 3-14).

MALARIA

Areas with malaria: All areas, including the city of Nouakchott.

Estimated relative risk of malaria for US travelers: High.

Drug resistance[4]: Chloroquine.

Malaria species: *P. falciparum* >85%, *P. ovale* 5%–10%, *P. vivax* rare.

Recommended chemoprophylaxis: Atovaquone-proguanil, doxycycline, or mefloquine.

MAURITIUS

YELLOW FEVER

Requirements: Required if traveling from a country with risk of YFV transmission and ≥1 year of age,

including transit >12 hours in an airport located in a country with risk of YFV transmission.[1]

Recommendations: None.

MALARIA

No malaria transmission.

MAYOTTE (FRANCE)

YELLOW FEVER

Requirements: Required if traveling from a country with risk of YFV transmission and ≥1 year of age, including transit >12 hours in an airport located in a country with risk of YFV transmission.[1]

Recommendations: None.

MALARIA

Areas with malaria: Rare cases.

Estimated relative risk of malaria for US travelers: No data.

Drug resistance[4]: Chloroquine.

Malaria species: *P. falciparum* 93%, *P. vivax* 5%, *P. malariae* and *P. ovale* 2%.

Recommended chemoprophylaxis: Mosquito avoidance only.

MEXICO *(see Map 3-32.)*

YELLOW FEVER

No requirements or recommendations.

MALARIA

Areas with malaria: Present in Campeche, Chiapas, Chihuahua, Nayarit, and Sinaloa. Rare cases in Durango, Jalisco, Oaxaca, Sonora, and Tabasco. Rare cases in the municipality of Othón P. Blanco in the southern part of Quintana Roo bordering Belize. No malaria along the US-Mexico border (see Map 3-32).

Estimated relative risk of malaria for US travelers: Very low.

Drug resistance[4]: None.

Malaria species: *P. vivax* 100%.

Recommended chemoprophylaxis:

States of Campeche, Chiapas, Chihuahua, Nayarit, and Sinaloa: Atovaquone-proguanil, chloroquine, doxycycline, mefloquine, or primaquine[5].

States of Durango, Jalisco, Oaxaca, Sonora, Tabasco, and Othón P. Blanco municipality of Quintana Roo: Mosquito avoidance only.

MICRONESIA, FEDERATED STATES OF; INCLUDES YAP, POHNPEI, CHUUK, AND KOSRAE ISLANDS

YELLOW FEVER

No requirements or recommendations.

MALARIA

No malaria transmission.

*All footnotes are located on page 424.

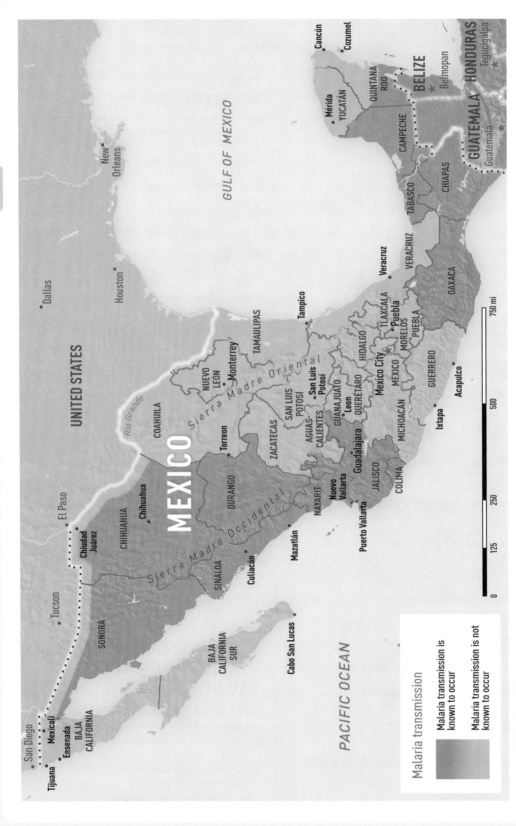

MAP 3-32. Malaria in Mexico

Malaria transmission

Malaria transmission is known to occur

Malaria transmission is not known to occur

MOLDOVA

YELLOW FEVER
No requirements or recommendations.

MALARIA
No malaria transmission.

MONACO

YELLOW FEVER
No requirements or recommendations.

MALARIA
No malaria transmission.

MONGOLIA

YELLOW FEVER
No requirements or recommendations.

MALARIA
No malaria transmission.

MONTENEGRO

YELLOW FEVER
No requirements or recommendations.

MALARIA
No malaria transmission.

MONTSERRAT (UK)

YELLOW FEVER
Requirements: Required if traveling from a country with risk of YFV transmission and ≥1 year of age.[1]
Recommendations: None.

MALARIA
No malaria transmission.

MOROCCO

YELLOW FEVER
No requirements or recommendations.

MALARIA
No malaria transmission.

MOZAMBIQUE

YELLOW FEVER
Requirements: Required if traveling from a country with risk of YFV transmission and ≥9 months of age, including transit >12 hours in an airport located in a country with risk of YFV transmission.[1] This requirement includes São Tomé and Príncipe, Somalia, and Tanzania and excludes Argentina, French Guiana, Paraguay, and South Sudan.
Recommendations: None.

MALARIA
Areas with malaria: All.
Estimated relative risk of malaria for US travelers: Moderate.
Drug resistance[4]: Chloroquine.
Malaria species: *P. falciparum* >90%, *P. malariae, P. ovale, P. vivax* rare.

*All footnotes are located on page 424.

Recommended chemoprophylaxis: Atovaquone-proguanil, doxycycline, or mefloquine.

MYANMAR *(see: Burma)*

NAMIBIA

YELLOW FEVER
Requirements: Required if traveling from a country with risk of YFV transmission. The countries or parts of countries included in the endemic zones in Africa and South America are regarded as areas with risk of YFV transmission.[1] Travelers on scheduled flights that originated outside the countries with risk of YFV transmission, but who have been in transit through these areas, are not required to possess a certificate provided that they remained at the airport or in the adjacent town during transit. All travelers whose flights originated in countries with risk of YFV transmission or who have been in transit through these countries on unscheduled flights are required to possess a certificate. The certificate is not required for children <1 year of age, but such infants may be subject to surveillance.
Recommendations: None.

MALARIA
Areas with malaria: Present in the provinces of Kavango (East and West), Kunene, Ohangwena, Omusati, Oshana, Oshikoto, Otjozondjupa and Zambezi. Rare cases in other parts of the country. No malaria in the city of Windhoek.
Estimated relative risk of malaria for US travelers: Low.
Drug resistance[4]: Chloroquine.
Malaria species: *P. falciparum* >90%; *P. malariae, P. ovale, P. vivax* rare.
Recommended chemoprophylaxis:
Kavango (East and West), Kunene, Ohangwena, Omusati, Oshana, Oshikoto, Otjozondjupa, and Zambezi: Atovaquone-proguanil, doxycycline, or mefloquine.
Other parts of the country with rare cases: Mosquito avoidance only.

NAURU

YELLOW FEVER
Requirements: Required if traveling from a country with risk of YFV transmission and ≥1 year of age.[1]
Recommendations: None.

MALARIA
No malaria transmission.

NEPAL

YELLOW FEVER
Requirements: Required if traveling from a country with risk of YFV transmission and ≥1 year of age, including transit >12 hours in an airport located in a country with risk of YFV transmission.[1]
Recommendations: None.

MALARIA

Areas with malaria: Present throughout the country at altitudes <2,000 m (6,562 ft). None in Kathmandu and on typical Himalayan treks.

Estimated relative risk of malaria for US travelers: Low.

Drug resistance[4]: Chloroquine.

Malaria species: *P. vivax* 85%, *P. falciparum* 15%.

Recommended chemoprophylaxis: Atovaquone-proguanil, doxycycline, or mefloquine.

NETHERLANDS, THE

YELLOW FEVER

No requirements or recommendations.

MALARIA

No malaria transmission.

NEW CALEDONIA (FRANCE)

YELLOW FEVER

Requirements: Required if traveling from a country with risk of YFV transmission and ≥1 year of age, including transit >12 hours in an airport located in a country with risk of YFV transmission.[1] *Note:* In the event of an epidemic threat to the territory, a specific vaccination certificate may be required.

Recommendations: None.

MALARIA

No malaria transmission.

NEW ZEALAND

YELLOW FEVER

No requirements or recommendations.

MALARIA

No malaria transmission.

NICARAGUA *(see Map 3-33.)*

YELLOW FEVER

No requirements or recommendations.

MALARIA

Areas with malaria: Present in Región Autónoma Atlántico Norte (RAAN) and Región Autónoma Atlántico Sur (RAAS). Rare cases in Boaco, Chinandega, Esteli, Jinotega, Leon, Matagalpa, and Nueva Segovia. No malaria in the city of Managua (see Map 3-33).

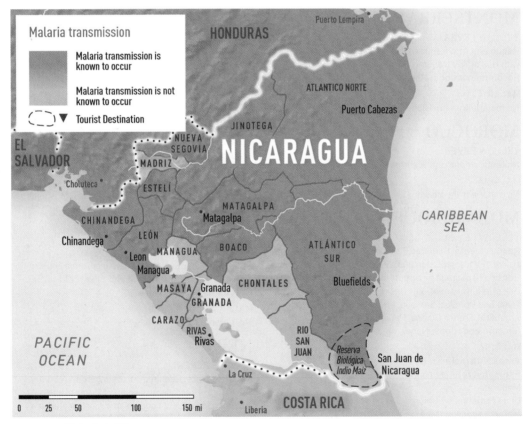

MAP 3-33. Malaria in Nicaragua

*All footnotes are located on page 424.

Estimated relative risk of malaria for US travelers: Low.

Drug resistance[4]: None.

Malaria species: *P. vivax* 90%, *P. falciparum* 10%.

Recommended chemoprophylaxis:
Región Autónoma Atlántico Norte (RAAN) and Región Autónoma Atlántico Sur (RAAS): Atovaquone-proguanil, chloroquine, doxycycline, or mefloquine.
Other areas with malaria: Mosquito avoidance only.

NIGER

YELLOW FEVER

Requirements: Required for arriving travelers from all countries if traveler is ≥1 year of age. The government of Niger recommends vaccine for travelers departing Niger.

Recommendations:

Recommended for all travelers ≥9 months of age traveling to areas south of the Sahara Desert (see Map 3-14).

Not recommended for travelers whose itineraries are limited to areas in the Sahara Desert (see Map 3-14).

MALARIA

Areas with malaria: All.

Estimated relative risk of malaria for US travelers: High.

Drug resistance[4]: Chloroquine.

Malaria species: *P. falciparum* 85%, *P. ovale* 5%–10%, *P. vivax* rare.

Recommended chemoprophylaxis: Atovaquone-proguanil, doxycycline, or mefloquine.

NIGERIA

YELLOW FEVER

Requirements: Required if traveling from a country with risk of YFV transmission and ≥1 year of age.[1]

Recommendations: ***Recommended*** for all travelers ≥9 months of age.

MALARIA

Areas with malaria: All.

Estimated relative risk of malaria for US travelers: High.

Drug resistance[4]: Chloroquine.

Malaria species: *P. falciparum* >85%, *P. ovale* 5%–10%, *P. vivax* rare.

Recommended chemoprophylaxis: Atovaquone-proguanil, doxycycline, or mefloquine.

NIUE (NEW ZEALAND)

YELLOW FEVER

Requirements: Required if traveling from a country with risk of YFV transmission and ≥9 months of age.[1]

Recommendations: None.

MALARIA

No malaria transmission.

*All footnotes are located on page 424.

NORFOLK ISLAND (AUSTRALIA)

YELLOW FEVER

Requirements: Required if traveling from a country with risk of YFV transmission and ≥1 year of age, including transit >12 hours in an airport located in a country with risk of YFV transmission.[1] This requirement excludes Galápagos Islands in Ecuador and the island of Tobago and is limited to Misiones Province in Argentina.

Recommendations: None.

MALARIA

No malaria transmission.

NORTH KOREA

YELLOW FEVER

Requirements: Required if traveling from a country with risk of YFV transmission and ≥1 year of age.[1]

Recommendations: None.

MALARIA

Areas with malaria: Present in southern provinces.

Estimated relative risk of malaria for US travelers: No data.

Drug resistance[4]: None.

Malaria species: Presumed to be 100% *P. vivax*.

Recommended chemoprophylaxis: Atovaquone-proguanil, chloroquine, doxycycline, mefloquine, or primaquine[5].

NORTHERN MARIANA ISLANDS (US), INCLUDES SAIPAN, TINIAN, AND ROTA ISLANDS

YELLOW FEVER

No requirements or recommendations.

MALARIA

No malaria transmission.

NORWAY

YELLOW FEVER

No requirements or recommendations.

MALARIA

No malaria transmission.

OMAN

YELLOW FEVER

Requirements: Required if traveling from a country with risk of YFV transmission and ≥9 months of age, including transit in an airport located in a country with risk of YFV transmission.[1]

Recommendations: None.

MALARIA

Areas with malaria: Sporadic transmission in Dakhliyah, North Batinah, and North and South Sharqiyah.

Estimated relative risk of malaria for US travelers: Very low.

Drug resistance[4]: Chloroquine.

Malaria species: *P. falciparum* and *P. vivax*.

Recommended chemoprophylaxis: Mosquito avoidance only.

PAKISTAN

YELLOW FEVER

Requirements: Required if traveling from a country with risk of YFV transmission and ≥1 year of age, including transit >12 hours in an airport located in a country with risk of YFV transmission.[1]

Recommendations: None.

MALARIA

Areas with malaria: All areas (including all cities) <2,500 m (8,202 ft).

Estimated relative risk of malaria for US travelers: Moderate.

Drug resistance[4]: Chloroquine.

Malaria species: *P. vivax* 70%, *P. falciparum* 30%.

Recommended chemoprophylaxis: Atovaquone-proguanil, doxycycline, or mefloquine.

PALAU

YELLOW FEVER

No requirements or recommendations.

MALARIA

No malaria transmission.

PANAMA *(see Maps 3-34 and 3-35.)*

YELLOW FEVER

Requirements: No requirements.

Recommendations:

Recommended for all travelers ≥9 months of age traveling to all mainland areas east of the area surrounding the canal (the entire provinces of Darién, Emberá, and Kuna Yala [also spelled Guna Yala] and areas of the provinces of Colón and Panamá that are east of the canal) (see Map 3-34).

Not recommended for travelers whose itineraries are limited to areas west of the canal, the city of Panama, the canal area itself, and the Balboa

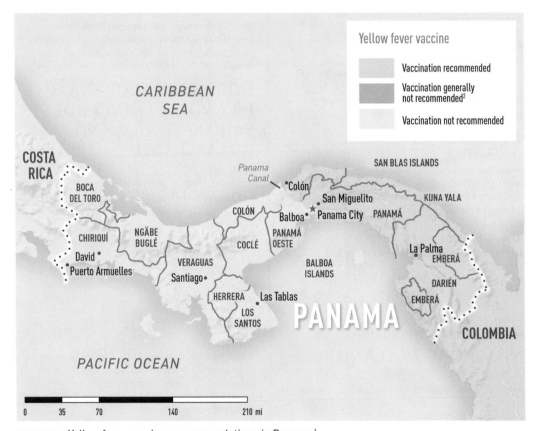

MAP 3-34. Yellow fever vaccine recommendations in Panama[1]

[1,2] See footnotes on page 424.

*All footnotes are located on page 424.

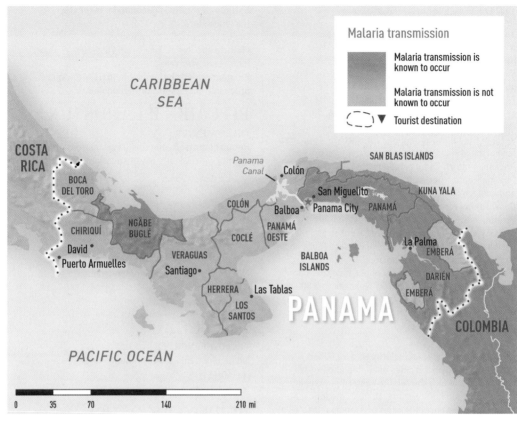

MAP 3-35. Malaria in Panama

Islands (Pearl Islands) and San Blas Islands (see Map 3-34).

MALARIA

Areas with malaria: Malaria is present in the provinces of Darien, Kuna Yala (also spelled Guna Yala), Ngäbe-Buglé, and eastern Panama province. None in Panama Oeste, the Canal Zone, and Panama City (see Map 3-35).

Estimated relative risk of malaria for US travelers: Low.

Drug resistance[4]: Chloroquine (east of the Panama Canal).

Malaria species: *P. vivax* 99%, *P. falciparum* 1%.

Recommended chemoprophylaxis:
Provinces of Darien, Guana Yala, and Panama Este: Atovaquone-proguanil, doxycycline, mefloquine, or primaquine[5].
Ngäbe-Buglé: Atovaquone-proguanil, chloroquine, doxycycline, mefloquine, or primaquine[5].

PAPUA NEW GUINEA

YELLOW FEVER

No requirements or recommendations.

MALARIA

Areas with malaria: Present throughout the country at altitudes <2,000 m (6,562 ft).

Estimated relative risk of malaria for US travelers: High.

Drug resistance[4]: Chloroquine (both *P. falciparum* and *P. vivax*).

Malaria species: *P. falciparum* 65%–80%, *P. vivax* 10%–30%, *P. malariae* and *P. ovale* rare.

Recommended chemoprophylaxis: Atovaquone-proguanil, doxycycline, or mefloquine.

PARAGUAY

YELLOW FEVER

Requirements: Required if traveling from a country with risk of YFV transmission and ≥9 months of age, including transit >12 hours in an airport located in a country with risk of YFV transmission.[1]

Recommendations:

Recommended for all travelers ≥9 months of age, except as mentioned below.

Generally not recommended for travelers whose itinerary is limited to the city of Asunción.

MALARIA
No malaria transmission

*All footnotes are located on page 424.

PERU *(see Maps 3-36 and 3-37.)*

YELLOW FEVER
Requirements: None.
Recommendations:
Recommended for all travelers ≥9 months of age going to the following areas at elevations below 2,300 m: the regions of Amazonas, Loreto, Madre de Dios, San Martin, Ucayali, Puno, Cusco, Junín, Pasco, and Huánuco, and designated areas (see Map 3-36) of the following regions: far north of Apurimac, far northern Huancavelica, far northeastern Ancash, eastern La Libertad, northern and eastern Cajamarca, northern and northeastern Ayacucho, and eastern Piura.
Generally not recommended for travelers whose itineraries are limited to the following areas west of the Andes: regions of Lambayeque and Tumbes and the designated areas (see Map 3-36) of western Piura and south, west, and central Cajamarca.
Not recommended for travelers whose itineraries are limited to the following areas: all areas above 2,300 m elevation, areas west of the Andes not listed above, the city of Cusco, the capital city of Lima, Machu Picchu, and the Inca Trail (see Map 3-36).

MALARIA
Areas with malaria: All departments <2,000 m (6,562 ft), including the cities of Iquitos and Puerto Maldonado and only the remote eastern regions of La Libertad and Lambayeque. None in the following areas: Lima Province; the cities of Arequipa, Ica, Moquegua, Nazca, Puno, and Tacna; the highland tourist areas (Cusco, Machu Picchu, and Lake Titicaca); and along the Pacific Coast (see Map 3-37).
Estimated relative risk of malaria for US travelers: Moderate.
Drug resistance[4]: Chloroquine.
Malaria species: *P. vivax* 85%, *P. falciparum* 15%.
Recommended chemoprophylaxis: Atovaquone-proguanil, doxycycline, or mefloquine.

PHILIPPINES

YELLOW FEVER
Requirements: Required if traveling from a country with risk of YFV transmission and ≥1 year of age, including transit in an airport located in a country with risk of YFV transmission.[1]
Recommendations: None.

MALARIA
Areas with malaria: Present in rural areas <600 m (1,969 ft) except none in the 22 provinces of Aklan, Albay, Benguet, Biliran, Bohol, Camiguin, Capiz, Catanduanes, Cavite, Cebu, Guimaras, Iloilo, Northern Leyte, Southern Leyte, Marinduque, Masbate, Eastern Samar, Northern Samar, Western Samar, Siquijor, Sorsogon, and Surigao Del Norte. None in metropolitan Manila and other urban areas.

Estimated relative risk of malaria for US travelers: Low.
Drug resistance[4]: Chloroquine.
Malaria species: *P. falciparum* 70%–80%, *P. vivax* 20%–30%, *P. knowlesi* rare.
Recommended chemoprophylaxis: Atovaquone-proguanil, doxycycline, or mefloquine.

PITCAIRN ISLANDS (UK)

YELLOW FEVER
Requirements: Required if traveling from a country with risk of YFV transmission and ≥1 year of age.[1]
Recommendations: None.

MALARIA
No malaria transmission.

POLAND

YELLOW FEVER
No requirements or recommendations.

MALARIA
No malaria transmission.

PORTUGAL

YELLOW FEVER
No requirements or recommendations.

MALARIA
No malaria transmission.

PUERTO RICO (US)

YELLOW FEVER
No requirements or recommendations.

MALARIA
No malaria transmission.

QATAR

YELLOW FEVER
No requirements or recommendations.

MALARIA
No malaria transmission.

RÉUNION (FRANCE)

YELLOW FEVER
Requirements: Required if traveling from a country with risk of YFV transmission and ≥1 year of age, including transit >12 hours in an airport located in a country with risk of YFV transmission.[1]
Recommendations: None.

MALARIA
No malaria transmission.

ROMANIA

YELLOW FEVER
No requirements or recommendations.

*All footnotes are located on page 424.

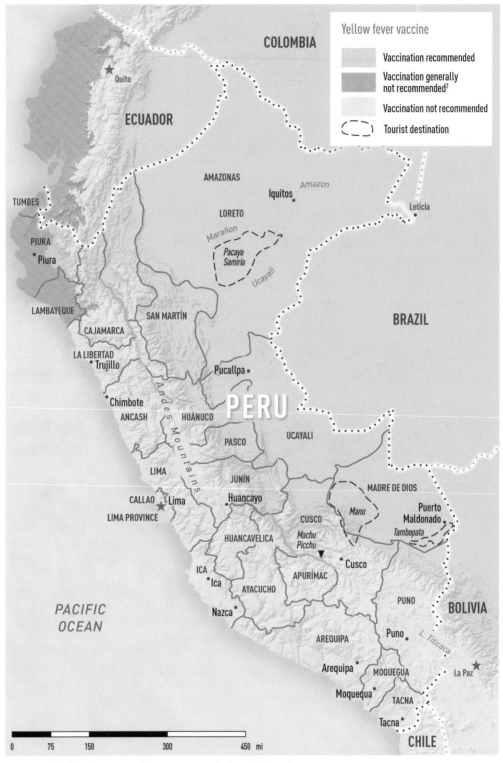

Yellow fever vaccine

- Vaccination recommended
- Vaccination generally not recommended[2]
- Vaccination not recommended
- Tourist destination

MAP 3-36. Yellow fever vaccine recommendations in Peru[1]

[1,2] See footnotes on page 424.

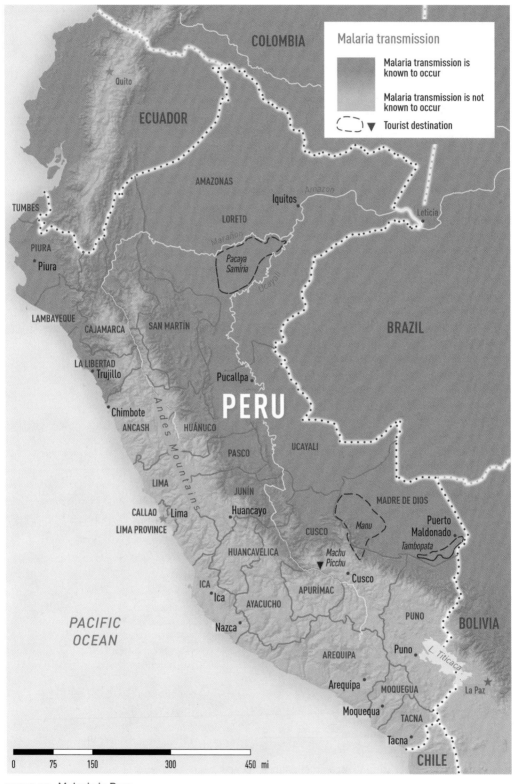

MAP 3-37. Malaria in Peru

MALARIA
No malaria transmission.

RUSSIA

YELLOW FEVER
No requirements or recommendations.

MALARIA
No malaria transmission.

RWANDA

YELLOW FEVER
Requirements: Required if traveling from a country with risk of YFV transmission and ≥1 year of age. Also required if traveling from a country with an active yellow fever outbreak. Further details available at http://moh.gov.rw/index.php?id=34&tx_ttnews%5btt_news%5d=633&cHash=31c90fd13b953240c27d812275643392.
Recommendations: *Generally not recommended* for travelers to Rwanda.

MALARIA
Areas with malaria: All.
Estimated relative risk of malaria for US travelers: Moderate.
Drug resistance[4]: Chloroquine.
Malaria species: *P. falciparum* 90%, *P. vivax* 5%, *P. ovale* 5%.
Recommended chemoprophylaxis: Atovaquone-proguanil, doxycycline, or mefloquine.

SABA

YELLOW FEVER
Requirements: Required if traveling from a country with risk of YFV transmission and ≥6 months of age.[1]
Recommendations: None.

MALARIA
No malaria transmission.

SAINT BARTHÉLEMY

YELLOW FEVER
Requirements: Required if traveling from a country with risk of YFV transmission and ≥1 year of age, including transit >12 hours in an airport located in a country with risk of YFV transmission.[1]
Recommendations: None.

MALARIA
No malaria transmission.

SAINT HELENA (UK)

YELLOW FEVER
No requirements or recommendations.

MALARIA
No malaria transmission.

SAINT KITTS (SAINT CHRISTOPHER) AND NEVIS (UK)

YELLOW FEVER
Requirements: Required if traveling from a country with risk of YFV transmission and ≥1 year of age, including transit >12 hours in an airport located in a country with risk of YFV transmission.[1]
Recommendations: None.

MALARIA
No malaria transmission.

SAINT LUCIA

YELLOW FEVER
Requirements: Required if traveling from a country with risk of YFV transmission and ≥1 year of age.[1]
Recommendations: None.

MALARIA
No malaria transmission.

SAINT MARTIN

YELLOW FEVER
Requirements: Required if traveling from a country with risk of YFV transmission and ≥1 year of age, including transit >12 hours in an airport located in a country with risk of YFV transmission.[1]
Recommendations: None.

MALARIA
No malaria transmission.

SAINT PIERRE AND MIQUELON (FRANCE)

YELLOW FEVER
No requirements or recommendations.

MALARIA
No malaria transmission.

SAINT VINCENT AND THE GRENADINES

YELLOW FEVER
Requirements: Required if traveling from a country with risk of YFV transmission and ≥1 year of age.[1]
Recommendations: None.

MALARIA
No malaria transmission.

SAMOA (FORMERLY WESTERN SAMOA)

YELLOW FEVER
Requirements: Required if traveling from a country with risk of YFV transmission and ≥1 year of age,

*All footnotes are located on page 424.

including transit >12 hours in an airport located in a country with risk of YFV transmission.[1]
Recommendations: None.

MALARIA
No malaria transmission.

SAN MARINO

YELLOW FEVER
No requirements or recommendations.

MALARIA
No malaria transmission.

SÃO TOMÉ AND PRÍNCIPE

YELLOW FEVER
Requirements: Required if traveling from a country with risk of YFV transmission and ≥1 year of age, including transit in an airport located in a country with risk of YFV transmission.[1]
Recommendations: *Generally not recommended* for travelers to São Tomé and Príncipe.

MALARIA
Areas with malaria: All.
Estimated relative risk of malaria for US travelers: Very low.
Drug resistance[4]: Chloroquine.
Malaria species: *P. falciparum* 85%; *P. malariae, P. ovale, P. vivax* 15% combined.
Recommended chemoprophylaxis: Atovaquone-proguanil, doxycycline, or mefloquine.

SAUDI ARABIA

YELLOW FEVER
Requirements: Required if traveling from a country with risk of YFV transmission and ≥1 year of age, including transit >12 hours in an airport located in a country with risk of YFV transmission.[1]
Recommendations: None.

MALARIA
Areas with malaria: Rare cases in Asir and Jazan emirates by border with Yemen. None in the cities of Jeddah, Mecca, Medina, Riyadh, and Ta'if.
Estimated relative risk of malaria for US travelers: Very low.
Drug resistance[4]: Chloroquine.
Malaria species: *P. falciparum* predominantly, remainder *P. vivax*.
Recommended chemoprophylaxis: Mosquito avoidance only.

SENEGAL

YELLOW FEVER
Requirements: Required if traveling from a country with risk of YFV transmission and ≥9 months of age, including transit in an airport located in a country with risk of YFV transmission.[1]

Recommendations: *Recommended* for all travelers ≥9 months of age.

MALARIA
Areas with malaria: All.
Estimated relative risk of malaria for US travelers: High.
Drug resistance[4]: Chloroquine.
Malaria species: *P. falciparum* >85%, *P. ovale* 5%–10%, *P. vivax* rare.
Recommended chemoprophylaxis: Atovaquone-proguanil, doxycycline, or mefloquine.

SERBIA

YELLOW FEVER
No requirements or recommendations.

MALARIA
No malaria transmission.

SEYCHELLES

YELLOW FEVER
Requirements: Required if traveling from a country with risk of YFV transmission and ≥1 year of age, including transit >12 hours in an airport located in a country with risk of YFV transmission.[1]
Recommendations: None.

MALARIA
No malaria transmission.

SIERRA LEONE

YELLOW FEVER
Requirements: Required for arriving travelers from all countries.
Recommendations: *Recommended* for all travelers ≥9 months of age.

MALARIA
Areas with malaria: All.
Estimated relative risk of malaria for US travelers: High.
Drug resistance[4]: Chloroquine.
Malaria species: *P. falciparum* >85%, *P. ovale* 5%–10%, *P. malariae* and *P. vivax* rare.
Recommended chemoprophylaxis: Atovaquone-proguanil, doxycycline, or mefloquine.

SINGAPORE

YELLOW FEVER
Requirements: Required for travelers who are ≥1 year of age who, within the preceding 6 days, have been in or have been in transit >12 hours in an airport located in a country with risk of YFV transmission.[1]
Recommendations: None.

MALARIA
No malaria transmission.

*All footnotes are located on page 424.

SINT EUSTATIUS

YELLOW FEVER

Requirements: Required if traveling from a country with risk of YFV transmission and ≥6 months of age.[1]
Recommendations: None.

MALARIA
No malaria transmission.

SINT MAARTEN

YELLOW FEVER

Requirements: Required if traveling from a country with risk of YFV transmission and ≥6 months of age.[1]
Recommendations: None.

MALARIA
No malaria transmission.

SLOVAKIA

YELLOW FEVER
No requirements or recommendations.

MALARIA
No malaria transmission.

SLOVENIA

YELLOW FEVER
No requirements or recommendations.

MALARIA
No malaria transmission.

SOLOMON ISLANDS

YELLOW FEVER

Requirements: Required if traveling from a country with risk of YFV transmission.[1]
Recommendations: None.

MALARIA
Areas with malaria: All.
Estimated relative risk of malaria for US travelers: High.
Drug resistance[4]: Chloroquine.
Malaria species: *P. falciparum* 60%, *P. vivax* 35%–40%, *P. ovale* <1%.
Recommended chemoprophylaxis: Atovaquone-proguanil, doxycycline, or mefloquine.

SOMALIA

YELLOW FEVER

Requirements: Required if traveling from a country with risk of YFV transmission and ≥9 months of age, including transit >12 hours in an airport located in a country with risk of YFV transmission.[1]
Recommendations:
Generally not recommended for travelers going to the following regions: Bakool, Banaadir, Bay, Galguduud, Gedo, Hiiraan, Lower Jubabada, Lower Shabelle, Middle Jubabada, and Middle Shabelle (see Map 3-14).
Not recommended for all other areas not listed above.

*All footnotes are located on page 424.

MALARIA
Areas with malaria: All.
Estimated relative risk of malaria for US travelers: High.
Drug resistance[4]: Chloroquine.
Malaria species: *P. falciparum* 90%, *P. vivax* 5%–10%, *P. malariae* and *P. ovale* rare.
Recommended chemoprophylaxis: Atovaquone-proguanil, doxycycline, or mefloquine.

SOUTH AFRICA *(see Map 3-38.)*

YELLOW FEVER

Requirements: Required if traveling from a country with risk of YFV transmission and ≥1 year of age, including transit >12 hours in an airport located in a country with risk of YFV transmission.[1]
Recommendations: None.

MALARIA
Areas with malaria: Present along the border with Zimbabwe and Mozambique. Specifically in Vembe and Mopane district municipalities of Limpopo Province; Ehlanzeni district municipality in Mpumalanga Province; and Umkhanyakude in Kwazulu-Natal Province. Present in Kruger National Park (see Map 3-38).
Estimated relative risk of malaria for US travelers: Low.
Drug resistance[4]: Chloroquine.
Malaria species: *P. falciparum* 90%, *P. vivax* 5%, *P. ovale* 5%.
Recommended chemoprophylaxis: Atovaquone-proguanil, doxycycline, or mefloquine.

SOUTH GEORGIA AND SOUTH SANDWICH ISLANDS (UK)

YELLOW FEVER
No requirements or recommendations.

MALARIA
No malaria transmission.

SOUTH KOREA

YELLOW FEVER
No requirements or recommendations.

MALARIA
Areas with malaria: Limited to the months of March–December in rural areas in the northern parts of Incheon, Kangwon-do, and Kyônggi-do Provinces, including the demilitarized zone (DMZ).
Estimated relative risk of malaria for US travelers: Low.
Drug resistance[4]: None.
Malaria species: *P. vivax* 100%.

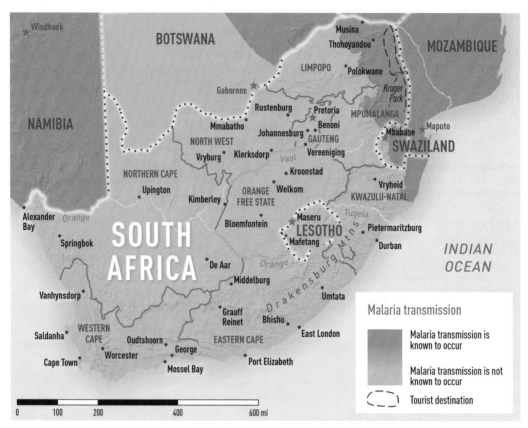

MAP 3-38. Malaria in South Africa

Malaria transmission

- Malaria transmission is known to occur
- Malaria transmission is not known to occur
- Tourist destination

0 100 200 400 600 mi

Recommended chemoprophylaxis: Atovaquone-proguanil, chloroquine, doxycycline, mefloquine, or primaquine[5].

SOUTH SUDAN, REPUBLIC OF

YELLOW FEVER

Requirements: None.
Recommendations: *Recommended* for all travelers ≥9 months of age.

MALARIA

Areas with malaria: All.
Estimated relative risk of malaria for US travelers: High.
Drug resistance[4]**:** Chloroquine.
Malaria species: *P. falciparum* 90%, *P. vivax* 5%–10%, *P. malariae* and *P. ovale* rare.
Recommended chemoprophylaxis: Atovaquone-proguanil, doxycycline, or mefloquine.

SPAIN

YELLOW FEVER

No requirements or recommendations.

*All footnotes are located on page 424.

MALARIA

No malaria transmission.

SRI LANKA

YELLOW FEVER

Requirements: Required if traveling from a country with risk of YFV transmission and ≥9 months of age, including transit >12 hours in an airport located in a country with risk of YFV transmission.[1]
Recommendations: None.

MALARIA

No malaria transmission.

SUDAN

YELLOW FEVER

Requirements: Required if traveling from a country with risk of YFV transmission and ≥1 year of age, including transit >12 hours in an airport located in a country with risk of YFV transmission.[1] A certificate may be required for travelers departing Sudan.
Recommendations:
Recommended for all travelers ≥9 months of age traveling to areas south of the Sahara Desert (see Map 3-14).

Not recommended for travelers whose itineraries are limited to areas in the Sahara Desert and the city of Khartoum (see Map 3-14).

MALARIA
Areas with malaria: All.
Estimated relative risk of malaria for US travelers: High.
Drug resistance[4]: Chloroquine.
Malaria species: *P. falciparum* 90%, *P. vivax* 5%–10%, *P. malariae* and *P. ovale* rare.
Recommended chemoprophylaxis: Atovaquone-proguanil, doxycycline, or mefloquine.

SURINAME

YELLOW FEVER
Requirements: Required if traveling from a country with risk of YFV transmission and ≥1 year of age, including transit >12 hours in an airport located in a country with risk of YFV transmission.[1]
Recommendations: *Recommended* for all travelers ≥9 months of age.

MALARIA
Areas with malaria: Present in the municipality of Tapanahony in Sipaliwini Province. Rare cases in Brokopondo Province and Boven Saramacca municipality in Sipaliwini Province. No malaria in Paramaribo.
Estimated relative risk of malaria for US travelers: Low.
Drug resistance[4]: Chloroquine.
Malaria species: *P. falciparum* >70%, *P. vivax* 15%–20%.
Recommended chemoprophylaxis:
Tapanohony municipality in Sipaliwini Province: Atovaquone-proguanil, doxycycline, or mefloquine.
Other areas with malaria: Mosquito avoidance only.

SWAZILAND

YELLOW FEVER
Requirements: Required if traveling from a country with risk of YFV transmission.[1]
Recommendations: None.

MALARIA
Areas with malaria: Present in eastern areas bordering Mozambique and South Africa, including all of Lubombo district and the eastern half of Hhohho, Manzini, and Shiselweni districts.
Estimated relative risk of malaria for US travelers: Very low.
Drug resistance[4]: Chloroquine.
Malaria species: *P. falciparum* 99%, *P. ovale* and *P. vivax* 1%.
Recommended chemoprophylaxis: Atovaquone-proguanil, doxycycline, or mefloquine.

SWEDEN

YELLOW FEVER
No requirements or recommendations.

MALARIA
No malaria transmission.

SWITZERLAND

YELLOW FEVER
No requirements or recommendations.

MALARIA
No malaria transmission.

SYRIA

YELLOW FEVER
No requirements or recommendations.

MALARIA
No malaria transmission.

TAIWAN

YELLOW FEVER
No requirements or recommendations.

MALARIA
No malaria transmission.

TAJIKISTAN

YELLOW FEVER
No requirements or recommendations.

MALARIA
Areas with malaria: Rare indigenous cases.
Estimated relative risk of malaria for US travelers: Very low.
Drug resistance[4]: Chloroquine.
Malaria species: *P. vivax* 90%, *P. falciparum* 10%.
Recommended chemoprophylaxis: Mosquito avoidance only.

TANZANIA

YELLOW FEVER
Requirements: Required if traveling from a country with risk of YFV transmission and ≥1 year of age, including transit >12 hours in an airport located in a country with risk of YFV transmission.[1]
Recommendations: *Generally not recommended* for travelers to Tanzania.

MALARIA
Areas with malaria: All areas <1,800 m (5,906 ft).
Estimated relative risk of malaria for US travelers: High.
Drug resistance[4]: Chloroquine.
Malaria species: *P. falciparum* >85%, *P. ovale* >10%, *P. malariae* and *P. vivax* rare.
Recommended chemoprophylaxis: Atovaquone-proguanil, doxycycline, or mefloquine.

*All footnotes are located on page 424.

THAILAND

YELLOW FEVER

Requirements: Required if traveling from a country with risk of YFV transmission and ≥9 months of age, including transit >12 hours in an airport located in a country with risk of YFV transmission.[1]
Recommendations: None.

MALARIA

Areas with malaria: Primarily in provinces that border Burma (Myanmar), Cambodia, and Laos and the provinces of Kalasin, Krabi (Plai Phraya district), Nakhon Si Thammarat, Narathiwat, Pattani, Phang Nga (including Phang Nga City), Rayong, Sakon Nakhon, Songkhla, Surat Thani, and Yala, especially the forest and forest fringe areas of these provinces. Rare to few cases in other parts of Thailand, including other parts of Krabi Province and the cities of Bangkok, Chiang Mai, Chiang Rai, Koh Phangan, Koh Samui, and Phuket. None in the islands of Krabi Province (Koh Phi Phi, Koh Yao Noi, Koh Yao Yai, and Ko Lanta) and Pattaya City.
Estimated relative risk of malaria for US travelers: Low.
Drug resistance[4]: Chloroquine and mefloquine.
Malaria species: *P. falciparum* 50% (up to 75% in some areas), *P. vivax* 50% (up to 60% in some areas), *P. ovale* and *P. knowlesi* rare.
Recommended chemoprophylaxis:
Provinces that border Burma (Myanmar), Cambodia, and Laos, the provinces of Kalasin, Plai Phraya district of Krabi, Nakhon Si Thammarat, Narathiwat, Pattani, Phang Nga (including Phang Nga City), Rayong, Sakon Nakhon, Songkhla, Surat Thani, and Yala: Atovaquone-proguanil or doxycycline.
All other areas of Thailand with malaria including the cities of Bangkok, Chiang Mai, Chiang Rai, Koh Phangan, Koh Samui, and Phuket: Mosquito avoidance only.

TIMOR-LESTE

YELLOW FEVER

Requirements: Required if traveling from a country with risk of YFV transmission and ≥1 year of age, including transit in an airport located in a country with risk of YFV transmission.[1]
Recommendations: None.

MALARIA

Areas with malaria: All.
Estimated relative risk of malaria for US travelers: Moderate.
Drug resistance[4]: Chloroquine.
Malaria Species: *P. falciparum* 50%, *P. vivax* 50%, *P. ovale* <1%, *P. malariae* <1%.
Recommended chemoprophylaxis: Atovaquone-proguanil, doxycycline, or mefloquine.

TOGO

YELLOW FEVER

Requirements: Required for arriving travelers from all countries if traveler is ≥9 months of age.
Recommendations: *Recommended* for all travelers ≥9 months of age.

MALARIA

Areas with malaria: All.
Estimated relative risk of malaria for US travelers: High.
Drug resistance[4]: Chloroquine.
Malaria species: *P. falciparum* 85%, *P. ovale* 5%–10%, remainder *P. vivax*.
Recommended chemoprophylaxis: Atovaquone-proguanil, doxycycline, or mefloquine.

TOKELAU (NEW ZEALAND)

YELLOW FEVER

No requirements or recommendations.

MALARIA

No malaria transmission.

TONGA

YELLOW FEVER

No requirements or recommendations.

MALARIA

No malaria transmission.

TRINIDAD AND TOBAGO

YELLOW FEVER

Requirements: Required if traveling from a country with risk of YFV transmission and ≥1 year of age, including transit in an airport located in a country with risk of YFV transmission.[1]
Recommendations:
Recommended for all travelers ≥9 months of age traveling to the island of Trinidad, except as mentioned below.
Generally not recommended for travelers whose itinerary is limited to the urban areas of the capital city of Port of Spain, cruise ship passengers who do not disembark from the ship, and airplane passengers in transit.
Not recommended for travelers whose itineraries are limited to the island of Tobago.

MALARIA

No malaria transmission.

TUNISIA

YELLOW FEVER

No requirements or recommendations.

MALARIA

No malaria transmission.

*All footnotes are located on page 424.

TURKEY

YELLOW FEVER

No requirements or recommendations.

MALARIA

No malaria transmission.

TURKMENISTAN

YELLOW FEVER

No requirements or recommendations.

MALARIA

No malaria transmission.

TURKS AND CAICOS ISLANDS (UK)

YELLOW FEVER

No requirements or recommendations.

MALARIA

No malaria transmission.

TUVALU

YELLOW FEVER

No requirements or recommendations.

MALARIA

No malaria transmission.

UGANDA

YELLOW FEVER

Requirements: Required for arriving travelers from all countries. Also, proof of yellow fever vaccination required of all travelers leaving Uganda.

Recommendations: *Recommended* for all travelers ≥9 months of age.

MALARIA

Areas with malaria: All.

Estimated relative risk of malaria for US travelers: High.

Drug resistance[4]: Chloroquine.

Malaria species: *P. falciparum* >85%; remainder *P. malariae, P. ovale,* and *P. vivax.*

Recommended chemoprophylaxis: Atovaquone-proguanil, doxycycline, or mefloquine.

UKRAINE

YELLOW FEVER

No requirements or recommendations.

MALARIA

No malaria transmission.

UNITED ARAB EMIRATES

YELLOW FEVER

No requirements or recommendations.

MALARIA

No malaria transmission.

*All footnotes are located on page 424.

UNITED KINGDOM, WITH CHANNEL ISLANDS AND ISLE OF MAN

YELLOW FEVER

No requirements or recommendations.

MALARIA

No malaria transmission.

UNITED STATES

YELLOW FEVER

No requirements or recommendations.

MALARIA

No malaria transmission.

URUGUAY

YELLOW FEVER

No requirements or recommendations.

MALARIA

No malaria transmission.

UZBEKISTAN

YELLOW FEVER

No requirements or recommendations.

MALARIA

No malaria transmission.

VANUATU

YELLOW FEVER

No requirements or recommendations.

MALARIA

Areas with malaria: All.

Estimated relative risk of malaria for US travelers: Moderate.

Drug resistance[4]: Chloroquine.

Malaria species: *P. falciparum* 60%, *P. vivax* 35%–40%, *P. ovale* <1%.

Recommended chemoprophylaxis: Atovaquone-proguanil, doxycycline, or mefloquine.

VENEZUELA *(see Maps 3-39 and 3-40.)*

YELLOW FEVER

Requirements: None.

Recommendations:

Recommended for all travelers ≥9 months of age, except as mentioned below.

Generally not recommended for travelers whose itinerary is limited to the following areas: the states of Aragua, Carabobo, Miranda, Vargas, and Yaracuy, and the Distrito Federal (see Map 3-39).

Not recommended for travelers whose itineraries are limited to the following areas: all areas >2,300m in elevation in the states of Merida, Tachira, and Trujillo;

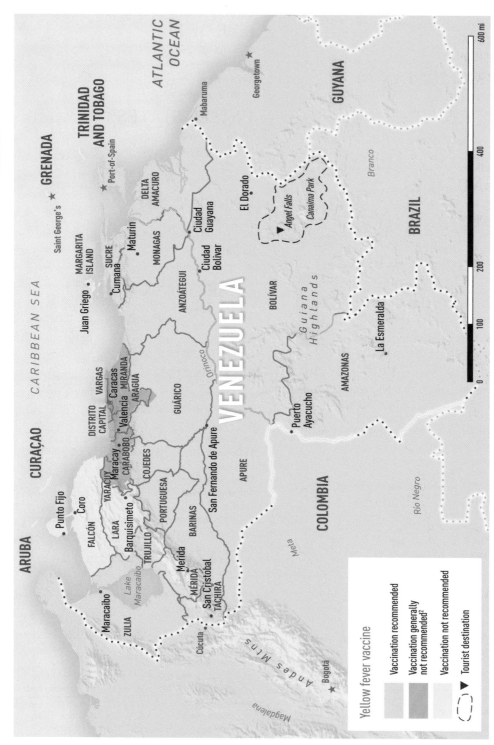

MAP 3-39. Yellow fever vaccine recommendations in Venezuela[1]

1,2 See footnotes on page 424.

Yellow fever vaccine

Vaccination recommended

Vaccination generally not recommended[2]

Vaccination not recommended

▼ Tourist destination

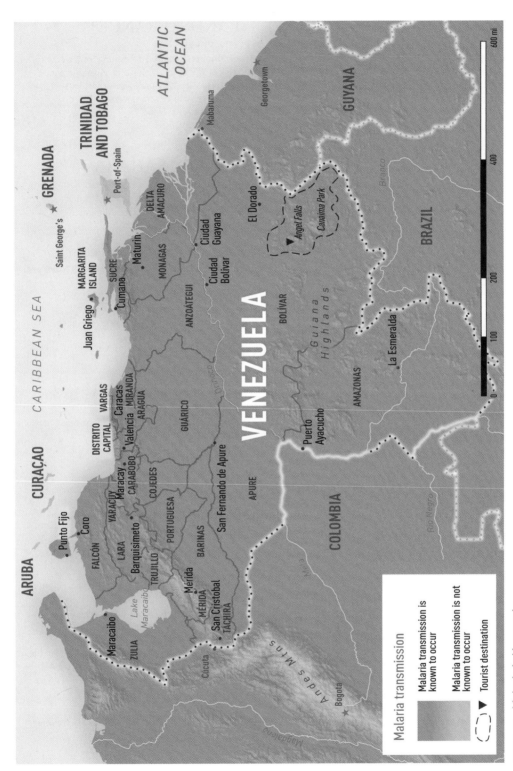

MAP 3-40. Malaria in Venezuela

Malaria transmission

Malaria transmission is known to occur

Malaria transmission is not known to occur

▼ Tourist destination

the states of Falcón and Lara; Margarita Island; the capital city of Caracas; and the city of Valencia (see Map 3-39).

MALARIA
Areas with malaria: All areas <1,700 m (5,577 ft). Present in Angel Falls (see Map 3-40).
Estimated relative risk of malaria for US travelers: Low.
Drug resistance[4]: Chloroquine.
Malaria species: *P. vivax* 83%, *P. falciparum* 17%.
Recommended chemoprophylaxis: Atovaquone-proguanil, doxycycline, or mefloquine.

VIETNAM

YELLOW FEVER
Requirements: Required if traveling from a country with risk of YFV transmission and ≥1 year of age.[1]
Recommendations: None.

MALARIA
Areas with malaria: Rural areas only. Rare cases in the Mekong and Red River Deltas. None in the cities of Da Nang, Haiphong, Hanoi, Ho Chi Minh City (Saigon), Nha Trang, and Qui Nhon.
Estimated relative risk of malaria for US travelers: Low.
Drug resistance[4]: Chloroquine and mefloquine.
Malaria species: *P. falciparum* 50%–90%, *P. vivax* 10%–50%, *P. knowlesi* rare.
Recommended chemoprophylaxis:
Southern part of the country in the provinces of Dac Lac, Gia Lai, Khanh Hoa, Kon Tum, Lam Dong, Ninh Thuan, Song Be, Tay Ninh: Atovaquone-proguanil or doxycycline.
Other areas with malaria except Mekong and Red River Deltas: Atovaquone-proguanil, doxycycline, or mefloquine.
Mekong and Red River Deltas: Mosquito avoidance only.

VIRGIN ISLANDS, BRITISH

YELLOW FEVER
No requirements or recommendations.

MALARIA
No malaria transmission.

VIRGIN ISLANDS, US

YELLOW FEVER
No requirements or recommendations.

MALARIA
No malaria transmission.

WAKE ISLAND, US

YELLOW FEVER
No requirements or recommendations.

MALARIA
No malaria transmission.

*All footnotes are located on page 424.

WALLIS AND FUTUNA ISLANDS (FRANCE)

YELLOW FEVER
Requirements: Required if traveling from a country with risk of YFV transmission and ≥1 year of age, including transit >12 hours in an airport located in a country with risk of YFV transmission.[1]
Recommendations: None.

MALARIA
No malaria transmission.

WESTERN SAHARA

YELLOW FEVER
Requirements: This territory has not stated its yellow fever vaccination certificate requirements.
Recommendations: None.

MALARIA
Areas with malaria: Rare cases.
Estimated relative risk of malaria for US travelers: No data.
Drug resistance[4]: Chloroquine.
Malaria species: Unknown.
Recommended chemoprophylaxis: Mosquito avoidance only.

YEMEN

YELLOW FEVER
No requirements or recommendations.

MALARIA
Areas with malaria: All areas <2,000 m (6,562 ft). None in Sana'a.
Estimated relative risk of malaria for US travelers: Low.
Drug resistance[4]: Chloroquine.
Malaria species: *P. falciparum* 95%; *P. malariae*, *P. vivax*, *P. ovale* 5% combined.
Recommended chemoprophylaxis: Atovaquone-proguanil, doxycycline, or mefloquine.

ZAMBIA *(see Map 3-41.)*

YELLOW FEVER
Requirements: Required if traveling from a country with risk of YFV transmission and ≥9 months of age, including transit >12 hours in an airport located in a country with risk of YFV transmission.[1]
Recommendations:
Generally not recommended for travelers going to the North West and Western Provinces (see Map 3-41).
Not recommended in all other areas not listed above.

MALARIA
Areas with malaria: All.
Estimated relative risk of malaria for US travelers: Moderate.
Drug resistance[4]: Chloroquine.

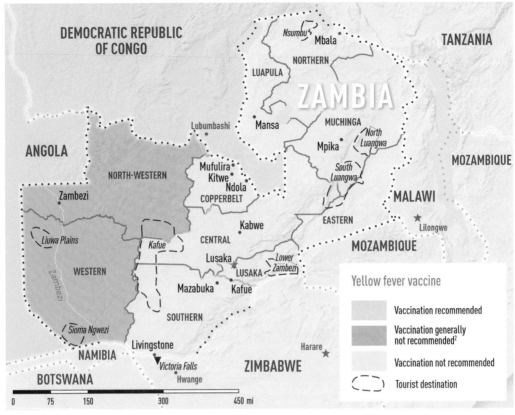

MAP 3-41. Yellow fever vaccine recommendations in Zambia[1]

[1,2] See footnotes on page 424.

Yellow fever vaccine

Vaccination recommended

Vaccination generally not recommended[2]

Vaccination not recommended

Tourist destination

Malaria species: *P. falciparum* >90%, *P. vivax* up to 5%, *P. ovale* up to 5%.
Recommended chemoprophylaxis: Atovaquone-proguanil, doxycycline, or mefloquine.

ZIMBABWE

YELLOW FEVER
Requirements: Required if traveling from a country with risk of YFV transmission and ≥9 months of age, including transit >12 hours in an airport located in a country with risk of YFV transmission.[1]
Recommendations: None.

MALARIA
Areas with malaria: All.
Estimated relative risk of malaria for US travelers: Moderate.
Drug resistance[4]: Chloroquine.
Malaria species: *P. falciparum* >90%, *P. vivax* up to 5%, *P. ovale* up to 5%.
Recommended chemoprophylaxis: Atovaquone-proguanil, doxycycline, or mefloquine.

*All footnotes are located on page 424.

FOOTNOTES

Yellow Fever

[1] The official WHO list of countries with risk of YFV transmission can be found in Table 3-22. Proof of yellow fever vaccination should be required only if traveling from a country on the WHO list, unless otherwise specified. The following countries, containing only areas with low potential for exposure to YFV, are not on the WHO list: Eritrea, Rwanda, São Tomé and Príncipe, Somalia, Tanzania, Zambia.

[2] An elevation of 2,300 m is equivalent to 7,546 ft.

Malaria

[3] This risk estimate is based largely on cases occurring in US military personnel who travel for extended periods of time with unique itineraries that likely do not reflect the risk for the average US traveler.

[4] Refers to *P. falciparum* malaria unless otherwise noted.

[5] Primaquine can cause hemolytic anemia in people with G6PD deficiency. Patients must be screened for G6PD deficiency before starting primaquine.

Yellow Fever Maps

[1] This map, which aligns with recommendations also published by the World Health Organization (WHO), is an updated version of the 2010 map created by the Informal WHO Working Group on the Geographic Risk of Yellow Fever.

[2] Yellow fever (YF) vaccination is generally not recommended in areas where there is low potential for YF virus exposure. However, vaccination might be considered for a small subset of travelers to these areas who are at increased risk for exposure to YF virus because of prolonged travel, heavy exposure to mosquitoes, or inability to avoid mosquito bites. Consideration for vaccination of any traveler must take into account the traveler's risk of being infected with YF virus, country entry requirements, and individual risk factors for serious vaccine-associated adverse events (such as age or immune status).

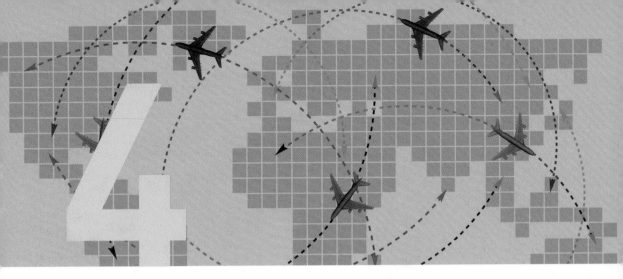

Select Destinations

RATIONALE FOR SELECT DESTINATIONS

Ronnie Henry

This chapter of the *Yellow Book* was created to allow experts who have lived in or have frequently visited particular destinations to share their insider's knowledge of these places. Each of these sections should be considered a personal perspective on the area discussed. They are editorial in nature, containing the author's expressed opinions; they should not be taken as a prescription for pretravel care. These sections are intended to help a travel health provider feel more comfortable giving advice about destinations that he or she may have never visited and to provide a level of detail about the attractions and risks that has not been provided elsewhere in this book.

The destination sections are among the most popular features of the *Yellow Book*. Space limitations prevent us from including all tourist destinations in this chapter, and the decision of what destinations to add or remove is guided by volume of US travel, uniqueness of health risks, and other factors. In this edition, we have added Cuba (reflecting the loosening of US travel restrictions) and Burma (reflecting its emergence as a tourist destination). To accommodate these new sections, we have removed Cambodia and Egypt & Nile River Cruises. Because these destinations remain relevant, these sections will continue to exist in the Yellow Book online (www.cdc.gov/yellowbook), along with other online-only sections: Guatemala and Belize, Iguaçu Falls, and Jamaica.

AFRICA & THE MIDDLE EAST

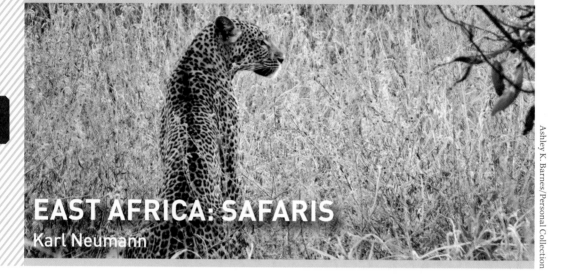

EAST AFRICA: SAFARIS
Karl Neumann

Ashley K. Barnes/Personal Collection

DESTINATION OVERVIEW

Arguably the ultimate in adventure travel, an African safari is also an easily doable family vacation, an experience of a lifetime for people of all ages, and, with a little research, not much more difficult to arrange than a week at a Caribbean resort. While the centerpiece of safari-going remains viewing majestic animals in their natural habitats, many tour operators now include programs on local culture, history, geology, and ecosystems and encourage travelers to get to know the local people not merely as subjects of photos. Safaris can also be differentiated by the topography, vegetation, and bird life of the region. There are safaris for families, honeymooners, and people with similar interests (serious photography, for example). Many safaris accept children as young as 6 years and have special age-appropriate programs for children and adolescents aged 6–16 years.

Animals can be viewed from open trucks, air-conditioned vans, private aircraft, hot air balloons, or while hiking (where animals are friendly). Trips need not be strenuous. Accommodations range from crawl-in tents to air-conditioned, walk-in tents with full bathrooms. There are even luxurious 5-star lodges with floodlit water holes to view animals at night. Lunch in the wilderness varies from prepackaged sandwiches eaten sitting on a tree stump to 3-course meals served on tables covered with linen cloths and matching napkins. Some safaris include side trips to exotic places—to see or climb Mount Kilimanjaro, or visit Zanzibar or Lake Victoria, for example.

Travelers on their first safari often choose game parks in Kenya and Tanzania, in East Africa. The most famous game park in Kenya is the Masai Mara National Reserve, which, in effect, is the northern continuation of the Serengeti National Park game reserve in Tanzania. Together they form the home of perhaps the grandest and most complete collection of the large wild animals for which Africa is famous. The Serengeti is the starting point of the annual migration of more than a million wildebeest and several hundred thousand zebras as they search for pasture and water. Tanzania also has the Ngorongoro Crater, a 100-square mile depression (caldera) formed when a giant volcano, perhaps the size of Mount Kilimanjaro, exploded and collapsed on itself millions of years ago. The crater has most of the same animals as the Masai Mara reserve. The major East African game parks are shown on Map 4-1.

Travelers should research the optimum time of the year for their safari. The wildebeest migration in the Serengeti is a seasonal event, for example, although the precise time of the migration may vary from year to year. Some parks have a dry season, offering better views of the animals, as the vegetation is sparser and animals gather where water is present, but roads are dustier. And many areas of Africa have times of the year that are more comfortable for visitors, with cooler weather, lower humidity, and less chance of rain.

HEALTH ISSUES

Health and safety issues that safari-goers are likely to encounter are mostly predictable and largely avoidable. The best insurance for carefree trips is a pretravel consultation with a travel health care provider, choosing an experienced and sophisticated tour operator, and taking along a small, personalized medical kit (see Chapter 2, Travel Health Kits).

Experienced tour operators generally require that clients buy medical evacuation insurance, supply clients with ample literature relating to local conditions, and employ knowledgeable guides who carry first aid kits and communication equipment to summon help, if necessary (see Chapter 2, Travel Insurance, Travel Health Insurance, & Medical Evacuation Insurance).

Health advice must be itinerary- and game park–specific. Immunizations and preventive medications necessary for one park may not be necessary for others. Parks may be long distances apart and located in countries with different health standards and dissimilar climates. Some

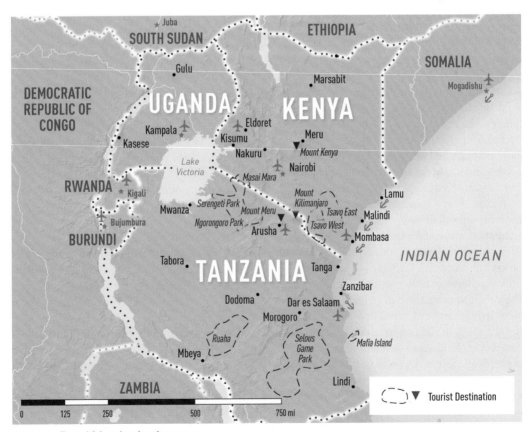

MAP 4-1. East Africa destination map

parks are located at higher elevations and close to the equator, making proper sun precautions imperative, including seeking shade when possible and avoiding the sun during midday hours. Significant sunburns can occur in less than an hour. Sunglasses are essential, in addition to protective clothing, hats, and use of a broad-spectrum sunscreen with SPF ≥15 that protects against both UVA and UVB.

Generally, proper preparations, common-sense precautions, the short duration of most trips (usually <2 weeks), experienced guides, and leaving the driving to others make safaris relatively low-risk undertakings for travelers of all ages.

Food and Water

Travelers' diarrhea appears to be the most common ailment, and most cases are mild. Sensible food and water selections may reduce the incidence (see Chapter 2, Food & Water Precautions). Illness may occur even on deluxe trips. Carrying medication for self-treatment is generally recommended (see Chapter 2, Travelers' Diarrhea).

Animals

Wild animals are unpredictable. Travelers should follow oral and written instructions provided by safari operators. Animal-related injuries are extremely rare and are usually the result of disregarding rules, for example approaching animals too closely to feed or photograph them.

Rabies exists throughout Africa. Although most cases result from dog bites, all mammals are susceptible and could transmit the virus. Wounds from mammals (except small rodents) should be considered a risk for rabies exposure unless proven otherwise. Licks can also result in rabies; the virus can enter through minor breaks in the skin. The incidence of rabies from bats seems to be increasing. In addition to rabies, bats may also transmit other diseases to humans, such as viral hemorrhagic fevers. Travelers should be encouraged to avoid entering caves where bats are known to be present. Cases of Marburg fever have occurred in travelers who visited a python cave in western Uganda.

Malaria

Malaria transmission occurs in most game parks. Most infections are caused by *Plasmodium falciparum*, and all *P. falciparum* in sub-Saharan Africa should be considered to be chloroquine-resistant. Safari activities often include sleeping in tents and observing animals at dusk or after dark, sometimes near water holes, all increasing the risk of being bitten by malaria-carrying mosquitoes. Taking preventive medication and using personal protection techniques—wearing long-sleeved shirts and pants, using insect repellents, and sleeping under permethrin-impregnated mosquito netting—are essential. Observing recommendations to prevent malaria helps minimize the risk of a host of other diseases spread by insects.

Yellow Fever

Travelers to East Africa must consult a travel medicine professional for the very latest information regarding yellow fever in that area. Yellow fever activity and vaccination recommendations can change frequently. Currently, yellow fever vaccination is recommended for much of East Africa (see Chapter 3, Yellow Fever & Malaria Information, by Country). In 2010, the World Health Organization and CDC reclassified a portion of East Africa to "low potential for exposure" to yellow fever virus and consequently downgraded the vaccination recommendation for these areas to "generally not recommended." This recommendation limits the need for vaccination to a small subset of travelers who are at increased risk for exposure to yellow fever virus (such as prolonged travel, heavy exposure to mosquitoes, or inability to avoid mosquito bites). These areas of East Africa where vaccine is generally not recommended include but are not limited to eastern Kenya, the cities of Nairobi and Mombasa, and all of Tanzania (see Chapter 3, Yellow Fever & Malaria Information, by Country).

However, some countries require proof of yellow fever vaccination in the form of a valid International Certificate of Vaccination or Prophylaxis (ICVP) as a condition of entry. Moreover, some safaris include more than one country.

4

Travelers must check the requirements of each country on their itinerary, including countries they only transit through on the way to their destination. Some countries may require a valid ICVP even if there is no yellow fever in the country travelers are leaving or entering.

Other Health Risks

African trypanosomiasis (sleeping sickness), a disease only rarely seen among travelers, is transmitted by day-biting tsetse flies (*Glossina*). Wearing light-colored clothing (and avoiding wearing blue) seems to deter the flies. Insect repellents are only partially effective. Symptoms include fever, eschar at the site of the bite, headache, and signs of central nervous system involvement. Several cases of trypanosomiasis (*rhodesiense*) have recently been reported in European tourists visiting the Masai Mara National Reserve in Kenya and wildlife reserves in Tanzania.

Dengue, filariasis, leishmaniasis, and onchocerciasis (river blindness) are other diseases carried by insects that occur in East Africa. Swimming in freshwater ponds, lakes, and rivers can result in schistosomiasis (bilharzia), a parasite found in freshwater snails and transmitted by exposure to water. All freshwater sources should be considered contaminated. Swimming in the ocean or well-chlorinated pools is safe.

Myiasis and tungiasis are rare skin diseases among travelers. Myiasis is caused by fly larvae penetrating the skin and causing a boil-like lesion with a central aperture. Eggs are usually laid on clothing left to dry outdoors, and the larvae enter the skin when the clothing is worn. Clothing should be dried indoors or ironed before wearing. Tungiasis is caused by direct penetration of skin by sand fleas, resulting in small, painful nodules, often on the foot adjacent to toenails. Prevention includes wearing closed-toed footwear and not walking barefoot.

Symptoms of many diseases acquired in Africa may surface weeks and occasionally months after exposure, sometimes long after the traveler has returned home. Patients should mention all travel to their health care provider if they become ill after a trip.

Other Safety Risks

Although being a crime victim is an unusual occurrence for those on safari, robberies, muggings, and carjackings may occur in major urban centers, notably Nairobi and Mombasa. Street muggings during the day and night are common. The rates of fatal motor vehicle crashes in sub-Saharan Africa are among the highest in the world. Travelers should fasten seat belts when riding in cars and wear a helmet when riding bicycles or motorbikes. Within game parks, serious motor vehicle crashes are rare, as the poor roads discourage speeding. However, travel in rural areas between parks is high risk, especially after dark. If at all possible, nighttime driving in sub-Saharan Africa should be avoided, and pedestrians should take extra care for speeding vehicles. Boarding an overcrowded bus should be avoided.

BIBLIOGRAPHY

1. Gobbi F, Bisoffi Z. Human African trypanosomiasis in travellers to Kenya. Eurosurveillance. 2012 Mar 8;17(10):pii=20109.

2. CDC. Yellow fever vaccine: recommendations of the Advisory Committee on Immunization Practices (ACIP). MMWR Recomm Rep. 2010 Jun 30;59(RR-7): 1–27.

3. Meltzer E, Artom G, Marva E, Assous MV, Rahav G, Schwartzt E. Schistosomiasis among travelers: new aspects of an old disease. Emerg Infect Dis. 2006 Nov;12(11):1696–700.

4. Thrower Y, Goodyer LI. Application of insect repellents by travelers to malaria endemic areas. J Travel Med. 2006 Jul-Aug;13(4):198–202.

5. Warne B, Weld LH, Cramer JP, Field VK, Grobusch MP, Caumes E, et al. Travel-related infection in European travelers, EuroTravNet 2011. J Travel Med 2014 Jul-Aug;21(4):248–54.

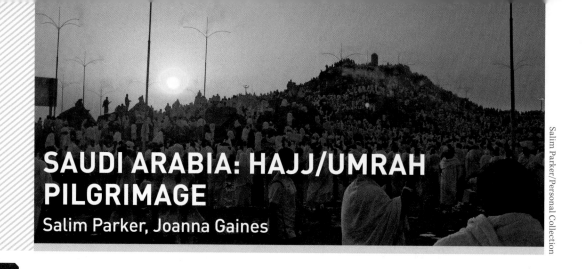

Salim Parker/Personal Collection

SAUDI ARABIA: HAJJ/UMRAH PILGRIMAGE

Salim Parker, Joanna Gaines

4

DESTINATION OVERVIEW

The Hajj and Umrah are religious pilgrimages to Mecca, Saudi Arabia. Islamic religious doctrine dictates that every able-bodied adult Muslim who can afford to do so is required to make Hajj at least once in his or her lifetime. Hajj takes place from the 8th through the 12th day of Dhul Hijah, the last month of the Islamic year. Because the Islamic calendar is lunar, the timing of Hajj varies with respect to the Gregorian calendar, occurring about 11 days earlier the following year (for example, it was held September 22–27 in 2015 and September 10–14 in 2016). Umrah is called the "minor pilgrimage," can be completed at any time of the year, and is not compulsory.

More than 2 million Muslims from over183 countries make Hajj each year (approximately 2.8 million in 2010); more than 11,000 pilgrims travel from the United States. The Kingdom of Saudi Arabia (KSA) continues to undertake engineering efforts to allow for an even greater number of pilgrims. Most international pilgrims fly into Jeddah or Medina and take a bus to Mecca. Pilgrims travel by foot or by bus approximately 5 miles (8 km) to the tent city of Mina, the largest temporary city in the world, where most pilgrims are housed in air-conditioned tents.

At dawn on the 9th day of Dhul Hijah, pilgrims begin a nearly 9 mile (14.4 km) walk, bus ride, or train ride to the plain of Arafat, passing Muzdalifah along the way (Map 4-2). Though the route features mist sprinklers to mitigate the oppressive daytime temperatures (which can reach 122°F [50°C]), the risk of heat-related illnesses during this part of the journey is still high. Ambulances and medical stations along the route are available for medical assistance. Hajj climaxes on the Plain of Arafat, a few miles east of Mecca. Pilgrims spend the day in supplication, praying and reading the Quran. The presence on Arafat, even if only for a few moments, on the ninth day of Dhul Hijah is an absolute rite of Hajj. If the pilgrim fails to reach the Plain of Arafat on that day, the Hajj is invalid and will have to be repeated. After sunset, pilgrims begin the 5.5 mile (9 km) journey back to Muzdalifah, where most sleep in the open air. Dust, inadequate and overcrowded washing and sanitation facilities, and the possibility of getting separated or lost are some potential problems pilgrims face.

At sunrise on the 10th day of Dhul Hijah, pilgrims collect small pebbles at Muzdalifah and carry them to Mina. This day's ritual is called the Stoning of the Devil at Jamaraat. During this ritual, pilgrims throw 7 tiny pebbles (specifically, no larger than a chickpea) at the largest of 3 white pillars. The crowded conditions at this site pose potential hazards; multiple deadly crowd crush disasters have occurred at and around Mina.

Traditionally after Jamaraat, pilgrims sacrifice an animal. Pilgrims have the option to purchase a "sacrifice voucher" in Mecca and have this sacrifice performed by proxy. Centralized, licensed abattoirs perform the sacrifice on behalf of the pilgrim, limiting the exposure of pilgrims to potential zoonotic diseases. However, some pilgrims

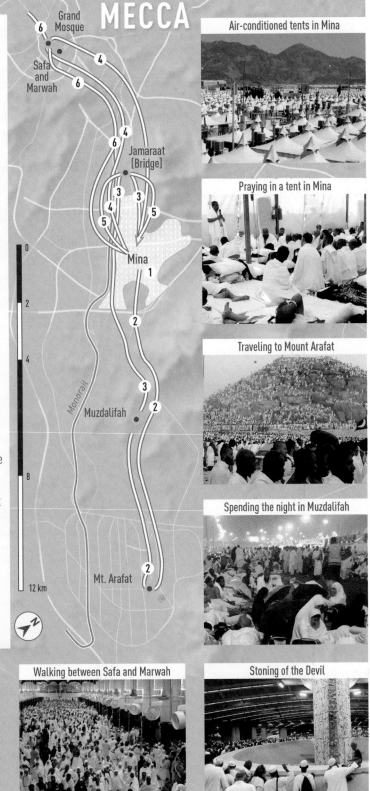

1 Most pilgrims arrive at **Mina** on foot or by bus and are housed in air-conditioned tents.

2 At dawn, pilgrims travel about 14 km on foot, by bus, or by train from **Mina** to **Mount Arafat**, where they spend the day praying and reading the Quran. After sunset, they travel 9 km on foot, or by bus or monorail, from **Mount Arafat** to Muzdalifah and a large number sleep in the open air.

3 At sunrise, pilgrims collect pebbles at **Muzdalifah** and carry them to **Mina**. During the ritual of Stoning of the Devil at **Jamaraat**, pilgrims throw 7 pebbles at the largest of 3 pillars representing Satan, before returning to **Mina** for the night.

4 Pilgrims travel from **Mina** to the **Grand Mosque** in Mecca and perform a *tawaf*, circling the Ka'aba 7 times. Pilgrims may also perform sa'i, walking or running 7 times between **Safa and Marwah,** before they return to **Mina**.

5 Pilgrims stay over at **Mina** and pelt all three representations of Satan with 7 pebbles each on either two or three days.

6 Pilgrims leave **Mina** for the final time, travel to the **Grand Mosque** for the last *tawaf*, after which they leave Mecca, ending Hajj.

MECCA

Grand Mosque

Safa and Marwah

Jamaraat [Bridge]

Mina

Monorail

Muzdalifah

Mt. Arafat

0
2
4
8
12 km

Air-conditioned tents in Mina

Praying in a tent in Mina

Traveling to Mount Arafat

Spending the night in Muzdalifah

Performing tawaf at Grand Mosque

Walking between Safa and Marwah

Stoning of the Devil

MAP 4-2. Hajj destination map

may visit farms where they either sacrifice an animal themselves or have it done by an appointed representative. The World Health Organization recommends travelers visiting farms or other areas where animals are present practice general hygiene measures, including regular handwashing before and after touching animals and avoiding contact with sick animals. Travelers should avoid the consumption of raw or undercooked animal products (including milk and meat).

After returning to Mecca, pilgrims go immediately to the Grand Mosque, which contains the Ka'aba, and perform a *tawaf*, which involves circling the Ka'aba 7 times counterclockwise. Because of the vast number of people (each floor of the 3-level mosque has a capacity of 750,000 people), performing a *tawaf* can take hours. In addition to *tawaf*, pilgrims may perform *sa'i*, walking (and running during certain parts) 7 times between the hills of Safa and Marwah, and then drinking water from the Well of Zamzam. This route is enclosed by the Grand Mosque and can be traversed via air-conditioned tunnels, with separate sections for walkers, runners, and disabled pilgrims. Pilgrims then return to Mina and pelt all three columns at the Jamaraat on the 11th and 12th of the month, with the option of repeating it on the 13th.

After performing a final *tawaf*, pilgrims leave Mecca, ending Hajj. Although it is not required as part of Hajj, many pilgrims extend their trips to travel to Medina. In Medina, pilgrims visit the Mosque of the Prophet, which contains the tomb of Mohammed. Physicians should query patients about their itineraries to ensure they have adequate medication and supplies for the length of their trip.

HEALTH ISSUES

The Kingdom of Saudi Arabia (KSA) sets medical requirements such as proof of vaccination as part of the visa application process for Hajj pilgrims. These vaccinations may include seasonal influenza, H1N1, and meningitis. Health experts in KSA currently advise that the elderly, the terminally ill, pregnant women, and children postpone their plans for Hajj and Umrah for safety reasons. KSA may also choose to limit issuance

of visas to travelers from countries experiencing infectious disease outbreaks. In 2012, Uganda was not permitted to send pilgrims due to an Ebola outbreak in that country, and the same restriction applied to Liberia, Guinea, and Sierra Leone in 2015. Multiple medical facilities are located in and around the holy sites; medical services are offered free of charge to pilgrims. An estimated 20,000 health care workers were in attendance during the 2012 Hajj.

Vaccine-Preventable Diseases

CDC recommends all travelers to Saudi Arabia be up-to-date with routine immunizations. In addition, hepatitis A vaccine is recommended for most travelers, and hepatitis B vaccine is recommended for travelers who might be exposed to blood or other body fluids. Travelers from yellow fever–endemic countries, or those who travel via these areas, must provide proof of yellow fever vaccination. Although a requirement for polio vaccine does not include adult pilgrims from the United States, it is best to ensure full vaccination against polio before travel. All pilgrims who travel from countries where polio is reported are required to show proof of polio vaccination at least 6 weeks prior to arrival in Saudi Arabia. In addition, a single dose of the polio vaccine is administered to all pilgrims in Saudi Arabia from countries where polio has been reported irrespective of previous immunization against the disease. The number of polio doses administered at ports of entry is about 500,000, representing more than 90% of eligible pilgrims.

MENINGOCOCCAL VACCINE

The Kingdom of Saudi Arabia will not issue Hajj or Umrah visas without proof of meningococcal vaccination at least 10 days and no more than 3 years before arrival for polysaccharide vaccine and no more than 8 years before arrival for conjugate vaccine. (CDC recommends revaccination with conjugate vaccine after 5 years for people at continued risk.) All pilgrims must have received a single dose of quadrivalent ACWY vaccine and must show proof of vaccination on a valid International Certificate of Vaccination or

Prophylaxis. Although the KSA Ministry of Health currently advises against travel to the Hajj for pregnant women or children, if they choose to travel these groups should receive meningococcal vaccination according to licensed indications for their age. These requirements are regularly updated on the Saudi Ministry of Hajj website and should be consulted before travel.

Current Hajj vaccination requirements are available from the following sources:

- Saudi Arabian Embassy (http://embassies. mofa.gov.sa/sites/usa/AR/Pages/default. aspx)

- Saudi Arabian Ministry of Hajj (http://haj. gov.sa/english/pages/default.aspx)

- Saudi Arabian Ministry of Health (www. moh.gov.sa/en/Hajj/HealthGuidelines/ HealthGuidelinesBeforeHajj/Pages/ default.aspx)

Respiratory Infections

Respiratory tract infections are common during Hajj, with pneumonia being the most common cause of hospital admission. These risks underscore the need to follow recommendations from the Advisory Committee on Immunization Practices for pneumococcal conjugate and polysaccharide vaccines for pilgrims aged ≥65 years and for younger travelers with comorbidities.

Seasonal influenza vaccine is strongly recommended for all pilgrims. Behavioral interventions such as hand hygiene, wearing a face mask, cough etiquette, social distancing, and contact avoidance may mitigate respiratory illness among pilgrims. Pretravel advice about common respiratory conditions should include a general assessment for respiratory fitness, necessary vaccinations, and prescription of adequate supplies of portable respiratory medications (inhalers are easier to transport than nebulizers).

The crowded conditions during Hajj increase the probability of tuberculosis transmission. Risk is estimated to be about 10% in those with high level of exposure. Many pilgrims come from highly endemic areas and some arrive for Hajj with active pulmonary disease. Pilgrims are advised to see their doctors if they develop signs of active tuberculosis.

Middle East respiratory syndrome (MERS) is caused by the MERS coronavirus, which was first identified in Saudi Arabia in 2012. Cases have been identified in and around the Arabian Peninsula, and cases have also been exported to other countries, including the United States. The most common symptoms include fever, cough, and shortness of breath. However, myalgia, diarrhea, vomiting, abdominal pain, thrombocytopenia, and leukopenia have also been reported. The severity of illness has ranged from mild to severe, and approximately 40% of reported cases have been fatal. The role of animal-to-human transmission is unclear, but the virus has been found in camels in this region. The diagnosis can be suspected on clinical grounds and confirmed by PCR testing. More information is available in Chapter 3, Middle East Respiratory Syndrome (MERS).

Other Health and Safety Risks
COMMUNICABLE DISEASES

Diarrheal disease is common during Hajj, and travelers should be educated on usual prevention measures and self-treatment. A pretravel visit should include discussions about prevention, oral rehydration strategies, antimotility agents, and emergency antibiotic use for treatment of travelers' diarrhea. More information can be found in Chapter 2, Travelers' Diarrhea.

Chafing caused by long periods of standing and walking in the heat can lead to fungal or bacterial skin infections. Clothing should be light, not restrictive, and changed often to maintain hygiene. Travelers should be advised to keep skin dry, use talcum powder, and be aware of any pain or soreness caused by garments. Any sores or blisters that develop should be disinfected and kept covered. Special attention should be paid to protect the feet, which are bare when inside the Grand Mosque. People with diabetes are at increased risk of skin infections.

Nasal ablution, called *istinshaaq*, is the practice of rinsing your nose with water before performing

4

some rituals during the Hajj. Medical literature has identified cases of primary amebic meningoencephalitis (PAM) caused by *Naegleria fowleri* transmitted as a result of nasal ablution. Nasal ablution is common during Hajj, and pilgrims are advised to use safe water to protect themselves from this potential risk (see Chapter 2, Water Disinfection for Travelers).

At the end of Hajj, Muslim men must shave their heads. The use of unclean blades can transmit bloodborne pathogens, such as hepatitis B virus, hepatitis C virus, and HIV. Licensed barbers are tested for these bloodborne pathogens and are required to use disposable, single-use blades. Unfortunately, unlicensed barbers continue to operate by the roadside, where they use nonsterile blades on multiple men. Male travelers should be advised to be shaved only at officially designated centers, which are clearly marked.

Aedes and *Anopheles* mosquitoes, which transmit dengue and malaria, respectively, are present in Saudi Arabia, and mosquito bite prevention measures are advisable. Dengue has been documented in Mecca but not during Hajj. Intensive insecticide spraying campaigns are undertaken before Hajj, and the housing units of pilgrims arriving from endemic areas are especially targeted before their arrival. Prophylaxis against malaria is not required.

NONCOMMUNICABLE DISEASES AND OTHER HAZARDS

Hajj is arduous even for young, healthy pilgrims, and many Muslims may wait until they are older before making Hajj. Travelers who are caught up in the experience of Hajj or Umrah may forget to take their usual medications. People with chronic medical conditions should undergo a functional assessment before leaving for Hajj. The medical provider should identify each traveler's unique risks and tailor a plan for how to reduce them. The provider should make any adjustments to the usual medical regimen, ensure that the traveler has an adequate supply of medications, and educate the traveler about symptoms that should prompt urgent medical attention.

Heat exhaustion and heatstroke are a threat to the health and well-being of travelers, can exacerbate chronic conditions, and are a leading cause of death, particularly when Hajj occurs during the summer months. Pilgrims should stay hydrated, wear sunscreen, and seek shade when possible. Umbrellas are frequently used to provide portable sun protection. Travelers should be counseled on minimizing the risk of heat-related injuries, as well as sun avoidance. Some rituals may also be performed at night to avoid daytime heat. Pilgrims can be reassured that religious leaders have deemed night rituals as legitimate. Except for the absolute presence on Arafat on the ninth of Dhul Hijah, most compulsory rituals can be postponed or done by proxy, or a penalty can be paid.

Fire is a potential risk at Hajj. In 1997, open stoves set tents on fire, and the resulting blaze killed 343 pilgrims and injured more than 1,500. As a result, makeshift tents were replaced with permanent fiberglass structures; pilgrims are not allowed to set up their own tents or prepare their own food. Cooking in the tents is also prohibited. In 2015, a hotel caught fire, leading to the evacuation of more than 1,000 pilgrims.

TRAUMA

Trauma is a major cause of injury and death during Hajj. Motor vehicle crashes are the primary risk for US travelers overseas, and pilgrims may walk long distances through or near dense traffic. In such dense crowds, crush disasters (or "stampedes") are also a risk. In 2004, after 251 pilgrims were killed and another 244 injured, the Saudi government replaced the round pillars with wide, elliptical columns to reduce crowd densities. After another crowd crush in 2006 that killed 280 pilgrims and injured 289, the single-tiered Jamaraat pedestrian bridge was demolished and replaced with a wider, multilevel bridge. In 2015, thousands of pilgrims were killed during a crush at Mina, making it the deadliest Hajj disaster on record. Death usually results from asphyxiation or head trauma, and large crowds limit the movement of emergency medical services, making prompt treatment difficult.

Special Health Considerations

MENSTRUATION

Menstruating women are not permitted to perform *tawaf* around the Ka'aba, one of the obligatory rituals. All other rituals are independent of menses. Pilgrims generally know well in advance that they will be making Hajj/Umrah and female pilgrims are advised to consult their doctors 2–3 months before the journey if they intend to manipulate their periods before the pilgrimage.

Chronic Health Conditions

Close to 64% of admissions to intensive care units and 46%–66% of deaths among pilgrims during Hajj are caused by cardiovascular conditions. Physicians should ensure any preexisting conditions are stabilized and advise travelers on prudent activities during the pilgrimage. Pilgrims with heart disease should carry a supply of all their medications, including copies of all prescriptions.

Diabetic pilgrims should carefully construct a diabetes management plan tailored to the physical challenges of the Hajj and the traveler's specific needs. Diabetic travelers should ensure adequate prescriptions for all medications, including syringes and needles. A diabetes emergency kit should include easily accessible carbohydrate sources to counter hypoglycemia, glucometer and test strips, urine ketone sticks to evaluate for ketoacidosis, a list of medications and care plans, and glucagon as indicated. Lastly, durable and protective footwear is necessary to avoid minor foot trauma that can lead to infections.

BIBLIOGRAPHY

1. Alsafadi H, Goodwin W, Syed A. Diabetes care during Hajj. Clin Med. 2011 Jun;11(3):218–21.

2. Alzahrani AG, Choudhry AJ, Al Mazroa MA, Turkistani AH, Nouman GS, Memish ZA. Pattern of diseases among visitors to Mina health centers during the Hajj season, 1429 H (2008 G). J Infect Public Health. 2012 Mar;5(1):22–34.

3. Assiri A, Al-Tawfiq JA, Al-Rabeeah AA, Al-Rabiah FA, Al-Hajjar S, Al-Barrak A, et al. Epidemiological, demographic, and clinical characteristics of 47 cases of Middle East respiratory syndrome coronavirus disease from Saudi Arabia: a descriptive study. Lancet Infect Dis. 2013 Sep;13(9):752–61.

4. Balaban V, Stauffer WM, Hammad A, Afgarshe M, Abd-Alla M, Ahmed Q, et al. Protective practices and respiratory illness among US travelers to the 2009 Hajj. J Travel Med. 2012 May-Jun;19(3):163–8.

5. Memish Z, Zumla A, Alhakeem R, Assiri A, Turkestani A, Al Harby KD, et al. Hajj: infectious disease surveillance and control. Lancet. 2014 Jun 14;383(9934):2073–82.

6. Memish ZA. The Hajj: communicable and non-communicable health hazards and current guidance for pilgrims. Euro Surveill. 2010 Sep 30;15(39):19671.

7. Memish ZA. Saudi Arabia has several strategies to care for pilgrims on the Hajj. BMJ. 2011;343:d7731.

8. Memish ZA, Al-Rabeeah AA. Health conditions of travellers to Saudi Arabia for the pilgrimage to Mecca (Hajj and Umra) for 1434 (2013). J Epidemiol Glob Health. 2013 Jun;3(2):59–61.

9. Shibl A, Tufenkeji H, Khalil M, Memish Z, Meningococcal Leadership Forum (MLF) Expert Group. Consensus recommendation for meningococcal disease prevention for Hajj and Umra pilgrimage/travel medicine. East Mediterr Health J 2013 Apr;19(4):389–92.

10. World Health Organization. Health conditions for travellers to Saudi Arabia pilgrimage to Mecca (Hajj). Wkly Epidemiol Rec. 2005 Dec 9;80(49-50):431–2.

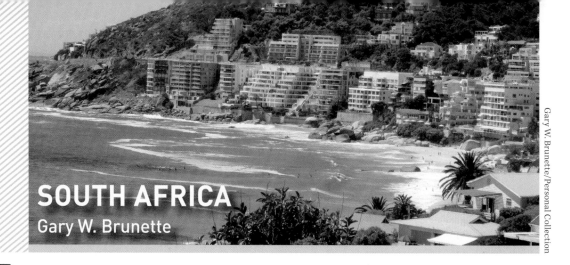

Gary W. Brunette/Personal Collection

SOUTH AFRICA
Gary W. Brunette

4

DESTINATION OVERVIEW

South Africa has been called "a world in one country." The epithet refers, in part, to the diversity in the geography, which includes lush subtropical regions, old hardwood forests, sweeping Highveld vistas, and the deep desert of the Kalahari; the splendor of the animal species found throughout the country and protected in expansive game reserves; the diverse origins of the locals (from Africa, Europe, India, and Southeast Asia); the cultural, artistic, and culinary variety; and access to the conveniences of a developed infrastructure amid the challenges of Africa.

South Africa has experienced a surge in tourism in the past 2 decades, with visitors from within the African continent as well as those from Europe and North America. Business travelers typically head to the commercial centers of Johannesburg, Cape Town, and Durban. Tourists may be attracted by the game reserves, the largest of which is Kruger National Park, located along the Mozambique border in the northeast (see Map 4-3). Kwa-Zulu Natal has a number of game parks (Hluhluwe-Umfolozi and Saint Lucia) set inland from Durban, and the Eastern Cape has parks (Addo Elephant Park and Shamwari) easily accessed from Port Elizabeth on the southern coast. Many smaller luxury reserves have emerged to cater to the high-end traveler. Visitors may be attracted to itineraries that include a trip from Cape Town along the south coast through the small scenic towns of Knysna and Plettenberg Bay; a tour

of the old gold-mining towns in Mpumalanga, many of which are in near-original condition; spectacular drives and fascinating tours of the old wineries along the wine routes in the Western Cape; or visits to the southernmost point of Africa at Cape Agulhas or Cape Point, where the Indian and Atlantic Oceans meet in a roar of foam.

South Africa is also a common destination for humanitarian workers, missionaries, and students. A sizable number of South Africans live outside the country and would be considered VFR travelers (visiting friends and relatives) when returning to the country for a visit (see Chapter 8, Immigrants Returning Home to Visit Friends & Relatives).

While there is a wide range of living standards in South Africa, most visitors experience standards comparable to those in developed countries. A smaller number of visitors may go to less developed areas, either the lower-income townships outside most towns and cities or to rural areas. Hikers, adventure-seekers, and missionaries will experience a wider range of living standards. Similarly, the quality and availability of health care are variable. Middle- and upper-income South Africans live in low-risk environments, have a standard of health comparable to that of North Americans, and have access to world-class medical facilities. Poorer South Africans live in areas with few amenities, are exposed to a wide range of diseases, and have limited access to adequate health care.

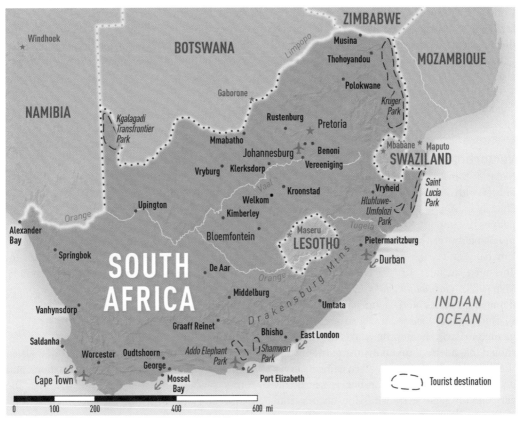

MAP 4-3. South Africa destination map

HEALTH ISSUES

Vaccine-Preventable Diseases

All travelers to South Africa should be up-to-date with their routine vaccinations. Infectious diseases such as measles and mumps are endemic in the region. In addition, hepatitis A vaccine is recommended for most travelers, and hepatitis B vaccine is recommended for travelers who might be exposed to blood or other body fluids, including through sexual contact. Travelers should also consider typhoid vaccine, especially those who are more adventuresome or staying in less sanitary surroundings.

YELLOW FEVER VACCINE REQUIREMENTS

South Africa requires a valid International Certificate of Vaccination or Prophylaxis (ICVP) documenting yellow fever vaccination ≥10 days before arrival in South Africa for all travelers aged ≥1 year who are traveling from or transiting for >12 hours through the airport of a country with risk of yellow fever virus transmission. Travelers not meeting this requirement can be refused entry to South Africa or be quarantined for up to 6 days. Unvaccinated travelers with a valid medical waiver should be allowed entry. South Africa considers an ICVP to be valid for life.

Travelers going to or transiting through South Africa are advised to seek the most current information by consulting the CDC Travelers' Health website (www.cdc.gov/travel), and also the website of the US embassy in South Africa (Pretoria) and the embassy of South Africa in Washington, DC.

HIV and Sexually Transmitted Diseases

South Africa has the largest estimated number of people living with HIV of any country in the world. The prevalence of HIV infection is approximately 19% among people aged 15–49 years, and the prevalence among sex workers is even higher. Other sexually transmitted diseases (STDs) are also present at high rates in this population. Travelers should be aware of STD risks and use condoms if they have sex with someone whose HIV or STD status is unknown.

Vectorborne Diseases

Malaria transmission only occurs along the border with Zimbabwe and Mozambique, specifically in Vembe and Mopane district municipalities of Limpopo Province, Ehlanzeni district municipality in Mpumalanga Province, and Umkhanyakude in Kwazulu-Natal Province. This area includes Kruger National Park (see Map 3-38). *Plasmodium falciparum* is the predominant species and is universally resistant to chloroquine. Visitors to these areas should be on a malaria chemoprophylaxis regimen and should be advised to take mosquito precautions. Malaria in the northeastern game reserves occurs throughout the year but is seasonally variable; the highest transmission occurs from September through May, peaking from February to early May. The risk to visiting travelers is low. Preventing mosquito bites is the first line of defense against malaria. The South African Department of Health recommends malaria chemoprophylaxis for all travelers visiting malaria risk areas from September through May and mosquito-avoidance measures for the rest of the year. CDC recommends chemoprophylaxis at all times of the year (see Chapter 3, Yellow Fever & Malaria Information, by Country).

Tick-bite fever caused by rickettsial species is common in South Africa. The incidence rate for visitors from Europe is estimated to be 4%–5%. The disease is characterized by an eschar at the bite site, regional adenopathy, and a maculopapular to petechial rash. Hikers and campers in rural areas who are exposed to ticks are especially at risk. Measures should be taken to prevent tick bites (see Chapter 2, Protection against Mosquitoes, Ticks, & Other Arthropods). Travelers who are taking doxycycline for malaria chemoprophylaxis may have some protection against tick-bite fever, but no studies exist to support or refute this viewpoint. Taking doxycycline only as prophylaxis for tick-bite fever (as opposed to taking it for malaria chemoprophylaxis) is not recommended.

Travelers' Diarrhea

As with most destinations, the risk of travelers' diarrhea depends on style of traveling and food choices. A fluoroquinolone, such as ciprofloxacin, can be considered for self-treatment of moderate to severe diarrhea.

Waterborne Diseases

Schistosomiasis, a common parasite throughout Africa, may be present in any body of freshwater, such as lakes, streams, and ponds. Travelers should avoid swimming in fresh, unchlorinated water.

Animal Avoidance

Although most travelers avoid wild animals in game reserves, rabies is common in dogs and other mammals throughout the country. The KwaZulu-Natal Province has the highest incidence of rabies. Travelers have no way of telling if a given animal is rabid and should avoid all contact with animals. Any bite or scratch from an animal should be washed with soap and water immediately and be evaluated as soon as possible by a clinician. Postexposure prophylaxis and medical care for rabies exposures can be obtained in South Africa. Rabies vaccine is available throughout South Africa, and human rabies immune globulin is available in major urban medical centers.

Safety and Security

South Africa has experienced a rise in violent crime, which includes armed robberies, carjackings, home invasions, and rape. Most of these incidents occur in lower income residential areas and, as such, most visitors will not be affected. However, awareness of personal safety and security should be stressed to all visitors. Travelers should rely on local guidance about the security precautions to take in specific areas.

Although South Africa has a modern road system, drivers should be alert for dangerous driving practices, stray animals, and poor roads in remote rural areas. Travelers should fasten seat belts when riding in cars and wear a helmet when riding bicycles or motorbikes.

BIBLIOGRAPHY

1. Blumberg LH, de Frey A, Frean J, Mendelson M. The 2010 FIFA World Cup: communicable disease risks and advice for visitors to South Africa. J Travel Med. 2010 May-Jun;17(3):150–2.

2. Durrheim DN, Braack LE, Waner S, Gammon S. Risk of malaria in visitors to the Kruger National Park, South Africa. J Travel Med. 1998 Dec;5(4):173–7.

3. Frean J, Blumberg L, Ogunbanjo GA. Tick bite fever in South Africa. SA Fam Pract. 2008 Mar-Apr;50(2):33–5.

4. Maharaj R, Raman J, Morris N, Moonasar D, Durrheim DN, Seocharan I, et al. Epidemiology of malaria in South Africa: from control to elimination. S Afr Med J. 2013 Oct;103(10 Pt2):779–83.

5. Probst C, Parry CD, Rehm J. Socio-economic differences in HIV/AIDS mortality in South Africa. Trop Med Int Health. 2016 Jul;21(7):846–55.

6. South African National Travel Health Network. SaNTHNet [homepage on the Internet]. Dunvegan (South Africa): South African National Travel Health Network; c2013 [cited 2016 Sep. 23]; Available from: http://www.santhnet.co.za/.

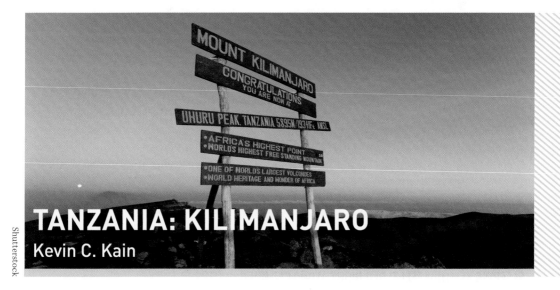

TANZANIA: KILIMANJARO
Kevin C. Kain

Shutterstock

DESTINATION OVERVIEW

As the highest mountain in Africa and one of the largest freestanding volcanoes in the world, Kilimanjaro remains a revered and classic image of East Africa. Its snow-capped peak rising 19,341 ft (5,895 m) above the tropical African savanna is an irresistible draw for trekkers, particularly since no technical climbing is required to reach the summit. Kilimanjaro is one of the "seven summits" representing the highest peaks on each continent. However, because it does not involve technical climbing, the difficulties are often misjudged. Climbing Kilimanjaro is a serious undertaking, requiring serious preparation. Despite being higher than classic trekking destinations in Nepal, such as Kala Pattar (18,450 ft; 5,625 m) or Everest base camp (17,598 ft; 5,364 m), typical ascent rates on Kilimanjaro are considerably faster (4–6 days vs 8–12 days).

The classic route up Kilimanjaro is the Marangu route (40 miles; 64 km), usually sold as a 5-day, 4-night trip. Marangu is frequently nicknamed the "Coca-Cola" route, since accommodation and food are provided in bunkhouses, and the trail is wide and relatively easy compared with other routes. There are at least 9 alternative routes (Map 4-4), including the stunningly beautiful Machame route (the so-called "whiskey" route, since the days are generally longer with tougher climbs). Machame and other routes involve camping but are usually sold as 6- to 9-day packages, providing more opportunity to acclimatize and a greater chance to successfully summit. Kilimanjaro can be climbed throughout the year (March–April are often the wettest months), but

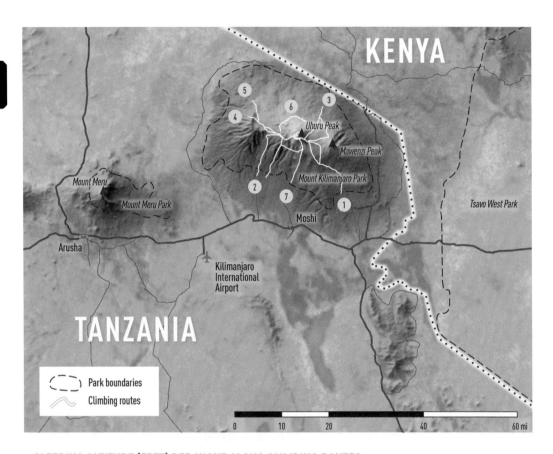

SLEEPING ALTITUDE (FEET) PER NIGHT ALONG CLIMBING ROUTES

	Route	Night 1	Night 2	Night 3	Night 4	Night 5	Night 6	Night 7	Night 8	Night 9
1	MARANGU	8,858	12,205	14,160	15,430	12,205	6,046	N/A	N/A	N/A
2	MACHAME	9,350	12,500	13,044	13,106	15,331	10,065	5,380	N/A	N/A
3	RONGAI	9,300	11,811	14,160	14,160	15,430	12,205	6,046	N/A	N/A
4	LEMOSHO	9,498	11,500	13,800	13,044	13,106	15,331	10,065	5,380	N/A
5	SHIRA	11,800	12,500	13,044	13,106	15,331	10,065	5,380	N/A	N/A
6	NORTHERN	9,498	11,500	12,500	13,580	13,200	12,700	15,600	10,065	5,380
7	UMBWE	9,514	13,044	13,106	15,331	10,065	5,380	N/A	N/A	N/A

MAP 4-4. Kilimanjaro destination map

the weather is unpredictable, and the climber must be prepared for extreme weather and rain at any time of the year. A 2011 review of UK companies arranging high-altitude trekking reported that only 16 of 93 (17%) companies offering Kilimanjaro treks complied with Wilderness Medical Society guidelines on ascending to altitude, compared with 92% of treks to Everest base camp. Moreover, fewer than half of these companies carry medications to prevent or treat altitude illness, so trekkers should be prepared to carry and understand how and when to use these medications.

Climbing Kilimanjaro is a dream for many who visit Africa. However, a large number of travelers are ill-prepared, ascend too quickly, and consequently fail to summit. With due preparation and more reasonable ascent rates, climbing "Kili" is an aspiration that can be successfully and safely accomplished by many.

HEALTH ISSUES

The main medical issues for those attempting to climb Kilimanjaro include the prevention and treatment of altitude illness and the potential for drug interactions between medications used for altitude illness and antimalarial or antidiarrheal agents commonly used by travelers to Tanzania.

Altitude and Acute Mountain Sickness (AMS)

Altitude illness is a problem on Kilimanjaro and a major contributor to the reason that only 50% of those attempting the standard 4- to 5-day Marangu route reach the crater rim, known as Gilman's Point (18,652 ft; 5,685 m), and as few as 10% reach the summit, known as Uhuru (Freedom) Peak (19,341 ft; 5,895 m). Prevalence rates of AMS were 75%–77% in recent studies of 4- and 5-day ascents on the Marangu route. Those using acetazolamide were significantly less likely to develop AMS on the 5-day ascents, but 40%–50% of those taking acetazolamide may still report AMS symptoms.

Every hiker on Kilimanjaro should receive pretravel advice on AMS, be able to recognize symptoms, and know how to prevent and treat

it. People with certain underlying medical conditions, including pregnancy, significant underlying lung or cardiac disease, and ocular and neurologic conditions, may be more susceptible to altitude-associated problems or may be taking medications that may interact with altitude medications, and should consult a travel health provider with knowledge of altitude illness before travel.

Enjoying the experience and successfully reaching the summit can be enhanced by allowing more time to acclimatize:

- If Ngorongoro crater is part of the planned combined safari/Kilimanjaro hike itinerary, try to spend the last few nights of the safari there, because its elevation (7,500 ft; 2,286 m) will aid acclimatization for the Kilimanjaro trek.

- It is strongly encouraged to add at least an extra day or two to the ascent of Kilimanjaro, regardless of the route, but especially on routes normally promoted as 4- to 6-day trips.

- If possible, before attempting Kilimanjaro travelers may acclimatize by hiking nearby Mount Meru (14,978 ft; 4,565 m) or Mount Kenya (to Point Lenana, 16,355 ft; 4,895 m). A number of combined climbing trips for Mount Kenya and Kilimanjaro are now offered commercially.

For those with a past history of susceptibility to AMS and for those in whom adequate acclimatization is not possible (most "Kili" clients), the use of medications such as acetazolamide to prevent altitude illness is recommended. Acetazolamide accelerates acclimatization, is effective in preventing (beginning the day before ascent) and treating AMS, and is safe in children.

For those who are intolerant of or allergic to acetazolamide, dexamethasone is an alternative for prevention of AMS, but there are cautions involved in using dexamethasone for ascent. Consideration should be given to carrying a treatment course of dexamethasone for high-altitude cerebral edema (HACE). Travelers with symptoms of altitude illness must not continue to ascend and need to descend if symptoms are worsening at the same altitude. A flexible itinerary and having an extra guide who can accompany any member of the group down the mountain if he or she becomes ill are considerations. See Chapter 2, Altitude Illness, for more information about prevention and treatment of altitude illness.

Malaria

Kilimanjaro is unique in that its tropical malaria-endemic location means that many trekkers will be on antimalarial drugs and may need to continue them after their climb, particularly if they are also visiting game parks and staying overnight at altitudes <5,906 ft (1,800 m). Malaria prophylaxis is recommended for Tanzania (even if only for a short trip). If a traveler flew directly into Kilimanjaro International Airport (2,932 ft; 894 m) and went the same day to an altitude above 1,800 m, there would be no risk of malaria. However, most people will be on safari or traveling before or after their Kilimanjaro trip and therefore will be on prophylaxis.

Kilimanjaro is also a unique destination in that high altitude will affect everyone, and possible interactions should be considered between drugs commonly used for malaria prophylaxis or treatment of AMS, high-altitude pulmonary edema, or HACE, such as acetazolamide, dexamethasone, and nifedipine. Fortunately, there are few reported clinically significant drug interactions between common malaria prophylaxis agents (atovaquone-proguanil, doxycycline, or mefloquine) and acetazolamide or dexamethasone. Nifedipine is metabolized by the CYP3A4 enzyme, and concurrent use of CYP3A4 inhibitors such as doxycycline could lead to elevated plasma levels of nifedipine and potentially lower blood pressure. Therefore, it would not be advised to take nifedipine for altitude illness prophylaxis concurrently with doxycycline.

Treatment of Travelers' Diarrhea

There are no reported drug interactions between acetazolamide and the fluoroquinolones (ciprofloxacin, levofloxacin) or macrolides (azithromycin) commonly used to treat travelers' diarrhea. There is a potential increased risk of tendon rupture when dexamethasone is used with fluoroquinolones. Avoid concurrent use of macrolides and nifedipine.

Remote Travel

Kilimanjaro treks are physically demanding and require a good level of fitness and preparation for the elements. Kilimanjaro weather is characterized by extremes; travelers should be prepared for tropical heat, heavy rains, and bitter cold. Gear, especially sleeping bags, should be kept in waterproof bags. Travelers should have adequate health insurance, including medical evacuation insurance, and make sure their medical care and medical evacuation policies will cover any potential costs for a rescue or evacuation from the top of the mountain.

Travelers should carry a first aid kit that includes bandages, tape, blister kit, antibacterial and antifungal cream, antibiotics for travelers' diarrhea, antimalarials, antiemetics, oral rehydration salts, antihistamines, analgesics, throat lozenges, and medications for altitude illness (see Chapter 2, Travel Health Kits).

BIBLIOGRAPHY

1. Bartsch P, Gibbs JS. Effect of altitude on the heart and the lungs. Circulation. 2007 Nov 6;116(19): 2191–202.

2. Baumgartner RW, Siegel AM, Hackett PH. Going high with preexisting neurological conditions. High Alt Med Biol. 2007 Summer;8(2):108–16.

3. Davies AJ, Kalson NS, Stokes S, Earl MD, Whitehead AG, Frost H, et al. Determinants of summiting success and acute mountain sickness on Mt Kilimanjaro (5895 m). Wilderness Environ Med. 2009 Winter;20(4):311–7.

4. Jackson SJ, Varley J, Sellers C, Josephs K, Codrington L, Duke G, et al. Incidence and predictors of acute mountain sickness among trekkers on Mount Kilimanjaro. High Alt Med Biol. 2010 Fall;11(3):217–22.

5. Low EV, Avery AJ, Gupta V, Schedlbauer A, Grocott MP. Identifying the lowest effective dose of acetazolamide for the prophylaxis of acute mountain

4

sickness: systematic review and meta-analysis. BMJ. 2012 Oct;345:e6779.

6. Luks AM, Swenson ER. Travel to high altitude with pre-existing lung disease. Eur Respir J. 2007 Apr;29(4):770–92.

7. Luks AM, Swenson ER. Medication and dosage considerations in the prophylaxis and treatment of high-altitude illness. Chest. 2008 Mar;133(3):744–55.

8. Rimoldi SF, Sartori C, Seiler C, Delacretaz E, Mattle HP, Scherrer U, et al. High-altitude exposure in patients with cardiovascular disease: risk assessment and practical recommendations. Prog Cardiovasc Dis. 2010 May-Jun;52(6):512–24.

9. Ritchie ND, Baggott AV, Andrew Todd WT. Acetazolamide for the prevention of acute mountain sickness—a systematic review and meta-analysis. J Travel Med. 2012 Sep-Oct;19(5):298–307.

10. Shah NM, Windsor JS, Meijer H, Hillebrandt D. Are UK commercial expeditions complying with wilderness medical society guidelines on ascent rates to altitude? J Travel Med. 2011 May-Jun;18(3):214–6.

4

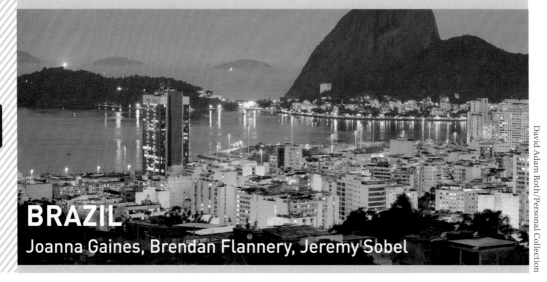

THE AMERICAS & THE CARIBBEAN

4

David Adam Roth/Personal Collection

BRAZIL

Joanna Gaines, Brendan Flannery, Jeremy Sobel

DESTINATION OVERVIEW

Brazil is the fifth largest country in the world and the largest country in South America, occupying nearly half the land area of the continent. With a population of more than 200 million, Brazil has the world's largest Portuguese-speaking population. Brazil has the world's seventh largest economy and is classified as an upper-middle-income country. The population is highly urbanized, with 84% living in urban areas.

Tourism is an important part of the Brazilian economy, and Brazil is receiving an increasing number of international visitors. In 2011, more than 5 million international visitors traveled to Brazil. Brazil hosted the World Cup in 2014 and the Summer Olympic and Paralympic Games in 2016. Brazil's beaches and natural areas are popular tourist destinations. Rio de Janeiro is Brazil's second-largest city (with a population of >6 million) and most frequently visited tourist destination for its beaches, landmarks, and annual Carnival celebration. Many of Brazil's major cities, including Salvador, Recife, Florianópolis, Fortaleza, and Natal, are tourist destinations for their beaches and regional culture. Brazil has a number of UNESCO World Heritage sites, including Iguaçu National Park in Paraná (the largest waterfalls in the Americas), historic towns of Olinda (Pernambuco), Ouro Preto (Minas Gerais), Salvador (Bahia) and Saõ Luis (Maranhão), the modern capital of Brasília, and natural areas of the Amazon forest, Pantanal Conservation Area (Mato Grosso and Mato Grosso do Sul), Atlantic forests (Rio de Janeiro and São Paulo), and the archipelago of Fernando de Noronha in the Atlantic Ocean (see Map 4-5). São Paulo, one of the world's largest cities (>20 million people in the metropolitan area), is the economic center of Brazil and the most visited destination for business travel.

HEALTH ISSUES

Vaccine-Preventable Diseases

Travelers to Brazil should be up-to-date on routine vaccines. Hepatitis A vaccination is recommended. Hepatitis B vaccination should be considered for most travelers and is recommended for those who might be exposed to blood or other body fluids, including through sexual

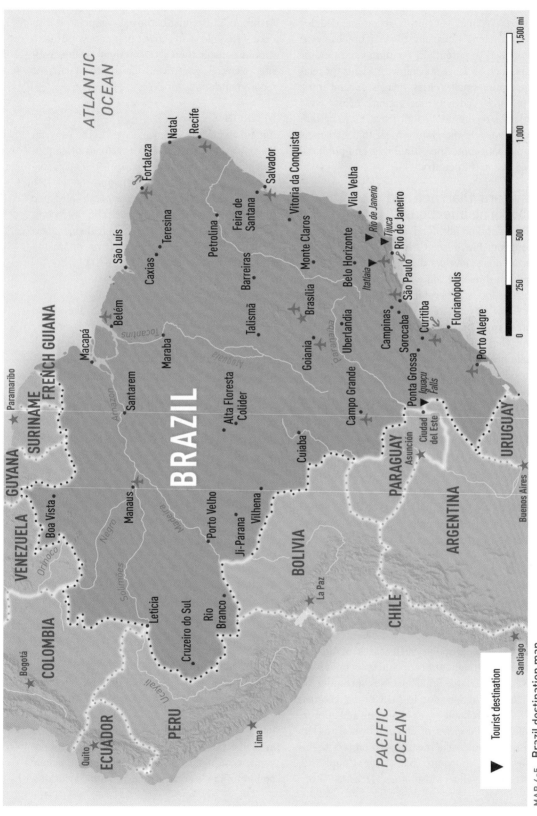

MAP 4-5. Brazil destination map

contact. Typhoid vaccine is recommended for most travelers, especially those more likely to be exposed to potentially contaminated food or water, such as those staying with friends or relatives; visiting smaller cities, villages, or rural areas; or prone to "adventurous eating." Yellow fever vaccine is recommended for travelers to certain areas, and it is therefore critical that clinicians ask patients about their itineraries and potential travel within the country.

Travelers' Diarrhea and Foodborne Infections

Travelers should take food and water precautions throughout Brazil (see Chapter 2, Food & Water Precautions). Travelers' diarrhea is the most common travel-related ailment, and travelers who consume foods or beverages from street vendors, raw fruits or vegetables, or unpasteurized dairy products are at increased risk for foodborne infections. Oral rehydration salts are available from public health clinics and in almost all pharmacies in Brazil. Clinicians may wish to prescribe an antibiotic for self-treatment of moderate to severe diarrhea (see Chapter 2, Travelers' Diarrhea).

Vectorborne Diseases

CHIKUNGUNYA, DENGUE, AND ZIKA

Vectorborne diseases, including mosquitoborne diseases, are present in many areas in Brazil; these infections are the leading causes of febrile illness among travelers returning from South America. Chikungunya, dengue, and Zika are all transmitted by *Aedes* mosquitoes, and risk is considered high in many Brazilian states because of high indices of *Aedes* infestation. Some of these vectorborne diseases are new to Brazil: chikungunya was first detected in Brazil in 2014, and Zika was first detected in Brazil in 2015.

From 2000 through 2010, cases of dengue increased throughout Brazil, and epidemics were reported from large Brazilian cities, including Rio de Janeiro and Salvador. In 2015, Brazil recorded 1.6 million probable cases of dengue and approximately 21,000 cases of chikungunya. Travelers to Brazil should take measures to protect themselves from mosquito bites (see Chapter 2, Protection against Mosquitoes, Ticks, & Other

Arthropods). Because of the risks associated with Zika virus infection during pregnancy, travelers should consult the CDC Travelers' Health website (www.cdc.gov/travel) for the most current recommendations for Zika.

Malaria

Almost all malaria in Brazil occurs in the Amazon Basin, although the mosquito vector is present in much of Brazil. *Plasmodium vivax* is the main species of malaria parasite, although approximately 15% of cases are caused by *P. falciparum*. Prophylactic treatment with antimalarial medication is recommended for travelers to malaria-endemic areas in Brazil (see Chapter 3, Yellow Fever & Malaria Information, by Country, and Map 3-21).

Yellow Fever

Yellow fever virus circulates in monkeys and is transmitted by mosquitoes throughout the Amazon Basin and in forested regions along all major river basins in Brazil, including Iguaçu Falls and as far south as Rio Grande do Sul. Vaccination against yellow fever is recommended for all travelers aged >9 months going to areas at risk of yellow fever. (See Chapter 3, Yellow Fever & Malaria Information, by Country, and Map 3-20.)

Rickettsial Disease

Several tickborne rickettsial diseases have been identified in Brazil, including febre maculosa and Brazilian spotted fever, caused by the etiologic agent of Rocky Mountain spotted fever, *Rickettsia rickettsii*. Travelers should take precautions to avoid flea and tick bites both indoors and outdoors. For more detailed information, see Chapter 2, Protection against Mosquitoes, Ticks, & Other Arthropods.

Other Infections

SEXUALLY TRANSMITTED DISEASES (STDS)

In Brazil, condoms are distributed free of charge by the government and are available in health clinics, tourist service centers, and other distribution points in many cities. Male condoms are available throughout Brazil in pharmacies, convenience stores, and large supermarkets; female condoms are also available in some locations.

4

Travelers, particularly those at high risk for acquiring HIV infection (such as men who have sex with men), may consider discussing preexposure prophylaxis with their health care provider (www.cdc.gov/hiv/prep).

RESPIRATORY DISEASES

Peak influenza circulation occurs from April through September in most of Brazil but may occur throughout the year in tropical areas. Seasonal influenza vaccination is recommended at least 2 weeks before travel. Pneumococcal vaccination is recommended for the elderly and younger adults with chronic medical conditions to prevent pneumonia complications.

A number of fungal diseases endemic to parts of Brazil, including coccidioidomycosis, histoplasmosis, paracoccidioidomycosis, and cryptococcosis, are caused by inhalation of fungal spores typically present in soil, resulting in respiratory illness and occasionally more severe disease such as meningitis or bone infection. Travelers should exercise caution before disturbing soil, particularly if it is contaminated by bird or bat feces, and should beware of bat guano in caves.

LEPTOSPIROSIS

Outbreaks of leptospirosis have occurred in urban areas in Brazil following heavy flooding. Travelers participating in recreational water activities are at increased risk, particularly after heavy rainfall or flooding.

PARASITIC INFECTIONS

Chagas' disease has been eliminated in most Brazilian states through insecticide spraying. Although risk to travelers is extremely low, outbreaks associated with contaminated food or drink have been reported, including locally prepared juice containing açái, an Amazonian fruit eaten throughout Brazil. Travelers and ecotourists staying in poor-quality housing may be at higher risk.

Schistosomiasis is found in freshwater lakes and rivers in many states of Brazil, especially in the northeast. Swimming, bathing, and wading in fresh, unchlorinated water can result in infection. Schistosomiasis is not acquired by contact with saltwater (oceans or seas).

Both cutaneous and visceral leishmaniasis occur in Brazil and are most common in the Amazon and northeast regions. The risk is highest from dusk to dawn because sand flies typically feed (bite) at night and during twilight hours. Ecotourists and adventure travelers might have an increased risk, but even short-term travelers in endemic areas have developed leishmaniasis.

RABIES

Preexposure rabies vaccination is recommended for prolonged stays, particularly for children and those planning rural travel. For shorter stays, rabies vaccination is recommended for adventure travelers, those who may be occupationally exposed to animals, and those staying in locations >24 hours from access to rabies immune globulin.

TUBERCULOSIS (TB)

Tuberculosis is prevalent in Brazil, but short-term travelers are not considered at high risk for infection unless they will be spending time in specific crowded environments. Travelers who anticipate possible prolonged exposure to people with TB because they will routinely come into contact with clinic, hospital, prison, or homeless shelter populations should have a tuberculin skin test or TB blood test before leaving the United States. If the test is negative, the traveler should have a repeat test 8–10 weeks after returning from Brazil.

Other Health and Safety Risks

As in many foreign countries, motor vehicle accidents are among the leading causes of injury and death of US citizens in Brazil. Road conditions in Brazil differ significantly from those in the United States, and driving at night can be dangerous. The national toll-free number for emergency roadside assistance is 193 (in Portuguese only). It is illegal to drive after drinking alcohol, even in small quantities. Seat belt use is mandatory in vehicles, and children aged ≤10 years must be seated in the back seat. Brazilian federal law requires car seats for all children under the age of 7.5 years. Travelers with small children (weighing <40 lb) should travel with car or booster seats, since safety seats may be limited or unavailable. Helmets are required for motorcycles.

Travelers to Brazil should familiarize themselves with climatic conditions at their destinations before travel. Temperatures >104°F (40°C) are common from October through January in some Brazilian cities (see Chapter 2, Problems with Heat & Cold).

Poisonous snakes are hazards in many locations in Brazil, although deaths from snakebites are rare. Travelers should be advised to seek immediate medical attention any time a bite wound breaks the skin or when snake venom is ejected into the eyes. Specific antivenoms are available for some snakes in some areas of Brazil, so trying to ascertain the species of snake that bit the victim may be critical.

Although travel in Brazil is generally safe, crime remains a problem in urban areas and has increased in rural areas. The incidence of crime against tourists is higher in areas surrounding beaches, hotels, nightclubs, and other tourist destinations. Drug-related violence has resulted in violent clashes with police in tourist areas. Political demonstrations may disrupt public and private transportation. Department of State advisories should be monitored for alerts in areas where travelers plan to visit. Several Brazilian cities have established specialized tourist police units to patrol areas frequented by tourists.

Health Care in Brazil

Good health care is available in most sizable Brazilian cities. Brazilian public health services are free. Foreign visitors who have health problems can seek treatment in the emergency care network of Brazil's public health system, known as the Unified Health System or by its acronym, SUS, or through private facilities. The toll-free emergency number for ambulance services throughout Brazil is 192. The website of the Brazilian Ministry of Health provides information for international visitors in English (http://portalsaude.saude.gov.br/index.php?option=com_content&view=article&id=9652&Itemid=509), including a list of reference hospitals for mass events in Brazil.

Brazil has a growing number of private clinics that offer medical procedures using advanced technologies and cater to international clientele. Travel to Brazil for cosmetic surgery, assisted reproductive technology, or other elective medical procedures has increased in recent years (see Chapter 2, Medical Tourism) and is a major medical industry in Brazil. Although Brazil has many cosmetic surgery facilities that are on par with those found in the United States, the quality of care varies widely. Patients seeking to undergo cosmetic surgery or other elective procedures in Brazil should be advised to make sure that emergency medical facilities are available.

BIBLIOGRAPHY

1. Gaines J, Sotir MJ, Cunningham TJ, Harvey KA, Lee CV, Stoney RJ, et al. Health and safety issues for travelers attending the World Cup and Summer Olympic and Paralympic Games in Brazil, 2014 to 2016. JAMA Intern Med. 2014 Aug;174(8): 1383–90.

2. Jentes ES, Poumerol G, Gershman MD, Hill DR, Lemarchand J, Lewis RF, et al. The revised global yellow fever risk map and recommendations for vaccination, 2010: consensus of the Informal WHO Working Group on Geographic Risk for Yellow Fever. Lancet Infect Dis. 2011 Aug;11(8):622–32.

3. Malaria Atlas Project. The spatial limits of *Plasmodium vivax* malaria transmission map in 2010 in Brazil. [cited 2016 Sep. 23]; Available from: http://www.map.ox.ac.uk/explore/countries/BRA/.

4. Nobrega AA, Garcia MH, Tatto E, Obara MT, Costa E, Sobel J, et al. Oral transmission of Chagas disease by consumption of acai palm fruit, Brazil. Emerg Infect Dis. 2009 Apr;15(4):653–5.

5. Oliveira-Ferreira J, Lacerda MV, Brasil P, Ladislau JL, Tauil PL, Daniel-Ribeiro CT. Malaria in Brazil: an overview. Malar J. 2010 Apr 30;9:115.

6. Teixeira MG, Siqueira JB Jr, Ferreira GL, Bricks L, Joint G. Epidemiological trends of dengue disease in Brazil (2000–2010): a systematic literature search and analysis. PLoS Negl Trop Dis. 2013 Dec 19;7(12):e2520.

7. Wilson ME, Chen LH, Han PV, Keystone JS, Cramer JP, Segurado A, et al. Illness in travelers returned from Brazil: the GeoSentinel experience and implications for the 2014 FIFA World Cup and the 2016 Summer Olympics. Clin Infect Dis 2014 May;58(10):1347–56.

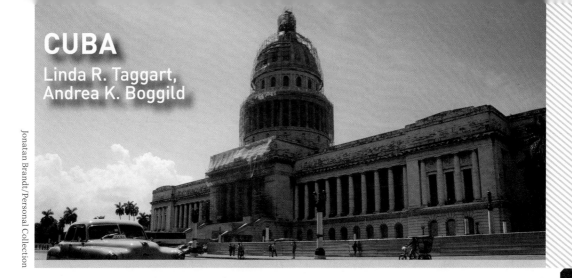

Jonatan Brandt/Personal Collection

CUBA
Linda R. Taggart,
Andrea K. Boggild

4

DESTINATION OVERVIEW

The Republic of Cuba is a Caribbean island located between the Caribbean Sea and the North Atlantic Ocean, approximately 90 miles (145 km) south of Key West, Florida. It is the largest country in the Caribbean and has a population of 11 million people. The official language is Spanish. The climate is tropical, with a dry season from November to April and a rainy season from May to October. Originally inhabited by a native Amerindian population, it was colonized by the Spanish in the 15th century. In 1898, Cuba gained independence from Spain, with the assistance of the United States, and then gained independence from the United States in 1902. In 1959, a revolutionary army under Fidel Castro overthrew the government and established a communist state. A US embargo has been in place since 1961; however, since December 2014, efforts have been made by the United States to reestablish diplomatic relations with Cuba. Although tourist travel to Cuba is still prohibited under US law, 12 categories of travel are now authorized, including family visits, professional research and meetings, and humanitarian projects.

Although out of reach of most US citizens for years, Cuba has long been a popular travel destination for Canadians and Europeans. The largest and most popular resort area is in Varadero, a peninsula with a vast, 13-mile stretch of sandy beach and more than 50 hotels. Those seeking to experience Cuban culture often travel to the nearby capital city of Havana to explore the streets of La Habana Vieja (Old Havana) or walk along the sea wall, the Malecon. Another popular destination is Trinidad, a colonial city known for its cobblestone streets (see Map 4-6). Throughout the country, tourists can enjoy the sight of vintage cars and sample Cuban cigars, rum, and mojitos.

HEALTH ISSUES

Vaccine-Preventable Diseases

Travelers should confirm that routine vaccinations are up-to-date, including seasonal influenza vaccine. Hepatitis A vaccine is recommended for non-immune travelers. Vaccination against hepatitis B should also be considered for most travelers, especially those who may be exposed to blood or body fluids, including those intending to do medical work or those who may seek medical treatment, obtain tattoos or piercings, use injection drugs, or have sex. Typhoid vaccination is recommended for most travelers, especially visitors of friends and relatives, those traveling to rural areas, and those likely to partake in "adventurous eating." Rabies vaccine is recommended for travelers who may be in contact with dogs, bats, or other mammals; travelers who expect to have occupational exposure to animals; and long-term travelers. Although extremely rare in travelers, cholera is a possible risk in parts of Cuba. Cholera vaccine is recommended for adult travelers visiting areas with cholera activity within the last year that are prone to recurrence of cholera epidemics.

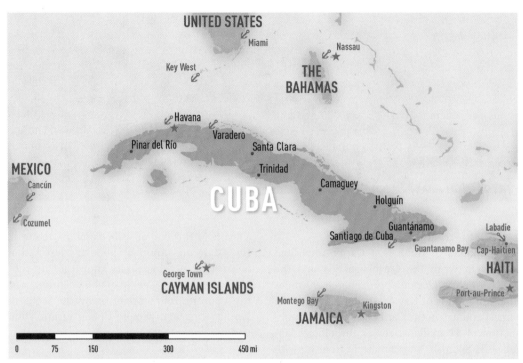

MAP 4-6. Cuba destination map

Vectorborne Diseases

Dengue is a risk in Cuba, and travelers should take precautions against mosquitoes, which include using insect repellents and wearing pants and long-sleeved shirts (see Chapter 2, Protection against Mosquitoes, Ticks, & Other Arthropods). Despite the large chikungunya outbreak that started in late 2013 and involved the entire region, Cuban authorities did not report any cases of local transmission. The first cases of local vectorborne Zika virus transmission were reported in Cuba in 2016, which emphasizes the need for mosquito precautions. Because of the risks to pregnancy, travelers should consult the CDC Travelers' Health website for the most current recommendations for Zika.

Other Health and Safety Risks

FOOD AND WATER SAFETY

Those traveling to Cuba are at risk of travelers' diarrhea, even when staying at resorts. Travelers should be reminded to avoid raw or undercooked meat and seafood as well as unpasteurized dairy products. Salads and uncooked vegetables should be avoided, and fruit should only be eaten if washed in clean water or peeled by the traveler. Travelers should drink only bottled water or water that has been boiled, filtered, or treated. Consideration should also be given to prescribing an antibiotic for self-treatment of moderate to severe diarrhea, especially given the lack of easy accessibility of these drugs in Cuba. Cholera spread to Cuba in 2012 as a result of the outbreak in Haiti that began in 2010. There continue to be cases reported, including at least 65 in 2015. The risk to travelers is low; however, food and water precautions should be followed, and cholera vaccine may be considered. Ciguatera fish poisoning is found in tropical and subtropical areas surrounded by coral reefs and is known to occur in Cuba. Travelers should be advised to avoid or limit consumption of large reef fish, including their viscera, especially species such as grouper, snapper, barracuda, jack, sturgeon, sea bass, and moray eel.

SUN, SAND, AND WATER HAZARDS

Care should be taken to avoid excess sun exposure. Visitors should apply sunscreen of SPF ≥15 that protects against both UVA and UVB, wear protective clothing, and seek shade when possible. Travelers to the Caribbean are at risk of cutaneous larva migrans from lying or walking on soil, including sandy beaches. Risk can be minimized by wearing shoes and avoiding lying directly on sand. Marine envenomations by jellyfish, microscopic cnidarians causing sea bather's eruption, sea urchins, and stingrays can occur in the warm shallow waters surrounding many resort areas.

SAFETY AND SECURITY

Road conditions are often dangerous. The Carretera Central (main east-west highway) is in good condition but lacks lighting, and road signs are often inadequate or confusing. Travelers should avoid driving outside urban areas at night. Cars in Cuba are often old and may lack basic safety features such as reliable brakes and turn signals. Tourist company buses and radio-dispatched taxis are generally safe and reliable. Travelers should fasten seat belts when riding in cars and wear a helmet when riding bicycles or motorbikes. Unlicensed taxis and yellow 3-wheeled "coco taxis" should be avoided. Thefts may occur, especially in crowded locations such as beaches, markets, Old Town Havana, and the Prado neighborhood. These are usually nonviolent, but there is some concern that violent crime is increasing, and travelers should not resist if confronted.

MEDICAL CARE

Health care may not meet American standards. Medical professionals are generally well trained; however, medical supplies and certain medications may be unavailable. Travelers should bring adequate supplies of prescription and nonprescription medications. Personal hygiene products are also not as readily available as they are elsewhere in the Caribbean.

BIBLIOGRAPHY

1. Boggild AK, Geduld J, Libman M, Ward BJ, McCarthy AE, Doyle PW, et al. Travel-acquired infections and illnesses in Canadians: surveillance report from CanTravNet surveillance data, 2009–2011. Open Med. 2014 Feb 11;8(1):e20–32.

2. Fillion K, Mileno MD. Cholera in travelers: shifting tides in epidemiology, management, and prevention. Curr Infect Dis Rep. 2015 Jan;17(1):455.

3. Morrison K, Aguiar Prieto P, Castro Domínguez A, Waltner-Toews D, FitzGibbon J. Ciguatera fish poisoning in La Habana, Cuba: a study of local social–ecological resilience. EcoHealth. 2008 Sep;5(3):346–59.

4. The World Factbook. Central Intelligence Agency; 2016 [updated Feb. 2016; cited 2016 Feb. 13]; Available from: https://www.cia.gov/library/publications/the-world-factbook/.

5. U.S. Department of State. US passport and international travel: Cuba. 2015 [updated Oct. 2015; cited 2016 Jan. 31]; Available from: https://travel.state.gov/content/passports/en/country/cuba.html.

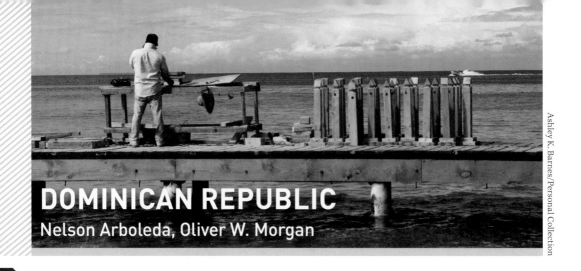

DOMINICAN REPUBLIC

Nelson Arboleda, Oliver W. Morgan

Ashley K. Barnes/Personal Collection

4

DESTINATION OVERVIEW

The Dominican Republic covers the eastern two-thirds of the Caribbean island of Hispaniola; the other third is covered by Haiti. It is the second largest Caribbean nation, both by area and population. The capital city, Santo Domingo, is located on the southern coast of the island (see Map 4-7). Spanish is the official language, although English is spoken in most tourist areas. More than 100,000 American citizens live in the Dominican Republic, and in 2015 it was the most visited destination in the Caribbean, with more than 5 million foreign tourists including approximately 3 million from the United States or Canada.

The Dominican Republic offers a diverse geography of beaches, mountain ranges (including the highest point in the Caribbean, Pico Duarte [10,164 ft; 3,098 m]), sugar cane and tobacco plantations, and farming areas. The average temperature ranges from 73.5°F (23°F) in January to 80°F (26.5°F) in August. The island receives more rain from May through November, and tropical storms or hurricanes are a possibility. Most of the tourism is concentrated in the east of the country around Punta Cana, which offers all-inclusive beach resorts. Whale watching is popular seasonally near the northeastern area in Samana, and kite- and wind-surfing attract visitors to the northern areas of Puerto Plata, Sosua, and Cabarete. A small number of travelers visit other parts of the country, where tourist infrastructure is limited or nonexistent. The capital city, Santo Domingo, has an attractive colonial district that contains many historical sites dating back to Christopher Columbus's arrival in the New World. A highway completed in 2014 connects Punta Cana to Santo Domingo and is expected to increase tourism in the capital.

HEALTH ISSUES

Vaccine-Preventable Diseases

All travelers should be up-to-date on routine vaccinations, including seasonal influenza. Cases of vaccine-preventable diseases have been reported among the local population and unvaccinated tourists from Europe and other parts of the world.

Travelers should also be vaccinated against hepatitis A and, depending upon the traveler's itinerary and activities, typhoid—especially those who are staying with friends or family. Hepatitis B vaccine is recommended for people who might be exposed to blood through needles or medical procedures or bodily fluids during sexual intercourse with a new partner.

Cases of rabies among animals continue to be reported in the Dominican Republic, and several human cases of rabies have been reported over the past few years. In 2015, there were 80 cases of animal rabies and 2 human rabies cases. Travelers potentially at risk for animal bites (such as those undertaking outdoor pursuits, working with or around animals, taking long trips or moving to the Dominican Republic, or children who may play with animals) should be vaccinated against rabies before travel.

Although cholera was reintroduced to the Dominican Republic in 2010, disease transmission is mostly limited to poor, urban areas or certain rural communities. Although extremely

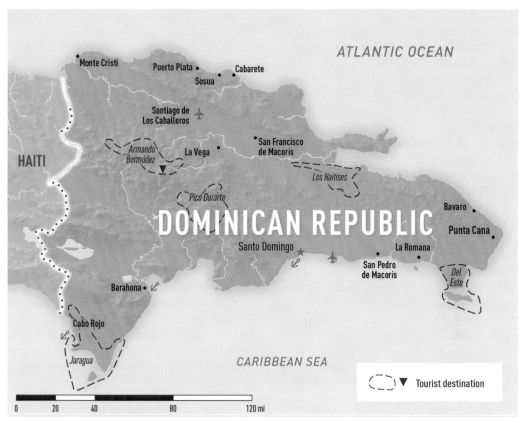

MAP 4-7. Dominican Republic destination map

rare in travelers, cholera is a possible risk in parts of the Dominican Republic. Cholera vaccine is recommended for adult travelers visiting an area with cholera activity within the last year that is prone to recurrence of cholera epidemics.

HIV and Other Sexually Transmitted Diseases

Commercial sex work occurs throughout the Dominican Republic, and some locations, such as Sosua and Puerto Plata, are known as sex tourism destinations. HIV prevalence among female commercial sex workers is as high as 6% in some areas; syphilis (12%), hepatitis B virus (2.4%), and hepatitis C virus (0.9%) are also concerns. Among men who have sex with men, HIV prevalence is as high as 6.9% and active syphilis as high as 13.9%. Travelers should avoid sexual intercourse with commercial sex workers and always use condoms with any partner whose HIV or sexually transmitted disease status is unknown.

Vectorborne Diseases

Zika, chikungunya, dengue, and malaria are potential concerns for travelers to the Dominican Republic. All travelers should take precautions to prevent mosquito bites by wearing long-sleeved shirts and long pants and using insect repellent. See Chapter 2, Protection against Mosquitoes, Ticks, & Other Arthropods for more information.

The malaria in the Dominican Republic is not drug-resistant. CDC recommends that travelers to the Dominican Republic take malaria chemoprophylaxis unless they are only visiting the urban areas of Santiago or Santo Domingo. Dengue is widespread throughout the Dominican Republic; 16,871 cases were reported in 2015, of which 103 were fatal (case-fatality ratio, 0.61). Although cases of dengue are reported year-round, transmission frequently increases during the rainy season from May through November. The mosquito vector for dengue is found in urban as well as rural areas. Chikungunya was introduced to the Dominican Republic in 2014.

The first cases of local vectorborne Zika virus transmission were reported in the Dominican Republic in 2016, which emphasizes the need for mosquito precautions. Because of the risks to pregnancy, travelers should consult the CDC Travelers' Health website (www.cdc.gov/travel) for the most current recommendations for Zika.

Food and Water Safety

Travelers should only drink water that is purified or bottled. Ice served in well-established tourist locations is usually made from purified water and safe to consume. However, ice may not be safe in remote or nontourist areas. Food hygiene at large, all-inclusive, and popular tourist locations has improved over the last few years. However, travelers' diarrhea continues to be the most common problem for visitors to the Dominican Republic. Food purchased on the street or sold on beaches by informal sellers presents a higher risk of illness. Tourists are advised not to eat raw or undercooked seafood in the Dominican Republic.

Sun and Heat Safety

Visitors to the Dominican Republic often underestimate the strength of the sun and the dehydrating effect of the humid environment. Visitors should take precautions to avoid sunburn by wearing hats and suitable clothing, along with proper application of a broad-spectrum sunscreen with an SPF ≥15 that protects against both UVA and UVB. Travelers should also drink plenty of fluids throughout the day.

Safety and Security

Driving in the Dominican Republic is hazardous. Traffic laws are rarely enforced, and drivers commonly drive while intoxicated, text while driving, exceed speed limits, do not respect red lights or stop signs, and drive without seatbelts or helmets. The Dominican Republic has among the highest number of traffic deaths per capita in the world (41.7 per 100,000 population). Many fatal or serious traffic crashes involve motorcycles and pedestrians. Motorcycle taxis, which are used throughout the country, including in tourist areas, frequently carry 2 or more passengers without helmets. Visitors should avoid motorcycle taxis, use only licensed taxis, and always wear a seatbelt.

Foreign tourists may become victims of crime in the Dominican Republic. The risks are similar to most major US cities. Although much crime affecting tourists involves robbery or pickpocketing, more serious assaults occasionally occur, and criminals may react violently if resisted. Visitors to the Dominican Republic should follow normal precautions such as going out in groups, especially at night; using only licensed taxi drivers; drinking alcohol in moderation; and being cautious of strangers. Criminal activity is often higher in the Christmas and New Year season, and additional caution is advised during those months.

MEDICAL TOURISM

The market for medical tourism, including plastic surgery and dental care, is growing in the Dominican Republic and attracts thousands of patients each year to access medical services that cost a fraction of what they do in the United States. Several companies and clinics offer package deals that include postsurgical recovery at a tourist resort. Most health care facilities catering to medical tourists in the Dominican Republic have not met the standards required by international accreditation organizations. Outbreaks of health care–associated infections, medical malpractice, and even deaths have been reported among foreign visitors traveling to the Dominican Republic for medical tourism. People considering traveling to the Dominican Republic for medical procedures, including plastic surgery or dental care, should consult with a health care provider before travel and consider whether foreign health care providers meet quality standards of care (see Chapter 2, Medical Tourism).

BIBLIOGRAPHY

1. Banco Central de la República Dominicana [Internet]. Estadísticas económicas: sector turismo. Santo Domingo (Dominican Republic): Banco Central de la República Dominicana.; c2012 [cited 2016 Sep. 23]; Available from: http://www.bancentral.gov.do/estadisticas_economicas/turismo/.

2. CDC. Dengue fever among US travelers returning from the Dominican Republic – Minnesota and Iowa, 2008. MMWR Morb Mortal Wkly Rep. 2010 Jun 4;59(21):654–6.

3. CDC. Notes from the field: rapidly growing nontuberculous *Mycobacterium* wound infections among medical tourists undergoing cosmetic surgeries in the Dominican Republic—multiple states, March 2013–February 2014. MMWR Morb Mortal Wkly Rep. 2014 Mar 7;63(9):201–2.

4. CONAVIHSIDA (Consejo Nacional para el VIH y sida). Segunda encuesta de vigilancia de comportamiento con vinculación serológica en poblaciones claves. Gais, trans y hombres que tienen sexo con hombres (GTH) trabajadoras sexuales (TRSX) usuarios de drogas (UD), 2012. Santo Domingo (Dominican Republic): CONAVIHSIDA; 2014 [cited 2016 Sep. 23]; Available from: http://countryoffice.unfpa.org/dominicanrepublic/drive/CONAVIHSIDASegundaEncuestaVigiliancia.pdf. Spanish.

5. Dirección General de Epidemiología [Internet]. Sistema nacional de vigilancia epidemiológica, boletín semanal 2013. Santo Domingo (Dominican Republic)2014 [updated Sep. 2014 ; cited 2016 Sep. 23]; Available from: http://digepisalud.gob.do/boletines/boletines-semanales/cat_view/34-boletines-semanales/108-2013.html. Spanish.

6. World Health Organization. Global status report on road safety 2013: supporting a decade of action. Geneva: 2013 Sep 22. Available from: http://www.who.int/violence_injury_prevention/road_safety_status/2013/en/.

4

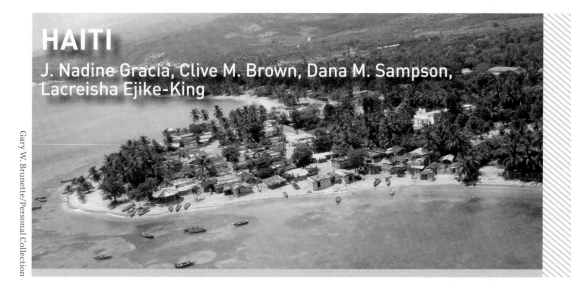

HAITI

J. Nadine Gracia, Clive M. Brown, Dana M. Sampson, Lacreisha Ejike-King

Gary W. Brunette/Personal Collection

DESTINATION OVERVIEW

Nestled between the Caribbean Sea and the Atlantic Ocean, the Republic of Haiti occupies the western third of the island of Hispaniola, with the Dominican Republic on the eastern two-thirds of the island (Map 4-8). Originally inhabited by the native Taíno, *Ayiti* ("land of high mountains") was introduced to European influence through periods of Spanish and French colonization from the 15th through 18th centuries. After a successful slave rebellion in 1804, Haiti became the first independent black republic in the Western Hemisphere, the first independent state in the Caribbean, and the second independent state in the Western Hemisphere after the United States.

Although it was once the wealthiest French colony in the Caribbean because of its natural resources and products such as sugar, rum, coffee, cotton,

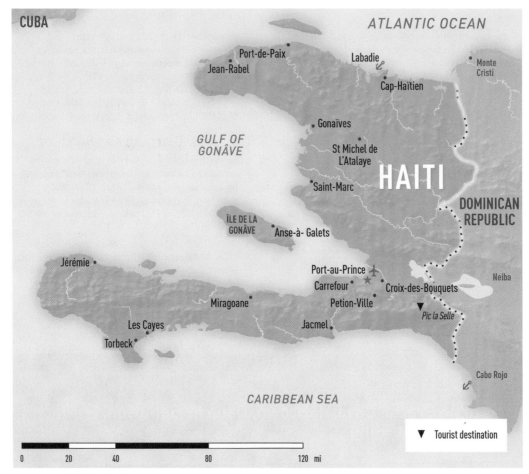

MAP 4-8. Haiti destination map

wood, and lumber, Haiti has experienced considerable environmental degradation due to deforestation, poor agricultural practices, and soil erosion. It is reported to be the poorest country in the Western Hemisphere, having suffered from political and economic instability for most of its history.

French and Creole are the official languages of the country. French is the principal written and administratively authorized language. It is the medium of instruction in most schools. Most (approximately 90%) of Haiti's 10.3 million people, however, use Creole as their primary language. Because of the mix of indigenous, African, and European influences, Haiti possesses a "mosaic culture" that is reflected in local art, music, and cuisine.

Once called the Pearl of the Antilles because of its natural beauty, Haiti is home to a vibrant and diverse landscape that includes beaches, waterfalls, caves, and the most mountains of any nation in the Caribbean. The people of Haiti are known for their resilience, strength, and warm and kind spirit, leaving travelers to often say after a visit to Haiti that they have fallen in love with the country and its people.

HEALTH ISSUES

Haiti has suffered significant environmental degradation, contributing to poor sanitation and water quality. As a result, various public health risks exist for Haitians and for people traveling to Haiti.

Vaccine-Preventable Diseases

All people traveling to Haiti should be up-to-date on routine vaccinations, including seasonal influenza and booster doses to protect against tetanus and diphtheria. Diphtheria is endemic in Haiti, and the number of reported cases has increased in recent years. Additionally, hepatitis A vaccine and typhoid are strongly recommended, especially if travelers are staying with friends or relatives or visiting smaller cities or rural areas. Providers should also consider administering hepatitis B vaccine. Rabies affects Haiti more than any other nation in the Americas. Prevention efforts have decreased the number of human cases of rabies transmitted by dogs, but deaths continue to be reported in Haiti. Rabies vaccination is recommended for travelers anticipating contact with animals. Yellow fever vaccination is required for people traveling from countries where the disease is endemic. Although extremely rare in travelers, cholera is a possible risk in parts of Haiti. Cholera vaccine is recommended for adult travelers visiting areas with cholera activity within the last year that are prone to recurrence of cholera epidemics.

Vectorborne Diseases

Vectorborne diseases are common in Haiti and include *Plasmodium falciparum* malaria, dengue, chikungunya, and Zika. Travelers to Haiti should take measures to protect themselves from mosquito bites (see Chapter 2, Protection against Mosquitoes, Ticks, & Other Arthropods).

MALARIA

P. falciparum malaria is endemic in Haiti. The incidence of malaria in Haiti is approximately 1,278 per 100,000 people annually. Highest transmission rates are reported to occur after the rainy seasons from March through May and October through November. Travelers are advised to begin malaria prophylaxis before travel. Suggested prophylactic medications for people traveling to Haiti include atovaquone-proguanil, chloroquine, doxycycline, or mefloquine.

DENGUE, CHIKUNGUNYA, AND ZIKA

Dengue is endemic in the Caribbean, including Haiti. Cases of dengue have been reported among military personnel and US missionaries; 240 cases were reported in 2014 alone. Chikungunya virus transmission was first reported in Haiti in May 2014, and the incidence rate is reported as 627 per 100,000 population.

Local transmission of Zika virus was confirmed in January 2016. Because of the serious consequences of Zika infection during pregnancy, travelers should consult the CDC Travelers' Health website (www.cdc.gov/travel) to obtain the most current recommendations for travel to Haiti.

Travelers' Diarrhea and Food- or Water-Related Diseases

Travelers to Haiti will want to experience the local, flavorful cuisine, such as rice with red beans, plantains, *griot* (seasoned, fried pork), and a variety of fish and shellfish, including conch. While enjoying the incredible Haitian cuisine, travelers should select food and beverages carefully (see Chapter 2, Food & Water Precautions). Travelers' diarrhea is a significant risk in Haiti, and travelers are at additional risk of contracting hepatitis A and typhoid fever.

CHOLERA

A severe cholera outbreak followed the earthquake in 2010, causing 700,000 cases of illness and 8,500 deaths that year. Incidence and mortality rates have declined each subsequent year as a result of improved access to clean water and sanitation, as well as the operations of cholera treatment centers. In 2014, there were 27,750 reported cholera cases and 296 reported deaths. Use of oral cholera vaccine has also been implemented as part of a complementary set of ongoing treatment and control measures. Travelers are urged to adhere to food and water precautions, and cholera vaccine may be considered.

LEPTOSPIROSIS

Leptospirosis is endemic in the Caribbean. Haiti may pose a higher risk than other areas because of recurring natural disasters such as tropical storms or flooding. Many cases have been reported in Haiti since the 2010 earthquake. The incidence of leptospirosis is highest during the rainy season. The disease can be transmitted from contact with the urine or tissues of an infected animal or with water or soil tainted by the urine of an infected animal. Travelers are advised to avoid freshwater (such as streams or lakes) that may be contaminated by animal urine.

4

Physical Concerns for the Traveler

MOTOR VEHICLE SAFETY

Motor vehicle crashes are the most common cause of death for healthy Americans traveling abroad. The risk of death from road injuries in Haiti is high; the 2013 rate was 945 per 100,000 population, compared with an average rate of 721 for the region. Road conditions in Haiti are significantly different from those in the United States: roads and lanes are generally unmarked, speed limits are seldom posted or adhered to, right of way is not widely observed, a variety of people and objects may appear on roads (such as carts, animals, and vendors), and roads may be unpaved or have large potholes. The main roads have been cleared of rubble from the 2010 earthquake, although some rubble remains in certain areas. Traffic is usually chaotic and congested in urban areas. *Tap taps* (vibrantly painted buses or pick-up trucks that serve as share taxis in Haiti but are open-air vehicles that are often overloaded with passengers and not mechanically sound) are a common form of public transportation for Haitians but are not recommended for visitors to the country because of safety concerns (such as crashes, robbery, or kidnapping). Travelers can exercise safety while traveling in Haiti by keeping alert when traveling on foot, choosing safe vehicles, and observing safety practices when operating vehicles. Travelers should fasten seat belts when riding in cars and wear a helmet when riding bicycles or motorbikes.

CRIME

The crime rate in Haiti is high, particularly in the capital of Port-au-Prince, which presents persistent safety concerns for travelers. Although much of the violent crime is perpetuated by Haitians on other Haitians, American citizens have also been victims of crime. Travelers arriving from US flights have been targeted for attack and robbery. Crime, disorderly conduct, and general congestion of local areas increase during Carnival. Travelers are advised to exercise caution throughout their trip including keeping valuables well hidden, ensuring possessions are not left in parked vehicles, keeping doors and windows in homes and vehicles closed and locked, avoiding nighttime travel, and remaining alert.

NATURAL DISASTERS

Natural disasters common to Haiti include tropical storms, flooding, hurricanes, and earthquakes. Haiti experiences 2 rainy seasons, from April through June and from October through November. Hurricane season lasts from June through November. In 2008, Haiti experienced a series of 4 hurricanes and tropical storms within 2 months.

In January 2010, Haiti experienced a 7.0 magnitude earthquake. More than 220,000 people died, and 1.5 million people were displaced from their homes. Multiple powerful aftershocks added to the widespread devastation and destruction. As a result, the health, emergency response, and safety infrastructure in the nation was significantly weakened; the country's infrastructure remains largely underdeveloped after the earthquake.

DISCLOSURE

Lacreisha Ejike-King is an employee of the US Food and Drug Administration (FDA); views expressed in this chapter are those of the authors and do not necessarily reflect the official policy or position of the FDA.

BIBLIOGRAPHY

1. Brown C, Ripp J, Kazura J. Perspectives on Haiti two years after the earthquake. Am J Trop Med Hyg. 2012 Jan;86(1):5–6.

2. CDC. Malaria in post-earthquake Haiti: CDC's recommendations for prevention and treatment. Atlanta: CDC; 2010 [cited 2016 Sep. 23]; Available from: http://www.cdc.gov/malaria/resources/pdf/new_info/2010/malaria-1-pager_dec3v1_508.pdf.

3. CDC. Dengue virus infections among travelers returning from Haiti—Georgia and Nebraska, October 2010. MMWR Morb Mortal Wkly Rep. 2011 Jul 15;60(27):914–7.

4. Dowell SF, Tappero JW, Frieden TR. Public health in Haiti—challenges and progress. N Engl J Med. 2011 Jan 27;364(4):300–1.

5. Institute for Health Metrics and Evaluation. Country Profile: Haiti. IHME; [cited 2016 Mar. 10]; Available from: http://www.healthdata.org/haiti.

6. Pan American Health Organization/World Health Organization (PAHO/WHO), Epidemiological Week/

EW 52. Number of reported cases of chikungunya fever in the Americas, by country or territory 2013–2014. Washington, DC: 2014 Dec 29. Available from: http://www.paho.org/hq/index.php?option=com_topics&view=readall&cid=5927&Itemid=40931&lang=en.

7. Pan American Health Organization/World Health Organization (PAHO/WHO), Health Information and Analysis Project (HSD/HA). Health situation in the Americas: basic indicators, 2014. Washington, DC: 2014. Available from: http://www.paho.org/hq/index.php?option=com_docman&task=doc_view&gid=27299&Itemid=721.

8. United Nations Development Programme (UNDP) Human Development Report Office. Human development report 2013. The rise of the South: human progress in a diverse world. New York: 2013 Sep 22. Available from: http://hdr.undp.org/en/2013-report.

9. World Food Programme [Internet]. Haiti overview. Port au Prince (Haiti): World Food Programme; c2014 [cited 2016 Sep. 23]; Available from: http://www.wfp.org/countries/haiti/overview.

10. World Health Organization. Countries: Haiti Country Profile. WHO; [cited 2016 Sep. 23]; Available from: http://www.who.int/countries/hti/en/.

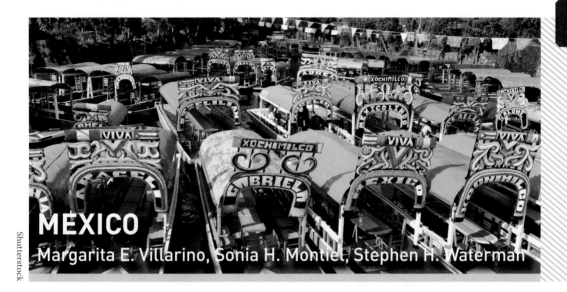

4

MEXICO
Margarita E. Villarino, Sonia H. Montiel, Stephen H. Waterman

Shutterstock

DESTINATION OVERVIEW

Mexico, the second most populous country in Latin America, has a population of more than 120 million, and 78% live in urban areas. The United States' second-largest agricultural trading partner and third-largest trading partner overall, Mexico is now considered a middle-income country with the world's 15th-largest economy. Mexico has a rich history and proud culture that reflect its pre-Columbian civilizations and Hispanic heritage. With one-fifth the area of the United States (about 3 times the size of Texas), Mexico has diverse geographic features within its 32 states. The Sonoran desert is in the northwest, beautiful beaches are available on both coasts, and forested mountain ranges traverse the western and eastern mainland. Impressive volcanic peaks rise up to 18,000 feet above the high central plateau. The

Yucatán Peninsula and southern regions are tropical. The Copper Canyon in the northwestern state of Chihuahua is larger than the US Grand Canyon. (See Map 4-9).

Mexico City is one of the world's largest cities, with a population of more than 20 million. Despite increasing national prosperity, Mexico's large cities contain much poverty. Extensive migration has taken place from the poor rural south to the northern border for jobs in bustling border cities, such as Ciudad Juárez and Tijuana.

Mexico has the most foreign visitors of any Latin American country and is the country most frequently visited by US tourists. Travel to beach resorts such as Acapulco, Ixtapa, Cancún, Puerto Peñasco, Cozumel, Puerto Vallarta, Nuevo Vallarta, and Cabo San Lucas, along with cruise ship tours, makes up a large

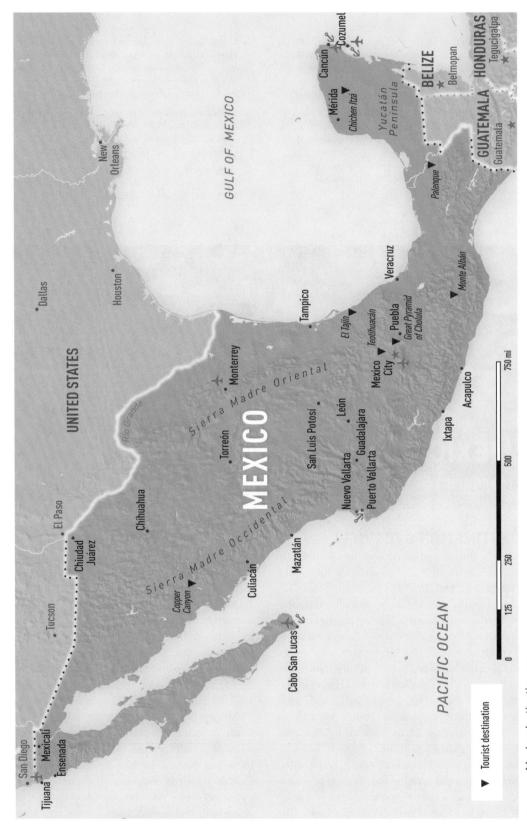

MAP 4-9. Mexico destination map

portion of tourism to Mexico. Also common are day trips to northern border cities and longer cultural trips to historical and World Heritage sites. Popular pre-Columbian anthropologic destinations include Teotihuacan outside Mexico City, Great Pyramid of Cholula in Puebla, Tulum and Cobá in Quintana Roo, El Tajín in Veracruz, Chichen Itzá in Yucatán, Monte Alban in Oaxaca, and Palenque in Chiapas. Baja California offers whale watching on the Pacific Coast and sports fishing in the Gulf of California.

A large number of US residents travel to Mexico to receive health services (medical tourism). Only Thailand sees a higher number of US travelers for this purpose. The main services sought are dental services, eye care, and cosmetic surgery in the border cities. Increasingly, a complete range of services and specialized procedures are offered in cities with large medical services infrastructure, such as Mexico City, Monterrey, Mérida, Cancún, and Guadalajara (see Chapter 2, Medical Tourism).

HEALTH ISSUES

Vaccine-Preventable Diseases

All travelers should be up-to-date with their routine immunizations. Hepatitis A is endemic in Mexico, and all travelers should be immunized with at least the first dose of hepatitis A vaccine before travel to Mexico. Hepatitis B vaccine should be considered for all travelers and is recommended especially for those with expected long-term stays (≥6 months), those who plan to use medical services, or who might be exposed to blood or other body fluids (including through sexual contact). Other vaccines, such as typhoid and rabies, may be considered, especially for those visitors (such as field biologists, nature adventure tourists) who will be traveling to less developed, remote areas of the country.

RABIES

Travelers should be educated on how to avoid animal bites to reduce the risk of rabies. In Mexico, the most common animal species that carry rabies are unvaccinated dogs or cats and wild animals such as bats, coatis, coyotes, foxes, and skunks. Preexposure rabies vaccination should be considered for travelers who are likely to come into contact with these animals or those who will be traveling to areas with limited access to medical care.

Travelers' Diarrhea and Other Foodborne and Waterborne Infections

Travelers' diarrhea is common among visitors to Mexico. In addition to practicing food and water precautions, travelers should consider bringing an antibiotic for self-treatment of diarrhea (see the Food & Water Precautions and Travelers' Diarrhea sections in Chapter 2). Travelers should keep in mind that tap water is not potable and should avoid consuming raw dairy products, undercooked meat or fish, leafy greens, or raw vegetables. Foodborne infections that are a risk in Mexico include amebiasis, cysticercosis, brucellosis, listeriosis, and infections with *Mycobacterium bovis*. Cholera is considered a low risk in Mexico; however, travelers should adhere to food and water precautions.

Vectorborne Diseases

DENGUE, CHIKUNGUNYA, AND ZIKA

Dengue is endemic throughout Mexico, and large outbreaks of dengue have been reported. Dengue virus transmission should be considered a risk year-round. Chikungunya was first reported in Mexico in 2014, and Zika was first reported in 2015. Travelers should take steps to prevent mosquito bites by using insect repellent, wearing long-sleeved shirts and long pants, and staying in accommodations that are well screened or air conditioned (see Chapter 2, Protection against Mosquitoes, Ticks, & Other Arthropods). Because of the risks to pregnancy, travelers should consult the CDC Travelers' Health website (www.cdc.gov/travel) for the most current recommendations for Zika.

MALARIA

Malaria incidence has decreased dramatically in recent decades in Mexico, and risk of infection with *Plasmodium vivax* among US travelers is considered very low. Major resorts are free of malaria, as is the US–Mexico border region. Malaria prophylaxis is recommended for travelers to Campeche, Chiapas, Chihuahua, Nayarit, and Sinaloa. Mosquito avoidance but not chemoprophylaxis is recommended for travelers to Durango, Jalisco, Oaxaca, Sonora, Tabasco, and Othón P. Blanco municipality of Quintana Roo.

RICKETTSIAL DISEASE

Rickettsial diseases found in Mexico include Rocky Mountain spotted fever, which is potentially fatal unless treated promptly with antibiotics, and fleaborne typhus, which usually causes symptoms that are similar to dengue. Travelers should take precautions to avoid flea and tick bites both indoors and outside. Rocky Mountain spotted fever associated with *Rhipicephalus sanguineus*, the brown dog tick, has been identified recently in northern Mexico in urban and rural areas with large stray dog populations.

PARASITIC INFECTIONS

Cutaneous leishmaniasis, transmitted by sand flies, is found in focal areas of coastal and southern Mexico. The risk is higher for ecotourists, field biologists, and long-term travelers. Travelers should prevent fly bites, which includes avoiding outdoor activities at night. Travelers to beach areas may be at risk for cutaneous larva migrans (CLM), a creeping skin eruption most commonly associated with dog hookworm infection. CLM can be prevented by wearing shoes and avoiding direct skin contact with sand. Chagas disease is endemic throughout Mexico.

Other Infections

RESPIRATORY DISEASES

Influenza virus strains similar to those in the United States circulate in Mexico, as was demonstrated by the emergence of pandemic influenza A (H1N1) in North America in the spring of 2009. Coccidioidomycosis, a fungal respiratory disease caused by inhaling spores in the soil, is endemic in northwestern Mexico. Several outbreaks of coccidioidomycosis have been reported among missionary groups from the United States doing construction projects in this region. Histoplasmosis, another fungal respiratory disease agent found in soil, is endemic in other regions of Mexico, mainly the central and southeast regions. Although cases of legionellosis are reported worldwide, CDC has investigated travel-associated clusters of legionellosis in association with hotels and resorts in Mexico. Legionellosis should be considered in elderly and immunocompromised travelers who develop pneumonia within 14 days of travel.

TUBERCULOSIS (TB)

Mexico's TB incidence is lower than rates in Asia, Africa, and Eastern Europe, but is 5 times that of the United States. The potential risk of exposure and infection with *M. tuberculosis* should be discussed with travelers planning long-term stays (≥6 months) or those who may be exposed to patients with untreated TB (such as those working in health care settings, homeless shelters, or prisons).

Other Health and Safety Risks

Good health care is available in most Mexican cities, and hotels in tourist resorts usually have well-trained physicians available. Travelers should be aware that payment up front (cash or credit card) may be required before receiving any care. Also, most providers do not accept US domestic health insurance or Medicare/Medicaid plans. Injuries, rather than infectious diseases, pose the largest risk of death among healthy travelers to Mexico. In one review, the leading cause of death to all US travelers to Mexico was injuries (51%), and 18% of deaths resulted from motor vehicle crashes.

Mexico's highway system and roads have become increasingly modernized over the years. Toll highways are often of high quality. Nevertheless, driving in traffic in cities and at night through the countryside can be dangerous. Travelers should fasten seat belts when riding in cars and wear a helmet when riding bicycles or motorbikes. Although travel in Mexico is generally safe, drug-related violence has continued to increase in parts of the country. Department of State advisories should be monitored for relevant safety and security alerts.

Air pollution in Mexico City, while decreased in recent years, can be particularly severe during the dry winter months and can exacerbate asthma and chronic lung and heart conditions. Both healthy travelers from lower elevations and people

4

with lung and heart conditions should cautiously acclimate to Mexico City's altitude.

Most injuries and deaths caused by poisonous *Centruroides* genus scorpions are reported from states in the Pacific Coast (from Sonora to Oaxaca) and in the center states of Morelos, State of Mexico, Guanajuato, and Durango. Travelers should exercise caution when visiting Mexico's rural areas and when participating in outdoor activities, especially during spring and summer.

BIBLIOGRAPHY

1. Brathwaite DO, San Martin JL, Montoya RH, del Diego J, Zambrano B, Dayan GH. The history of dengue outbreaks in the Americas. Am J Trop Med Hyg. 2012 Oct;87(4):584–93.

2. CDC. Update: novel influenza A (H1N1) virus infection – Mexico, March–May, 2009. MMWR Morb Mortal Wkly Rep. 2009 Jun 5;58(21):585–9.

3. CDC. Human rabies from exposure to a vampire bat in Mexico—Louisiana, 2010. MMWR Morb Mortal Wkly Rep. 2011 Aug 12;60(31):1050–2.

4. CDC. Notes from the field: outbreak of *Vibrio cholerae* Serogroup O1, Serotype Ogawa, Biotype El Tor Strain – La Huasteca Region, Mexico, 2013. MMWR Morb Mortal Wkly Rep. 2013;63(25):552–3.

5. Fitchett JR, Vallecillo AJ, Espitia C. Tuberculosis transmission across the United States–Mexico border. Rev Panam Salud Publica. 2011 Jan;29(1):57–60.

6. Flores-Figueroa J, Okhuysen PC, von Sonnenburg F, DuPont HL, Libman MD, Keystone JS, et al. Patterns of illness in travelers visiting Mexico and Central America: the GeoSentinel experience. Clin Infect Dis. 2011 Sep;53(6):523–31.

7. Laniado-Laborin R. Coccidioidomycosis and other endemic mycoses in Mexico. Rev Iberoam Micol. 2007 Dec 31;24(4):249–58.

8. Leparc-Goffart I, Nougairede A, Cassadou S, Prat C, de Lamballerie X. Chikungunya in the Americas. Lancet. 2014 Feb 8;383(9916):514.

9. Spradling PR, Xing J, Phippard A, Fonseca-Ford M, Montiel S, Guzman NL, et al. Acute viral hepatitis in the United States-Mexico border region: data from the Border Infectious Disease Surveillance (BIDS) Project, 2000–2009. J Immigr Minor Health. 2013 Apr;15(2):390–7.

4

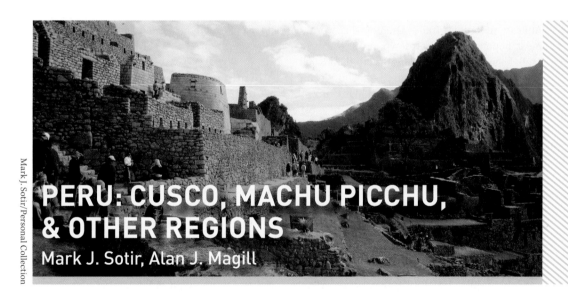

Mark J. Sotir/Personal Collection

PERU: CUSCO, MACHU PICCHU, & OTHER REGIONS
Mark J. Sotir, Alan J. Magill

DESTINATION OVERVIEW

Peru is a country almost twice the size of the state of Texas, with a population of 30 million people. Thousands of tourists are drawn to Peru every year to enjoy the country's magnificent geographic, biologic, and cultural diversity. A primary destination for most travelers is the remarkable Incan ruins of Machu Picchu, named a UNESCO World Heritage site in 1983 and voted one of the New Seven Wonders of the World in

2007. Machu Picchu is located in southern Peru and stands in the middle of a tropical mountain forest, in an extraordinarily picturesque setting. It was probably the most amazing urban creation of the Inca Empire at its height; its giant walls, terraces, and ramps seem as if they have been cut naturally in the continuous rock escarpments. The natural setting, on the eastern slopes of the Andes, is in the upper Amazon Basin, with its rich diversity of flora and fauna.

A visit to Peru will likely begin in the capital city of Lima, a sprawling megacity that is home to approximately one-third of Peru's population. Interestingly, many people think Lima is a high-altitude Incan city, but it is actually located on the Pacific coast at sea level (Map 4-10). From Lima, one can take an hour-long flight to Cusco, the gateway to Machu Picchu and a worthwhile destination of its own. Tourists can visit multiple Inca-era ruins, both in Cusco and mountain villages and markets in the Valle Sagrado (Sacred Valley), before taking the train to Machu Picchu. From the train there are multiple ways to reach the actual site, varying from buses up the mountain to Machu Picchu from the nearby town of Aguas Calientes to multiple-day hikes across Andean mountain trails. One of the world's most popular and best-known treks, the Inca Trail, begins at an elevation of more than 8,000 ft (>2,500 meters) on the Cusco–Machu Picchu railway. This moderate 26-mile (43-km) trek is usually done in 4 days and 3 nights, and most fit people should be able to complete the hike. Nevertheless, it is quite challenging, with 3 high mountain passes; the highest is Warmiwañusca at 13,796 ft (4,205 m), before ending at the ruins of Machu Picchu (7,970 ft; 2,430 m).

Many people also wish to add a tropical rainforest experience to their Cusco trip and take the 30-minute flight from Cusco to Puerto Maldonado, 34 miles (55 km) west of the Bolivian border, at the confluence of the Rio Tambopata with the Madre de Dios River, a major tributary of the Amazon River. Most travelers take a boat up the Rio Tambopata to one of several rustic lodges. Visitors wanting to see the Amazon rainforest may also go to the more remote Manu National Park in the south, also reached via Cusco.

Other popular tourist destinations in Peru include the northern Amazon rainforest in Loreto, which can be visited by traveling to the lodges around Iquitos or by journeying on the increasingly popular Amazon River cruises that go both upstream and downstream from Iquitos. Also, Peru is home to the Cordillera Blanca, a hundred-mile range of spectacular snow-covered peaks that form the backbone of the Andes Mountains in Peru. The Cordillera Blanca boasts 33 peaks >18,040 ft (5,500 m) and has an international reputation for its spectacular trekking and world-class mountaineering. Puno and Lake Titicaca, which has been called the highest navigable lake in the world, in southern Peru near the Bolivian border are also popular with tourists, with itineraries that include visitations to islands on the lake. Another tourist destination south of Lima is the Nazca Desert, home of the ancient geoglyphs known as the Nazca Lines.

HEALTH ISSUES

Important pretravel information for Peru includes advice on preventing high-altitude illness, the risk for cutaneous leishmaniasis in certain jungle areas, the risk of vectorborne illnesses, including malaria, and the use of yellow fever vaccine in some areas.

Altitude and Acute Mountain Sickness

Travelers to Machu Picchu will arrive and transit through Cusco, which is 11,200 ft (3,400 m) above sea level. A recent study of travelers to Cusco found that three-quarters flew directly from sea level. Most will quickly note shortness of breath on gathering luggage and making their way to local hotels on the hilly streets. Many arriving travelers, maybe as many as half, will find that Cusco's elevation leads to some degree of acute mountain sickness (AMS), with the initial symptoms of headache, nausea, and loss of appetite beginning 4–8 hours after arrival. The hypoxemia of high altitude can also affect the quality of sleep in the first few nights in Cusco, causing restless sleep, frequent awakening, and periodic breathing (irregular breathing patterns, often alternating periods of deep breathing and shallow breathing), even in those who appear

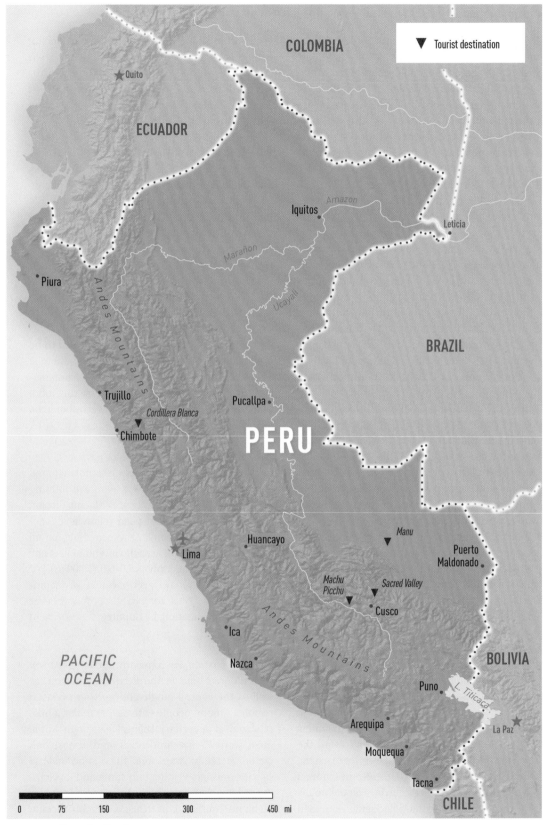

MAP 4-10. Peru destination map

to be doing well during the day. Some travelers may progress to severe forms of altitude illness, including high-altitude pulmonary edema and high-altitude cerebral edema. The symptoms of AMS can markedly impair the traveler and prevent enjoyment of the sights of Cusco. People with underlying lung disease may not be the best candidates for travel to this destination. Expert pretravel medical consultation is advised. (See Chapter 2, Altitude Illness)

Surveys have shown that most travelers arrive in Cusco with limited or no knowledge of AMS or the fact that AMS can be prevented to a large degree by prophylactic use of acetazolamide. Every traveler to Cusco should be counseled about AMS before travel and be prepared to prevent or self-treat AMS with acetazolamide. Travelers to other parts of Peru may also require counseling about AMS; other common travel destinations at high elevation include the Cordillera Blanca (peaks >18,040 ft; 5,500 m), Puno (12,556 ft; 3,830 m) and Lake Titicaca. (More information about prevention and treatment of altitude illness can be found in Chapter 2, Altitude Illness.) Locals refer to AMS as *soroche* and will almost always offer the new arrival a cup of hot coca tea (*mate de coca*) when checking in to the hotel. Although many believe *mate de coca* can prevent and treat *soroche*, no data support its use in the prevention or treatment of AMS. Perhaps of concern to some who may experience random drug screening as a condition of employment, people who drink a single cup of coca tea will test positive for cocaine metabolites in standard drug toxicology screens for several days. However, sitting quietly and resting while enjoying a cup of tea is a most civilized activity and a pleasant memory.

New arrivals may also find it helpful to transit directly from Cusco to the Valle Sagrado of the Rio Urubamba (Sacred Valley) to spend the first few days and nights at a somewhat lower altitude. This spectacular river valley begins 15 miles (24 km) northeast of Cusco in the town of Pisac (9,751 ft; 2,972 m), known for its colorful Sunday markets, and continues downstream toward the northwest for another 37 miles (60 km) to reach the town of Ollantaytambo (9,160 ft; 2,792 m). One can board the train to Machu Picchu in Ollantaytambo, at the northwest end of the Valle Sagrado and then visit Cusco on the return from Machu Picchu, when people are better acclimatized. The train follows the Rio Urubamba north and northwest (downstream) to Aguas Calientes (6,693 ft; 2,040 m). Machu Picchu (7,972 ft; 2,430 m) is located on a ridge above the town.

Cutaneous Leishmaniasis

Many areas in the Pacific valleys of the Andes and the Amazon tropical rainforest are endemic for cutaneous leishmaniasis (CL), a parasitic infection transmitted by bites of sand flies (see Chapter 3, Leishmaniasis, Cutaneous). While this disease is widespread in southeastern Peru, the highest risk for travelers seems to be in the Manu Park area in Madre de Dios. In Manu, CL is most often caused by *Leishmania braziliensis*, and there is a risk of both localized ulcerative CL and mucosal leishmaniasis. There is no visceral leishmaniasis in Peru. Travelers should be counseled to be meticulous about vector precautions, as there is no vaccine or prophylaxis to prevent leishmaniasis. Any person with a skin lesion persisting more than a few weeks after return from Peru should be evaluated for CL.

Yellow Fever

Proof of yellow fever vaccination is not required for entry into Peru. Travelers who are limiting their itineraries to Lima, Cusco, Machu Picchu, and the Inca Trail do not need yellow fever vaccination. Peru recommends vaccination for all travelers >9 months of age who intend to visit any jungle areas of the country <7,546 ft (2,300 m). For complete CDC yellow fever vaccination recommendations for Peru, see Chapter 3, Yellow Fever & Malaria Information, by Country.

Malaria

Both *Plasmodium vivax* malaria and *P. falciparum* malaria are found in the Peruvian Amazon, as well as the central jungle and northern coastal regions. Among people with severe malaria hospitalized at a tertiary referral center in Lima, most were *P. vivax* infections, and almost half were infected in Amazonia. There is no malaria risk for travelers visiting only Lima and its vicinity, coastal areas south of Lima, or the popular highland tourist areas (Cusco, Machu Picchu, and Lake Titicaca). The malaria-endemic areas for most tourists are the neotropical rainforests of the Amazon (see Map 3-37). Malaria in the Peruvian Amazon is unpredictable from season to season; *P. falciparum* epidemics occasionally occur in the Loreto region. The city of Iquitos in the northern rainforest is a frequent arrival destination for those traveling to jungle lodges around the city or for boarding river cruise boats for rainforest travel. Malaria transmission occurs in the areas in and around Iquitos. Malaria transmission occurs throughout the year but is seasonally variable, with peak activity between January and May that correlates with the rainy season. Prophylaxis is recommended for most travelers.

The city of Puerto Maldonado is a 30-minute flight from Cusco and a popular arrival destination for those visiting the rainforest lodges on the Rio Tambopata. Newly arrived travelers usually transit directly from the airport to the boats that take them up the river to numerous lodges. Peruvian Ministry of Health data document that malaria transmission occurs in Puerto Maldonado. Most cases reported in the region occur in local loggers and gold miners in the forests.

Other Infectious Diseases

Typical travelers' diarrhea is relatively common. Fluoroquinolone-resistant *Campylobacter* gastrointestinal infections can occur and should be suspected in anyone with a gastrointestinal illness with fever and systemic symptoms and failure to clinically improve in 12–24 hours after initial empiric fluoroquinolone treatment. Azithromycin can be used for people who do not respond to empiric treatment of acute gastroenteritis with a fluoroquinolone. Cyclosporiasis, an intestinal illness caused by the parasite *Cyclospora cayetanensis*, is also common in Peru. This diagnosis should be considered in people with watery diarrhea, loss of appetite, weight loss, cramping, and bloating that persist for days to weeks. Treatment is with trimethoprim-sulfamethoxazole.

Dengue is common in the neotropical areas of Peru and the northern coast. Mayaro virus, an alphavirus found in the Amazon Basin and transmitted by mosquitoes, causes a dengue-like illness. As with other alphaviruses, Mayaro can result in lengthy and debilitating arthralgia. Chikungunya, another alphavirus that can cause arthralgia, has also been reported in Peru. The first cases of local vectorborne Zika virus transmission were reported in Peru in 2016. Because of the risks to pregnancy, travelers should consult the CDC Travelers' Health website (www.cdc.gov/travel) for the most current recommendations for Zika. Travelers to Peru should take measures to protect themselves from daytime mosquito bites to prevent vectorborne illnesses (see Chapter 2, Protection against Mosquitoes, Ticks, & Other Arthropods). Physicians treating patients with signs and symptoms of a denguelike illness and a recent history of travel to the Amazon should consider Mayaro, chikungunya, and Zika in the differential diagnosis.

BIBLIOGRAPHY

1. Cabada MM, Maldonado F, Quispe W, Serrano E, Mozo K, Gonzales E, et al. Pretravel health advice among international travelers visiting Cuzco, Peru. J Travel Med. 2005 Mar-Apr;12(2):61–5.

2. Llanos-Chea F, Martínez D, Rosas A, Samalvides F, Vinetz JM, Llanos-Cuentas A. Characteristics of travel-related severe Plasmodium vivax and Plasmodium falciparum malaria in individuals hospitalized at a tertiary referral center in Lima, Peru. Am J Trop Med Hyg. 2015 Dec;93(6):1249–53.

3. Mazor SS, Mycyk MB, Wills BK, Brace LD, Gussow L, Erickson T. Coca tea consumption causes positive urine cocaine assay. Eur J Emerg Med. 2006 Dec;13(6):340–1.

4. Neumayr A, Gabriel M, Fritz J, Gunther S, Hatz C, Schmidt-Chanasit J, et al. Mayaro virus infection in traveler returning from Amazon Basin, northern Peru. Emerg Infect Dis. 2012 Apr;18(4):695–6.

5. Salazar H, Swanson J, Mozo K, White ACJ, Cabada MM. Acute mountain sickness impact among travelers to Cusco, Peru. J Travel Med 2012 Jul;19(4):220–5.

6. Shaw MT, Harding E, Leggat PA. Illness and injury to students on a school excursion to Peru. J Travel Med. 2014 May-Jun;21(3):183–8.

7. Steinhardt LC, Magill AJ, Arguin PM. Review: Malaria chemoprophylaxis for travelers to Latin America. Am J Trop Med Hyg. 2011 Dec;85(6):1015–24.

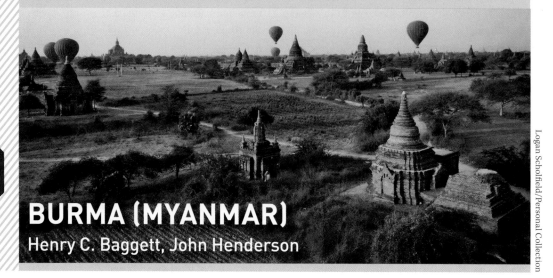

Logan Scholfield/Personal Collection

ASIA

4

BURMA (MYANMAR)

Henry C. Baggett, John Henderson

DESTINATION OVERVIEW

Burma offers visitors a mix of traditional and modern culture. Nearly all of the estimated 5 million travelers passing through the country in 2016 went to see the classic golden temples in Rangoon, Burma's biggest city. A growing number also took advantage of improving domestic bus and air service to explore cultural traditions or nature in other parts of the country. International flights to Mandalay are also now available from neighboring China, India, and Thailand.

Burma's varied geography includes highlands, plains, beaches, and more than 800 islands. Many climate zones are found along its river basins and mountain ranges. That diversity extends to languages, which number more than 100. Of the country's more than 56 million people, about two-thirds can speak or understand Burmese. English is widely spoken in popular visitor destinations.

Religious sites and ancient cities, with their temples and festivals, attract many of Burma's tourists. Unique architecture and heritage combine at places like Bagan, Kyaiktiyo, and Mrauk U. Nature-based activities such as boating, trekking, and cycling are easily arranged around Inle in hilly Shan State. River cruises along the Ayeyarwady begin or end in Mandalay (see Map 4-11). Ecotourism destinations are developing at the country's edges. Meditation retreats are also widespread.

In Rangoon, besides visiting the pagodas, tourists enjoy strolls among colonial-era parks and buildings and shopping at Bogyoke Aung San Market. The city's influences include British, Chinese, and Indian. Those wanting a glimpse of rural life get it with a short ferry ride across the Rangoon River to Dala or by riding the circle train that makes a loop just north of the city.

Climate varies depending on season and elevation. During the dry months between November and February, Yangon and southern Burma average 80°F (27°C) during the day. Further north in that season, nighttime temperatures can drop to 45°–50°F (8°–10°C). Hot season (March to June) and wet season (July to October) are well named.

Local dishes such as *mohinga* (rice noodles in fish soup), curries, and salads appeal to many visitors, but food hygiene caution is advised. Sanitation and clean water access are improving, but in secondary towns and rural areas they may be inadequate.

Though the country is slowly moving away from decades of authoritarian rule, economic isolation, and ethnic conflict, its governance and people mostly remain poor. While enjoying Burma's colorful and rustic aspects, visitors may

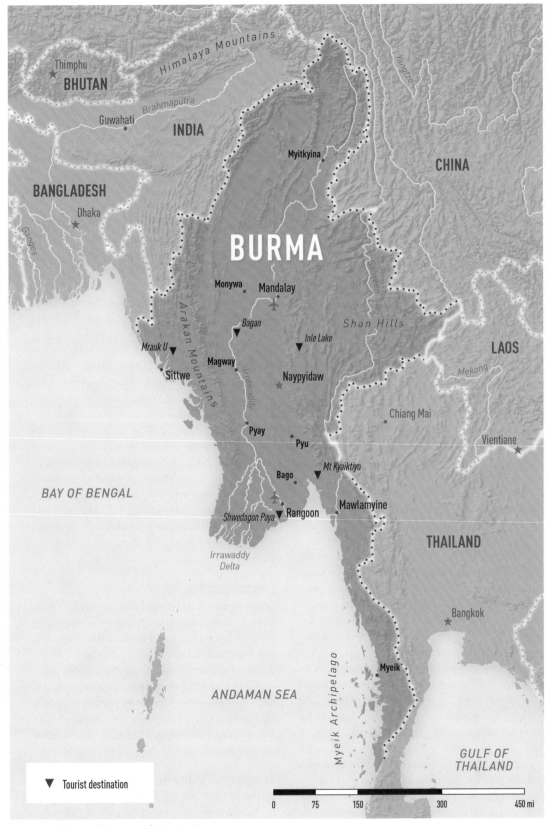

MAP 4-11. Burma (Myanmar) destination map

do well to attempt an understanding of the country's society, human rights, and environment, and tourism's potential impact on them.

HEALTH ISSUES

Vaccine-Preventable Diseases

ROUTINE IMMUNIZATIONS

Travelers to Burma should be up-to-date on routine vaccines, including vaccines for tetanus and influenza. Influenza exhibits a seasonal pattern with peaks occurring from June through September, overlapping with the typical rainy season.

OTHER VACCINATIONS

Hepatitis A is transmitted by contaminated food or water and is endemic in Burma; all nonimmune travelers should be vaccinated. Travelers can also reduce the risk of hepatitis A infection by following recommendations for safe food and water (see Chapter 2, Food & Water Precautions). Based on data from US-bound refugees, the prevalence of hepatitis B infection in Burma is high. Hepatitis B vaccination is recommended for most travelers before departure, especially those who might engage in activities that increase risk to body fluid exposure, such as unprotected sexual contact, injection drug use, tattooing, or providing medical care.

Typhoid and other diseases transmitted by contaminated food and water are common, and typhoid vaccine is recommended.

Rabies vaccination is recommended for travelers participating in extensive outdoor activities, such as camping or caving, that could increase their risk of animal bites. Vaccination is also recommended for travelers working with animals, such as veterinarians, and for young children, for whom it can be difficult to prevent interaction with dogs or other animals.

Japanese encephalitis (JE) is presumed to be endemic throughout Burma, so travelers should take precautions to avoid mosquito bites (see Chapter 2, Protection against Mosquitoes, Ticks, & Other Arthropods). Travelers should consider obtaining JE vaccine if they will be in Burma for >1 month or if their itineraries include higher-risk activities such as spending substantial time in rural areas, especially in the evening or at night; outdoor activities (such as camping, hiking, or farming); or staying in accommodations without air conditioning, window or door screens, or bed nets.

Malaria and Other Vectorborne Diseases

Malaria is present in all areas of Burma below altitudes of 3,281 ft (1,000 m), including Bagan, and the risk to travelers is considered moderate. The incidence of malaria in Burma is higher than that of neighboring countries in the Greater Mekong Subregion and is concentrated in and around forested areas. Drug-resistant malaria has been and continues to be a concern in Burma, and chemoprophylaxis recommendations vary accordingly. For travelers to Bago, Kachin, Kayah, Kayin, Shan, and Tanintharyi, atovaquone-proguanil or doxycycline is recommended but not mefloquine; for other malaria risk areas, atovaquone-proguanil, doxycycline, or mefloquine can be used. Other vectorborne infections endemic in Burma include dengue and chikungunya.

Zika is endemic in Burma; the risk to travelers is unknown but believed to be low. Because of the risk of birth defects in babies born to women who were infected with Zika while pregnant, women who are pregnant or planning to become pregnant should not travel to Burma. If they decide to travel, they should strictly follow steps to prevent mosquito bites. Travelers should consult the CDC Travelers' Health website (www.cdc.gov/travel) for the most current recommendations for Zika.

Leptospirosis

Leptospirosis is a bacterial disease usually transmitted through contact with water contaminated with the urine of infected animals (see Chapter 3, Leptospirosis). It occurs most commonly during the rainy season. Travelers should avoid contact with soil and water that could be contaminated, and cover any open wounds to prevent exposure. Skin wounds that have been contaminated with soil or water should be immediately and thoroughly cleaned.

Travelers' Diarrhea

Travelers' diarrhea is common among visitors to Burma (see Chapter 2, Travelers' Diarrhea).

4

Travelers should follow safe food and water recommendations, including eating food that is cooked and served hot and drinking only bottled water. Oral rehydration solution is helpful in severe cases of diarrhea and is usually available in pharmacies.

Other Health and Safety Risks

ROAD TRAFFIC INJURIES

Vehicular crashes are a leading cause of injury and death among travelers to Burma. Visitors should use only reputable taxi or public transportation companies and always wear seat belts. Motorcycles account for a high percentage of road traffic deaths and should be avoided. Pedestrians and bicyclists are also commonly victims of road traffic deaths and should exercise caution; right-of-way rules and infrastructure improvements (such as crosswalks or bike lanes) to protect these groups are often not followed or not in place.

HEAT-RELATED ILLNESSES

Average high temperatures in the hot season (March to June) can exceed 95°F (35°C) in many parts of Burma, including popular tourist destinations such as Rangoon, Mandalay, and Bagan. Prolonged heat exposure, especially for travelers in poor physical condition, elderly or very young travelers, and those not accustomed to heat, poses a risk for heat-related illnesses such as heat exhaustion or heat stroke. During periods of high heat, travelers should take precautions to reduce risk of heat-related illnesses, including drinking ample water and wearing lightweight, loose, and light-colored clothing (see Chapter 2, Problems with Heat & Cold).

HEALTH CARE ACCESS

Travelers with chronic medical conditions should not rely on being able to purchase or refill medications in Burma; counterfeit and substandard medications are common. International-standard medical care is rarely available, so treatment of chronic disease exacerbations or severe injuries can be suboptimal. Travelers should strongly consider medical evacuation insurance.

BIBLIOGRAPHY

1. Agency CI. The World FactBook: Burma. Central Intelligence Agency; 2016 [updated 2016 Sep.; cited 2016 Sep. 23]; Available from: https://www.cia.gov/library/publications/the-world-factbook/geos/bm.html.

2. Cheng AC, Currie BJ. Melioidosis: epidemiology, pathophysiology, and management. Clin Microbiol Rev. 2005 Apr;18(2):383–416.

3. Cui L, Yan G, Sattabongkot J, Cao Y, Chen B, Chen X, et al. Malaria in the Greater Mekong Subregion: heterogeneity and complexity. Acta Trop. 2012 Mar;121(3):227–39.

4. Dapat C, Saito R, Kyaw Y, Naito M, Hasegawa G, Suzuki Y, et al. Epidemiology of human influenza A and B viruses in Myanmar from 2005 to 2007. Intervirology 2009;52(6):310–20.

5. Hills SL, Rabe BR, Fischer M. Infectious diseases related to travel. Atlanta, GA: CDC; 2016 [updated 2015 July; cited 2016 Sep. 24]; Available from: http://wwwnc.cdc.gov/travel/yellowbook/2016/infectious-diseases-related-to-travel/japanese-encephalitis.

6. Hotez PJ, Bottazzi ME, Strych U, Chang LY, Lim YA, Goodenow MM, et al. Neglected tropical diseases among the Association of Southeast Asian Nations (ASEAN): overview and update. PLoS Negl Trop Dis 2015;9(4):e0003575.

7. Lo E, Nguyen J, Oo W, Hemming-Schroeder E, Zhou G, Yang Z, et al. Examining Plasmodium falciparum and P. vivax clearance subsequent to antimalarial drug treatment in the Myanmar-China border area based on quantitative real-time polymerase chain reaction. BMC Infect Dis 2016 Apr 16;16(1):154.

8. Mixson-Hayden T, Lee D, Ganova-Raeva L, Drobeniuc J, Stauffer WM, Teshale E, et al. Hepatitis B virus and hepatitis C virus infections in United States-bound refugees from Asia and Africa. Am J Trop Med Hyg 2014 Jun;90(6):1014–20.

9. Republic of the Union of Myanmar. The 2014 Myanmar population and housing census: highlights of the main results. Census Report. Nay Pyi Taw: Department of Population MoIaP; 2015 May. Available from: http://myanmar.unfpa.org/sites/asiapacific/files/pub-pdf/Census%20Highlights%20Report%20-%20ENGLISH%20(1).pdf.

10. U.S. Department of State. U.S. Passport & International Travel: Burma (Myanmar). USDS; [cited 2016 May 7]; Available from: https://travel.state.gov/content/passports/en/country/burma.html.

11. World Health Organization. Global status report on road safety 2013. WHO; 2013 [cited 2016 May 7]; Available from: http://www.who.int/violence_injury_prevention/road_safety_status/2013/en/.

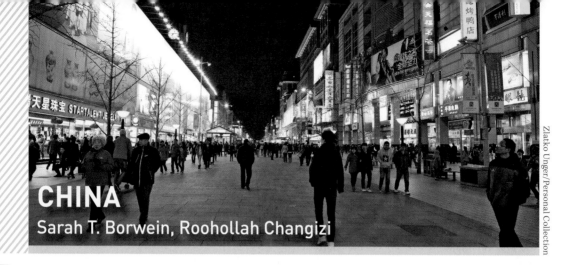

Zlatko Unger/Personal Collection

CHINA

Sarah T. Borwein, Roohollah Changizi

DESTINATION OVERVIEW

China, with >1.3 billion people, is the world's most populous country and the fourth largest geographically, behind Russia, Canada, and the United States. It shares a border with 14 other countries and has approximately 11,000 miles (18,000 km) of coastline. China is divided into 23 provinces, 5 autonomous regions, and 4 municipalities (Map 4-12). This large landmass is home to diverse topography, languages, and customs. The climate varies from tropical in the south to subarctic in the north, with wide variations between regions and seasons. Natural hazards include typhoons along the southern and eastern seaboards, dust storms in the north, floods, earthquakes, and landslides. Six of the 10 deadliest natural disasters in history occurred in China, including the 1556 Shaanxi earthquake, which is thought to have killed more than 800,000 people, making it the most lethal earthquake in history. Chinese superstition holds that natural disasters foretell the death of a ruler or the end of a dynasty, and indeed Mao Tse-tung died only 6 weeks after the 1976 Tangshan earthquake, the death toll of which was also in the hundreds of thousands. More recently, devastating earthquakes have struck the western provinces of Sichuan in 2008 and Qinghai in 2010. Torrential rain, floods, and landslides plagued large areas of China in the summer of 2010, as well as drought and dust storms in the north.

China has one of the world's oldest continuous civilizations, dating back >5,000 years. It has the world's longest continuously used written language system and is the source of many major inventions, including the "four great inventions of Ancient China": paper, the compass, gunpowder, and printing. Today, China is considerably more advanced (with the ability to put people in space, for example) and wealthier than many other developing countries, yet rural poverty and underdevelopment are still problems, particularly in the western part of the country.

Approximately 700 million Chinese people live in rural areas. Urban areas are growing rapidly, however, and China is now home to many of the world's largest megacities. Shanghai and Beijing each have close to 20 million inhabitants, and Chongqing, with a metropolitan population of more than 30 million, is among the fastest-growing urban centers in the world. Rivers play a central role in China's economy, history, and culture. The Yangtze River Basin, stretching 4,000 miles (6,400 km) from the Tibetan plateau to the East China Sea near Shanghai, is home to more than 5% of the world's population.

In 2015, more than 120 million tourists visited China. Tourism to China has grown at an extraordinary pace over the past decade, although numbers have leveled off slightly in the past few years. What is even more striking is the rapid growth in Chinese outbound tourism, from 29 million in 2004 to 120 million in 2015.

China's long history and varied natural beauty can be traced through its 48 UNESCO World Heritage sites, from the imperial grandeur of the Forbidden City and the Temple of Heaven to the marvel of the Great Wall, the Terracotta Warriors in Xi'an, and the spectacular mountainous sanctuaries of the west. The most recent additions are the Tusi tribal

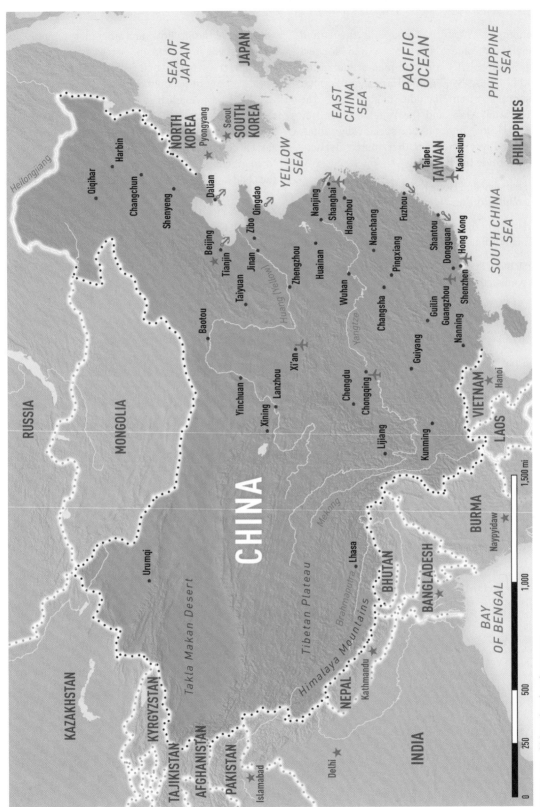

MAP 4-12. China destination map

domains in Western China and the Grand Canal, the oldest (468 BCE) and longest (1,115 miles; 1,794 km) man-made canal in the world, linking Beijing and Hangzhou. Popular itineraries often include Beijing and the Great Wall, Xi'an, and the Yangtze River (see Box 4-1 for information specifically about Yangtze River cruises). Other tourist destinations include the following:

- Shanghai and Hong Kong, with their futuristic architecture and East-meets-West mystique

- Lijiang in the province of Yunnan, where many ethnic minorities are concentrated

- Sichuan Province, home to China's iconic symbol, the panda

- Guilin, famous for its uniquely shaped limestone karst mountains that are often featured in Chinese paintings

- Tibet, accessible now by the world's highest railroad directly to Lhasa, with a maximum altitude of 16,640 ft (5,072 m)

Specialized itineraries are increasingly being offered, including hiking, mountain climbing, village tours, the Silk Road, and other more remote regions. Aside from tourism, increasing numbers of people travel to China to visit friends and relatives, to study, or to adopt children. These groups may be at particularly high risk of illness because they underestimate their risks, are less likely to seek pretravel advice, and stay in more local or rural accommodations. People traveling to China to adopt children often worry about the health of the child but neglect their own health.

HEALTH ISSUES

Although China is now the world's second-largest economy, per capita income is still below the world average, with wide disparity in wealth and development between rural and urban as well as east and west. Health risks vary accordingly.

Air Pollution

China's rapid economic expansion has resulted in tremendous increases in emissions of air pollutants, particularly in the megacities. Although aggressive efforts are underway to control pollution, 16 of the 20 most polluted cities in the world are in China, and Beijing regularly tops the list. On peak pollution days, the levels of particulate

---

BOX 4-1. Cruising down the Yangtze: what to consider

The Yangtze River is the third longest river in the world and one of the world's busiest (and most polluted) waterways. Yangtze River cruises are popular with tourists, and there are several health considerations for this trip:

- At least 1 case of Japanese encephalitis has been documented in a tourist whose 3-week trip to rural and urban China included a Yangtze River cruise, and documented cases are likely to be an underestimate.
- Malaria is not a substantial risk on this itinerary; only

insect bite precautions are recommended.

- Schistosomiasis—*Schistosoma japonicum*—exists in the Yangtze River basin. Swimming is ill-advised.
- Motion sickness is rare on Yangtze cruises, since much of it takes place on a calm reservoir. However, susceptible travelers should carry antiemetic medication.
- Excursions off the boat often involve steep climbs, many stairs, and long walking distances and may not be appropriate for physically infirm tourists.

- Air pollution can be a problem on Yangtze River cruises and can cause eye and throat irritation as well as respiratory problems in susceptible travelers. September and October are said to be the clearest months.
- Most non-Chinese-speaking tourists will prefer a 4- or 5-star "luxury" cruise. First class on a Chinese tourist boat may not meet expectations for cleanliness, and English may not be spoken.
- Food and water precautions apply, even on a luxury boat.

matter in the air can exceed 40 times the limit considered safe by the World Health Organization. Short-term exposure to these levels of air pollution can irritate the eyes and throat, and those with underlying cardiorespiratory illness, including asthma, chronic obstructive pulmonary disease, or congestive heart failure, may find their condition exacerbated. In addition, exposure to high levels of air pollution significantly increases the risk of respiratory tract infections, including sinusitis, otitis, bronchitis, and pneumonia. Children and the elderly are the most vulnerable to these effects.

Although surgical-style face masks have become increasingly fashionable in the big cities of China, especially Beijing and Shanghai, they provide no protection from air pollution and are not recommended. Properly fitted N95 masks can filter out particulates but not gaseous pollutants and can sometimes actually compound breathing problems, so are not routinely recommended.

Vaccine-Preventable Diseases

Routine vaccinations should be up-to-date, including seasonal influenza. In addition, hepatitis A and B and typhoid vaccinations are usually recommended. Since the Xinjiang Uygur Autonomous Region borders Pakistan, a polio-endemic country, adults traveling to this region who will be working in health care settings, refugee camps, or humanitarian aid settings should be vaccinated against polio, including a single lifetime booster dose of polio vaccine (IPV). Measles and rubella immunity is particularly important, and although a massive vaccination campaign begun in September 2010 has decreased the number of reported measles cases, there were still more than 100,000 cases reported in 2014. A few travelers have made news headlines by triggering outbreaks in their home countries after returning from China. Although limited data exist on rubella in China, it was not part of the national immunization program until 2008, and incidence is believed to be high.

China is making considerable advances in vaccination, with the objective of developing their own locally made vaccines. There have, however, been many well-publicized issues with counterfeit and improperly stored vaccines. In addition, vaccine shortages are frequent; adult tetanus vaccines were out of stock from 2014 through the time of writing. Travelers are unlikely to be able to complete unfinished vaccination series once in China and may be unable to access tetanus vaccine if injured while there. All travelers should have an up-to-date tetanus-containing vaccine before going to China. Hong Kong functions under different rules, and international vaccines are in use there.

HEPATITIS B

Hepatitis B infection is endemic in China. Nearly one-third of the 350 million people worldwide infected with the hepatitis B virus (HBV) reside in China. Hepatitis B vaccination and other preventive measures should be discussed with nonimmune travelers.

JAPANESE ENCEPHALITIS

Japanese encephalitis (JE) occurs in all regions except Qinghai, Xinjiang, and Xizang (Tibet) (see Map 3-8 and Table 3-7). China has greatly reduced the incidence of JE through vaccination and, as of 2008, included JE in its expanded national immunization program; however, the disease remains a threat to unimmunized travelers. Although the JE season varies by region, most cases in local residents are reported from June through October. The risk of JE for most travelers to China is low but varies based on season, destination, duration, and activities. Risk is highest among travelers to rural areas during the transmission season. JE vaccine is recommended for travelers who plan to spend ≥1 month in endemic areas during June through October. It should be considered for shorter-term travelers if they plan to travel to rural areas and will have an increased risk for JE virus exposure based on their activities or itineraries, such as spending substantial time outdoors or staying in accommodations without air conditioning, screens, or bed nets. However, rare sporadic cases have occurred on an unpredictable basis in short-term travelers, including in periurban Beijing and Shanghai.

RABIES

Rabies is a serious problem in China, as in much of Asia, with more than 3,000 reported human deaths per year. Mammal bites in any area of China, including urban areas, must be considered high risk for rabies. As rabies immune globulin is generally unavailable, animal bites are often trip-enders, requiring evacuation to Hong Kong, Bangkok, or home for postexposure prophylaxis. Bites are surprisingly common in tourists. For example, dog bites were the most common dermatologic problem seen after China travel in an analysis of data from the GeoSentinel Surveillance Network. Rabies risk and prevention should be discussed in pretravel consultations, and a strategy for dealing with a possible exposure should be developed. Long-term travelers and expatriates living in China should consider the preexposure vaccination series. Travel health insurance, including medical evacuation insurance, should be encouraged (see Chapter 2, Travel Insurance, Travel Health Insurance, & Medical Evacuation Insurance).

Vectorborne Diseases

MALARIA

Malaria risk is very low for travelers to China, with the exception of those visiting rural parts of southern Yunnan Province. For this area, chemoprophylaxis should be considered. Mefloquine resistance in southern Yunnan means that travelers should be given doxycycline or atovaquone-proguanil for travel in this area.

DENGUE

In 2014, southern China experienced its worst dengue outbreak in decades; Guangdong province reported more than 40,000 cases in just 2 months. Travelers should practice daytime mosquito precautions in the summer months.

Other Health Risks

FOODBORNE ILLNESSES

The risk for travelers' diarrhea appears to be low in deluxe accommodations in China but moderate elsewhere. Usual food and water precautions should apply, and travelers should consider bringing an antibiotic for self-treatment of moderate to severe diarrhea. Since highly quinolone-resistant *Campylobacter* is a problem in China, azithromycin may be a good choice. Tap water is not safe to drink even in major cities. Most hotels provide bottled or boiled water, and bottled water is easily available. In addition, there have been several well-publicized episodes of contamination of food with pesticides and other substances. Travelers should strictly avoid undercooked fish and shellfish and unpasteurized milk.

SEXUALLY TRANSMITTED DISEASES

Sexually transmitted diseases, including syphilis, HIV, gonorrhea, and chlamydia, are a growing problem in China, particularly along the booming eastern seaboard. Travel is associated with loosened inhibitions and increased casual sexual liaisons. Travelers should be aware of STD risks and use condoms if they have sex with someone whose HIV or STD status is unknown. Hepatitis B vaccination before travel should be considered.

ROAD TRAFFIC INJURIES

Traffic in China is often chaotic, and the rate of traffic crashes, including fatal ones, is among the highest in the world. Driving is on the right side of the road in mainland China but on the left in Hong Kong and Macau. In practice, many people drive down the middle of the road. Child safety seats, rear seat belts, and bicycle or motorcycle helmets are rarely seen and not widely available. Electronic bicycles (E-bikes) are popular and do not have to be registered. They often travel in pedestrian and bicycle lanes as well as with traffic. Because E-bikes are quiet (no engine noise), they can be hard to avoid. Motor vehicles and E-bikes often drive with no lights, making night travel dangerous. Traffic crashes, even minor ones, can create major traffic jams and sometimes turn into violent altercations, particularly when foreigners are involved. China has not signed the convention that created the International Driving Permit, and travelers require a Chinese license to drive in China. For all of these reasons, it is often simpler and safer to hire a local driver than to drive oneself. It is also advisable to avoid driving at night or when weather conditions are bad, and not to assume that traffic rules or right-of-way will be respected. Travelers should fasten seat belts when riding in cars and wear a helmet when riding bicycles or motorbikes.

VITAMIN D DEFICIENCY

Vitamin D deficiency is a major issue in the northern provinces of China, where smog often blocks out sunlight, causing inadequate absorption of vitamin D through the skin even in the summer months. If the traveler will be spending more than 6 months in China, vitamin D supplementation is recommended.

Medical Care in China

Western-style medical facilities that meet international standards are available in Beijing, Shanghai, and Hong Kong. Some hospitals in other cities have "VIP wards" (*gaogan bingfang*), which may have English-speaking staff. The standard of care in such facilities is somewhat unpredictable, and cultural and regulatory differences can cause difficulties for travelers. In rural areas, only rudimentary medical care may be available. Hepatitis B virus transmission from poorly sterilized medical equipment remains a risk outside major centers.

Ambulances are not staffed with trained paramedics and often have little or no medical equipment. Therefore, injured travelers may need to take taxis or other immediately available vehicles to the nearest major hospital rather than waiting for ambulances to arrive.

Pharmacies often sell prescription medications over the counter. Such medications have sometimes been counterfeit, substandard, or even contaminated. Travelers should bring all their regular medications in sufficient quantity; if more or other medications are required, it is advisable to visit a reputable clinic or hospital.

Some travelers wish to try traditional Chinese medicine and acupuncture. Although most do so uneventfully, there is a risk of bloodborne and skin infections from acupuncture needles, and traditional medicine products may be contaminated with heavy metals or pharmaceutical agents. Acupressure may be preferable to acupuncture.

Travelers are strongly advised to purchase travel health and medical evacuation insurance before travel. Most hospitals will not directly accept foreign medical insurance, however, and patients will often be expected to pay a deposit before care to cover the expected cost of the treatment.

BIBLIOGRAPHY

1. Custer B, Sullivan S, Hazlet TK, Iloeje U, Veenstra DL, Kowdley KV. Global epidemiology of hepatitis B virus. J Clin Gastroenterol. 2005 Nov-Dec;38(10 Suppl):S158–68.

2. Cutfield NJ, Anderson NE, Brickell K, Hueston L, Pikholz C, Roxburgh RH. Japanese encephalitis acquired during travel in China. Intern Med J. 2005 Aug;35(8):497–8.

3. Davis XM, MacDonald S, Borwein S, Freedman DO, Kozarsky PE, von Sonnenburg F, et al. Health risks in travelers to China: the GeoSentinel experience and implications for the 2008 Beijing Olympics. Am J Trop Med Hyg. 2008 Jul;79(1):4–8.

4. Hills SL, Griggs AC, Fischer M. Japanese encephalitis in travelers from non-endemic countries, 1973–2008. Am J Trop Med Hyg. 2010 May;82(5):930–6.

5. Shaw MT, Leggat PA, Borwein S. Travelling to China for the Beijing 2008 Olympic and Paralympic games. Travel Med Infect Dis. 2007 Nov;5(6):365–73.

6. United Nations World Tourism Organization. UNWTO tourism highlights. Madrid: United Nations World Tourism Organization; 2012 [cited 2016 Sep. 24]. Available from: http://mkt.unwto.org/en/publication/unwto-tourism-highlights-2012-edition.

7. World Health Organization. Hepatitis B Surveillance and control. WHO; [updated 2016 July; cited 2016 Sep. 24]; Available from: www.who.int/mediacentre/factsheets/fs204/en/.

8. World Health Organization. Measles bulletin: Western Pacific region. Geneva: World Health Organization; 2010 [cited 2016 Sep. 24]; Available from: http://www.wpro.who.int/entity/immunization/documents/docs/MeasBulletinVol4Issue1_F840.pdf.

9. Xia J, Min L, Shu J. Dengue fever in China: an emerging problem demands attention. Emerg Microbes Infect. 2015 Jan;4(1):e3

10. Zhang J, Jin Z, Sun GQ, Zhou T, Ruan S. Analysis of rabies in China: transmission dynamics and control. PLoS One. 2011;6(7):e20891.

11. Zhang YZ, Xiong CL, Xiao DL, Jiang RJ, Wang ZX, Zhang LZ, et al. Human rabies in China. Emerg Infect Dis. 2005 Dec;11(12):1983–4.

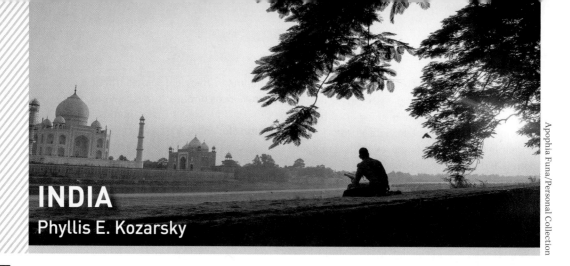

Apophia Funa/Personal Collection

INDIA

Phyllis E. Kozarsky

DESTINATION OVERVIEW

India is approximately one-third the size of the United States and has 4 times the population (almost 1.3 billion people). This makes it the second most populous country in the world, behind China. Rich in history, vibrant culture, and diversity, India is the birthplace of 4 world religions: Hinduism, Buddhism, Jainism, and Sikhism. Despite the growth of megacities such as Mumbai and Delhi (both more than 20 million people), India's rural population is still twice that of its urban population. Although India is one of the fastest-growing economies in the world, the literacy rate varies by state (64%–94%), the level of poverty is high, and the life expectancy is about 66 years. The topography is varied, ranging from tropical beaches to foothills, deserts, and the Himalayan mountains. The north has a more temperate climate, while the south is more tropical year-round. Many travelers prefer India during the winter—November through March, when the temperatures are more agreeable—although some, particularly families with children, must travel during the summer vacation time.

India is becoming more popular for US travelers, and rates of travel from the United States are increasing. International businesses are flourishing in India; tourists are flocking to the temples, beaches, and the Taj Mahal. For some new US residents, India remains their homeland, and they make frequent visits to family and friends. In addition, India has a large and growing medical tourism sector.

Because tourists could not possibly visit all the sites in India during a 2-week holiday, they usually select a part of India for any given trip. A typical itinerary in the north of India includes Delhi, Agra, Varanasi, and cities in Rajasthan, such as Jaipur (the Pink City) and Udaipur. Agra is the home of the Taj Mahal, a breathtaking monument to lost love. Along the northern travel circle, one can stop to enjoy the magnificent bird sanctuary at Keoladeo Ghana and the tiger reserve at Ran Thambore (see Map 4-13). Varanasi, sacred to Hindus, Buddhists, and Jains, welcomes Hindu pilgrimages and boasts extraordinary experiences along the Ganges. A more southern route might swing through Goa and its beautiful beaches along the western coast, a destination in the past forming the backdrop for great parties and old-time hippies, which has now become a haven for writers and artists boasting a chic new culture. Mumbai, a common entry point to India, hosts Bollywood, the largest film industry in the world. Kolkata (Calcutta) is considered the cultural capital of the country. Bengaluru (Bangalore) in the south-central region is both the garden city and India's Silicon Valley. The old seaside town of Kochi (Cochin) shows evidence of its Portuguese heritage, and Hyderabad shows off its old granite fort, many mosques, and bazaars. Despite the many and varied itineraries, most health recommendations for travelers to India are similar. The incidences of some illnesses, such as those transmitted by mosquitoes, increase during the monsoon season (May–October) with the high temperatures, heavy rains, and the risk of flooding.

Some of the most important health considerations of travel to India are those for travelers who are visiting friends and relatives (VFRs). These travelers often do not seek pretravel health advice, since they are returning to their land of origin. Such travelers may stay in rural areas often not visited by tourists or business people, live in homes, and eat and drink with their families, and

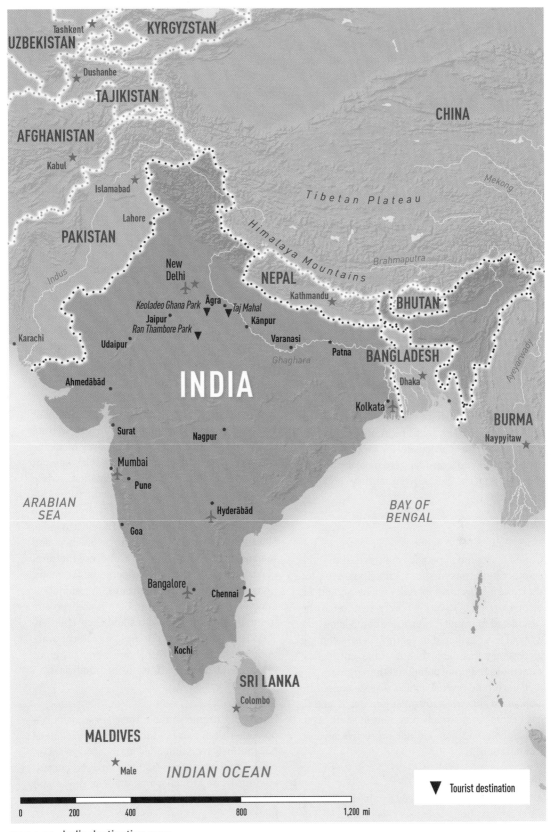

MAP 4-13. India destination map

thus are at higher risk of many travel-related illnesses (see Chapter 8, Immigrants Returning Home to Visit Friends and Relatives [VFRs]).

HEALTH ISSUES

Vaccine-Preventable Diseases

All travelers to India should be up-to-date with their routine immunizations and are advised to consider hepatitis B vaccine. Particularly important is making sure that the traveler is immune to measles. India has not had a case of wild poliovirus since early 2011, obtained its polio-free certification from the World Health Organization in March 2014, and celebrated 5 years of being polio-free in January 2016. Polio vaccine is no longer recommended for US travelers. However, all travelers (residents and nationals) from countries reporting cases of polio should check to see if there is a requirement for a dose of polio vaccine prior to entry into India.

HEPATITIS A

All travelers to India should be protected against hepatitis A. Although some assume that those born in India would have been exposed to hepatitis A in childhood and thus be immune, this may no longer be true, particularly for younger people. Providers should consider serologic testing for hepatitis A IgG in VFR travelers, or they should be immunized.

TYPHOID

More than 80% of typhoid fever cases in the United States are in people who traveled to India or other countries in south Asia. Thus, even for short-term travel, a typhoid vaccine should be recommended. Patients who are hesitant to be vaccinated may find it even more compelling that typhoid fever acquired in south Asia is becoming increasingly resistant to quinolone antibiotics, sometimes requiring parenteral therapy.

Paratyphoid fever, a similar disease caused by *Salmonella enterica* serovar Paratyphi A, B, and C, has become increasingly prevalent in south Asia, but typhoid vaccines are not protective against this infection.

JAPANESE ENCEPHALITIS

Although there has never been a published case of a traveler acquiring Japanese encephalitis (JE) in India, the disease is present in many parts of the country. Risk is highest during the monsoon season from May through October; however, the season may be extended or year-round in some areas, especially in the south. Vaccination is not recommended for the typical 2-week trip most travelers take to see the major tourist sites in urban areas. However, vaccination is recommended for travelers who plan to spend ≥1 month in endemic areas during the JE virus transmission season and should be considered for short-term travelers as well, if they plan repeated travel or travel to peri-urban areas and have an increased risk for JE virus exposures (see Chapter 3, Japanese Encephalitis). Publicized outbreaks in recent years have not been in typical tourist destinations.

RABIES

India has the highest burden of rabies in the world, with estimates of 18,000–20,000 human cases per year. Dogs roam in packs in many areas of the country. Unfortunately, human rabies immune globulin is not readily available except in some clinics in major cities. Information about such clinics can be obtained from the website of the International Society of Travel Medicine (www.istm.org). Otherwise, if a traveler has not received preexposure rabies vaccination, a bite may result in having to leave the country for postexposure prophylaxis. Even so, a preexposure series is not recommended for all travelers to India. However, education about bite avoidance and management should be a part of every pretravel consultation. Cost is a consideration for many. Long-term travelers, expatriates, missionaries, and volunteers may want to obtain preexposure immunization for themselves and their children. Travelers may want to purchase a medical evacuation insurance policy that will cover travel for recommended rabies postexposure prophylaxis.

CHOLERA

Although extremely rare in travelers, cholera is a possible risk in parts of India. Cholera vaccine is not routinely recommended for most travelers on typical tourist itineraries, but it may be considered for those at higher risk, such as those who are visiting friends and relatives or traveling for humanitarian aid work in disaster areas.

4

MALARIA

Although the intensity of malaria transmission may be related to the season, unlike other countries in Asia malaria is holoendemic in India (except at altitudes >6,562 ft [2,000 m]) and occurs in both rural and urban areas. Rates of *Plasmodium falciparum* have increased in the last few decades, and thus chemoprophylaxis is recommended for all destinations. Travelers should be reminded that malaria-transmitting mosquitoes primarily bite between dusk and dawn.

Other Infections

MULTIDRUG-RESISTANT BACTERIA

Strains of bacteria that are resistant to most antibiotics have been carried by travelers from India to many other countries, including the United States. High rates of resistance to multiple antibiotics have been shown among gram-negative (such as, *Escherichia coli, Klebsiella* spp., and *Salmonella* spp.) and gram positive (such as *Staphylococcus aureus*) bacteria in India. In particular, bacterial resistance to carbapenems, third-generation cephalosporins, fluoroquinolones, and even colistin are becoming more common.

DENGUE

Dengue is endemic in all of India except at high elevation in mountainous regions. It is poorly reported at the local and national levels, and large outbreaks continue to occur, including in many urban areas. The incidence is highest during the wet summer season, which includes the monsoon season (May–October). Travelers to India should take measures to protect themselves from daytime mosquito bites to prevent dengue (see Chapter 2, Protection against Mosquitoes, Ticks, & Other Arthropods).

CHIKUNGUNYA

During the last several years there have been outbreaks of chikungunya, which is transmitted by day- and night-biting mosquitoes. Symptoms are similar to those of dengue and malaria, although often with severe and persistent arthralgia.

HEPATITIS E

Hepatitis E is being recognized more frequently in travelers to India. A traveler who develops symptomatic hepatitis despite being immunized against hepatitis A will likely have hepatitis E.

ANIMAL BITES AND WOUNDS

In addition to rabies, other diseases can be transmitted by animal bites and wounds. Cellulitis, fasciitis, and wound infections may result from scratches or bites of any animal. B virus is carried by Old World monkeys and may be transmitted by active macaques that are kept as pets, inhabit many of the temples, and scatter themselves in many tourist gathering places (see Chapter 3, B virus). Monkeys can be aggressive and often seek food from travelers. When visiting temple areas that have monkeys, travelers should not carry any food in their hands, pockets, or bags. It is important to stress to travelers that monkeys and other animals should not be approached or handled at all. If travelers are bitten, they should seek medical care.

TRAVELERS' DIARRHEA

The risk for travelers' diarrhea is moderate to high in India, with an estimated 30%–50% likelihood of developing diarrhea during a 2-week journey. Travelers should practice safe food and water precautions (see Chapter 2, Food & Water Precautions). Providers should discuss with the traveler when it may be appropriate to self-treat for diarrheal illness (see Chapter 2, Travelers' Diarrhea).

TUBERCULOSIS (TB)

India has among the highest prevalences of TB; approximately one-fourth of all TB cases worldwide occur there. Roughly 2%–3% of newly diagnosed cases are estimated to be multidrug-resistant, and a smaller percentage are extensively drug-resistant. Travelers who anticipate possible prolonged exposure to people with TB because they will routinely come in contact with clinic, hospital, prison, or homeless shelter populations should have a tuberculin skin test or TB blood test before leaving the United States. If the test is negative, they should have a repeat test 8–10 weeks after returning from India. Travelers who plan to work in high-risk settings or in crowded institutions (such as medical clinics, hospitals, prisons, or homeless shelters) should consult their health care providers about measures for prevention and testing before and after travel. Use of bacillus Calmette-Guérin (BCG) vaccine in health care workers who will have increased risk of tuberculosis during travel has recently been proposed, although this recommendation remains controversial (see Chapter 3, Tuberculosis). Access to vaccine and lack of expertise in administering the vaccine are also barriers.

Other Issues

Arrival in India for the first time may be shocking to travelers who have never ventured into the developing world. The crowds, the intense colors, heat, and smells are striking and invade all the senses at once. It is difficult to enjoy the beauty without being touched by the enormity of the poverty. The close juxtaposition of the old and new is noteworthy. At times this can be overwhelming.

Transportation in India remains problematic. While traveling through India, travelers should be advised to carry food and beverages with them in the event of delays, which are almost inevitable no matter the mode of transport. Traveling by train can be harrowing, particularly having to force one's way through the crowd and onto the train. Travelers should make sure to keep passports and valuables safe while in a crowd. Roadways are some of the most hazardous in the world, and India has a large number of traffic-related deaths, including pedestrian deaths. Animals, rickshaws, motor scooters, people, bicycles, trucks, and overcrowded buses compete for space in an unregulated free-for-all.

Fasten seat belts when riding in cars and wear a helmet when riding bicycles or motorbikes. Avoid overcrowded buses, travel by bus into the interior or on curving, mountainous roads, and long-distance travel at night. Rural nighttime driving should be discouraged, even when a paid driver has been hired. Air pollution is a problem in the major cities, so those with chronic lung disease or asthma may consider spending time outdoors when there is less traffic or staying in facilities outside major cities.

Medical tourism is a growing industry in India. Many newer medical facilities have recently opened for travelers desiring cardiac, orthopedic, dental, or plastic surgery or transplantations at a substantially lower cost than in the United States. The benefits and hazards require careful examination (see Chapter 2, Medical Tourism). Health care is quite variable in India and dependent on the location.

In general, travelers feel safe while in India. Peddlers and promoters are aggressive with tourists, however, and may require a firm "no." Travelers may want to avoid making eye contact with a peddler or his goods, or they may risk having someone follow them down the street trying to sell them something. The stress of negotiating one's way through India makes this destination a place where having a close traveling companion is important.

It is always wise to pay attention to Department of State advisories in case of issues that arise at some borders, or occasional increases in religious tensions or terrorist activities.

BIBLIOGRAPHY

1. Baggett HC, Graham S, Kozarsky PE, Gallagher N, Blumensaadt S, Bateman J, et al. Pretravel health preparation among US residents traveling to India to VFRs: importance of ethnicity in defining VFRs. J Travel Med. 2009 Mar-Apr;16(2):112–8.

2. Buhl MR, Lindquist L. Japanese encephalitis in travelers: review of cases and seasonal risk. J Travel Med. 2009 May;16:217–9.

3. Epelboin L, Robert J, Tsyrina-Kouyoumdjian E, Laouira S, Meyssonnier V, Caumes E, et al. High rate of multidrug-resistant gram-negative bacilli carriage and infection in hospitalized returning travelers: a cross-sectional cohort study. J Travel Med. 2015 Sep-Oct;22(5):292–9.

4. Jensenius M, Han PV, Schlagenhauf P, Schwartz E, Parola P, Castelli F, et al. Acute and potentially life-threatening tropical diseases in western travelers—a GeoSentinel multicenter study, 1996–2011. Am J Trop Med Hyg. 2013 Feb;88(2):397–404.

5. Kumarasamy KK, Toleman MA, Walsh TR, Bagaria J, Butt F, Balakrishnan R, et al. Emergence of a new antibiotic resistance mechanism in India, Pakistan, and the UK: a molecular, biological, and epidemiological study. Lancet Infect Dis. 2010 Sep;10(9):597–602.

6. Laxminarayan R, Chaudhury RR. Antibiotic Resistance in India: Drivers and Opportunities for Action. PLoS Med. 2016 Mar 2;13(3):e1001974.

7. Leder K, Torresi J, Brownstein JS, Wilson ME, Keystone JS, Barnett E, et al. Travel-associated illness trends and clusters, 2000–2010. Emerg Infect Dis. 2013 Jul;19(7):1049–73.

8. Lynch MF, Blanton EM, Bulens S, Polyak C, Vojdani J, Stevenson J, et al. Typhoid fever in the United States, 1999–2006. JAMA. 2009 Aug 26;302(8): 859–65.

9. Shaw MT, Leggat PA, Chatterjee S. Travelling to India for the Delhi XIX Commonwealth Games 2010. Travel Med Infect Dis. 2010 May;8(3):129–38.

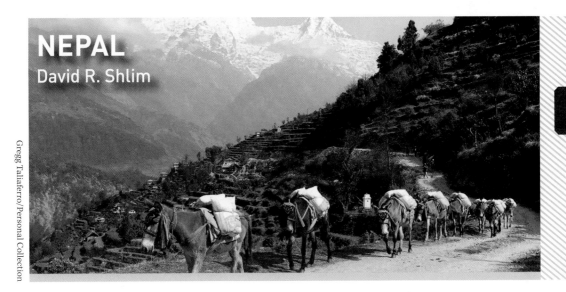

NEPAL
David R. Shlim

4

Gregg Taliaferro/Personal Collection

DESTINATION OVERVIEW

Nepal is a country of more than 28 million people that stretches for 500 miles (805 km) along the Himalayan mountains that form the border of Nepal and Tibet (see Map 4-14). The topography rises from low plains with an altitude of 200 ft (70 m) to the highest point in the world at 29,029 ft (8,848 m), the summit of Mount Everest. Approximately 30% of tourists come to Nepal to trek into the mountains, while others come to experience the culture and stunning natural beauty. Kathmandu is the capital city, with a population of more than 2 million people. It sits in a lush valley at 4,344 ft (1,324 m) in altitude. Nepal's latitude of 28°N (the same as Florida) means that the nonmountainous areas are temperate year-round. Most of the annual rainfall comes during the monsoon season (June through September). The main tourist seasons are in the spring (March to May) and fall (October and November). The winter months, December through February, are pleasant in the lowlands but can be too cold to make trekking enjoyable in the high mountains.

In April 2015, a major earthquake caused extensive damage and killed more than 9,000 people. However, most of the damage occurred in nontourist areas, and the infrastructure for tourists has largely been repaired. The Mount Everest region east of Kathmandu and the Annapurna region to the west are the destination for most trekkers. The Langtang valley trekking area, north of Kathmandu, was destroyed by a major landslide after the earthquake, and tourist services have not yet been restored.

Trekkers into the Mount Everest region routinely sleep at altitudes of 14,000–16,000 ft (4,267–4,876 m) and hike to altitudes >18,000 ft (5,486 m). This prolonged exposure to very high altitudes means that tourists must be knowledgeable about the risks of altitude illness and may need to carry specific medications to prevent and treat the problem (see Chapter 2, Altitude Illness). Most trekkers into the Mount Everest region arrive there by flying to a tiny airstrip at Lukla at 9,383 ft (2,860 m). The following day they reach Namche Bazaar at 11,290 ft (3,440 m).

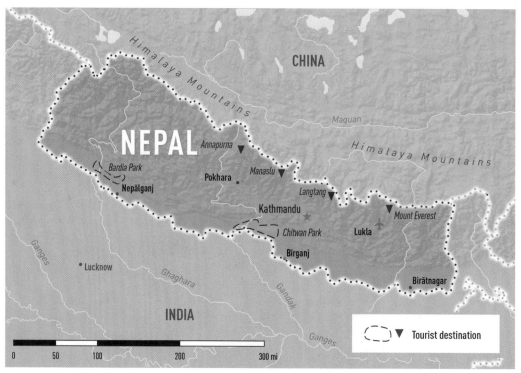

MAP 4-14. **Nepal destination map**

Acetazolamide prophylaxis can substantially decrease the chances of developing acute mountain sickness in Namche.

In the Annapurna region, short-term trekkers may choose to hike to viewpoints in the foothills without reaching any high altitudes. Others may undertake a longer trek around the Annapurna massif, going over a 17,769-ft (5,416-m) pass (the Thorung La). Roads have been constructed up the 2 major valleys of this trek, shortening the overall trekking distance and changing the nature of the experience (cars and motorcycles may be encountered along the trek). The total exposure to high altitude is less in this region than in the Everest region. The Langtang region has a high point of 14,000 ft (4,200 m).

In addition to trekking, Nepal has some of the best rafting and kayaking rivers in the world. Jungle lodges in Chitwan National Park allow tourists to view a wide range of wildlife, including tigers, rhinoceroses, bears, and crocodiles, and a huge variety of exotic birds. It is also possible to travel by road to comfortable lodges in the foothills that afford panoramic views of the Himalayas.

HEALTH ISSUES
Vaccine-Preventable Diseases

Travelers to Nepal are at high risk for enteric diseases. Hepatitis A vaccine and typhoid vaccine are the 2 most important immunizations. The risk of typhoid fever and paratyphoid fever among travelers to Nepal is among the highest in the world, and the prevalence of fluoroquinolone resistance is high.

JAPANESE ENCEPHALITIS

Japanese encephalitis (JE) is endemic in Nepal, with highest disease risk occurring in the Terai region during and immediately after the monsoon season (June through October). JE has been identified in local residents of the Kathmandu Valley, but no cases of JE acquired in Nepal have been reported in tourists or expatriates. JE vaccine is not routinely recommended for those trekking in higher altitude areas or spending short periods in Kathmandu or Pokhara en route to such treks (see Chapter 3, Japanese Encephalitis).

RABIES

Rabies is highly endemic among dogs in Nepal, but in recent years there are fewer stray dogs in Kathmandu. Half of all tourist exposures to a possibly rabid animal occur near Swayambunath, a beautiful hilltop shrine also known as the monkey temple. Tourists should be advised to be extra cautious with dogs and monkeys in this area. The monkeys can be aggressive if approached and can jump on a person's back if they smell food in a backpack. Clinics in Kathmandu that specialize in the care of foreigners almost always have complete postexposure rabies prophylaxis, including human rabies immune globulin. Trekkers who are bitten in the mountains should be able to return to Kathmandu within an average of 5 days.

CHOLERA

Although extremely rare in travelers, cholera is a possible risk in parts of Nepal. Cholera vaccine is recommended for adult travelers visiting areas with cholera activity within the last year that are prone to recurrence of cholera epidemics.

Malaria

Malaria is not a risk for most travelers to Nepal. There is no transmission of malaria in Kathmandu, and all the main trekking routes in Nepal are free of malaria transmission. Chitwan National Park is a popular tourist destination for wildlife viewing in the Terai. Although the Nepalese Ministry of Health and other regional organizations regard the Terai to be a malaria transmission area, this author, in 30 years of treating travelers in Nepal, has not seen a single case of malaria in a traveler to Chitwan, including foreign workers living in the park. Nepal has been targeted for the complete elimination of malaria within the next 10 years.

Other Health and Safety Risks

GASTROINTESTINAL ISSUES

Cyclospora cayetanensis is an intestinal protozoal pathogen that is highly endemic in Nepal. The risk for infection is distinctly seasonal: transmission occurs almost exclusively from May through October, with a peak in June and July. Because this is outside the main tourist seasons, the primary effect is on expatriates who stay through the monsoon. In addition to watery diarrhea, profound anorexia and fatigue are the hallmark symptoms of *Cyclospora* infection. The treatment of choice is trimethoprim-sulfamethoxazole; no highly effective alternatives have been identified.

Travelers' diarrhea is a risk, and the risk in the spring trekking season (March through May) is double that in the fall trekking season (October and November). Since many tourists are heading to remote areas that do not have medical care available, they should be provided with medications for self-treatment. Extensive resistance to fluoroquinolones has been documented among bacterial diarrheal pathogens in Nepal, and moderate to severe diarrhea should be empirically treated with azithromycin. Hepatitis E virus is endemic in Nepal, and several cases each year are diagnosed in tourists or expatriates. There is no vaccine commercially available against hepatitis E.

RESPIRATORY ISSUES

The Kathmandu Valley often has air pollution problems. People with underlying cardiorespiratory illness, including asthma, chronic obstructive pulmonary disease, or coronary heart failure may suffer exacerbations in Kathmandu, particularly after a viral upper respiratory infection. Short-term exposure to these levels of air pollution can irritate the eyes and throat. In addition, exposure to high levels of air pollution significantly increases the risk of respiratory tract infections, including sinusitis, otitis, bronchitis, and pneumonia. Children and the elderly are the most vulnerable.

Viral upper respiratory infections are extremely common, and the percentage of these that lead to bacterial sinusitis or bronchitis is high. Trekkers should consider carrying an antibiotic such as azithromycin to empirically treat a respiratory infection that lasts >7 days with no sign of improvement. More treks may have been ruined by prolonged respiratory infection than by gastrointestinal illness.

EVACUATION AND MEDICAL CARE

Helicopter evacuation from most areas is readily available. Communication has improved from remote areas because of satellite and cellular telephones, and private helicopter companies accept credit cards and are eager to perform evacuations for profit. Evacuation can often take place on the same day as the request, if weather permits. Helicopter rescue is usually limited to morning hours because of afternoon winds in the mountains. Helicopter rescue is billed at $4,000 per hour, with an average total cost of $8,000 to $10,000.

Two main clinics in Kathmandu specialize in the care of foreigners in Nepal. Contact information is available on the International Society of Travel Medicine website (www.istm.org). Hospital facilities have improved steadily over the years, and general and orthopedic emergency surgery are reliable and available in Kathmandu. The closest evacuation point for definitive care is Bangkok.

THE POLITICAL SITUATION

The political situation in Nepal has been in transition since 1990, when a mainly peaceful democratic revolution led to a multiparty parliamentary system under a constitutional monarch. Frustration with the rate of progress in rural areas led to a Maoist insurrection and 10 years of low-grade but violent civil war. A peace agreement was reached and the monarchy abolished in 2008, but an effective government has yet to remain in place. The main effect on tourists can be disruptions to their schedule by demonstrations and strikes, but none of the political tension has been aimed at foreigners; Nepal remains a safe destination to visit. However, visitors should monitor the political situation while planning their journey.

BIBLIOGRAPHY

1. Cave W, Pandey P, Osrin D, Shlim DR. Chemoprophylaxis use and the risk of malaria in travelers to Nepal. J Travel Med. 2003 Mar-Apr;10(2):100–5.

2. Hoge CW, Shlim DR, Echeverria P, Rajah R, Herrmann JE, Cross JH. Epidemiology of diarrhea among expatriate residents living in a highly endemic environment. JAMA. 1996 Feb 21;275(7):533–8.

3. Schwartz E, Shlim DR, Eaton M, Jenks N, Houston R. The effect of oral and parenteral typhoid vaccination on the rate of infection with *Salmonella typhi and Salmonella paratyphi* A among foreigners in Nepal. Arch Intern Med. 1990 Feb;150(2):349–51.

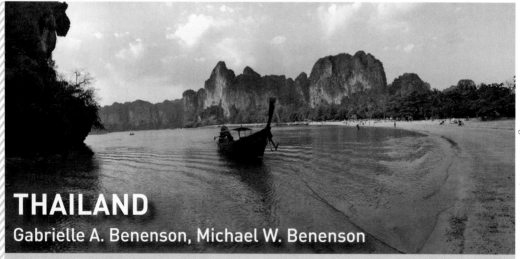

Logan Scholfield/Personal Collection

THAILAND
Gabrielle A. Benenson, Michael W. Benenson

DESTINATION OVERVIEW

Known as "the Land of Smiles," Thailand is a popular destination because of its warm and welcoming reception of tourists and expatriates, beautiful beaches, delicious cuisine, excellent shopping, fabulous golf courses, exciting nightlife, and exotic adventure opportunities. Many travelers also visit Thailand for business, and the country has become a regional business hub. In 2015 more than 29 million visitors spent more than

1 night in Thailand, and the number of visitors continues to grow. Thai is a melodic, tonal language that can be difficult to learn. Luckily, English is commonly spoken at most popular destinations in Thailand. Road signs, maps, and tourist guides provide information in English and Thai.

With close to 68 million people and 76 political provinces, Thailand is a geographically diverse country a little smaller than the state of Texas (Map 4-15). Because Thailand is close to the equator, the climate is tropical and often hot and humid. Flooding is always a possibility in Thailand, and various regions are prone to flash floods. Monsoon rains fall from July through October and can last until cooler, drier weather comes in November, making November through February a popular time of year to visit. Thailand's central location and major international airport in Bangkok make it an easy access point for other destinations in Asia.

More than 9 million people live in the capital city of Bangkok, a major metropolis and center of commerce. Bangkok is a mix of old and new—skyscrapers and waterways, bustling city streets full of people, vendors, dogs, uneven sidewalks, and lots of traffic, in contrast to the fast, quiet, and modern monorail and subway systems. Tourists visit historic sites of glittering grandeur such as one of Bangkok's many Buddhist temples or the Grand Palace to catch a glimpse of the Emerald Buddha. The main artery of Bangkok is the Chao Phraya River and its canals, which provide access to tourist sites, boat tours, the floating market, and restaurants. Bangkok is a paradise of culinary delights, from local fare at a sidewalk noodle stand to a fancy 5-star meal in a restaurant. Rounding off a visit to Bangkok, many tourists will enjoy the pleasures of Thai nightlife, which includes a variety of bars and pubs, dance clubs, drag shows, and the famous red-light districts of Soi Cowboy, Nana, and Patpong.

Visitors to Thailand will also likely visit Chiang Mai in northern Thailand. The city, surrounded by a moat and defensive wall, has more than 300 temples, a popular night bazaar for great shopping, and easy access to the handicraft villages, elephant nature parks, and outdoor adventures that are popular in the region.

Over the years, medical tourism to Thailand has increased, as the costs for treatment are much lower and the quality of care is generally good. In addition, Thailand has a large expatriate community and has also become a popular destination for retirees from around the world. The warm climate and low cost of living make Thailand an attractive place to live.

HEALTH ISSUES
Vaccine-Preventable Diseases
All travelers should be up-to-date on their routine vaccinations. In addition, travelers to Thailand should also be vaccinated against hepatitis A and hepatitis B. Typhoid and Japanese encephalitis vaccines should be considered based on potential risk.

RABIES
Government-sponsored mass vaccination campaigns for dogs and cats have reduced the prevalence of rabies in Thailand, but rabies is still a small risk. Preexposure vaccination is only recommended for travelers who have an occupation that puts them at risk for exposure (such as veterinarians) or who will be traveling in areas where it will be difficult to get immediate access to care, including biologics (see Chapter 3, Rabies). Hospitals and clinics in Bangkok cater to the expatriate community and medical tourists, and rabies vaccine is readily available for preexposure and postexposure prophylaxis, although not all hospitals in Thailand carry human rabies immune globulin.

JAPANESE ENCEPHALITIS
Japanese encephalitis (JE) is endemic throughout Thailand (see Chapter 3, Japanese Encephalitis). Transmission occurs year-round, with seasonal epidemics from May through October in the northern provinces. JE vaccine is recommended for travelers who plan to visit Thailand for ≥1 month and should be considered for those visiting for a shorter period but who have an increased risk of JE virus exposure due to their itineraries or activities. The highest rates of human disease have been reported from the Chiang Mai Valley. Several cases have been

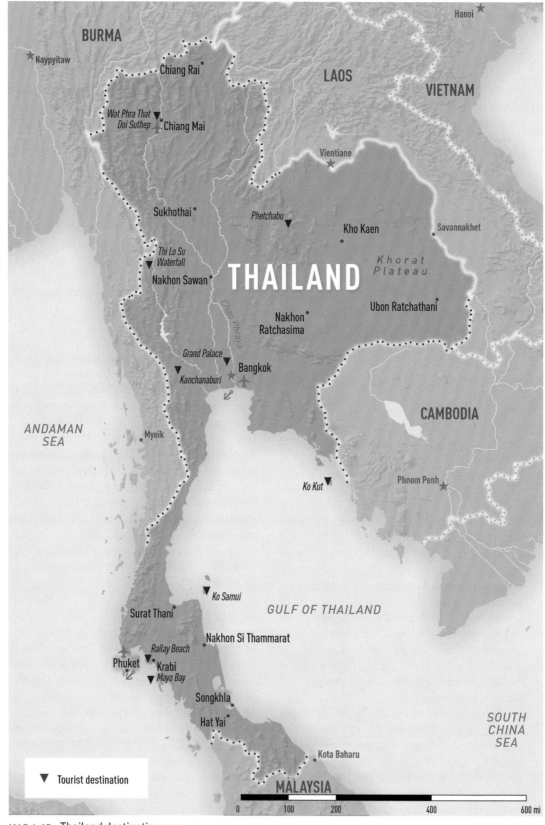

MAP 4-15. Thailand destination map

reported among travelers who visited resort or coastal areas of southern Thailand.

CHOLERA

Although extremely rare in travelers, cholera is a possible risk in parts of Thailand. Cholera vaccine is not routinely recommended for most travelers on typical tourist itineraries, but it is recommended for adult travelers visiting an area with cholera activity within the last year that are prone to recurrence of cholera epidemics.

Vectorborne Diseases

MALARIA

Malaria is endemic in specific areas of Thailand, particularly the rural, forested areas that border Burma (Myanmar), Cambodia, and Laos and the provinces of Kalasin, Krabi (Plai Phraya district), Nakhon Si Thammarat, Narathiwat, Pattani, Phang Nga (including Phang Nga City), Rayong, Sakon Nakhon, Songkhla, Surat Thani, and Yala, especially the forest and forest fringe areas of these provinces. Prophylaxis is recommended for travelers visiting any of these areas (see Chapter 3, Malaria). Transmission in Thailand occurs year-round, and most cases are due to *Plasmodium falciparum*, with the rest due to *P. vivax* or mixed infection. Atovaquone-proguanil or doxycycline are the recommended antimalarial drugs for travelers in Thailand.

DENGUE

Dengue is endemic throughout Thailand (see Chapter 3, Dengue) with large epidemics that occur every several years. Peak transmission occurs during the rainy season, although cases occur year-round even in non-epidemic years. Travelers to Thailand should take measures to protect themselves from daytime mosquito bites to prevent dengue (see Chapter 2, Protection against Mosquitoes, Ticks, & Other Arthropods).

ZIKA

Zika is endemic in Thailand, but the risk to travelers is believed to be low. Because of the risk of birth defects in babies born to women who were infected with Zika while pregnant, women who are pregnant should not travel to Thailand.

If they decide to travel to Thailand, they should strictly follow steps to prevent mosquito bites. Travelers should consult the CDC Travelers' Health website (www.cdc.gov/travel) for the most current recommendations for Zika. See Chapter 3, Zika.

Travelers' Diarrhea

Although the Thai government and several nongovernmental organizations are leading projects to provide clean water across Thailand, and some hotels use their own filtration systems, water and food may still contain harmful bacteria and other contaminants. Travelers should practice food and water precautions and bring an antibiotic for self-treatment of moderate to severe diarrhea. Because fluoroquinolone resistance is widespread in Thailand and other areas of Southeast Asia, azithromycin may be preferred (see Chapter 2, Travelers' Diarrhea).

Water and Soil Diseases

Melioidosis is highly endemic in northeast Thailand, and the highest number of leptospirosis cases can be found in the southern and northeastern regions of the country. For both diseases, most cases occur during the rainy season from July through October. Adventure travelers may be at increased risk because of their exposure to water and soil. Travelers who visit endemic areas should avoid contact with soil and water that could be contaminated and ensure that any open wounds are covered to prevent exposure. When contact cannot be avoided, travelers should wear protective clothing and footwear to reduce the risk of exposure. Skin lacerations, abrasions, or burns that have been contaminated with soil or surface water should be immediately and thoroughly cleaned.

Other Health and Safety Risks

MEDICAL TOURISM

Thailand is among the top medical tourist destinations worldwide. Travelers who plan to seek medical care in Thailand should be advised to research facilities and develop a plan before departure, learn about health insurance coverage, and evaluate their health before making the trip (see Chapter 2, Medical Tourism).

SEXUALLY TRANSMITTED DISEASES AND HIV/AIDS

Thailand is a popular destination for sex tourism (see Chapter 3, *Perspectives*: Sex & Tourism) and, although illegal, sex work is practiced openly across the country. A 100% condom program with sex workers helped slow the spread of HIV and other sexually transmitted diseases; however, approximately 450,000 people were living with HIV/AIDS in Thailand in 2014. Although the number of new HIV infections has been decreasing, HIV remains concentrated in key populations. Travelers should be aware of these risks and always use condoms during sex with partners whose HIV status is unknown.

SAFETY AND SECURITY

Approximately 14,000 people are killed on the roads in Thailand each year, and a substantial proportion (73% in 2012) are killed in motorcycle crashes. Motorcycles are a cheap, easy, and popular mode of transportation, but they are also the most vulnerable vehicles on the road (see Chapter 2, Injury Prevention). Travelers should avoid riding motorcycles. If they must ride, they should wear a helmet. Travelers should fasten seat belts when riding in cars.

Thailand has experienced intermittent periods of political unrest throughout the country and ethnonationalist violence in the southern provinces. In 2014, a caretaker military government was established to maintain peace, develop a constitution, and facilitate democratic elections. However, the country remains politically divided, and travelers should be aware of the possibility of demonstrations, pay attention to the local news, and monitor the US embassy website (http://bangkok.usembassy.gov) and social media outlets to find out if and where protests and demonstrations may occur. Travelers should avoid these locations, since no one can predict whether protests will stay peaceful or turn violent.

BIBLIOGRAPHY

1. Bureau of Epidemiology, Ministry of Public Health, Thailand. National disease surveillance (report 506): Leptospirosis. Bangkok: 2014 2014 Sep 22. Available from: http://www.boe.moph.go.th/boedb/surdata/506wk/y57/en/d43_0957_en.pdf

2. Central Intelligence Agency. The World Fact Book 2013-14. Washington, DC: CIA; 2013 [updated 2016 Sep; cited 2016 Apr. 9]; Available from: https://www.cia.gov/library/publications/the-world-factbook/geos/th.html.

3. Chanlett-Avery E, Dolven B. Thailand: background and US relations. Washington, DC: 2014 2014 Sep 22. Report No.: RL32593.

4. Department of Tourism, Ministry of Tourism and Sports. International tourist arrivals to Thailand in 2015. Bangkok, Thailand: Ministry of Tourism and Sports; 2015 [cited 2016 Apr. 2]; Available from: http://www.tourism.go.th/home/details/11/221/24710.

5. Gongal G, Wright AE. Human rabies in the WHO Southeast Asia Region: forward steps for elimination. Adv Prev Med. 2011;Article ID 383870:1–5.

6. Joint Commission International (JCI) [Internet]. JCI-accredited organizations. Oak Brook (IL): JCI; 2016 [cited 2016 Sep. 25]; Available from: www.jointcommissioninternational.org/about-jci/jci-accredited-organizations/.

7. National AIDS Committee, Royal Thai Government. Thailand ending AIDS: Thailand AIDS response progress report 2015. Geneva: UNAIDS, 2015 Apr 2.

8. World Health Organization. Global status report on road safety 2015. Geneva: 2015 2016 Apr 9. Report No. 978 92 4 156506 6.

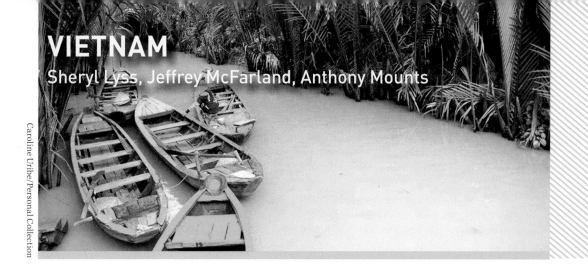

VIETNAM

Sheryl Lyss, Jeffrey McFarland, Anthony Mounts

Caroline Uribe/Personal Collection

DESTINATION OVERVIEW

Vietnam has a population of approximately 94 million people, of whom about two-thirds live in rural areas. The total size of Vietnam is 127,243 mi^2 (331,114 km^2), slightly larger than New Mexico. It is located in Southeast Asia and borders China, Laos, and Cambodia. Vietnam is divided into 63 provinces. The terrain and climate vary, particularly between the north and the south and the mountainous and coastal areas. Once among the poorest countries in the world, Vietnam has since achieved lower-middle income status.

Vietnam is an increasingly popular travel destination for business and tourism. Travelers often try to get a flavor for the entire country with a trip of at least 10 days or combine their Vietnam travels with other nearby Southeast Asia destinations such as Angkor Wat in Cambodia or Luang Prabang in Laos. There is no shortage of attractions in Vietnam, regardless of whether a traveler is interested in touring historical sites, shopping in ethnic markets or traditional trade villages, trekking or biking in hills or valleys, seeing native wildlife, cruising on the Mekong River or Ha Long Bay, scuba diving in the sea, relaxing at a spa resort, visiting art galleries, or taking cooking lessons to understand the regional variations of Vietnam's cuisine.

A typical itinerary might start in the north and include visiting the capital, Hanoi; touring the UNESCO World Heritage site, Ha Long Bay, aboard a junk boat; and exploring the rice fields in Sapa or Mai Chau. In the coastal region, travelers often go to Hue, Hoi An, Da Nang, and Nha Trang, each with its own charms and unique personality. In the south, travelers often choose to see Vietnam's largest, busiest, and most modern city, Ho Chi Minh City. From there, Phu Quoc Island,

Dalat, the Cu Chi tunnels, and floating markets of the Mekong Delta are easy trips (see Map 4-16).

HEALTH ISSUES

Vaccine-Preventable Diseases

Travelers to Vietnam should be up-to-date on routine vaccines, including seasonal influenza. Travelers should also protect themselves by getting vaccinated against typhoid and hepatitis A. Hepatitis B protection is advised, especially for long-term travelers and expatriates, given the high prevalence of chronic HBV infection in the population.

JAPANESE ENCEPHALITIS

Because Japanese encephalitis (JE) is endemic throughout Vietnam, JE vaccination is recommended for all travelers who spend ≥1 month in the country and should be considered for short-term travelers who plan on spending time outside urban areas and may be involved in activities that expose them to the mosquitoes that transmit JE virus. Such activities may include camping, hiking, biking or other outdoor activities, or staying in accommodations without air conditioning, screens, or bed nets (see Chapter 3, Japanese Encephalitis). JE has seasonal peaks from May through October, and the highest rates of JE disease occur in the northern provinces around Hanoi and the northwestern and northeastern provinces bordering China. Personalized advice during a thorough pretravel consultation is important.

Malaria

Malaria in Vietnam is caused by *Plasmodium falciparum* and *P. vivax*. Cases and deaths have decreased substantially in the past 15 years, and ongoing local transmission is primarily a concern in rural, forested areas that are not included in most tourist itineraries. There are rare cases in the Mekong Delta and Red River Delta. There are no cases in cities of Da Nang, Haiphong, Hanoi, Ho Chi Minh City (Saigon), Nha Tran, and Qui Nhon. Travelers to the Mekong Delta should take precautions to avoid mosquito bites, such as wearing loose-fitting clothing (long pants and long-sleeved shirts) and using insect repellent (see Chapter 2, Protection against Mosquitoes, Ticks, & Other Arthropods) but do not need to take antimalarial drugs. Travelers the southern part of the country in the provinces of Dac Lac, Gia Lai, Khanh Hoa, Kon Tum, Lam Dong, Ninh Thuan, Song Be, and Tay Ninh should take atovaquone-proguanil or doxycycline. Travelers to other areas with malaria should take atovaquone-proguanil, doxycycline, or mefloquine (see Chapter 3, Malaria).

Dengue and Zika

Dengue is endemic in Vietnam and, although peak transmission occurs during the summer rainy season, dengue virus transmission occurs year-round. Zika is also endemic in Vietnam, but the risk to travelers is believed to be low. Because of the risk of birth defects in babies born to women infected with Zika while pregnant, women who are pregnant should not travel to Vietnam. If they decide to travel to Vietnam, they should strictly follow steps to prevent mosquito bites. Travelers should consult the CDC Travelers' Health website (www.cdc.gov/travel) for the most current recommendations for Zika.

Avian Influenza

Vietnam has reported sporadic cases of human infection with avian influenza A (H5N1) virus. H5N1 is endemic in domestic poultry in Vietnam, with continued sporadic and geographically dispersed poultry outbreaks.

A novel avian influenza A (H7N9) virus was identified in China in 2013, including in a province bordering Vietnam. To date, no animals or humans have been identified in Vietnam with this strain of avian influenza virus.

To avoid infection with avian influenza viruses, travelers to an area affected by avian influenza should avoid direct contact with birds, including poultry (such as chickens and ducks) and wild birds; avoid touching surfaces that have bird droppings (feces) or other bird fluids on them; and avoid places where live birds are raised, kept, or sold, such as live bird markets.

Travelers should eat only bird meat or products that have been thoroughly cooked. Any dishes that contain uncooked (raw) or undercooked bird meat or products such as eggs and poultry blood should be avoided. For example, egg yolks should not be runny or liquid. Travelers should also practice healthy habits to help stop the spread of germs by washing hands often with soap and clean water or using an alcohol-based hand sanitizer (containing at least 60% alcohol) when soap and clean water are not available and hands are not visibly dirty.

Other Health and Safety Risks

FOODBORNE ILLNESSES

Drinking tap water should be avoided, as should beverages with ice. Travelers should avoid eating raw or undercooked meat or seafood, uncooked vegetables, and raw fruits that cannot be peeled by the traveler. Travelers should be cautious about eating food or drinking beverages from street vendors. Travelers with seafood allergies should be particularly cautious in Vietnam, given the common use of fish and other seafood sauces in many dishes.

Travelers should be particularly careful not to consume dishes containing uncooked blood of pigs or other animals because of the risk of trichinellosis and *Streptococcus suis* infections (meningitis or septicemia). One popular traditional Vietnamese dish, *tiet canh*, is made of coagulated, fresh, raw blood mixed with cooked pieces of meat. It can be difficult to know just by looking if a dish contains uncooked blood. Ask, and when in doubt do not eat it.

ENVIRONMENTAL EXPOSURES

Skin rashes may result from fungal infections or the combination of heat and humidity. Sunstroke, sunburn, and dehydration can be problems for travelers. Efforts should be made to keep clothes, shoes, and linens clean and dry. Use of a broad-spectrum sunscreen with SPF ≥15 that protects against both UVA and UVB is recommended; travelers should keep well hydrated and minimize sun exposure by using clothing, hats, and umbrellas.

Travelers with allergies or asthma may find their conditions are exacerbated because of high

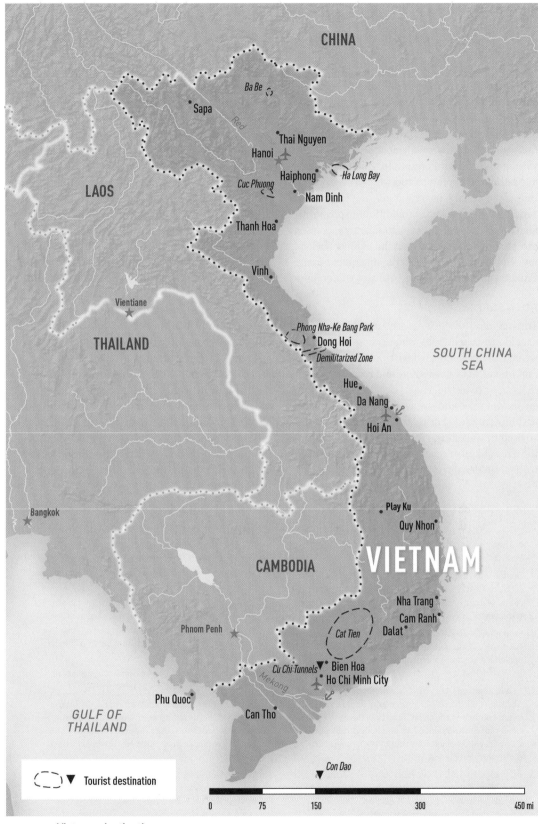

MAP 4-16. Vietnam destination map

levels of particulate matter and indoor air pollution, especially in Hanoi and Ho Chi Minh City. The US Department of State in partnership with the US Environmental Protection Agency monitors air quality in Vietnam (https://airnow.gov/index.cfm?action=airnow.global_summary#Vietnam). Short-term exposure to these levels of air pollution can irritate the eyes and throat, and those with underlying cardiorespiratory illness, including asthma, chronic obstructive pulmonary disease, or coronary heart failure, may find their condition exacerbated. In addition, exposure to high levels of air pollution significantly increases the risk of respiratory tract infections, including sinusitis, otitis, bronchitis, and pneumonia. Children and the elderly are the most vulnerable.

ROAD SAFETY

To avoid motor vehicle–related injuries, travelers should fasten seat belts when riding in cars and wear a safety helmet when riding bicycles and motorbikes. Pedestrians may find road conditions in Vietnam to be challenging because of an apparent lack of rules and the large number of vehicles and motorcycles sharing the road. Travelers are advised to walk facing traffic and, when crossing the street, to proceed at a consistent walking pace with no sudden direction changes, such as quickly turning back. Pedestrians will observe that motorbikes and cars will go around them much like a school of fish will part when it encounters an object, and then regroup. Note that motorbikes and sometimes cars will travel on the wrong side of the street (against oncoming traffic) as well as on sidewalks, so travelers should be urged to always look in both directions and be particularly cautious when crossing at corners.

Medical Care in Vietnam

Several private medical practices, clinics, and hospitals that serve foreigners are available in Hanoi and Ho Chi Minh City. However, blood transfusion services, inpatient care, and specialty services are generally not of high quality. Thus, travelers should ensure that they have adequate medical evacuation insurance in case they need to be evacuated to Singapore or Bangkok where high-quality specialty services are provided (see Chapter 2, Travel Insurance, Travel Health Insurance, & Medical Evacuation Insurance). To ensure the quality of any needed medications, travelers may want to consider purchasing them through an expatriate or international travel clinic, even if the price is higher. If a traveler is taking prescription medicine, he or she should bring enough medication for the entire trip, in the original bottle, and with the prescription.

BIBLIOGRAPHY

1. Carrique-Mas JJ, Bryant JE. A review of foodborne bacterial and parasitic zoonoses in Vietnam. EcoHealth. 2013 Dec;10(4):465–89.

2. Central Intelligence Agency. The World Fact Book: Vietnam. CIA; 2016 [updated 2016 Sep.; cited 2016 Apr. 12]; Available from: https://www.cia.gov/library/publications/resources/the-world-factbook/geos/vm.html.

3. Cuong HQ, Vu NT, Cazelles B, Boni MF, Thai KT, Rabaa MA, et al. Spatiotemporal dynamics of dengue epidemics, southern Vietnam. Emerg Infect Dis. 2013 Jun;19(6):945–53.

4. Hsu A, Emerson J, Levy M, de Sherbinin A, Johnson L, Malik O, et al. The 2014 Environmental Performance Index: country profiles, Viet Nam. New Haven (CT): Yale Center for Environmental Law and Policy; 2014 [cited 2016 Sep. 25]; Available from: http://epi2012.yale.edu/epi/country-profile/viet-nam.

5. Huong VT, Hoa NT, Horby P, Bryant JE, Van Kinh N, Toan TK, et al. Raw pig blood consumption and potential risk for Streptococcus suis infection, Vietnam. Emerg Infect Dis. 2014 Nov;20(11):1895–8.

6. Manabe T, Yamaoka K, Tango T, Binh NG, Co DX, Tuan ND, et al. Chronological, geographical, and seasonal trends of human cases of avian influenza A (H5N1) in Vietnam, 2003–2014: a spatial analysis. BMC Infect Dis 2016 Feb 4;16(64):1391–8.

7. Phung D, Hien TT, Linh HN, Luong LM, Morawska L, Chu C, et al. Air pollution and risk of respiratory and cardiovascular hospitalizations in the most populous city in Vietnam. Sci Total Environ 2016 Jul 1;557-558(2016):322–30.

8. Roberts L. In Vietnam, an anatomy of a measles outbreak. Science. 2015 May 29;348(6238):962.

9. World Health Organization Western Pacific Region [Internet]. WHO representative office in Vietnam. Hanoi: World Health Organization; 2014 [cited 2016 Sep. 25]; Available from: http://www.wpro.who.int/vietnam/en.

10. Yen NT, Duffy MR, Hong NM, Hien NT, Fischer M, Hills SL. Surveillance for Japanese encephalitis in Vietnam, 1998–2007. Am J Trop Med Hyg. 2010 Oct;83(4):816–9.

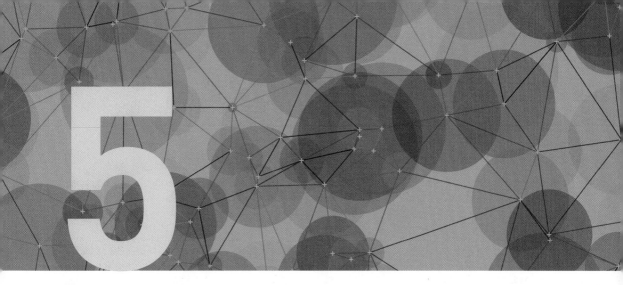

5

Post-Travel Evaluation

GENERAL APPROACH TO THE RETURNED TRAVELER

Jessica K. Fairley

THE POST-TRAVEL EVALUATION

Travel-related health problems have been reported in as many as 22%–64% of travelers to developing countries. Although most of these illnesses are mild, up to 8% of travelers are ill enough to seek care from a health care provider. Most post-travel infections become apparent soon after travel, but incubation periods vary, and some syndromes can present months to years after initial infection. When evaluating a patient with a probable travel-related illness, the clinician should consider the items summarized in Box 5-1.

The Severity of Illness

The severity of illness is not only important in order to triage the patient but also can distinguish certain infections from each other. Is this a potentially life-threatening infection, such as malaria?

A severe respiratory syndrome or signs of hemorrhagic fever are examples of cases that may also necessitate prompt involvement of public health authorities. See "Management" below for more details.

Travel Itinerary

The itinerary and activities in which the traveler participated are crucial to formulating a differential diagnosis, because potential exposures differ depending on the region of travel and behaviors. A febrile illness with nonspecific symptoms could be malaria, dengue, typhoid fever, or rickettsial disease, among others. Being able to exclude certain infections will avoid unnecessary testing. A 2013 study from the GeoSentinel Surveillance Network found a distinct pattern of diagnoses depending on the region of the world visited. In travelers

BOX 5-1. Important elements of a medical history in an ill returned traveler

- Severity of illness
- Travel itinerary and duration of travel
- Timing of onset of illness in relation to international travel
- Past medical history and medications
- History of a pretravel consultation
  - › Travel immunizations

- › Adherence to malaria chemoprophylaxis
- Individual exposures
  - › Type of accommodations
  - › Insect precautions taken (such as repellent, bed nets)
  - › Source of drinking water
  - › Ingestion of raw meat or seafood or unpasteurized dairy products

- › Insect or arthropod bites
- › Freshwater exposure (such as swimming, rafting)
- › Animal bites and scratches
- › Body fluid exposure (such as tattoos, sexual activity)
- › Medical care while overseas (such as injections, transfusions)

to sub-Saharan Africa presenting with fever, malaria was the most common specific diagnosis. On the other hand, febrile patients after travel to Latin America or Southeast Asia were much more likely to have dengue. The duration of travel is also important, since the risk of a travel-related illness increases with the length of the trip. A tropical medicine specialist can assist with the differential diagnosis and may be aware of outbreaks or the current prevalence of an infectious disease in an area. The 2014–2015 Ebola virus epidemic in West Africa highlighted the importance of epidemiologic factors and travel itineraries in managing patients and protecting staff and the community.

Timing of Illness in Relation to Travel

Most ill travelers will seek medical attention within 1 month of return from their destination, because most common travel-related infections have short incubation periods. Occasionally, however, infections such as schistosomiasis, leishmaniasis, or tuberculosis can manifest months or even years later. Therefore, in unusual cases, a detailed history that extends beyond a few months before presentation can be helpful. The most common travel-related infections with short incubation periods are listed in Table 5-1.

Underlying Medical Illness

Comorbidities can affect the susceptibility to infection, as well as the clinical manifestations and severity of illness. An increasing number of immunosuppressed people (due to organ transplants, immune-modulating medications, HIV infection, or other primary or acquired immunodeficiencies) are international travelers (see Chapter 8, Immunocompromised Travelers).

Vaccines Received and Prophylaxis Used

The history of vaccinations and malaria chemoprophylaxis should be reviewed when evaluating an ill returned traveler. Less than half of US travelers to developing countries seek pretravel medical advice and may not have received vaccines or taken antimalarial drugs. Although adherence to malaria chemoprophylaxis does not rule out the possibility of malaria, it reduces the risk and increases the likelihood of an alternative diagnosis. Fever and a rash in a traveler without measles vaccination would raise concern about measles. The most common vaccine-preventable diseases found in a large 2010 GeoSentinel study of returned travelers included enteric fever (typhoid and paratyphoid), viral hepatitis, and influenza. More than half of these patients with vaccine-preventable diseases were hospitalized.

Table 5-1. Illnesses associated with fever presenting in the first 2 weeks after travel

SYNDROME	POSSIBLE CAUSE
Systemic febrile illness with initial nonspecific symptoms	Malaria Dengue Typhoid fever Rickettsial diseases (such as scrub typhus, spotted fevers) East African trypanosomiasis Acute HIV infection Leptospirosis Ebola virus disease Viral hemorrhagic fevers
Fever with central nervous system involvement	Meningococcal meningitis Malaria Arboviral encephalitis (such as Japanese encephalitis virus, West Nile virus) East African trypanosomiasis Angiostrongyliasis Rabies
Fever with respiratory symptoms	Influenza Bacterial pneumonia Acute histoplasmosis or coccidioidomycosis *Legionella* pneumonia Q fever Malaria Tularemia Pneumonic plague Middle East respiratory syndrome (MERS)
Fever and skin rash	Dengue Chikungunya Zika Measles Varicella Spotted fever or typhus group rickettsiosis Typhoid fever Parvovirus B19 Mononucleosis Acute HIV infection

5

Individual Exposure History

Knowledge of the patient's exposures during travel, including insect bites, contaminated food or water, or freshwater swimming, can also assist with the differential diagnosis. In addition to malarial parasites, mosquitoes can transmit viruses (such as dengue virus, yellow fever virus, chikungunya virus, and Zika virus) and filarial parasites (such as *Wuchereria bancrofti*). Depending on the clinical syndrome, a history of a tick bite could suggest a diagnosis of tickborne encephalitis, African tick-bite fever, or other rickettsial infections. Tsetse flies are large, and their bites are painful and often recalled by the patient. They can carry *Trypanosoma brucei*, the protozoan that causes African sleeping sickness.

Freshwater swimming or other water contact can put the patient at risk for schistosomiasis, leptospirosis, and other diseases.

The activities during a trip and the type of accommodations can also influence the risk for acquiring certain diseases. Travelers who visit friends and relatives are at higher risk of malaria, typhoid fever, and certain other diseases, often because they stay longer, travel to more remote destinations, have more contact with local water sources, and do not seek pretravel advice (see Chapter 8, Immigrants Returning Home to Visit Friends & Relatives [VFRs]). Someone backpacking and camping in rural areas will also have a higher risk of certain diseases than those staying in luxury, air-conditioned hotels.

COMMON SYNDROMES

The most common clinical presentations after travel to developing countries include systemic febrile illness, diarrheal illness, and dermatologic conditions. These are described in more detail in the following sections of this chapter (Fever in Returned Travelers, Persistent Travelers' Diarrhea, and Skin & Soft Tissue Infections in Returned Travelers). Fever in a traveler returning from a malaria-endemic country needs to be evaluated immediately.

Respiratory Complaints

Respiratory complaints are frequent among returned travelers and are typically associated with common respiratory viruses (see Chapter 2, Respiratory Infections). Influenza is among the most common vaccine-preventable diseases associated with international travel. Severe respiratory symptoms—especially associated with fever—in a returned traveler should alert the physician to common infectious diseases such as seasonal influenza, bacterial pneumonia, and malaria but could also suggest more unusual entities, such as Legionnaires' disease. Emerging respiratory infections such as Middle East respiratory syndrome (MERS) and H7N9 avian influenza from China should be in the differential if the travel history is appropriate and respiratory symptoms do not have a clear alternative diagnosis. In these suspected cases, local public health authorities and CDC should be alerted immediately. See relevant sections in Chapter 3 for more information on these emerging infections.

Delayed onset and chronic cough after travel could be tuberculosis, especially in a long-term traveler or health care worker. Other uncommon infections causing respiratory illness after travel to specific regions are histoplasmosis, coccidioidomycosis, Q fever, plague, tularemia, and melioidosis. Helminth infections that produce pulmonary disease include strongyloidiasis, paragonimiasis, and schistosomiasis.

Eosinophilia

Eosinophilia in a returning traveler suggests a possible helminth infection. Allergic diseases, hematologic disorders, and a few other viral, fungal, and protozoan infections can also cause eosinophilia. Fever and eosinophilia can be present during pulmonary migration of parasites, such as hookworm, *Ascaris*, and *Strongyloides*. Acute schistosomiasis, or Katayama syndrome, is also a cause of fever and eosinophilia and can be associated with pulmonary infiltrates. Other parasitic infections associated with eosinophilia include chronic strongyloidiasis, visceral larval migrans, lymphatic filariasis, and acute trichinellosis. Findings in an outbreak of sarcocystosis in travelers returning from Tioman Island, Malaysia, included myalgia and eosinophilia. The affected travelers had eosinophilic myositis on muscle biopsy.

MANAGEMENT

Most post-travel illnesses can be managed on an outpatient basis, but some patients, especially those with systemic febrile illnesses, may need to be hospitalized. Furthermore, potentially severe, transmissible infections such as Ebola or MERS require enhanced infection control measures and may require higher levels of care. Severe presentations, such as acute respiratory distress, mental status change, and hemodynamic instability, require inpatient care. Clinicians should have a low threshold for admitting febrile patients if malaria is suspected. Confirmation of diagnosis can be delayed, and complications can occur rapidly. Management in an inpatient setting is especially important if the patient may not reliably follow up or when no one is at home to assist if symptoms worsen quickly. Consultation with an infectious diseases physician is recommended in severe travel-related infections, when management is complicated, or when the diagnosis remains unclear. A tropical medicine or infectious disease specialist should be involved in cases that require specialized treatment, such as neurocysticercosis, severe malaria, and leishmaniasis, among others. Public health authorities may need to be involved for transmissible, high-consequence infections. CDC provides on-call assistance with the diagnosis and management of parasitic infections at 404-718-4745 for parasitic infections other than malaria or 770-488-7788 (toll-free at 855-856-4713) for malaria, during business hours. After business hours, call the CDC Emergency Operations Center at 770-488-7100.

BIBLIOGRAPHY

1. Boggild AK, Castelli F, Gautret P, Torresi J, von Sonnenburg F, Barnett ED, et al. Vaccine preventable diseases in returned international travelers: results from the GeoSentinel Surveillance Network. Vaccine. 2010 Oct 28;28(46):7389–95.

2. CDC. Notes from the field: acute muscular sarcocystosis among returning travelers—Tioman Island, Malaysia, 2011. MMWR Morb Mortal Wkly Rep. 2012 Jan 20;61(2):37–8.

3. Chen LH, Wilson ME, Davis X, Loutan L, Schwartz E, Keystone J, et al. Illness in long-term travelers visiting GeoSentinel clinics. Emerg Infect Dis. 2009 Nov;15(11):1773–82.

4. Fairley JK, Kozarsky PE, Kraft CS, Guarner J, Steinberg JP, Anderson E, et al. Ebola or Not? Evaluating the ill traveler from Ebola-affected countries in West Africa. Open Forum Infect Dis. 2016 Jan 18;3(1ofw005).

5. Hamer DH, Connor BA. Travel health knowledge, attitudes and practices among United States travelers. J Travel Med. 2004 Jan–Feb;11(1):23–6.

6. Hendel-Paterson B, Swanson SJ. Pediatric travelers visiting friends and relatives (VFR) abroad: illnesses, barriers and pre-travel recommendations. Travel Med Infect Dis. 2011 Jul;9(4):192–203.

7. Leder K, Torresi J, Libman MD, Cramer JP, Castelli F, Schlagenhauf P, et al. GeoSentinel surveillance of illness in returned travelers, 2007–2011. Ann Intern Med. 2013 Mar 19;158(6):456–68.

8. Ryan ET, Wilson ME, Kain KC. Illness after international travel. N Engl J Med. 2002 Aug 15;347(7):505–16.

9. Schulte C, Krebs B, Jelinek T, Nothdurft HD, von Sonnenburg F, Loscher T. Diagnostic significance of blood eosinophilia in returning travelers. Clin Infect Dis. 2002 Feb 1;34(3):407–11.

10. Wilson ME, Weld LH, Boggild A, Keystone JS, Kain KC, von Sonnenburg F, et al. Fever in returned travelers: results from the GeoSentinel Surveillance Network. Clin Infect Dis. 2007 Jun 15;44(12):1560–8.

FEVER IN RETURNED TRAVELERS

Mary Elizabeth Wilson

INITIAL FOCUS

Fever commonly accompanies serious illness in returned travelers. Because it can signal a rapidly progressive infection such as malaria, the clinician must initiate early evaluation, especially in people who have visited areas with malaria in recent months (see Chapter 3, Malaria). The initial focus in evaluating a febrile returned traveler should be on identifying infections that are rapidly progressive, treatable, or transmissible. In some instances, public health officials must be alerted if the traveler may have been contagious while traveling or infected with a pathogen of public health importance (such as yellow fever or Ebola) at the origin or destination.

USE OF HISTORY, LOCATION OF EXPOSURE, AND INCUBATION TO LIMIT DIFFERENTIAL DIAGNOSIS

Often the list of potential diagnoses is long, but multiple recent studies help to identify more

Table 5-2. Common causes of fever, by geographic area

GEOGRAPHIC AREA	COMMON TROPICAL DISEASE CAUSING FEVER	OTHER INFECTIONS CAUSING OUTBREAKS OR CLUSTERS IN TRAVELERS
Caribbean	Chikungunya, dengue, malaria (Haiti), Zika	Acute histoplasmosis, leptospirosis
Central America	Chikungunya, dengue, malaria (primarily *Plasmodium vivax*), Zika	Leptospirosis, histoplasmosis, coccidioidomycosis
South America	Chikungunya, dengue, malaria (primarily *P. vivax*), Zika	Bartonellosis, leptospirosis, enteric fever, histoplasmosis
South-central Asia	Dengue, enteric fever, malaria (primarily non-falciparum)	Chikungunya
Southeast Asia	Dengue, malaria (primarily non-falciparum)	Chikungunya, leptospirosis
Sub-Saharan Africa	Malaria (primarily *P. falciparum*), tickborne rickettsiae (main cause of fever in southern Africa), acute schistosomiasis, dengue	African trypanosomiasis, chikungunya, enteric fever, filariasis

common diagnoses. A large proportion of illnesses in returned travelers is caused by common, cosmopolitan infections (such as bacterial pneumonia or pyelonephritis), so these must be considered along with unusual infections. Because the geographic area of travel determines the relative likelihood of major causes of fever, it is essential to identify where the febrile patient has traveled and lived (Table 5-2). Details about activities (such as freshwater exposure in schistosomiasis-endemic areas, animal bites, sexual activities, tattoos, or local medical care with injections) and accommodations in areas with malaria (bed nets, window screens, air conditioning) during travel may provide useful clues. Preparation before travel (such as hepatitis A vaccine or yellow fever vaccine) will markedly reduce the likelihood of some infections, so this is a relevant part of the history. A history of travel and residence should be an integral part of every medical history.

Because each infection has a characteristic incubation period (although the range is extremely wide with some infections), the time of exposures needs to be defined in different geographic areas (Table 5-3). This knowledge will allow the clinician to exclude some infections from the differential diagnosis. Most serious febrile infections manifest within the first month after return from tropical travel, yet infections related to travel exposures can occasionally occur months or even >1 year after return. In the United States, >90% of reported cases of *Plasmodium falciparum* malaria manifest within 30 days of return, but almost half of cases of *P. vivax* malaria manifest >30 days after return.

FINDINGS REQUIRING URGENT ATTENTION

Presence of associated signs, symptoms, or laboratory findings can focus attention on specific infections (Table 5-4). Findings that should prompt urgent attention include hemorrhage, neurologic impairment, and acute respiratory distress. Even if an initial physical examination is unremarkable, it is worth repeating the examination, as new findings may appear that will help in the diagnostic process (such as skin lesions or tender liver). Although most febrile illnesses in returned travelers are related to infections, the clinician should bear in mind that other problems, including pulmonary emboli and drug hypersensitivity reactions, can be associated with fever.

Table 5-3. Common infections, by incubation period

DISEASE	USUAL INCUBATION PERIOD (RANGE)	DISTRIBUTION
Incubation <14 Days		
Chikungunya	2–4 days (1–14 days)	Tropics, subtropics
Dengue	4–8 days (3–14 days)	Tropics, subtropics
Encephalitis, arboviral (Japanese encephalitis, tickborne encephalitis, West Nile virus, other)	3–14 days (1–20 days)	Specific agents vary by region
Enteric fever	7–18 days (3–60 days)	Especially in Indian subcontinent
Acute HIV infection	10–28 days (10 days to 6 weeks)	Worldwide
Influenza	1–3 days	Worldwide, can also be acquired while traveling
Legionellosis	5–6 days (2–10 days)	Widespread
Leptospirosis	7–12 days (2–26 days)	Widespread, most common in tropical areas
Malaria, *Plasmodium falciparum*	6–30 days (98% onset within 3 months of travel)	Tropics, subtropics
Malaria, *P. vivax*	8 days to 12 months (almost half have onset >30 days after completion of travel)	Widespread in tropics and subtropics
Spotted fever rickettsiosis	Few days to 2–3 weeks	Causative species vary by region
Zika virus infection	3–14 days	Widespread in Latin America, endemic through much of Africa, Southeast Asia, and Pacific Islands
Incubation 14 Days to 6 Weeks		
Encephalitis, arboviral; enteric fever; acute HIV; leptospirosis; malaria	See above incubation periods for relevant diseases	See above distribution for relevant diseases
Amebic liver abscess	Weeks to months	Most common in resource-poor countries
Hepatitis A	28–30 days (15–50 days)	Most common in resource-poor countries
Hepatitis E	26–42 days (2–9 weeks)	Widespread
Acute schistosomiasis (Katayama syndrome)	4–8 weeks	Most common in sub-Saharan Africa

(continued)

Table 5-3. Common infections, by incubation period (continued)

DISEASE	USUAL INCUBATION PERIOD (RANGE)	DISTRIBUTION
Incubation >6 Weeks		
Amebic liver abscess, hepatitis E, malaria, acute schistosomiasis	See above incubation periods for relevant diseases	See above distribution for relevant diseases
Hepatitis B	90 days (60–150 days)	Widespread
Leishmaniasis, visceral	2–10 months (10 days to years)	Asia, Africa, Latin America, southern Europe, and the Middle East
Tuberculosis	Primary, weeks; reactivation, years	Global distribution, rates and levels of resistance vary widely

Table 5-4. Common clinical findings and associated infections

COMMON CLINICAL FINDINGS	INFECTIONS TO CONSIDER AFTER TROPICAL TRAVEL
Fever and rash	Dengue, chikungunya, Zika, rickettsial infections, enteric fever (skin lesions may be sparse or absent), acute HIV infection, measles
Fever and abdominal pain	Enteric fever, amebic liver abscess
Undifferentiated fever and normal or low white blood cell count	Dengue, malaria, rickettsial infection, enteric fever, chikungunya, Zika
Fever and hemorrhage	Viral hemorrhagic fevers (dengue and others), meningococcemia, leptospirosis, rickettsial infections
Fever and arthralgia or myalgia, sometimes persistent	Chikungunya, dengue, Zika
Fever and eosinophilia	Acute schistosomiasis, drug hypersensitivity reaction, fascioliasis and other parasitic infections (rare)
Fever and pulmonary infiltrates	Common bacterial and viral pathogens, legionellosis, acute schistosomiasis, Q fever, leptospirosis
Fever and altered mental status	Cerebral malaria, viral or bacterial meningoencephalitis, African trypanosomiasis, scrub typhus
Mononucleosis syndrome	Epstein-Barr virus infection, cytomegalovirus infection, toxoplasmosis, acute HIV infection
Fever persisting >2 weeks	Malaria, enteric fever, Epstein-Barr virus infection, cytomegalovirus infection, toxoplasmosis, acute HIV infection, acute schistosomiasis, brucellosis, tuberculosis, Q fever, visceral leishmaniasis (rare)
Fever with onset >6 weeks after travel	*Plasmodium vivax* or *ovale* malaria, acute hepatitis (B, C, or E), tuberculosis, amebic liver abscess

Fever accompanied by any of the following syndromes deserves further scrutiny, because it may indicate a disease of public health importance:

- Skin rash with or without conjunctivitis
- Difficulty breathing
- Shortness of breath
- Persistent cough
- Decreased consciousness
- Bruising or unusual bleeding (without previous injury)
- Persistent diarrhea
- Persistent vomiting (other than air or motion sickness)
- Jaundice
- Paralysis of recent onset

People who travel to visit friends and relatives (VFRs) often do not seek pretravel medical advice and are at higher risk for some diseases than other travelers. A review of GeoSentinel Surveillance Network data showed that a larger proportion of immigrant VFRs than tourist travelers presented with serious (requiring hospitalization), potentially preventable travel-related illnesses.

CHANGE OVER TIME

Clinicians have access to resources on the Internet that provide information about geographic-specific risks, disease activity, and other useful information, such as drug-susceptibility patterns for pathogens. Infectious diseases are dynamic, as demonstrated by the introduction and spread of chikungunya virus in the Americas beginning in late 2013 and the rapid spread of Zika virus in the Americas in 2015 and 2016. In contrast, because of the wide use of vaccine, hepatitis A infection is now infrequently seen in travelers.

Common infections in returned travelers may be seen at unexpected times of the year. Because influenza transmission can occur throughout the year in tropical areas, and the peak season in the Southern Hemisphere is May to August, clinicians in the Northern Hemisphere must be alert to the possibility of influenza outside the usual US influenza season.

Travelers may acquire infections caused by common bacteria that are unusually resistant. Bacteria that produce extended-spectrum β-lactamases and carbapenem-resistant Enterobacteriaceae, including bacteria expressing the metalloprotease NDM-1, which confers resistance to many available antibiotics, have been found in infections acquired during travel, most often related to medical care (both elective and emergency). Enteric fever, the term used to describe either typhoid or paratyphoid fever, has also become increasingly resistant to fluoroquinolones (see Chapter 3, Typhoid & Paratyphoid Fever).

The tables in this section identify some common infections by presenting findings or other characteristics, by area of travel and by incubation periods. These highlight only the most common infections. The listed references and websites should be consulted for more detailed information. In most studies, a specific cause for fever is not identified in about 25% of returned travelers.

KEEP IN MIND

- Initial symptoms of life-threatening and self-limited infections can be identical.
- Fever in returned travelers is often caused by common, cosmopolitan infections, such as pneumonia and pyelonephritis, which should not be overlooked in the search for exotic diagnoses.
- Travelers may be infected with highly drug-resistant pathogens.
- Patients with malaria may be afebrile at the time of evaluation but typically give a history of fever or chills.
- Malaria is the most common cause of acute undifferentiated fever after travel to sub-Saharan Africa and to some other tropical areas.
- Malaria, especially *P. falciparum*, can progress rapidly. Diagnostic studies should be done promptly and treatment instituted immediately if malaria is diagnosed (see Chapter 3, Malaria).
- A history of taking malaria chemoprophylaxis does not exclude the possibility of malaria.

- Patients with malaria can have prominent respiratory (including acute respiratory distress syndrome), gastrointestinal, or central nervous system findings.

- Dengue is the most common cause of febrile illness among people who seek medical care after travel to Latin America or Asia.

- Other arboviral infections are emerging as causes of fever in travelers, including chikungunya and Zika.

- Viral hemorrhagic fevers are important to identify but are rare in travelers;

bacterial infections, such as leptospirosis, meningococcemia, and rickettsial infections, can also cause fever and hemorrhage and should be always be considered because of the need to institute prompt, specific treatment.

- Sexually transmitted diseases, including acute HIV, can cause acute febrile infections.

- Consider infection control, public health implications, and requirements for reportable diseases.

BIBLIOGRAPHY

1. Bottieau E, Clerinx J, Schrooten W, Van den Enden E, Wouters R, Van Esbroeck M, et al. Etiology and outcome of fever after a stay in the tropics. Arch Intern Med. 2006 Aug 14-28;166(15):1642–8.

2. Hassing RJ, Alsma J, Arcilla MS, van Genderen PJ, Stricker BH, Verbon A. International travel and acquisition of multidrug-resistant Enterobacteriaceae: a systematic review. Euro Surveill 2015;20(47):pii=30074. DOI: http://dx.doi.org/10.2807/1560-7917. ES.2015.20.47.30074.

3. Jensenius M, Davis X, von Sonnenburg F, Schwartz E, Keystone JS, Leder K, et al. Multicenter GeoSentinel analysis of rickettsial diseases in international travelers, 1996–2008. Emerg Infect Dis. 2009 Nov;15(11):1791–8.

4. Kumarasamy KK, Toleman MA, Walsh TR, Bagaria J, Butt F, Balakrishnan R, et al. Emergence of a new antibiotic resistance mechanism in India, Pakistan, and the UK: a molecular, biological, and epidemiological study. Lancet Infect Dis. 2010 Sep;10(9):597–602.

5. Leder K, Torresi J, Libman MD, Cramer JP, Castelli F, Schlagenhauf P, et al. GeoSentinel surveillance of illness in returned travelers, 2007–2011. Ann Intern Med. 2013 Mar 19;158(6):456–68.

6. Mendelson M, Han PV, Vincent P, von Sonnenburg F, Cramer JP, Loutan L, et al. Regional variation in travel-related illness acquired in Africa, March 1997–May 2011. Emerg Infect Dis. 2014 Apr;20(4):532–41.

7. Ryan ET. Troubling news from Asia about treating enteric fever: a coming storm. Lancet Infect Dis 2016 May;16(5):508–9.

8. Ryan ET, Wilson ME, Kain KC. Illness after international travel. N Engl J Med. 2002 Aug 15;347(7):505–16.

9. Wilson ME, Weld LH, Boggild A, Keystone JS, Kain KC, von Sonnenburg F, et al. Fever in returned travelers: results from the GeoSentinel Surveillance Network. Clin Infect Dis. 2007 Jun 15;44(12):1560–8.

PERSISTENT TRAVELERS' DIARRHEA

Bradley A. Connor

Although most cases of travelers' diarrhea are acute and self-limited, a certain percentage of travelers will develop persistent (>14 days) gastrointestinal symptoms (see Chapter 2, Travelers' Diarrhea). The pathogenesis of persistent travelers' diarrhea generally falls into one of the following broad categories: 1) persistent infection or coinfection with a second organism not targeted by initial therapy, 2) previously undiagnosed gastrointestinal disease unmasked by the enteric infection, or 3) a postinfectious phenomenon.

PERSISTENT INFECTION

Most cases of travelers' diarrhea are the result of bacterial infection and are short-lived and self-limited. Travelers may experience prolonged diarrheal symptoms if they are immunosuppressed, are infected sequentially with diarrheal pathogens, or are infected with protozoan parasites. Parasites as a group are the pathogens most likely to be isolated from patients with persistent diarrhea, and their probability relative to bacterial infections increases with increasing duration of symptoms. Parasites may also be the cause of persistent diarrhea in patients already treated for a bacterial pathogen.

Giardia is by far the most likely persistent pathogen to be encountered. Suspicion for giardiasis should be particularly high when upper gastrointestinal symptoms predominate. Untreated, symptoms may last for months, even in immunocompetent hosts. The diagnosis can often be made through stool microscopy, antigen detection, or immunofluorescence, but PCR-based diagnostics (particularly the multiplex DNA extraction PCR) are becoming the diagnostic method of choice to diagnose *Giardia* as well as other protozoan pathogens, including *Cryptosporidium, Cyclospora*, and *Entamoeba histolytica*. In the absence of diagnostics, however, and given the high prevalence of *Giardia* in persistent travelers' diarrhea, empiric therapy is a reasonable option in the clinical setting. Other intestinal parasites that may be rare causes of persistent symptoms include *Microsporidia, Dientamoeba fragilis*, and *Cystoisospora.*

Individual bacterial infections rarely cause persistence of symptoms, although persistent diarrhea has been reported in children infected with enteroaggregative or enteropathogenic *Escherichia coli* and among people with diarrhea due to *Clostridium difficile. C. difficile*–associated diarrhea may follow treatment of a bacterial pathogen with a fluoroquinolone or other antibiotic, or may even follow malaria chemoprophylaxis. This is especially important to consider in the patient with persistent travelers' diarrhea that seems refractory to multiple courses of empiric antibiotic therapy. The initial workup of persistent travelers' diarrhea should always include a *C. difficile* stool toxin assay. Treatment of *C. difficile* infection is with metronidazole, oral vancomycin, or fidaxomicin, although increasing reports of resistance to the first 2 drugs have been noted.

Persistent travelers' diarrhea has also been associated with tropical sprue and Brainerd diarrhea. These syndromes are suspected to result from infectious diseases, but specific pathogens have not been identified. Tropical sprue is associated with deficiencies of vitamins absorbed in the proximal and distal small bowel and most commonly affects long-term travelers to tropical areas. The incidence of tropical sprue appears to have declined dramatically over the past 2 decades and is rarely diagnosed in travelers. Investigation of an outbreak of Brainerd diarrhea among passengers on a cruise ship to the Galápagos Islands of Ecuador revealed that diarrhea persisted from 7 to more than 42 months and did not respond to antimicrobial therapy. Brainerd diarrhea is one of the persistent mysteries of ongoing diarrhea.

UNDERLYING GASTROINTESTINAL DISEASE

In some cases, persistence of gastrointestinal symptoms relates to chronic underlying gastrointestinal disease or susceptibility unmasked by the enteric infection. Most prominent among these is celiac disease, a systemic disease manifesting primarily with small bowel changes. In genetically susceptible people, villous atrophy and crypt hyperplasia are seen in response to exposure to antigens found in wheat, leading to malabsorption. The diagnosis is made by obtaining serologic tests, including tissue transglutaminase antibodies. A biopsy of the small bowel showing villous atrophy confirms the diagnosis. Treatment is with a gluten-free diet.

Idiopathic inflammatory bowel disease, both Crohn's disease and ulcerative colitis, may be seen after acute bouts of travelers' diarrhea. One prevailing hypothesis is that an initiating exogenous pathogen changes the person's microbiota, which triggers inflammatory bowel disease in genetically susceptible people.

Depending on the clinical setting and age group, it may be necessary to do a more comprehensive search for other underlying causes of chronic diarrhea. Colorectal cancer should be considered, particularly in patients passing occult or gross blood rectally or with the onset of a new iron-deficiency anemia.

POSTINFECTIOUS PHENOMENA

In a certain percentage of patients who present with persistent gastrointestinal symptoms, no specific source will be found. Patients may experience temporary enteropathy following an acute diarrheal infection, with villous atrophy, decreased absorptive surface area, and disaccharidase deficiencies. This can lead to osmotic diarrhea, particularly when large amounts of lactose, sucrose, sorbitol, or fructose are consumed. Use of antimicrobial medications during the initial days of diarrhea may also lead to alterations in intestinal flora and diarrhea symptoms.

Occasionally, the onset of symptoms of irritable bowel syndrome (IBS) can be traced to an acute bout of gastroenteritis. IBS that develops after acute enteritis has been termed postinfectious (PI)-IBS. To be labeled PI-IBS, symptoms should follow an episode of gastroenteritis or travelers' diarrhea if the work-up for microbial pathogens and underlying gastrointestinal disease is negative. Whether the use of antibiotics to treat acute TD decreases or increases the likelihood of PI-IBS is unknown.

EVALUATION

Diagnostics to determine specific microbial etiologies in cases of persistent diarrhea have advanced in the past number of years. Among the most useful tools in microbial diagnosis is the high-throughput multiplex DNA extraction PCR. This technology uses a single stool specimen to simultaneously detect multiple bacterial, parasitic, and viral enteropathogens. This may be particularly helpful when persistent diarrhea is caused by a parasite or *C. difficile*.

Overall, these assays have high sensitivity and specificity; however, the clinical and financial effect of these molecular panels has not yet been fully assessed, and molecular testing may, in some cases, detect colonization rather than infection, making it difficult for clinicians to interpret the results.

Traditional methods of microbial diagnosis have relied on the use of microscopy; 3 or more stool specimens should be examined for ova and parasites, including acid-fast stains for *Cryptosporidium, Cyclospora,* and *Cystoisospora,* as well as *Giardia* antigen testing; *C. difficile* toxin assay; and a D-xylose absorption test to determine if nutrients are being properly absorbed. If underlying gastrointestinal disease is suspected, an initial evaluation should include serologic tests for celiac and inflammatory bowel disease. Subsequently, other studies to visualize both the upper and lower gastrointestinal tracts, with biopsies, may be indicated.

MANAGEMENT

Dietary modifications may help those with malabsorption. If stools are bloody or when disease is caused by *C. difficile*, antidiarrheal medications such as loperamide or diphenoxylate should not be used in children and should be used cautiously, if at all, in adults. Probiotic medications have been shown to reduce the duration of persistent diarrhea among children in some settings. Antimicrobial medications may be useful in treating persistent diarrhea caused by parasites. Nonabsorbable antibiotics may help if small intestinal bacterial overgrowth accompanies the symptom complex.

BIBLIOGRAPHY

1. Connor BA. Sequelae of traveler's diarrhea: focus on postinfectious irritable bowel syndrome. Clin Infect Dis. 2005 Dec 1;41 (Suppl 8):S577–86.

2. Connor BA. Chronic diarrhea in travelers. Curr Infect Dis Rep. 2013 Jun;15(3):203–10.

3. Hanevik K, Dizdar V, Langeland N, Hausken T. Development of functional gastrointestinal disorders after *Giardia lamblia* infection. BMC Gastroenterol 2009 Apr. 21;9:27.

4. Libman MD, Gyorkos TW, Kokoskin E, Maclean JD. Detection of pathogenic protozoa in the diagnostic laboratory: result reproducibility, specimen pooling, and competency assessment. J Clin MIcrobiol. 2008 Jul;76(7):2200–5.

5. Mintz ED, Weber JT, Guris D, Puhr N, Wells JG, Yashuk JC, et al. An outbreak of Brainerd diarrhea among travelers to the Galapagos Islands. J Infect Dis. 1998 Apr;177(4):1041–5.

6. Norman FF, Perez-Molina J, Perez de Ayala A, Jimenez BC, Navarro M, Lopez-Velez R. *Clostridium difficile*-associated diarrhea after antibiotic treatment for traveler's diarrhea. Clin Infect Dis. 2008 Apr 1;46(7):1060–3.

7. Platts-Mills JA, Operario DJ, Houpt ER. Molecular diagnosis of diarrhea: current status and future potential. Curr Infect Dis Rep. 2012 Feb;14(1):41–6.

8. Porter CK, Tribble DR, Aliaga PA, Halvorson HA, Riddle MS. Infectious gastroenteritis and risk of developing inflammatory bowel disease. Gastroenterology. 2008 Sep;135(3):781–6.

9. Schwille-Kiuntke J, Mazurak N, Enck P. Systematic review with meta-analysis: post-infectious irritable bowel syndrome after travellers' diarrhoea. Aliment Pharmacol Ther 2015 Jul;41(11):1029–37.

10. Spiller R, Garsed K. Postinfectious irritable bowel syndrome. Gastroenterology. 2009 May;136(6):1979–88.

SKIN & SOFT TISSUE INFECTIONS IN RETURNED TRAVELERS

Jay S. Keystone

Skin problems are among the most frequent medical problems in returned travelers. A large case series of dermatologic problems in returned travelers from the GeoSentinel Surveillance Network showed that cutaneous larva migrans, insect bites, and bacterial infections were the most frequent skin problems in ill travelers who sought medical care, making up 30% of the 4,742 diagnoses (Table 5-5). A recent Canadian study of 1,076 returned travelers with dermatologic problems confirmed this finding. However, both of these studies are biased in that they do not include skin problems that were diagnosed and, in many cases, easily managed during travel or that were self-limited.

Skin problems generally fall into either of the following categories: (1) those associated with fever, usually a rash or secondary bacterial infection (cellulitis, lymphangitis, bacteremia, toxin-mediated) and (2) those not associated with fever. Most skin problems are minor and are not accompanied by fever. Diagnosis of skin problems in returned travelers is based on the following:

- Pattern recognition of the lesions: papular, macular, nodular, linear, or ulcerative

- Location of the lesions: exposed versus unexposed skin surfaces

- Exposure history: freshwater, ocean, insects, animals, or human contact

- Associated symptoms: fever, pain, pruritus

- Location and duration of travel

- Time of onset of lesions during or after travel

It is important to recognize that skin conditions in returned travelers may not have a travel-related cause.

PAPULAR LESIONS

Insect bites, the most common cause of papular lesions, may be associated with secondary infection or hypersensitivity reactions. Bed bug and flea bites may produce grouped papules (see Box 2-5 for more information about bed bugs). Flea bites tend to have hemorrhagic centers. Scabies infestation usually manifests as a generalized or regional pruritic, papular rash. Scabies burrows may present as papules or pustules in a short linear pattern on the skin, frequently in the web spaces of the fingers.

Onchocerciasis may occur in long-stay travelers living in rural sub-Saharan Africa and, rarely, Latin America. It usually manifests as a generalized pruritic, papular dermatitis.

NODULAR OR SUBCUTANEOUS LESIONS, INCLUDING BACTERIAL SKIN INFECTIONS

Bacterial skin infections may occur more frequently after bites and other wounds in the

Table 5-5. Ten most common skin lesions in returned travelers, by cause[1]

SKIN LESION	PERCENTAGE OF ALL DERMATOLOGIC DIAGNOSES (N = 4,742)
Cutaneous larva migrans	9.8
Insect bite	8.2
Skin abscess	7.7
Superinfected insect bite	6.8
Allergic rash	5.5
Rash, unknown origin	5.5
Dog bite	4.3
Superficial fungal infection	4.0
Dengue	3.4
Leishmaniasis	3.3
Myiasis	2.7
Spotted fever group rickettsiosis	1.5
Scabies	1.5
Cellulitis	1.5

[1] Modified from Lederman ER, Weld LH, Elyazar IR, et al. Dermatologic conditions of the ill returned traveler: an analysis from the GeoSentinel Surveillance Network. Int J Infect Dis. 2008;12(6):593–602.

tropics, particularly when good hygiene cannot be maintained. Organisms responsible are commonly *Staphylococcus aureus* or *Streptococcus pyogenes*. Drug-resistant organisms are frequently acquired in the tropics. The presentations can include pyoderma or impetigo, abscess formation, erysipelas, cellulitis, lymphangitis, or ulceration. Furunculosis, or recurrent pyoderma, may be the result of colonization of the skin and nasal mucosa with *S. aureus*. Boils may continue to occur weeks or months after a traveler returns and, if associated with *S. aureus*, definitive treatment usually involves decolonization with nasal mupirocin, a skin wash with an antimicrobial skin cleanser, and less often, an oral antibiotic combination including rifampin.

In addition to pyoderma, cellulitis or erysipelas may complicate excoriated insect bites or any trauma to the skin. Cellulitis and erysipelas manifest as areas of skin erythema, edema, and warmth in the absence of an underlying suppurative focus. Unlike cellulitis, erysipelas lesions are raised, there is a clear line of demarcation at the edge of the lesion, and the lesions are more likely to be associated with fever. Cellulitis, on the other hand, is more likely to be associated with lymphangitis. Cellulitis and erysipelas are usually caused by β-hemolytic streptococci (such as groups A, B, C, G, and F *Streptococcus*). *S. aureus* (including methicillin-resistant strains) and gram-negative aerobic bacteria may also cause cellulitis.

Another common bacterial skin infection, especially in children in the tropics, is impetigo due to *S. aureus* or *S. pyogenes*. Impetigo is a highly contagious superficial skin infection that generally appears on the arms, legs, or face as "honey-colored" or golden crusting formed from dried serum. Local care and a topical antibiotic such as mupirocin may be used, although a systemic antibiotic may be required. Emerging antibiotic resistance among staphylococci and streptococci complicates antimicrobial options.

Myiasis presents as a painful lesion similar to a boil. It is caused by infestation with the larval stage of the African tumbu fly (*Cordylobia anthropophaga*) or the Latin American bot fly (*Dermatobia hominis*). At the center of the lesion is a small punctum that allows the larva to breathe. Extraction of the fly larva can be difficult, especially of the bot fly; extraction may be facilitated by first asphyxiating the larva, usually with an occlusive dressing or covering (such as a bottle cap filled with petroleum jelly) for several hours and then squeezing the larva out.

Tungiasis is caused by a sand flea (*Tunga penetrans*). The female burrows into the skin, usually the foot, and produces a nodular, pale, subcutaneous lesion with a central dark spot. The painful or pruritic lesion expands as the female produces eggs in her uterus. Treatment involves extraction.

Loa loa filariasis occurs rarely in long-term travelers living in rural sub-Saharan Africa. The traveler may present with transient, migratory, subcutaneous, painful, or pruritic swellings produced by the adult nematode migration (Calabar swelling). Rarely, the worm can be visualized crossing the conjunctiva of the eye or eyelid. Eosinophilia is common. Loiasis can be diagnosed by finding microfilariae in blood collected during daytime; however, since microfilaremia may be absent, filarial serologic tests may be helpful.

Gnathostomiasis is a nematode infection found primarily in Southeast Asia and less commonly in Africa and Latin America. Infection results from eating undercooked or raw freshwater fish. Infected travelers may experience transient, migratory, subcutaneous, pruritic, or painful swellings that may occur weeks or even years after exposure. The symptoms are due to migration of the worm through the body, and the central nervous system may be involved. Eosinophilia is common, and a definitive diagnosis is often difficult.

MACULAR LESIONS

Macular lesions are common and often nonspecific and may be due to drug reactions or viral exanthems. Superficial mycoses, such as tinea versicolor and tinea corporis, may also present as macular lesions.

Tinea versicolor, due to *Malassezia furfur* (previously *Pityrosporum ovale*), is characterized by asymptomatic hypopigmented or hyperpigmented oval, slightly scaly patches measuring 1–3 cm that are found on the upper chest, neck, and back. Diagnosis may be made by examination with a Wood's lamp or by placing a drop of methylene blue on a slide onto which clear cellulose acetate tape is placed sticky side down, after it has been touched briefly to the skin lesions to pick up superficial scales. Detection of hyphae ("spaghetti") and spores ("meatballs") suggest the diagnosis. Treatment with topical or systemic azoles (ketoconazole, fluconazole), terbinafine, or selenium sulfide (present in some shampoos) is recommended.

Tinea corporis (ringworm) may be caused by a number of different superficial fungi. The lesion is often a single lesion with an expanding red, raised ring, with a central area of clearing in the middle. Treatment is usually several weeks' application of a topical antifungal agent or a short course of an oral antifungal agent.

Lyme disease, a tickborne infection with *Borrelia burgdorferi*, is common in North America, Europe, and Russia (see Chapter 3, Lyme Disease). An infected traveler may present with ≥1 large erythematous patches, with or without central clearing, often surrounding a prior tick bite. The patient may not have noticed the tick bite.

Leprosy (Hansen disease) frequently presents with hypopigmented or erythematous patches that are frequently hypoesthetic to pin prick and associated with peripheral nerve enlargement. This condition is almost exclusively found in immigrants from developing countries.

LINEAR LESIONS

Cutaneous larva migrans, a skin infection with the larval stage of dog or cat hookworm

(*Ancylostoma* spp.), manifests as an extremely pruritic, serpiginous, linear lesion that advances in the epidermis of the skin relatively slowly (see Chapter 3, Cutaneous Larva Migrans). A similar lesion that may be more urticarial and that rapidly progresses may be due to **larva currens** (running larva) due to cutaneous migration of filariform larvae of *Strongyloides stercoralis*.

Lymphocutaneous spread of infection occurs when organisms spread along superficial cutaneous lymphatics, producing raised, linear, cord-like lesions; nodules or ulcers may also be found. Examples include sporotrichosis, *Mycobacterium marinum* infection (associated with exposure to water), leishmaniasis, bartonellosis (cat-scratch disease), *Nocardia* infection, tularemia, melioidosis, and blastomycosis.

Phytophotodermatitis is a noninfectious condition that results from interaction of natural psoralens, most commonly from spilled lime juice, and ultraviolet radiation from the sun. The result is an exaggerated sunburn that gives rise to a linear, asymptomatic lesion that later develops hyperpigmentation. The hyperpigmentation may take weeks or months to resolve.

SKIN ULCERS

Ulcerated skin lesions may result from *Staphylococcus* infections or may be the direct result of an unseen spider bite. The necrotic ulcer of anthrax is often surrounded by edema and usually results from handling animal hides or products. Rarely, a painless destructive ulcer with undermining edges may result from infection with *Mycobacterium ulcerans* (Buruli ulcer). Of particular concern is the ulcer (or less commonly, nodule) caused by **cutaneous leishmaniasis**. The main areas of risk are Latin America, the Mediterranean, the Middle East, Asia, and parts of Africa. The lesion is a chronic, usually painless ulcer unless superinfected, with heaped-up margins on exposed skin surfaces. Special diagnostic techniques are necessary to confirm the diagnosis. Both topical and systemic treatments may be effective; the species of the infection often determines the treatment modality. If cutaneous leishmaniasis is suspected, clinicians can contact CDC

at 404-718-4745 or parasites@cdc.gov for further advice about diagnosis and treatment (see Chapter 3, Leishmaniasis, Cutaneous).

MISCELLANEOUS SKIN INFECTIONS

Skin Infections Associated with Water

Soft tissue infections can occur after both freshwater and saltwater exposure, particularly if there is associated trauma. Puncture wounds due to fishhooks and fish spines, lacerations from inanimate objects during wading and swimming, and bites or stings from fish or other sea creatures may be the source of the trauma leading to waterborne infections. Soft tissue infections associated with exposure to water or water-related animals include *M. marinum, Aeromonas* spp., *Plesiomonas* spp., *Edwardsiella tarda, Erysipelothrix rhusiopathiae*, and *Vibrio* spp. A variety of skin and soft tissue manifestations may occur in association with these infections, including cellulitis, abscess formation, ecthyma gangrenosum, and necrotizing fasciitis. Vibriosis infection may be especially severe in those with underlying liver disease and may manifest as a dramatic cellulitis with hemorrhagic bullae and sepsis. In general, infections caused by these organisms may be more severe in those who are immunosuppressed. Acute infections related to aquatic injury should be treated with an antibiotic that provides both gram-positive and gram-negative coverage (such as a fluoroquinolone or third-generation cephalosporin) until a specific organism has been identified. *M. marinum* lesions are usually indolent and usually appear as solitary nodules or papules on an extremity, especially on the dorsum of feet and hands; subsequent progression to shallow ulceration and scar formation may occur. Occasionally, "sporotrichoid" spread may occur as the lesions spread proximally along superficial lymphatics.

"Hot tub folliculitis" due to *Pseudomonas aeruginosa* may result from the use of inadequately disinfected swimming pools and hot tubs. Folliculitis typically develops 8–48 hours after exposure in contaminated water and consists of tender, pruritic papules, papulopustules, or nodules. Most patients have malaise, and some have low-grade fever. The condition is self-limited in 2–12 days; typically no antibiotic therapy is required.

Skin Infections Associated with Bites

Wound infections after dog and cat bites are caused by a variety of microorganisms. *S. aureus*; α-, β-, and γ-hemolytic streptococci; several genera of gram-negative organisms; and a number of anaerobic microorganisms have been isolated. The prevalence of *Pasteurella multocida* isolates from dog bite wounds is 20%–50%; *P. multocida* is a major pathogen in cat bite infections. Splenectomized patients are at particular risk of severe cellulitis and sepsis due to *Capnocytophaga canimorsus* after a dog bite. Management of dog and cat bites includes consideration of rabies postexposure prophylaxis, tetanus immunization, and antibiotic prophylaxis. Primary closure of puncture wounds and dog bites to the hand should be avoided. Antibiotic prophylaxis for dog bites is controversial, although most experts would treat splenectomized patients with amoxicillin-clavulanate prophylactically. Since *P. multocida* is a common accompaniment of cat bites, prophylaxis with amoxicillin-clavulanate or a fluoroquinolone for 3–5 days should be considered. Management of monkey bites includes wound care, tetanus immunization, rabies postexposure prophylaxis, and consideration of antimicrobial prophylaxis. Bites and scratches from Old World macaque monkeys have also been associated with fatal encephalomyelitis due to B virus infection in humans (see Chapter 3, B virus). Valacyclovir postexposure prophylaxis is recommended after a high-risk macaque exposure.

FEVER AND RASH

Fever and rash in returned travelers are most often due to a viral infection.

Dengue is caused by 1 of 4 strains of dengue viruses (see Chapter 3, Dengue). The disease is transmitted by an *Aedes* mosquito often found in urban areas, and its incidence continues to increase. The disease is characterized by the abrupt onset of high fever, frontal headache (often accompanied by retro-orbital pain), myalgia, and a faint macular rash (containing islands of pallor) that becomes evident on the second to fourth day of illness. A petechial rash may be found in classical dengue, as well as in severe dengue. Antigen and antibody detection tests, as well as PCR assays, are available to diagnose dengue; detecting IgM in the appropriate clinical scenario would support the diagnosis. Treatment is supportive.

Chikungunya, a virus transmitted by a primarily *Aedes* mosquito, has caused major outbreaks of illness in southeast Africa, South Asia, the Americas, and the Caribbean (see Chapter 3, Chikungunya). Chikungunya is similar to dengue clinically, including the rash, although hemorrhage, shock, and death are not typical of chikungunya. A major distinguishing feature is that arthritis or arthralgia is common with chikungunya (and may persist for months), whereas in dengue, myalgia is the major clinical feature. Similar to dengue, serologic tests are available. Treatment of the arthritis is with nonsteroidal anti-inflammatory drugs.

Zika, a virus also transmitted by *Aedes* mosquitoes has caused a major outbreak in the Western Hemisphere since May 2015 (see Chapter 3, Zika). Sexual transmission has been documented as well. The infection is characterized by fever, arthralgia, lymphadenopathy, maculopapular rash, and conjunctivitis. Microcephaly, brain and eye damage, and fetal loss have occurred as a result of fetal infection. An increased risk of Guillain-Barré syndrome has also been documented. Diagnosis is by molecular diagnostics and serologic testing. Treatment is supportive.

South African tick typhus, or African tick-bite fever (*Rickettsia africae*), is the most frequent cause of fever and rash in southern Africa. Transmitted by ticks, the disease is characterized by fever and a papular or vesicular rash associated with localized lymphadenopathy and the presence of an eschar (a mildly painful 1 to 2 cm black necrotic lesion with an erythematous margin). Satellite lesions may be present. Diagnosis is usually through clinical recognition and is confirmed by serologic testing. Treatment is with doxycycline. Other rickettsial infections such as rickettsialpox and scrub typhus may present with eschars or maculopapular, vesicular, and petechial rashes.

Rocky Mountain spotted fever (RMSF), although uncommon in travelers, is an important cause of fever and rash because of its potential severity and the need for early treatment. This tickborne infection is found in the United States, Mexico, and parts of Central and South America. Most patients with RMSF develop a rash between the 3rd and 5th days of illness. The typical rash of RMSF begins on the ankles and wrists and spreads both centrally and to the palms and soles. The rash commonly begins as a maculopapular eruption and then becomes petechial, although in some patients it begins with petechiae. Doxycycline is the treatment of choice.

The category of fever with rash is large, and providers caring for ill travelers should also consider the following diagnoses: enteroviruses, such as echovirus and coxsackievirus; hepatitis B virus; measles; Epstein-Barr virus; cytomegalovirus; typhus; leptospirosis; syphilis; and HIV.

BIBLIOGRAPHY

1. Aronson N, Herwaldt B, Libman M, Pearson R, Lopez-Velez R, Weina P, et al. Diagnosis and treatment of leishmaniasis: clinical practice guidelines by the Infectious Diseases Society of America (IDSA) and the American Society of Tropical Medicine and Hygiene (ASTMH). Clin Infect Dis. 2016 November: doi:10.1093/cid/ciw670

2. Hochedez P, Canestri A, Lecso M, Valin N, Bricaire F, Caumes E. Skin and soft tissue infections in returning travelers. Am J Trop Med Hyg. 2009 Mar;80(3):431–4.

3. Jensenius M, Davis X, von Sonnenburg F, Schwartz E, Keystone JS, Leder K, et al. Multicenter GeoSentinel analysis of rickettsial diseases in international travelers,1996–2008. Emerg Infect Dis. 2009 Nov;15(11):1791–8.

4. Kamimura-Nishimuraa K, Rudikoffb D, Purswania M, Hagmann S. Dermatological conditions in international pediatric travelers: epidemiology, prevention and management. Travel Med Infect Dis. 2013 Nov-Dec;11(6):350–6.

5. Klion AD. Filarial infections in travelers and immigrants. Curr Infect Dis Rep. 2008 Mar;10(1):50–7.

6. Lederman ER, Weld LH, Elyazar IR, von Sonnenburg F, Loutan L, Schwartz E, et al. Dermatologic conditions of the ill returned traveler: an analysis from the GeoSentinel Surveillance Network. Int J Infect Dis. 2008 Nov;12(6):593–602.

7. Nordlund JJ. Cutaneous ectoparasites. Dermatol Ther. 2009 Nov-Dec;22(6):503–17.

8. Nurjadi D, Friedrich-Jänicke B, Schäfer J, Van Genderen PJ, Goorhuis A, Perignon A, et al. Skin and soft tissue infections in intercontinental travellers and the import of multi-resistant *Staphylococcus aureus* to Europe. Clin Microbiol Infect. 2015 Jul;21(6):567.e1–10.

9. Stevens MS, Geduld J, Libman M, Ward BJ, McCarthy AE, Vincelette J, et al. Dermatoses among returned Canadian travellers and immigrants: surveillance report based on CanTravNet data, 2009–2012. CMAJ Open 2015 Jan 13;3(1):E119–26.

10. Zimmerman RF, Belanger ES, Pfeiffer CD. Skin infections in returned travelers: an update. Current infectious disease reports. 2015 Mar;17(3):467.

SCREENING ASYMPTOMATIC RETURNED TRAVELERS

Michael Libman

CDC has no official guidelines or recommendations for screening asymptomatic international travelers. (For recommendations regarding the screening of newly arrived immigrants and refugees, see Chapter 8, Newly Arrived Immigrants & Refugees.) Nevertheless, the screening of travelers returning from developing countries represents a substantial portion of the activity of many travel and tropical medicine clinics. The scientific literature on the cost-effectiveness of screening asymptomatic travelers is sparse. It is clear that asymptomatic travelers can harbor many infections acquired during travel, some of which have the potential to cause serious sequelae or have public health implications. In some cases, these will include pathogens rarely found in the traveler's country of origin. Local medical practitioners will have little familiarity with the associated diseases, and specific diagnostic tests may not be readily available or may have poorly defined operating characteristics. The decision to screen for particular pathogens will depend on the type of travel, itinerary, and exposure history. However, exposure history is often unreliable and poorly predictive of infection, the value of a detailed itinerary is limited by incomplete information on where pathogens are endemic, and the type of travel often does not provide a practical assessment of risk.

Screening traditionally has been viewed as a secondary prevention intervention, that is, an attempt to identify existing occult illnesses or health risks. The cost effectiveness of screening involves a consideration of the natural history of the problem, the predictive value of the test, the direct and indirect costs of the test, and the effectiveness of prevention or therapy. Because of convenience and the susceptibility to suggestion at the time of screening, the screening visit may also offer an opportunity to promote primary prevention by discussing behavioral or other risk factors predisposing to ill health. These may include, for example, counseling on sexual health or the avoidance of schistosomiasis or malaria.

PARASITIC INFECTION

Travelers are often most concerned with the possibility of occult parasitic infection. Unfortunately, when screening for parasitic disease, the literature shows that patient questionnaires and common laboratory testing have poor sensitivity and specificity. Studies have shown that even an exhaustive risk-factor history in asymptomatic patients is unable to reliably detect those who would or would not have evidence of parasitic infection. Physical examination is equally unrewarding.

Most commonly, a stool examination is performed, typically microscopy. Several molecular assays are commercially available; these detect a panel of viral, bacterial, and parasitic (protozoal) pathogens. In some cases these panels are more sensitive than traditional testing methods, and even asymptomatic people are often found to harbor pathogens. The clinical implications of asymptomatic carriage, sometimes at a low level, are unknown for most of these agents, and the risks and benefits of treatment are not well studied. Travelers are often concerned about "worms," by which they mean intestinal nematodes. However, probably because of hygiene and short duration of exposure for most travelers, infections with large numbers of the common nematodes, such as *Ascaris*, *Trichuris*, or hookworm, are rare. Questioning returning expatriates infected with intestinal helminths has disclosed no attributable symptoms compared with uninfected controls, although there have been case reports of complications, such as migration of *Ascaris* into the biliary system. The life cycles of almost all helminths preclude any real risk of ongoing transmission from asymptomatic hosts in developed countries. Helminths generally have a natural lifespan of months to a few years, which ensures eventual spontaneous clearance and are of limited clinical importance when present in low intensity infection, though in rare cases aberrant migration of *Ascaris* might result in clinical disease. The exception to this rule is *Strongyloides*. For this helminth, serious complications are well known, nonspecific symptoms may easily be overlooked, duration of carriage after infection is unlimited, and the original burden of infection is irrelevant. Unfortunately, diagnosis by stool examination is notoriously insensitive, and serologic methods are often required, as discussed below. Molecular panels for helminths are at the research stage of development.

The finding of pathogenic protozoa in asymptomatic patients is of questionable significance (with the possible exception of *Entamoeba histolytica*, a rare finding in these travelers). History of exposure to contaminated food or water has poor predictive value. There is no evidence to suggest that these asymptomatic carriers are likely to develop symptoms at a later time. Certainly, the medications used to treat pathogens have their own adverse effects. In theory, these carriers pose a public health risk, although transmission by asymptomatic travelers appears to be rare. This is further complicated by the fact that stool microscopy for protozoa is expensive, not very sensitive, and not highly reproducible, and many laboratories have limited expertise. *Entamoeba histolytica* cannot be distinguished from *E. dispar* by microscopy, requiring further specimen collection and testing. Studies reveal that most travelers with

Entamoeba on microscopy are carrying *E. dispar*. Antigen testing for *E. histolytica* and *Giardia* (among others) is fairly reliable but lacks the potential to screen for all intestinal parasites with a single test. Commercial molecular methods to screen stool specimens for multiple pathogens simultaneously typically include several protozoa, generally with sensitivity at least as good as microscopy, and offer rapid turnaround times of several hours, although costs remain high. Some of these panels are sensitive for questionably pathogenic organisms, such as *Blastocystis* and *Dientamoeba*. Identifying these may lead to patient anxiety and unnecessary treatment.

Among the helminths capable of causing eventual illness in asymptomatic travelers, most emphasis has been given to *Strongyloides* and the parasites that cause schistosomiasis and filariasis. There is no evidence that the low-burden schistosomal infections typically found in travelers are likely to lead to the types of complications commonly found in endemic areas, such as liver fibrosis or malignancy. Nevertheless, this possibility cannot be entirely ruled out, particularly in those who may have more intense exposures. Even brief exposures to freshwater lakes and rivers in known endemic foci in Africa are associated with substantial seroconversion rates. In addition, complications due to ectopic egg migration can occur in light infections and without warning. On the other hand, reports of travelers with late complications from asymptomatic filarial infections are virtually nonexistent. Traditional tests for the parasites that cause these infections, including stool examination for *Strongyloides* and *Schistosoma* spp., urine for *S. haematobium*, and blood or skin snips for microfilaria, all lack sensitivity, particularly in low-burden infection. For this reason, serologic testing has been advocated as the best screening tool. The problems with serologic screening include expense, lack of easy availability, and lack of standardization. Serologic tests are often designed to maximize sensitivity, typically at the expense of specificity. Unfortunately, specificity is almost impossible to define. Seropositivity in the absence of direct pathogen detection is common, and its clinical significance can be difficult to determine. Fortunately, for strongyloidiasis and schistosomiasis, treatment is cheap, easy,

and effective. The common antihelminthic agents, such as ivermectin, albendazole, and praziquantel, have excellent safety profiles. Nevertheless, rare but severe adverse events can occur when certain occult, unsuspected parasitoses are present, such as ivermectin and loiasis or albendazole and neurocysticercosis. While it is not clear who should be screened, it is logical to at least perform serologic tests on travelers with a high duration and risk of exposure and to treat all those found to be positive. Since asymptomatic filarial infections appear least likely to have sequelae, and treatment is often neither very effective nor easy, the threshold for filarial serology (or antigen testing in the case of *Wuchereria bancrofti*) should be higher. Serology usually only becomes positive after adult forms have matured, which means waiting for 3 months or so after exposure. Serology for these pathogens are available at the parasitic diseases laboratory at CDC (www.dpd.cdc.gov/dpdx; 404-718-4745; parasites@cdc.gov). Serology for filarial infection is available as well through the NIH laboratory (301-496-5398).

Screening for eosinophilia is a common test, since it is quick, universally available, and theoretically of value in detecting invasive helminths, if not protozoa. However, multiple studies have shown eosinophilia to have poor sensitivity. Specificity can be high; however, the low prevalence of infection in asymptomatic travelers means positive predictive value is low. In addition, the finding of eosinophilia may lead to an extensive and often fruitless search for a cause, generating high costs. Many cases of eosinophilia resolve spontaneously, possibly because of infection with nonpathogenic organisms or a noninfectious cause, such as allergy or drug reaction. Eosinophil counts may be repeated after several weeks or months before embarking on an extensive investigation. Counts may be highly variable, even within a single day, and are suppressed by endogenous or exogenous steroids. Evaluation of absolute counts, rather than by percentage of leukocytes, is more reproducible and predictive.

Immigrants with frequent and regular exposure to malaria may gradually develop partial immunity. This may result in low-level parasitemia with few or no symptoms. They may later recrudesce with more severe illness. This phenomenon is rare in other travelers. There is no justification for screening most asymptomatic travelers, whether by blood film, serologic tests, or molecular methods. No available tests can detect latent infections with *Plasmodium vivax* or *P. ovale*. Travelers should be reminded to seek evaluation for unexplained fever and notify practitioners of any recent travel.

Occult trypanosomiasis in asymptomatic travelers (as opposed to immigrants) appears to be extremely rare. Screening tests, such as serology and molecular diagnostics, are of unknown value. For travelers to endemic areas of Latin America, testing might be considered in cases of prolonged residence in primitive housing, such as mud walls and thatched roofs, especially if reduviid bugs have been seen. East African trypanosomiasis has affected travelers but typically causes symptoms. West African disease is generally not reported in travelers. Other parasitic infections rarely seen in returning travelers include neurocysticercosis, fascioliasis, paragonimiasis, and others. Primary care providers should refer patients suspected of having these infections to an infectious diseases specialist.

NONPARASITIC ILLNESS

Sexual activity and travel seem to be linked. High rates of contact with new partners, including sex workers, have been documented in volunteers, expatriate workers, backpackers, and military personnel. Of concern are the low rates of reported condom use. Returning travelers with acute HIV or hepatitis B infection pose public health risks. Travelers may be hesitant to volunteer a relevant history. Screening for sexually transmitted infections should always be considered.

The incidence of tuberculosis related to travel is difficult to estimate. Estimates of exposure based on skin test (Mantoux) conversions suggest rates of exposure of the same general magnitude as the local population. Work in high-prevalence settings such as health care institutions or refugee camps merits screening. Traditionally, this has been done using pre- and post-travel skin tests. This is cumbersome, requiring as many as 4 pretravel visits for a 2-step test and 2 visits after potential exposure. This number can be reduced by using the more expensive interferon-γ

release assay (IGRA), which also is less subject to false-positive results related to BCG vaccination. Unfortunately, recent data suggest that IGRA results show inadequate reproducibility, leading to false "conversions" on follow-up testing. In most patients born and raised in low-prevalence countries, a case can be made for omitting the pretravel test, because results are rarely positive.

For many long-term travelers, such as expatriate workers and some missionary and aid workers, the visits for asymptomatic screening may also be their only interludes from a continuing assignment abroad allowing for a general health evaluation. The usual recommendations for the periodic health exam, which may include screening for hypertension, diabetes, and malignancy, would apply. These visits also provide an opportune time to review vaccination status, malaria prophylaxis, and health behaviors.

SUMMARY

Recommendations for screening the asymptomatic traveler are necessarily based on opinion and common sense, rather than convincing evidence. The following may serve as a general guideline.

For the asymptomatic short stay (<3–6 months) traveler, the yield of screening is low and should be directed by specific risk factors revealed in the history. A history of prolonged (>2 weeks) digestive symptoms during travel can suggest protozoal infection. Exposure to fresh water in a region endemic for schistosomiasis, especially in Africa, merits serologic screening, with the addition of stool and urine examination in the case of high-intensity exposure. Serology for *Strongyloides* should be considered in those who have a high risk of skin exposure to soil likely to be contaminated with human feces, usually those with a history of frequently walking barefoot outdoors. A sexual history should be obtained, and screening for sexually transmitted and bloodborne infections is often warranted. Work in a health care setting or other area at high risk for TB may merit screening.

For longer-stay travelers, as the overall yield of screening increases it becomes less useful to rely on history for selective testing. The emphasis should be on those with the longest stays and the most problematic sanitary conditions. In some

5

cases, employers may require certain tests, partly for reasons of liability. Stool examinations are usually done, although they serve mostly to provide a psychological reassurance. Serologic testing for schistosomiasis and strongyloidiasis should be done in those with recent or remote travel histories to endemic areas and reporting some level of risk. Eosinophil counts are usually done, although results should be interpreted cautiously. Screening for sexually transmitted and bloodborne infections including HIV, hepatitis B and C, gonorrhea, chlamydia, and syphilis should be offered to all except those with the most convincing absence of risk. Mantoux or IGRA tests should be limited to those who have worked in a health care or similar setting, or who have had intimate and prolonged contact with residents of an endemic area for ≥6 months. Any other screening should be guided by exceptional exposures or knowledge about local outbreaks.

BIBLIOGRAPHY

1. Baaten GG, Sonder GJ, van Gool T, Kint JA, van den Hoek A. Travel-related schistosomiasis, strongyloidiasis, filariasis, and toxocariasis: the risk of infection and the diagnostic relevance of blood eosinophilia. BMC Infect Dis. 2011 Apr 5;11:84.

2. MacLean JD, Libman M. Screening returning travelers. Infect Dis Clin North Am. 1998 Jun;12(2):431–43.

3. Soonawala D, van Lieshout L, den Boer MA, Claas EC, Verweij JJ, Godkewitsch A, et al. Post-travel screening of asymptomatic long-term travelers to the tropics for intestinal parasites using molecular diagnostics. Am J Trop Med Hyg. 2014 May;90(5):835–9.

4. Yansouni CP, Merckx J, Libman MD, Ndao M. Recent advances in clinical parasitology diagnostics. Curr Infect Dis Rep 2014 Nov;16(11):434.

5

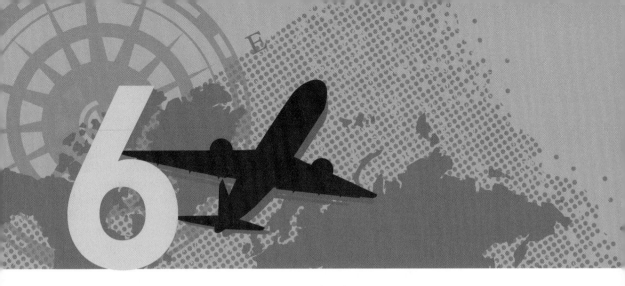

6

Conveyance & Transportation Issues

AIR TRAVEL

Susan A. Lippold, Tina Objio, Phyllis E. Kozarsky

Worldwide, >2.8 billion people travel by commercial aircraft every year, and this number continues to rise. Travelers often have concerns about the health risks of flying in airplanes. Those with underlying illness need to be aware that the entire point-to-point travel experience, including buses, trains, taxis, public waiting areas, and even movement within the airport, can pose challenges. Although illness may occur as a direct result of air travel, it is uncommon; the main concerns are:

- Exacerbations of chronic medical problems due to changes in air pressure and humidity

- Relative immobility during flights (risk of thromboembolic disease, see Chapter 2, Deep Vein Thrombosis & Pulmonary Embolism)

- Close proximity to other passengers with certain communicable diseases.

PREFLIGHT MEDICAL CONSIDERATIONS

During flight, the aircraft cabin pressure is usually maintained at the equivalent of 6,000–8,000 ft (1,829–2,438 m) above sea level. Most healthy travelers will not notice any effects. However, for travelers with cardiopulmonary diseases (especially those who normally require supplemental oxygen), cerebrovascular disease, anemia, or sickle cell disease, conditions in an aircraft can exacerbate underlying medical conditions. Aircraft cabin air is typically dry, usually 10%–20% humidity, which can cause dryness of the mucous membranes of the eyes and airways.

The new Boeing 787 and Airbus A 350 boast innovative changes: a greater number of temperature zones, a higher humidity of 25%, a faster time to refresh cabin air, lower ambient noise, and multiple shades of LED lighting. These, along with a cabin air pressure equivalent to an altitude of only 2,000 ft, promise to insure greater comfort and ease jet lag.

The Aerospace Medical Association (www.asma.org) recommends evaluating chronic medical conditions and addressing instabilities prior to travel, particularly in those who have underlying cardiovascular disease, a history of deep venous thrombosis or pulmonary embolism, chronic lung disease, surgical conditions, seizures, stroke, mental illness, and diabetes.

For information on contraindications and precautions related to flying during pregnancy, see Chapter 8, Pregnant Travelers. Specific information for travelers with disabilities and medical conditions that may affect security screening can be found at www.tsa.gov/travel/special-procedures. For those who require supplemental in-flight oxygen, the following must be taken into consideration:

- Travelers must arrange their own oxygen supplies while on the ground, at departure, during layovers, and upon arrival.

- Federal regulations prohibit airlines from allowing passengers to bring their own oxygen onboard; passengers requiring in-flight supplemental oxygen should notify the airline ≥72 hours before departure.

- Airlines might not offer in-flight supplemental oxygen on all aircraft or flights; some airlines permit only Federal Aviation Administration (FAA)-approved portable oxygen concentrators. Information to assist people who require supplemental oxygen during travel and FAA-approved portable oxygen concentrators can be found at the FAA website: www.faa.gov/about/initiatives/cabin_safety/portable_oxygen.

- Information regarding the screening of portable oxygen concentrators at airports in the United States can be found at www.tsa.gov/node/1754.

For more information, see Chapter 8, Travelers with Chronic Illnesses.

BAROTRAUMA DURING FLIGHT

Barotrauma may occur when the pressure inside an air-filled, enclosed body space (such as the middle ear, sinuses, or abdomen) is not the same as the air pressure inside the aircraft cabin. It most commonly occurs during rapid changes in environmental pressure, such as during ascent, when cabin pressure rapidly decreases, and during descent, when cabin pressure rapidly increases. Barotrauma most commonly affects the middle ear; it occurs when the eustachian tube is blocked and thus unable to equalize the air pressure in the middle ear with the outside cabin pressure. Middle ear barotrauma is usually not severe or dangerous and can usually be prevented or self-treated. It may rarely cause complications such as a perforated tympanic membrane, dizziness, permanent tinnitus, or hearing loss. The following suggestions may help avoid potential barotrauma:

- People with ear, nose, and sinus infections or severe congestion may wish to temporarily avoid flying to prevent pain or injury.

- Oral or nasal decongestants may alleviate symptoms.

- Travelers with allergies should continue their regular allergy medications.

- Travelers should stay hydrated to help avoid irritation of nasal passages and pharynx and to promote better function of the eustachian tubes.

- Travelers sensitive to abdominal bloating should avoid carbonated beverages and foods that can increase gas production.

- People who have had recent surgery, particularly intra-abdominal, neurologic, intrapulmonary, or intraocular procedures, should consult with their physicians before flying.

VENTILATION AND AIR QUALITY

All commercial jet aircraft built after the late 1980s, and a few modified older aircraft, recirculate 10%–50% of the air in the cabin, mixed with outside air. The recirculated air passes through a series of filters 20–30 times per hour. In most newer-model airplanes, the recycled air passes through high-efficiency particulate air (HEPA) filters, which capture 99.9% of particles (bacteria, fungi, and larger viruses or virus clumps) 0.1–0.3 µm in diameter. Furthermore, air generally circulates in defined areas within the aircraft, thus limiting the distribution of pathogens spread by small-particle aerosols beyond a small number of rows. As a result, the cabin air environment is not conducive to the spread of most infectious diseases.

Some diseases may be spread by contact with infected secretions, such as when an ill person sneezes or coughs and the secretions or droplets land on someone's face (mouth, nose, eyes), or by touching a contaminated surface and then touching one's face with contaminated hands. Practicing good handwashing and respiratory hygiene (covering mouth when coughing or sneezing) decreases the risk of disease spread by direct or indirect contact.

IN-FLIGHT MEDICAL EMERGENCIES

The increasing number of travelers combined with an aging flying population make the incidence of onboard medical emergencies likely to increase. Medical emergencies occur in approximately 1 in 600 flights; this is approximately 16 medical emergencies per 1 million passengers. The most commonly encountered in-flight medical events are:

- Syncope or presyncope (37%)
- Respiratory symptoms (12%)
- Nausea or vomiting (10%)
- Cardiac symptoms (8%)
- Seizures (6%)

Although in-flight medical emergencies occur, serious illness or death onboard a commercial aircraft is rare. Deaths onboard commercial aircraft have been estimated at 0.3 per 1 million passengers; approximately two-thirds of these are caused by cardiac conditions. Most commercial airplanes that fly within the United States are required to carry at least 1 approved automatic external defibrillator (AED) and an emergency medical kit.

Flight attendants are trained in basic first aid procedures such as CPR, and use of AED machines but are generally not certified in emergency medical response. Many airlines use ground-based medical consultants to assist flight crew and volunteer passenger responders in managing medical cases. In nearly one-half of in-flight emergencies, physician volunteers have provided assistance. The Aviation Medical Assistance Act, passed in 1998, provides some protection from liability to providers who respond to in-flight medical emergencies.

The goal of managing in-flight medical emergencies is to stabilize the passenger until ground-based medical care can safely be reached. When considering diversion to a closer airport, the captain must consider the needs of the ill passenger, as well as other safety concerns such as weather, landing conditions, and terrain. Certain routes, such as transoceanic flights, and availability of definitive medical care may restrict diversion options.

IN-FLIGHT TRANSMISSION OF COMMUNICABLE DISEASES

Communicable diseases may be transmitted to other travelers during air travel; therefore, people who are acutely ill, or still within the infectious period for a specific disease, should delay their travel until they are no longer contagious. For example, otherwise healthy adults can transmit influenza to others for 5–7 days. Travelers should be up-to-date on routine vaccinations and receive destination-specific vaccinations before travel. Travelers should be reminded to wash their hands frequently and thoroughly (or use an alcohol-based hand sanitizer containing ≥60% alcohol), especially after using the toilet and before preparing or eating food, and to cover their noses and mouths when coughing or sneezing.

Aircraft contact investigations may be conducted for certain serious communicable diseases (see CDC's webpage "Protecting Travelers' Health from Airport to Community: Investigating Contagious Diseases on Flights" at www.cdc.gov/quarantine/contact-investigation.html). If a passenger with a serious communicable disease was infectious during a flight, passengers who may have been exposed may be contacted by public health authorities for possible screening or prophylaxis. When necessary, public health authorities will obtain contact information from the airline for potentially exposed travelers so they may be contacted and offered an intervention.

For information regarding CDC's travel restrictions, see www.cdc.gov/quarantine/qas-frn-travel-restriction.html. To request a consultation, public health authorities may contact the CDC quarantine station of jurisdiction (see www.cdc.gov/quarantine/quarantinestationcontactlistfull.html) or the CDC Emergency Operations Center by calling 770-488-7100.

Tuberculosis (*Mycobacterium tuberculosis*)

Tuberculosis (TB) is transmitted from person to person via airborne respiratory droplet nuclei. Although the risk of transmission onboard aircraft is low, CDC recommends conducting passenger contact investigations for flights ≥8 hours if the person with TB has sputum that is smear-positive for acid-fast bacilli and cavitation on chest radiograph or has multidrug-resistant TB. People known to have active TB disease should not travel by commercial air (or any other commercial means) until they are determined to be noninfectious. State health department TB controllers are valuable resources for advice to determine when a person can be considered non-infectious (www.tbcontrollers.org/community/statecityterritory).

Meningococcal disease (*Neisseria meningitidis*)

Meningococcal disease caused by *N. meningitidis* is transmitted by direct contact with respiratory droplets and secretions and can be rapidly fatal. Therefore, close contacts of ill travelers need to be quickly identified and provided with prophylactic antimicrobial agents. Antimicrobial prophylaxis should be considered for any of the following:

- Household members traveling with the ill traveler

- Travel companions with prolonged close contact

- Travelers seated directly next to the ill traveler on flights ≥8 hours (gate to gate) or who have

had direct contact with respiratory secretions or vomitus.

Measles (Rubeola)

Measles is a viral illness transmitted by respiratory droplets, direct contact, or airborne routes. Most measles cases diagnosed in the United States are imported from countries where measles is endemic. An ill traveler is considered infectious during a flight of any duration if he or she traveled during the 4 days before rash onset through 4 days after rash onset. Flight-related contact investigations are initiated as quickly as possible so postexposure prophylaxis may be provided to susceptible travelers. If indicated, MMR (measles, mumps, and rubella) vaccine given within 72 hours of exposure or immune globulin, given within 6 days of exposure, may prevent measles or decrease its severity in people who are not immune.

DISINSECTION

To reduce the accidental spread of mosquitoes and other vectors via airline cabins and luggage compartments, a number of countries require disinsection of all inbound flights or flights from certain areas. Although disinsection, when done appropriately, was declared safe by the World Health Organization (WHO) in 1995, there is still much debate about the safety of the agents and the effectiveness of disinsection as a public health measure to prevent the spread of vectorborne diseases. Although CDC reserves the right to require disinsection to control importation and spread of a vectorborne infectious disease, it is not currently required for aircraft arriving at US airports. WHO information on aircraft disinsection, including available procedures, can be found at www.who.int/ith/mode_of_travel/aircraft_disinsection/en. An updated list of countries that require disinsection, and the types of methods used, is available at the Department of Transportation website: www.transportation.gov/office-policy/aviation-policy/aircraft-disinsection-requirements.

INFORMATION FOR AIR CREW

In preparation for a healthy journey, flight crew can refer to Chapter 8, Advice for Air Crews and to the CDC Travelers' Health website (www.cdc.gov/travel). If flight crew encounter passengers with potentially infectious diseases, see the CDC Airline Guidance webpage: www.cdc.gov/quarantine/air. Requirements and tools for reporting are also provided.

BIBLIOGRAPHY

1. Aerospace Medical Association Air Transport Medicine Committee. Medical guidelines for airline travel. Alexandria, VA: Aerospace Medical Association; 2014 [cited 2016 Mar. 24]; Available from: https://www.asma.org/publications/medical-publications-for-airline-travel/medical-considerations-for-airline-travel.
2. Bagshaw M, Barbeau DN. The aircraft cabin environment. In: Keystone JS, Freedman DO, Kozarsky PE, Connor BA, Nothdurft HO, editors. Travel Medicine. 3rd ed. Philadelphia: Saunders Elsevier; 2013. pp. 405–12.
3. Huizer YL, Swaanm CM, Leitmeyer KC, Timen A. Usefulness and applicability of infectious disease control measures in air travel: a review. Travel Med Infect Dis. 2015 Jan-Feb;13(1):19–30.
4. Illig PA. Passenger health. In: Curdt-Christiansen C, Draeger J, Kriebel J, Antunano M, editors. Principles and Practice of Aviation Medicine. Hackensack, NJ: World Scientific; 2009. pp. 667–708.
5. Marienau KJ, Cramer EH, Coleman MS, Marano N, Cetron MS. Flight related tuberculosis contact investigations in the United States: comparative risk and economic analysis of alternate protocols. Travel Med Infect Dis. 2014 Jan-Feb;12(1):54–62.
6. Nable JV, Tupe CL, Gehle BD, Brady WJ. In-Flight medical emergencies during commercial travel. N Engl J Med 2015 Sep 3;375(10):939–45.
7. Neatherlin J, Cramer EH, Dubray C, Marienau KJ, Russell M, Sun H, et al. Influenza A(H1N1)pdm09 during air travel. Travel Med Infect Dis. 2013 Mar-Apr;11(2):110–8.
8. Nelson K, Marienau K, Schembri C, Redd S. Measles transmission during air travel, United States, December 1, 2008–December 31, 2011. Travel Med Infect Dis. 2013 Mar-Apr;11(2):81–9.
9. Peterson DC, Martin-Gill C, Guyette FX, Tobias AZ, McCarthy CE, Harrington ST, et al. Outcomes of medical emergencies on commercial airline flights. N Engl J Med. 2013 May 5;368(22):2075–83.
10. World Health Organization. Tuberculosis and air travel: guidelines for prevention and control. Geneva: World Health Organization; 2008 [cited 2016 Sep 26]; 3rd ed. Available from: http://www.who.int/tb/publications/2008/WHO_HTM_TB_2008.399_eng.pdf.

CRUISE SHIP TRAVEL

Joanna J. Regan, Kara Tardivel, Susan A. Lippold, Krista Kornylo Duong

INTRODUCTION

Cruise ship travel presents a unique combination of health concerns. Travelers from diverse regions brought together in often crowded, semi-enclosed environments onboard ships can facilitate the spread of person-to-person, foodborne, or waterborne diseases. Outbreaks on ships can be sustained for multiple voyages by transmission among crew members who remain onboard or by persistent environmental contamination. Port visits can expose travelers to local vectorborne diseases. The remote location of the travelers at sea means that they may need to rely on the medical capabilities and supplies available onboard the ship for extended periods of time, and cruise travelers and their physicians should be aware of ships' medical limitations and prepare accordingly. Certain groups, such as pregnant women, the elderly, or those with chronic health conditions or who are immunocompromised, require special consideration when considering cruise travel.

CRUISE SHIP MEDICAL CAPABILITIES

Medical facilities on cruise ships can vary widely depending on ship size, itinerary, length of cruise, and passenger demographics. Generally, shipboard medical clinics can provide medical care comparable to that of ambulatory care centers.

Although no agency officially regulates medical practice aboard cruise ships, consensus-based guidelines for cruise ship medical facilities were published by the American College of Emergency Physicians (ACEP) in 1995 and most recently updated in 2013. ACEP guidelines (www.acep. org/content.aspx?id=29500), which are followed by most major cruise lines, state that the cruise ship medical facilities should maintain the following minimum capabilities:

- Provide emergency medical care for passengers and crew

- Stabilize patients and initiate reasonable diagnostic and therapeutic interventions

- Facilitate the evacuation of seriously ill or injured patients

ILLNESSES AND INJURY ABOARD CRUISE SHIPS

Cruise ship medical clinics deal with a wide variety of illnesses and injuries. Approximately 3%–11% of conditions reported to cruise ship infirmaries are urgent or an emergency. Approximately 95% of illnesses are treated or managed onboard, and 5% require evacuation and shoreside consultation for medical, surgical, or dental problems. Roughly half of passengers who seek medical care are older than 65 years of age. Most infirmary visits are due to acute illnesses, of which respiratory illnesses (19%–29%); seasickness (10%–25%); injuries from slips, trips, or falls (12%–18%); and gastrointestinal (GI) illness (9%–10%) are the most frequently reported diagnoses. Death rates for cruise ship passengers, most often from cardiovascular events, range from 0.6 to 9.8 deaths per million passenger-nights.

The most frequently reported cruise ship outbreaks involve respiratory infections, GI infections (norovirus), and vaccine-preventable diseases other than influenza, such as varicella (chickenpox). To reduce the risk of onboard introduction of communicable diseases by embarking passengers, ships may conduct medical screening during embarkation to identify ill passengers, preventing them from boarding or requiring isolation if they are allowed to board.

The following measures should be encouraged to limit the introduction and spread of communicable diseases on cruise ships:

- Passengers and their clinicians should consult CDC's Travelers' Health website (www.cdc. gov/travel) before travel for updates on outbreaks and travel health notices.

- Passengers ill with communicable diseases before a voyage should delay travel until they are no longer contagious.

- Passengers who become ill during the voyage should seek care in the ship's infirmary to receive clinical management, facilitate infection control measures, and maximize reporting of potential public health events.

SPECIFIC HEALTH RISKS

GI Illness

From 2008 through 2014, rates of GI illness among passengers on voyages lasting 3–21 days decreased from 27.2 to 22.3 cases per 100,000 travel days. Despite this decrease, GI illness outbreaks continue to occur. Updates on these outbreaks involving ships with US ports of call can be found at www.cdc.gov/nceh/vsp/surv/gilist.htm.

More than 90% of GI outbreaks with a confirmed cause are due to norovirus. Characteristics of norovirus that facilitate outbreaks are a low infective dose, easy person-to-person transmissibility, prolonged viral shedding, no long-term immunity, and the organism's ability to survive routine cleaning procedures. From 2010 through 2015, 8–16 outbreaks of norovirus infections occurred on cruise ships each year. GI outbreaks on cruise ships from food and water sources have also been associated with *Salmonella* spp., enterotoxigenic *Escherichia coli*, *Shigella* spp., *Vibrio* spp., *Staphylococcus aureus*, *Clostridium perfringens*, *Cyclospora cayetanensis*, and hepatitis A and E viruses.

To protect themselves from infections and reduce the spread of GI illnesses on cruise ships, passengers should be counseled on the following:

- Passengers should wash their hands with soap and water often, especially before eating and after using the restroom.

6

- Passengers who develop a GI illness, even if symptoms are mild, should promptly call the ship's medical center (or the ship's master, if no medical center exists) and follow cruise ship guidance regarding isolation and other infection control measures (see Chapter 3, Norovirus).

- Additional information on cruise ship outbreaks is available at www.cdc.gov/nceh/vsp.

Respiratory Illness

INFLUENZA

Respiratory illnesses are the most common medical complaint, and influenza is the most commonly reported vaccine-preventable illness on cruise ships. Since passengers and crew originate from all regions of the world, shipboard outbreaks of influenza A and B can occur year-round, and travelers on cruise ships can be exposed to strains circulating in different parts of the world. Using 2008–2011 surveillance data, CDC found a mean rate of influenzalike illness (defined as temperature ≥100°F plus cough or sore throat) of 0.065 cases per 1,000 person-nights, without a detectable seasonal pattern.

Given the cruise ship environment, population, and variable medical capabilities, the following measures are recommended year round to protect travelers from influenza:

- Clinicians should provide cruise travelers, particularly those at high risk for influenza complications, with the current seasonal influenza vaccine (if available) ≥2 weeks before travel.

- Passengers at high risk for influenza complications should discuss antiviral treatment and chemoprophylaxis with their health care provider before travel.

- Passengers should practice good respiratory hygiene and cough etiquette.

- Passengers should report their respiratory illness to the infirmary promptly and follow isolation recommendations, if indicated.

Additional guidance on the prevention and control of influenza on cruise ships is available at www.cdc.gov/quarantine/cruise/management/guidance-cruise-ships-influenza-updated.html. For more information, see Chapter 3, Influenza.

LEGIONNAIRES' DISEASE

Although it is not a common cause of respiratory illness on cruise ships, Legionnaires' disease is a treatable infection that can result in severe pneumonia leading to death. More than 20% of all Legionnaires' disease cases reported to CDC are travel-associated. Clusters of Legionnaires' disease associated with hotel or cruise ship travel are difficult to identify because travelers often disperse from the source of infection before symptoms begin. A total of 83 ship-associated cases of Legionnaires' disease were reported in the literature from 1977 through 2012. The cases involved outbreaks on 8 ships, with a median of 4 cases per outbreak (range, 2–50 cases); 6 cases resulted in death.

In general, Legionnaires' disease is not transmitted person to person but is contracted by inhaling or aspirating warm, aerosolized water contaminated with *Legionella* organisms. Person-to-person transmission may be possible in rare cases. Contaminated ships' hot tubs are the most commonly implicated sources of shipboard *Legionella* outbreaks; potable water supply systems have also been implicated. Improvements in ship design and standardization of water disinfection have reduced the risk of *Legionella* growth and colonization.

Most cruise ships have health care personnel who can perform *Legionella* urine antigen testing. People with suspected Legionnaires' disease require prompt antibiotic treatment. See Chapter 3, Legionellosis (Legionnaires' Disease & Pontiac Fever) for more information.

In evaluating cruise travelers for Legionnaires' disease, clinicians should do the following:

- Obtain a thorough travel history of all destinations from 10 days before symptom onset (to assist in the identification of potential source of exposure).

- Collect urine for antigen testing.

- Culture lower respiratory secretions on selective media, which is essential to identify the species or serogroup.

- Inform CDC of any travel-associated Legionnaires' disease cases by sending an email to travellegionella@cdc.gov. Cases of Legionnaires' disease should be quickly reported to public health officials in order to determine if there are links to previously reported clusters and to stop potential clusters and new outbreaks.

Vaccine-Preventable Diseases (VPDs)

Although most cruise ship passengers are from countries with routine vaccination programs (such as the United States and Canada), many crew members originate from developing countries with low immunization rates. Outbreaks of measles, rubella, meningococcal disease and, most commonly, varicella have been reported on cruise ships. Preventive measures to reduce the spread of VPDs onboard cruise ships should be followed:

- Crew members should have documented proof of immunity to VPDs (see Chapter 2, General Recommendations for Vaccination & Immunoprophylaxis).

- Passengers, especially older passengers (>65 years of age) and immunocompromised people, should be up-to-date with routine vaccinations before travel, as well as any required or recommended vaccinations specific for their destinations.

- Women of childbearing age should be immune to varicella and rubella before cruise ship travel.

Vectorborne Diseases

Cruise ship port visits may include countries where vectorborne diseases such as malaria, dengue, yellow fever, Japanese encephalitis, and Zika are endemic. New diseases might surface in unexpected locations. For example, chikungunya was reported in late 2013 for the first time in the Caribbean (with subsequent spread throughout the Caribbean and numerous North, Central, and South American countries and territories). Zika virus was first reported in Brazil in 2015 and subsequently spread across the Caribbean and Latin America. See Chapter 3 for additional information on specific vectorborne diseases.

Passengers should follow recommendations for avoiding mosquito bites and vectorborne infections:

- Use an effective insect repellent (see Chapter 2, Protection against Mosquitoes, Ticks, & Other Arthropods).

- Treat clothing and gear with permethrin or purchase permethrin-treated items.

- While indoors, remain in well-screened or air-conditioned areas.

- When outdoors, wear long-sleeved shirts, long pants, boots, and hats.

- Obtain yellow fever vaccination if recommended or required.

- Take antimalarial chemoprophylaxis if needed (see Chapter 3, Yellow Fever & Malaria Information, by Country).

Other Health Concerns

Stresses of cruise ship travel include varying weather and environmental conditions, as well as unaccustomed changes in diet and physical activity. Foreign travel may increase the likelihood of risk-taking behaviors such as alcohol misuse, drug use, and unsafe sex. In spite of modern stabilizer systems, seasickness is a common complaint (affecting up to one-fourth of travelers) (see Chapter 2, Motion Sickness). Cruise lines may not allow women to board after the 24th week of pregnancy, and pregnant women should contact the cruise line for specific policies and recommendations before booking (for additional information, see Chapter 8, Pregnant Travelers).

PREVENTIVE MEASURES FOR CRUISE SHIP TRAVELERS

Cruise ship travelers often have complex itineraries due to multiple, short port visits. Although most of these port visits do not include overnight stays off the cruise ship, some trips have options for travelers to venture off the ship for ≥1 night. Therefore, cruise ship travelers may be uncertain

6

about potential exposures and which antimicrobial prophylaxis, immunizations, and preventive measures should be considered. Box 6-1 summarizes recommendations for cruise travelers and clinicians advising cruise travelers in pretravel preparation and healthy behaviors during travel. Travelers with special medical needs, such as wheelchairs, oxygen tanks, or dialysis, should inform their cruise line before traveling. Travelers with health conditions should carry a written summary of essential health information (electrocardiogram, chest radiograph, if abnormal, blood type, chronic conditions, allergies, treating physician contact information, and medication list) that would facilitate their care during a medical emergency. In addition, all prospective cruise travelers should verify coverage with their health insurance carriers and, if not included, consider

BOX 6-1. Cruise travel health precautions

ADVICE FOR CLINICIANS GIVING PRETRAVEL CRUISE CONSULTATIONS

Risk Assessment and Risk Communication

- Discuss itinerary, including season, duration of travel, and activities at port stops.
- Review the traveler's medical and immunization history, allergies, and special health needs.
- Discuss relevant travel-specific health hazards and risk reduction.
- Provide the traveler with documentation of his or her medical history, immunizations, and medications.

Immunization and Risk Management

- Provide immunizations that are routinely recommended (age-specific), required (yellow fever), and recommended based on risk.
- Discuss food and water precautions and insect-bite prevention.
- Older travelers, especially those with a history of heart disease, should carry a baseline electrocardiogram to facilitate onboard or overseas medical care.

Medications Based on Risk and Need

- Consider malaria chemoprophylaxis if itinerary includes port stops in malaria-endemic areas.
- Consider motion sickness medications for self-treatment (see Chapter 2, Motion Sickness).

PRECAUTIONS FOR CRUISE SHIP TRAVELERS

Pretravel

- Evaluate the type and length of the planned cruise in the context of personal health requirements.
- Consult medical and dental providers before cruise travel.
- Notify cruise line of special needs (such as wheelchair access, dialysis, oxygen tank).
- Consider additional insurance for overseas health care and medical evacuation.
- Carry prescription medications in their original containers, with a copy of the prescription and accompanying physician's letter.
- Bring insect repellent and sunscreen and consider treating clothes and gear with permethrin.
- Defer travel while acutely ill.

- Consult wwwnc.cdc.gov/travel/notices for travel health notices.
- Check www.cdc.gov/nceh/vsp/surv/gilist.htm for gastrointestinal outbreaks.

During Travel

- Wash hands frequently with soap and water. If soap and water are not available, use an alcohol-based sanitizer that contains ≥60% alcohol.
- Follow safe food and water precautions when eating off the ship at ports of call.
- Use measures to prevent insect bites during port visits, especially in malaria- or dengue-endemic areas or areas where outbreaks of vectorborne diseases, such as chikungunya and Zika, are occurring.
- Use sun protection.
- Maintain good fluid intake, but avoid excessive alcohol consumption.
- Avoid contact with ill people.
- If sexually active, practice safe sex.
- Report illness to ship's infirmary and follow medical recommendations.

6

purchasing additional insurance to cover medical evacuation and health services in foreign countries (see Chapter 2, Travel Insurance, Travel Health Insurance, & Medical Evacuation Insurance).

REPORTING ILLNESS AFTER TRAVEL

Travelers who become ill after returning home should inform their health care providers of where they have traveled. Clinicians should report suspected communicable diseases in recently returned cruise ship travelers to public health authorities:

- Report GI illnesses related to cruise ship travel to the CDC VSP by calling 800-CDC-INFO (800-232-4636) or by visiting www.cdc.gov and clicking on "Contact CDC-INFO" in the bottom right hand corner.

- Inform CDC of any travel-associated Legionnaires' disease cases by sending an e-mail to travellegionella@cdc.gov.

- Report communicable diseases to their local public health authority. Health departments should notify the CDC quarantine station of jurisdiction (www.cdc.gov/quarantine/quarantinestationcontactlistfull.html) for communicable diseases of public health concern during travel.

BIBLIOGRAPHY

1. Cramer EH, Slaten DD, Guerreiro A, Robbins D, Ganzon A. Management and control of varicella on cruise ships: a collaborative approach to promoting public health. J Travel Med. 2012 Jul;19(4):226–32.

2. Freeland AL, Vaughan GHJ, Banerjee SN. Acute gastroenteritis on cruise ships—United States, 2008–2014. MMWR Morb Mortal Wkly Rep. 2016 Jan 15;65(1):1–5.

3. Guyard C, Low DE. *Legionella* infections and travel associated legionellosis. Travel Med Infect Dis. 2011 Jul;9(4):176–86.

4. Hill CD. Cruise ship travel. In: Keystone JS, Freedman DO, Kozarsky PE, Connor BA, Nothdurft HD, editors. Travel Medicine. 3rd ed. Philadelphia: Saunders Elsevier; 2013. pp. 349–55.

5. Lanini S, Capobianchi MR, Puro V, Filia A, Del Manso M, Karki T, et al. Measles outbreak on a cruise ship in the western Mediterranean, February 2014, preliminary report. Euro Surveill. 2014 Mar 13;19(10):2–6.

6. Millman AJ, Kornylo Duong K, Lafond K, Green NM, Lippold SA, Jhung MA. Influenza outbreaks among passengers and crew on two cruise ships: a recent account of preparedness and response to an ever-present challenge. J Travel Med. 2015 Sep-Oct;22(5):306–11.

7. Mouchtouri VA, Rudge JW. Legionnaires' disease in hotels and passenger ships: a systematic review of evidence, sources, and contributing factors. J Travel Med. 2015 Sep-Oct;22(5):325–37.

8. Neri A, Fazio C, Ciammaruconi A, Anselmo A, Fortunato A, Palozzi A, et al. Draft genome sequence of C:P1.5-1,10-8:F3-6:ST-11 meningococcal clinical isolate associated with a cluster on a cruise ship. Genome Announc. 2014 Dec 4;2(6).

9. Peake DE, Gray CL, Ludwig MR, Hill CD. Descriptive epidemiology of injury and illness among cruise ship passengers. Ann Emerg Med. 1999 Jan;33(1):67–72.

10. Tomaszewski R, Nahorski WL. Interpopulation study of medical attendance aboard a cruise ship. Int Marit Health. 2008;59(1-4):61–8.

DEATH DURING TRAVEL

Nicole J. Cohen, Megan R. Reynolds, G. Gale Galland

OBTAINING US DEPARTMENT OF STATE ASSISTANCE

When a US citizen dies outside the United States, the deceased person's family members, domestic partner, or legal representative should notify US consular officials at the Department of State. Consular personnel are available 24 hours a day, 7 days a week, to provide assistance to US citizens for overseas emergencies.

- If a family member, domestic partner, or legal representative is in the foreign country with the deceased US citizen, he or she should contact the nearest US embassy or consulate for assistance. Contact information for US embassies, consulates, and consular agencies overseas may be found at the Department of State website (www.usembassy.gov).

- If a family member, domestic partner, or legal representative is located in the United States or Canada, he or she should call the Department of State's Office of Overseas Citizens Services in Washington, DC, from 8 AM to 8 PM Eastern Time, Monday through Friday, at 888-407-4747 (toll-free) or 202-501-4444. For emergency assistance after working hours or on weekends and holidays, call the Department of State switchboard at 202-647-4000 and ask to speak with the Overseas Citizens Services duty officer. In addition, the US embassy closest to or in the country where the US citizen died can provide assistance (www.usembassy.gov).

Emergency services provided by US consular officials can include advising the family, domestic partner, or legal representative about disposing of the remains and personal effects of the deceased. Preparing and returning human remains to the United States can be an expensive and lengthy process. The Department of State does not pay for these expenses; they are the responsibility of the deceased person's family, domestic partner, or legal representative. Consular officials may also serve as provisional conservators of the deceased person's estate, if no other legal representative is present in the foreign country where the death occurred.

IMPORTATION OF HUMAN REMAINS FOR INTERMENT OR CREMATION

General Guidance

Except for cremated remains, human remains intended for interment (placement in a grave or tomb) or cremation after entry into the United States must be accompanied by a death certificate stating the cause of death. A death certificate is an official document signed by a coroner, health care provider, or other official authorized to make a declaration of cause of death. Death certificates written in a language other than English must be accompanied by an English translation. Any requirements of the country of origin, air carrier, US Customs and Border Protection, and the Transportation Security Administration must also be met.

Remains of a Person Known or Suspected to Have Died from a Quarantinable Communicable Disease

Federal quarantine regulations (42 CFR Part 71.55) state that the remains of a person who is known or suspected to have died from a quarantinable communicable disease may not be brought into the United States unless the remains are cremated, properly embalmed and placed in a hermetically sealed casket, or accompanied by a CDC permit to allow importation of human remains, issued by the CDC director.

Information about communicable diseases for which federal isolation and quarantine are authorized is available at www.cdc.gov/quarantine/aboutlawsregulationsquarantineisolation.html.

A hermetically sealed casket is one that is airtight and secured against the escape of microorganisms. It should be accompanied by valid documentation certifying that it is hermetically sealed.

If a CDC permit is obtained to allow importation of human remains, CDC may impose additional conditions for importation. Permits for the importation of human remains of a person known or suspected to have died from a quarantinable communicable disease may be obtained from CDC's Division of Global Migration and Quarantine by calling the CDC Emergency Operations Center at 770-488-7100. A copy of the CDC permit must accompany the human remains at all times during shipment.

Remains of a Person Who Died of Any Cause Other than a Quarantinable Communicable Disease

When the cause of death is anything other than a quarantinable communicable disease, the remains may be cleared, released, and authorized for entry into the United States if 1 of the following conditions is met:

1. The remains meet the standards for importation found in 42 CFR 71.55: the remains are cremated or properly embalmed and placed in a hermetically sealed casket or are accompanied by a permit issued by the CDC director.

2. The remains are shipped in a leakproof container. A leakproof container is one that is puncture resistant and sealed so that there is no leakage of fluids outside the container during handling, storage, transport, or shipping.

CDC may also require additional measures, including detention, disinfection, disinfestation, fumigation, or other related measures, if there is evidence that the human remains are or may be infected or contaminated with a communicable disease and that such measures are necessary to prevent the introduction, transmission, or spread of communicable diseases into the United States.

EXPORTATION OF HUMAN REMAINS

CDC does not regulate the exportation of human remains outside the United States, although other state and local regulations may apply. Exporters of human remains and travelers taking human remains out of the United States should be aware that the importation requirements of the destination country and the air carrier must be met. Information regarding these requirements may be obtained from the appropriate foreign embassy or consulate (www.state.gov/s/cpr/rls) and the air carrier.

BIBLIOGRAPHY

1. Bureau of Consular Affairs, U.S. State Department. Death abroad. Washington, DC: US Department of State; 2014 [cited 2016 Apr. 11]; Available from: https://travel.state.gov/content/passports/en/abroad/events-and-records/death.html.

2. Bureau of Consular Affairs, U.S. State Department. Return of remains of deceased US citizens. Washington, DC: US Department of State; 2014 [cited 2016 Apr. 11]; Available from: http://travel.state.gov/content/passports/english/abroad/events-and-records/death/return-remains.html.

3. CDC. Quarantine station contact list, map, and fact sheets. Atlanta: CDC; 2013 [cited 2016 Apr. 11]; Available from: http://www.cdc.gov/quarantine/quarantinestationcontactlistfull.html.

4. CDC. Guidance for importation of human remains into the United States for interment or subsequent cremation. Atlanta: CDC; 2014 [cited 2016 Apr. 11]; Available from: http://www.cdc.gov/quarantine/human-remains.html.

5. CDC. Specific laws and regulations governing the control of communicable diseases. Atlanta: CDC; 2014 [cited 2016 Apr. 11]; Available from: http://www.cdc.gov/quarantine/SpecificLawsRegulations.html.

6. National Funeral Directors Association. Shipping remains from the United States to a foreign country. Brookfield, WI: National Funeral Directors Association; c2014 [cited 2016 Apr. 11]; Available from: http://nfda.org/additional-tools-shipping/2257-shipping-remains-from-the%20united-states%20to%20a%20foreign-country.html.

7. US Customs and Border Protection. Requirements for importing bodies in coffins/ashes in urns. Washington, DC: US Department of Homeland Security; 2015 [cited 2016 Apr. 11]; Available from: https://help.cbp.gov/app/answers/detail/a_id/237/kw/importation%20of%20human%20remains.

TAKING ANIMALS & ANIMAL PRODUCTS ACROSS INTERNATIONAL BORDERS

G. Gale Galland, Robert J. Mullan, Heather Bair-Brake

TRAVELING ABROAD WITH A PET

Travelers planning to take a companion animal to a foreign country must meet the entry requirements of the destination country and transportation guidelines of the airline. To obtain destination country information, travelers should contact the country's embassy in Washington, DC or the nearest consulate (see www.state.gov/s/cpr/rls/fco). Airline guidelines may be obtained from specific companies. Travelers should be aware that long flights can be hard on pets, particularly older animals with chronic health conditions, very young dogs, or breeds such as bulldogs that may be predisposed to respiratory stress. Additionally, upon reentering the United States, pets that traveled abroad are subject to the same import requirements as animals that have never lived in the United States.

REQUIREMENTS FOR ENTERING THE UNITED STATES

CDC restricts the importation of animals and animal products that might pose an infectious disease threat to humans. Any animal or animal product can be restricted from entry if there is reasonable knowledge or suspicion that it poses a human health risk. However, CDC has explicit restrictions for specific animals such as dogs, cats, turtles, nonhuman primates, African rodents, civets, and bats, as well as products made from them. Importers must meet stringent requirements in order to import these animals and items into the United States. Many of these animals are also regulated by other federal agencies or by individual state governments. Travelers should check with the Department of Agriculture (USDA), the Fish and Wildlife Service (FWS), and their destination state for specific rules about importation. Importers should research applicable requirements as soon as they know they will be importing an animal or animal product into the United States. Veterinary exams or certifications, vaccinations, or permits may be needed.

ANIMAL HEALTH CERTIFICATES

CDC regulations do not require general health certificates for animals entering the United States. However, some states may require health certificates for entry, and some airlines may require these certificates for transport. Before departure, travelers should check with the departments of health and of agriculture in their destination states and with the airline for any certificate requirements. The department of environmental protection or department of natural resources of some states and local governments may have additional requirements.

INTERNATIONAL PET RESCUE AND ADOPTION

Although done with the best of intentions, rescuing and importing stray animals from foreign countries can create human health risks. Travelers are at an increased risk for possible bites and scratches from fearful and stressed animals, which may result in injury or exposure to infectious disease. Animals that are infected with zoonotic diseases might not show any outward signs of being ill. Therefore, all rescued animals should be examined by a licensed veterinarian both before departure and after arrival in the United States. If the intent of travel is to rescue animals, participants should discuss rabies preexposure prophylaxis with their health care providers.

IMPORTATION OF LIVE ANIMALS

Dogs

Dogs are subject to inspection upon entry into the United States if they have evidence of being infected with a communicable disease or if they have not been vaccinated against rabies. If a dog appears to be ill, further examination by a licensed veterinarian may be required before entry is permitted. If necessary, this examination will be at the owner's expense.

Rabies vaccination is required for all dogs entering the United States from a country where rabies is present. Dogs must be accompanied by a current, valid rabies vaccination certificate that includes the following information:

- Name and address of owner

- Breed, sex, age, color, markings, and other identifying information for the dog

- Date of rabies vaccination and vaccine product information

- Date of expiration of vaccination

- Name, license number, address, and signature of veterinarian

- Rabies certificates have expiration dates that range from 1 to 3 years from the date of vaccination, depending on the type of vaccine given. All dogs must be ≥12 weeks of age before receiving their first rabies vaccination. Rabies vaccinations must occur at least 30 days before the date of arrival, as it takes 30 days for these vaccines to be fully effective.

- Routine rabies vaccination of dogs is recommended in the United States and required by most state and local health authorities in the United States. Check with state authorities at the final destination to determine any state requirements for rabies vaccination. State-specific information is found at www.aphis.usda.gov/wps/portal/aphis/ourfocus/animalhealth/sa_import_into_us/sa_entry_requirements/ct_us%20state_and_territory_animal_import_regulations.

- People seeking to import dogs that do not meet CDC's requirements should contact CDC in advance at CDCAnimalImports@cdc.gov to discuss their particular situation.

Cats

Cats are subject to inspection at US ports of entry and may be denied entry into the United States if they have evidence of being infected with a communicable disease. If a cat appears to be ill, further examination by a licensed veterinarian may be required before entry is permitted. This examination, if necessary, is conducted at the owner's expense. CDC does not require cats to have proof of rabies vaccination for importation into the United States. However, many states have rabies vaccination requirements for cats. Check with state and local health authorities at the final destination to determine any state requirements for rabies vaccination of cats. For more information about importing cats, see www.cdc.gov/animalimportation/cats.html.

All dogs and cats arriving in the state of Hawaii and the territory of Guam, even from the US mainland, are subject to locally imposed quarantine requirements. For more information about animal importation in Hawaii, consult http://hdoa.hawaii.gov or call 808-483-7151. For more information about animal importation in Guam, see www.guamcourts.org/CompilerofLaws/GAR/09GAR/09GAR001-1.pdf.

Nonhuman Primates

Nonhuman primates can transmit a variety of serious diseases to humans, including Ebola virus disease and tuberculosis. Nonhuman primates may only be imported into the United States by a CDC-registered importer and only for scientific, educational, or exhibition purposes. All nonhuman primates are considered endangered or threatened and require additional FWS permits for importation. Nonhuman primates that leave the United States may only return through a registered importer and only for the purpose of science, education, or exhibition. Nonhuman primates may not be imported as pets. Nonhuman primates that are kept as pets in the United States and travel outside of the United States will not be allowed to reenter the United States as pets. For more information on CDC's importation requirements, see www.cdc.gov/importation/bringing-an-animal-into-the-united-states/monkeys.html.

Turtles

Although often kept as pets, turtles can transmit *Salmonella* to humans. For this reason, CDC restricts the importation of some turtles. A person may import up to 6 viable turtle eggs or live turtles with a shell length of <4 in (10 cm) for noncommercial purposes. More live turtles or viable turtle eggs may be imported with CDC permission but only for science, education, or exhibition. CDC does not restrict the importation of live turtles with a shell length >4 inches. Check with USDA or FWS regarding additional requirements to import turtles. More information is available at www.cdc.gov/importation/bringing-an-animal-into-the-united-states/turtles.html.

African Rodents

African rodents are a known source of communicable diseases, such as monkeypox. Thus, CDC does not allow the importation of these animals. Exceptions may be made for animals imported for science, education, or exhibition purposes, with permission from CDC. Check with USDA or FWS regarding additional requirements to import African rodents. For additional information, see www.cdc.gov/importation/bringing-an-animal-into-the-united-states/african-rodents.html.

Civets and Related Animals

To reduce the risk of introducing severe acute respiratory syndrome (SARS) coronavirus, civets and related animals (family Viverridae) may not be imported into the United States. Exceptions may be made for animals imported for science, education, or exhibition purposes, with permission from CDC. Check with USDA or FWS regarding additional requirements to import civets and related animals. For more information, see www.cdc.gov/importation/bringing-an-animal-into-the-united-states/civets.html.

Bats and Other Vectors

Bats are reservoirs of many viruses that can infect humans, including rabies virus, Nipah virus, and SARS coronavirus. To reduce the risk

of introducing these viruses, the importation of all live bats requires a CDC permit. Many bats require additional permits issued by FWS. The application for a CDC import permit for bats can be found at www.cdc.gov/importation/bringing-an-animal-into-the-united-states/bats.html.

In some circumstances, known vectors of human disease such as ticks or mosquitoes may be imported into the United States with a permit from CDC for science, education, or exhibition. For additional information, see www.cdc.gov/phpr/ipp/index.htm.

Other Animals

Travelers planning to import horses, ruminants, swine, poultry or other birds, or dogs used for handling livestock should contact National Import Export Services, a part of USDA's Animal Plant Health Inspection Service, at 301-851-3300 or visit www.aphis.usda.gov to learn about additional requirements.

Travelers planning to import fish, reptiles, spiders, wild birds, rabbits, bears, wild members of the cat family, or other wild or endangered animals should contact FWS at 800-344-9453 (toll-free general number), 703-358-1949 (FWS Office of Law Enforcement), or visit www.fws.gov/le/travelers.html.

IMPORTATION OF ANIMAL PRODUCTS

Trophies and Animal Products

Travelers often want to import animal skins, hunting trophies, or other items made from animals when returning from a trip. Many of these items must either be rendered noninfectious (see www.cdc.gov/animalimportation/animalproducts.html) or be accompanied by an import permit. CDC restricts products made from nonhuman primates, African rodents, civets, and bats. These products may also be regulated by other US federal agencies. CDC has the right to restrict other items known to carry infectious diseases. For example, CDC restricts goatskin souvenirs, such as Haitian goatskin drums, from entry into the United States because they have been associated with cases of anthrax in humans. Travelers who want to import hunting trophies or other

6

products made from animals should check with CDC, USDA, and FWS to make sure they are complying with federal regulations.

Bushmeat

Animal products may also include items intended for human consumption. Bushmeat, for example, is an animal product that is an important aspect of West and Central African culture. This product, generally raw, smoked, or partially processed meat from wild animals, might harbor infectious and zoonotic agents that can cause human and animal disease. Bushmeat has been linked to deadly diseases including Ebola. Recent studies have found evidence of simian foamy viruses, which are known to cause infections in humans but have not been associated with human disease. As people migrate around the world, bushmeat has become a growing commodity in the global wildlife trade. CDC prohibits the importation of bushmeat into the United States from CDC-restricted species. Bushmeat importation may also be restricted under USDA or FWS regulations. In addition to the human and animal health risks, many of the wild animals commonly hunted for bushmeat are threatened or endangered species protected by international wildlife laws and treaties such as the Convention on International Trade of Endangered Species (CITES).

For additional information about importing animals and animal products into the United States and for permit applications, travelers should visit www.cdc.gov/importation/index.html or contact 1-800-CDC INFO (1-800-232-4636). To request CDC permission to import a CDC-regulated animal or product, send a message to CDCAnimalImports@cdc.gov.

BIBLIOGRAPHY

1. Bair-Brake H, Bell T, Higgins A, Bailey N, Duda M, Shapiro S, et al. Is that a rodent in your luggage? A mixed method approach to describe bushmeat importation into the United States. Zoonoses Public Health. 2014 Mar;61(2):97–104.

2. CDC. Multistate outbreak of monkeypox—Illinois, Indiana, and Wisconsin, 2003. MMWR Morb Mortal Wkly Rep. 2003 Jun 13;52(23):537–40.

3. CDC. Rabies in a dog imported from Iraq—New Jersey, June 2008. MMWR Morb Mortal Wkly Rep. 2008 Oct 3;57(40):1076–8.

4. DeMarcus TA, Tipple MA, Ostrowski SR. US policy for disease control among imported nonhuman primates. J Infect Dis. 1999 Feb;179 Suppl 1:S281–2.

5. Dobson AP. What links bats to emerging infectious diseases? Science. 2005 Oct 28;310(5748):628–9.

6. Editorial: bongo-drum disease. Lancet. 1974 Jun 8;1(7867):1152.

7. McQuiston JH, Wilson T, Harris S, Bacon RM, Shapiro S, Trevino I, et al. Importation of dogs into the United States: risks from rabies and other zoonotic diseases. Zoonoses Public Health. 2008 Oct;55(8-10):421–6.

8. National Association of State Public Health Veterinarians, Inc. Compendium of animal rabies prevention and control, 2009. MMWR Recomm Rep. 2009;58(RR-1):1–15.

9. Stam F, Romkens TE, Hekker TA, Smulders YM. Turtle-associated human salmonellosis. Clin Infect Dis. 2003 Dec 1;37(11):e167–9.

10. Wu D, Tu C, Xin C, Xuan H, Meng Q, Liu Y, et al. Civets are equally susceptible to experimental infection by two different severe acute respiratory syndrome coronavirus isolates. J Virol. 2005 Feb;79(4):2620–5.

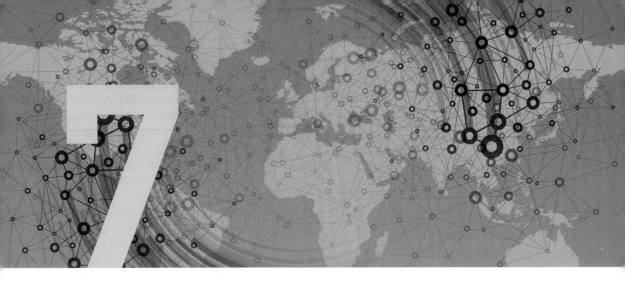

International Travel with Infants & Children

TRAVELING SAFELY WITH INFANTS & CHILDREN

Nicholas Weinberg, Michelle S. Weinberg, Susan A. Maloney

OVERVIEW

The number of children who travel or live outside their home countries has increased dramatically. In 2014, an estimated 2.44 million international travelers from the United States were children or adults traveling with children. Although data about the incidence of pediatric illnesses associated with international travel are limited, the risks that children face while traveling are likely similar to those their parents face. However, children are less likely to receive pretravel advice. In a review of children with post-travel illnesses seen at clinics in the GeoSentinel Surveillance Network, only 51% of all children and 32% of the children visiting

friends and relatives (VFRs) had received pretravel medical advice, compared with 59% of adults. The most commonly reported health problems among child travelers are as follows:

- Diarrheal illnesses
- Dermatologic conditions, including animal and arthropod bites, cutaneous larva migrans, and sunburn
- Systemic febrile illnesses, especially malaria
- Respiratory disorders

Motor vehicle and water-related injuries are also major health problems for child travelers. In assessing a child who is planning international travel, clinicians should:

- Review routine childhood and travel-related vaccinations. The pretravel visit is an opportunity to ensure that children are up-to-date on routine vaccinations.

- Assess all anticipated travel-related activities.

- Provide preventive counseling and interventions tailored to specific risks, including special travel preparations and treatment that may be required for infants and children with underlying conditions, chronic diseases, or immunocompromising conditions. Adolescents traveling in a student group or program may require counseling about disease prevention and the risks of sexually transmitted infections, empiric treatment and management of common travel-related illnesses, sexual assault, and drug and alcohol use during international travel (see Chapter 8, Study Abroad & Other International Student Travel).

- Give special consideration to the risks of children who are VFR travelers in developing countries. Conditions may include increased risk of malaria, intestinal parasites, and tuberculosis.

- Consider counseling adults traveling with children and older children to take a course in basic first aid before travel.

DIARRHEA

Diarrhea and associated gastrointestinal illness are among the most common travel-related problems affecting children. Infants and children with diarrhea can become dehydrated more quickly than adults. The etiology of travelers' diarrhea (TD) in children is similar to that in adults (see Chapter 2, Travelers' Diarrhea).

Prevention

For infants, breastfeeding is the best way to reduce the risk of foodborne and waterborne illness. Infant formulas available abroad may not have the same nutritional composition or be held to the same safety standards as in the United States; parents feeding their child formula should consider whether they need to bring formula from home.

Water served to young children, including water used to prepare infant formula, should be disinfected (see Chapter 2, Water Disinfection for Travelers). In some parts of the world, bottled water may also be contaminated and should be disinfected before consumption.

Similarly, food precautions should be followed diligently. Foods served to children should be thoroughly cooked and eaten while still hot; fruits eaten raw should be peeled by the caregiver immediately before consumption. Additionally, caution should be used with fresh dairy products, which may not be pasteurized and may be diluted with untreated water. For short trips, parents may want to bring a supply of safe snacks from home for times when the children are hungry and the available food may not be appealing or safe. See Chapter 2, Food & Water Precautions for more information.

Scrupulous attention should be paid to handwashing and cleaning bottles, pacifiers, teething rings, and toys that fall to the floor or are handled by others; water used to clean these items should be potable. Parents should be particularly careful to wash hands well after diaper changes, especially for infants with diarrhea, to avoid spreading infection to themselves and other family members. When proper handwashing facilities are not available, an alcohol-based hand sanitizer (containing ≥60% alcohol) can be used as a disinfecting agent. However, because alcohol-based hand sanitizers are not effective against certain pathogens, hands should be washed with soap and water as soon as possible. Additionally, alcohol does not remove organic material; visibly soiled hands should be washed with soap and water.

Chemoprophylaxis with antibiotics is not generally used in children.

Treatment

ANTIEMETICS AND ANTIMOTILITY DRUGS

Because of potential side effects, antiemetics are generally not recommended for self- or family-administered treatment of children with vomiting and TD. Because of the association between salicylates and Reye syndrome, bismuth subsalicylate (BSS), the active ingredient in both Pepto-Bismol and Kaopectate, is not generally recommended to treat diarrhea in children aged <12 years. However, some clinicians use it off-label with caution in certain circumstances. Caution should be taken in administering BSS to children with viral infections, such as varicella or influenza, because of the risk for Reye syndrome. BSS is not recommended for children aged <3 years. A recent Cochrane Collaboration Review of the use of antiemetics for reducing vomiting related to acute gastroenteritis in children and adolescents showed some benefits with ondansetron, metoclopramide, or dimenhydrinate. However, the routine use of these medications for emesis associated with TD has not yet been determined and is not generally recommended.

Antimotility drugs, such as loperamide and diphenoxylate, are rarely given to small children. Loperamide is not recommended for children aged <6 years. Diphenoxylate and atropine combination tablets are not recommended for children aged <2 years. These drugs should be used with caution in children because of potential side effects (see Chapter 2, Travelers' Diarrhea).

ANTIBIOTICS

Few data are available regarding empiric treatment of TD in children. The antimicrobial options for empiric treatment of TD in children are limited. In practice, when an antibiotic is indicated for moderate to severe diarrhea, some clinicians prescribe azithromycin as a single daily dose (10 mg/kg) for 3 days. Clinicians can prescribe unreconstituted azithromycin powder before travel, with instructions from the pharmacist for mixing it into an oral suspension if it becomes necessary to use it. Although resistance breakpoints have not yet been determined, elevated minimum inhibitory concentrations for azithromycin have been reported for some gastrointestinal pathogens. Therefore, parents should be counseled to seek medical attention for their children if they do not improve after empiric treatment. Clinicians should review possible contraindications, such as QT prolongation and cardiac arrhythmias with azithromycin, before prescribing medications for empiric treatment of TD.

Although fluoroquinolones are frequently used for the empiric treatment of TD in adults,

they are not approved by the Food and Drug Administration for this purpose among children aged <18 years because of cartilage damage seen in animal studies. The American Academy of Pediatrics suggests that fluoroquinolones be considered for the treatment of children with severe infections caused by multidrug-resistant strains of *Shigella* species, *Salmonella* species, *Vibrio cholerae*, or *Campylobacter jejuni*. Clinicians should be aware that fluoroquinolone resistance in gastrointestinal organisms has been reported from some countries, particularly in Asia. Routine use of fluoroquinolones for chemoprophylaxis or empiric treatment for TD among children is not recommended.

Fluid and Nutrition Management

The biggest threat to the infant with diarrhea and vomiting is dehydration. Fever or increased ambient temperature increases fluid loss and speeds dehydration. Adults traveling with children should be counseled about the signs and symptoms of dehydration and the proper use of oral rehydration salts (ORS). Medical attention may be required for an infant or young child with diarrhea who has the following:

- Signs of moderate to severe dehydration

- Bloody diarrhea

- Temperature >101.5°F (38.6°C)

- Persistent vomiting (unable to maintain oral hydration)

The mainstay of management of TD is adequate hydration.

ORS USE AND AVAILABILITY

Parents should be advised that dehydration is best prevented and treated by use of ORS in addition to the infant's usual food. ORS should be provided to the infant by bottle, cup, oral syringe (often available in pharmacies), or spoon while medical attention is being obtained. Low-osmolarity ORS is the most effective in preventing dehydration, although other formulations are available and may be used if they are more acceptable to young children. Homemade sugar-salt solutions are not recommended. Adults traveling with children should be counseled that sports drinks, which are designed to replace water and electrolytes lost through sweat, do not contain the same proportions of electrolytes as the solution recommended by the World Health Organization for rehydration during diarrheal illness. However, if ORS is not readily available, children should be offered whatever safe, palatable liquid they will take until ORS is obtained. Breastfed infants should continue to be breastfed.

ORS packets are available at stores or pharmacies in almost all developing countries. ORS is prepared by adding 1 packet to boiled or treated water (see Chapter 2, Water Disinfection for Travelers). Travelers should be advised to check packet instructions carefully to ensure that the salts are added to the correct volume of water. ORS solution should be consumed or discarded within 12 hours if held at room temperature or 24 hours if kept refrigerated.

A dehydrated child will usually drink ORS avidly; travelers should be advised to give it to the child as long as the dehydration persists. As dehydration lessens, the child may refuse the salty-tasting ORS solution, and another safe liquid can be offered. An infant or child who has been vomiting will usually keep ORS down if it is offered by spoon or oral syringe in small sips; these small amounts must be offered frequently, however, so the child can receive an adequate volume of ORS. Older children will often drink well by sipping through a straw. Severely dehydrated children, however, often will be unable to drink adequately. Severe dehydration is a medical emergency that usually requires administration of fluids by intravenous or intraosseous routes.

In general, children weighing <22 lb (10 kg) who have mild to moderate dehydration should be administered 2–4 oz (60–120 mL) ORS for each diarrheal stool or vomiting episode. Children who weigh ≥22 lb (10 kg) should receive 4–8 oz (120–240 mL) of ORS for each diarrheal stool or vomiting episode. The American Academy of Pediatrics provides detailed guidance on rehydration for vomiting and diarrhea; see www.healthychildren.org/English/health-issues/conditions/abdominal/Pages/Treating-Dehydration-with-Electrolyte-Solution.aspx.

ORS packets are available in the United States from Jianas Brothers Packaging Company (816-421-2880; http://rehydrate.org/resources/jianas. htm). ORS packets may also be available at stores that sell outdoor recreation and camping supplies. In addition, Cera Products (843-842-2600 or 706-221-1542; www.ceraproductsinc.com) markets a rice-based, rather than glucose-based, product.

DIETARY MODIFICATION

Breastfed infants should continue nursing on demand. Formula-fed infants should continue their usual formula during rehydration. They should receive a volume that is sufficient to satisfy energy and nutrient requirements. Lactose-free or lactose-reduced formulas are usually unnecessary. Diluting formula may slow resolution of diarrhea and is not recommended. Older infants and children receiving semisolid or solid foods should continue to receive their usual diet during the illness. Recommended foods include starches, cereals, pasteurized yogurt, fruits, and vegetables. Foods that are high in simple sugars, such as soft drinks, undiluted apple juice, gelatins, and presweetened cereals, can exacerbate diarrhea by osmotic effects and should be avoided. In addition, foods high in fat may not be tolerated because of their tendency to delay gastric emptying.

The practice of withholding food for ≥24 hours is not recommended. Early feeding can decrease changes in intestinal permeability caused by infection, reduce illness duration, and improve nutritional outcome. Highly specific diets (such as the BRAT [bananas, rice, applesauce, and toast] diet) have been commonly recommended; however, similar to juice-based and clear fluid diets, such severely restrictive diets have no scientific basis and should be avoided.

MALARIA

Malaria is among the most serious and life-threatening infections that can be acquired by pediatric international travelers. Pediatric VFR travelers are at particularly high risk for acquiring malaria if they do not receive chemoprophylaxis.

Children with malaria can rapidly develop high levels of parasitemia. They are at increased risk for severe complications of malaria, including shock, seizures, coma, and death. Initial symptoms of malaria in children may mimic many other common causes of pediatric febrile illness and therefore may result in delayed diagnosis and treatment. Among 33 children with imported malaria diagnosed at 11 medical centers in New York City, 11 (32%) had severe malaria and 14 (43%) were initially misdiagnosed. Clinicians should counsel adults traveling with children in malaria-endemic areas to use preventive measures, be aware of the signs and symptoms of malaria, and seek prompt medical attention if they develop.

Antimalarial Drugs

Pediatric doses for malaria chemoprophylaxis are provided in Table 3-10. All dosing should be calculated on the basis of body weight. Medications used for infants and young children are the same as those recommended for adults, except under the following circumstances:

- Doxycycline should not be given to children aged <8 years because of the risk of teeth staining.

- Atovaquone-proguanil should not be used for prophylaxis in children weighing <11 lb (<5 kg) because of lack of data on safety and efficacy.

Chloroquine, mefloquine, and atovaquone-proguanil have a bitter taste. Before departure, pharmacists can be asked to pulverize tablets and prepare gelatin capsules with calculated pediatric doses. Mixing the powder in a small amount of food or drink can facilitate the administration of antimalarial drugs to infants and children. Additionally, any compounding pharmacy can alter the flavoring of malaria medication tablets so that children are more willing to take them. Assistance with finding a compounding pharmacy is available on the Compounder Connect section of the International Academy of Compounding Pharmacists' website (www.iacprx. org; 800-927-4227). Because overdose of antimalarial drugs, particularly chloroquine, can be fatal, medication should be stored in childproof containers and kept out of the reach of infants and children.

Personal Protective Measures and Repellent Use

Children should sleep in rooms with air conditioning or screened windows, or sleep under bed nets when available. Mosquito netting should be used over infant carriers. Children can reduce skin exposed to mosquitoes by wearing long pants and long sleeves while outdoors in areas where malaria is transmitted. Clothing and mosquito nets can be treated with insect repellents such as permethrin, a repellent and insecticide that repels and kills ticks, mosquitoes, and other arthropods. Permethrin remains effective through multiple washings. Clothing and bed nets should be retreated according to the product label. Permethrin should not be applied to the skin. Although permethrin provides longer duration of protection, recommended repellents that can be applied to skin can also be used on clothing and mosquito nets. See Chapter 2, Protection against Mosquitoes, Ticks, & Other Arthropods for more details about these protective measures.

CDC recommends the use of repellents containing one of the following active ingredients, which are registered with the Environmental Protection Agency, according to the product labels: DEET [N,N-diethyl-m-toluamide], picaridin, oil of lemon eucalyptus [OLE] or PMD [para-menthane-3,8-diol], and IR3535 (http://cfpub.epa. gov/oppref/insect). Most repellents can be used on children aged >2 months, with the following considerations:

- Products containing OLE specify that they should not be used on children aged <3 years.

- Repellent products must state any age restriction. If none is stated, the Environmental Protection Agency has not required a restriction on the use of the product.

- Many repellents contain DEET as the active ingredient. The concentration of DEET varies considerably among products. The duration of protection varies with the DEET concentration; higher concentrations protect longer. Products with DEET concentration above 50% do not offer a marked increase in protection time. The American Academy of Pediatrics recommends that

> ≤30% DEET should be used on children aged >2 months.
> Repellents with DEET should not be used on infants aged <2 months.

Repellents can be applied to exposed skin and clothing; however, they should not be applied under clothing. Repellents should never be used over cuts, wounds, or irritated skin. Young children should not be allowed to handle the product. When using repellent on a child, an adult should apply it to his or her own hands and then rub them on the child, with the following considerations:

- Avoid the child's eyes and mouth, and apply sparingly around the ears.

- Do not apply repellent to children's hands, since children tend to put their hands in their mouths.

- Heavy application and saturation are generally unnecessary for effectiveness. If biting insects do not respond to a thin film of repellent, then apply a bit more.

- After returning indoors, wash treated skin with soap and water or bathe. This is particularly important when repellents are used repeatedly in a day or on consecutive days.

Products that contain both repellents and sunscreen are generally not recommended, because instructions for use are different and sunscreen may need to be reapplied more often and in larger amounts than repellent alone. In general, apply sunscreen first, and then apply repellent. Mosquito coils should be used with caution in the presence of children to avoid burns and inadvertent ingestion. For more information about repellent use and other protective measures, see Chapter 2, Protection against Mosquitoes, Ticks, & Other Arthropods.

DENGUE AND OTHER ARBOVIRUSES

Pediatric VFR travelers who may have frequent and prolonged travel may have risk similar to children living in areas where dengue or other arboviruses (such as chikungunya, Japanese encephalitis, yellow fever, or Zika viruses) are endemic or epidemic. Among 8 children who were diagnosed with acute dengue infection after visiting friends and relatives in the Caribbean, 3 developed severe dengue. Children traveling to areas with dengue or other arboviruses should use the same mosquito protection measures described for malaria. However, families should be counseled that, unlike the mosquitoes that transmit malaria, the *Aedes* mosquitoes that transmit dengue, chikungunya, yellow fever, and Zika are aggressive daytime biters and can also bite at night. Clinicians should consider dengue or other arboviral infections in children with fever if they have recently been in an endemic or epidemic area.

INFECTION AND INFESTATION FROM SOIL CONTACT

Children are more likely than adults to have contact with soil or sand and therefore may be exposed to diseases caused by infectious stages of parasites present in soil, including ascariasis, hookworm infestation, cutaneous or visceral larva migrans, trichuriasis, and strongyloidiasis. Children and infants should wear protective footwear and play on a sheet or towel rather than directly on the ground. Clothing should not be dried on the ground. In countries with a tropical climate, clothing or diapers dried in the open air should be ironed before use to prevent infestation with fly larvae.

ANIMAL EXPOSURES AND RABIES

Worldwide, rabies is more common in children than adults. In addition to the potential for increased contact with animals, children are also more likely to be bitten on the head or neck, leading to more severe injuries. Children and their families should be counseled to avoid all stray or unfamiliar animals and to inform adults of any contact or bites. Bats throughout the world are considered to have the potential to transmit rabies virus. Animal bites and scratches should be washed thoroughly with water and soap (and povidone iodine if available); for mammal bites and scratches, the child should be evaluated promptly to assess the need

7

for rabies postexposure prophylaxis. Because rabies vaccine and rabies immune globulin may not be available in certain destinations, families should seriously consider purchasing medical evacuation insurance.

AIR TRAVEL

Although air travel is safe for healthy newborns, infants, and children, a few issues should be considered in preparation for travel. Children with chronic heart or lung problems may be at risk for hypoxia during flight, and a clinician should be consulted before travel. Making sure that children can be safely restrained during a flight is a safety consideration. Severe turbulence or a crash can create enough momentum that a parent cannot hold onto a child:

- Children should be placed in a rear-facing Federal Aviation Authority–approved child-safety seat until they are aged ≥1 year and weigh ≥20 lb (9 kg).

- Children aged ≥1 year and 20–40 lb (9–18 kg) should use a forward-facing Federal Aviation Authority–approved child-safety seat.

- Children who weigh >40 lb (18 kg) can be secured in the aircraft seat belt.

Ear pain can be troublesome for infants and children during descent. Pressure in the middle ear can be equalized by swallowing or chewing:

- Infants should nurse or suck on a bottle.

- Older children can try chewing gum.

- Antihistamines and decongestants have not been shown to be of benefit.

There is no evidence that air travel exacerbates the symptoms or complications associated with otitis media. Travel to different time zones, jet lag, and schedule disruptions can disturb sleep patterns in infants and children, as well as in adults (Chapter 2, Jet Lag).

INJURIES

Vehicle-Related

Vehicle-related injuries are the leading cause of death in children who travel. While traveling in automobiles and other vehicles, children weighing ≤40 lb (18 kg) should be restrained in age-appropriate car seats or booster seats, as described above. These seats often must be carried from home, since availability of well-maintained and approved seats may be limited abroad. In general, children are safest traveling in the rear seat; no one should ever travel in the bed of a pickup truck. Families should be counseled that in many developing countries, cars may lack front or rear seatbelts. They should attempt to arrange transportation in vehicles or rent vehicles with seatbelts and other safety features.

Drowning and Water-Related Illness and Injuries

Drowning is the second leading cause of death in young travelers. Children may not be familiar with hazards in the ocean or in rivers. Swimming pools may not have protective fencing to keep toddlers from falling into the pool. Close supervision of children around water is essential. Water safety devices such as life vests may not be available abroad, and families should consider bringing these from home. Protective footwear is important to avoid injury in many marine environments. Schistosomiasis is a risk to children and adults in endemic areas. While in schistosomiasis-endemic areas (Map 3-12), children should not swim in fresh, unchlorinated water such as lakes or ponds.

Accommodations

Conditions at hotels and other lodging may not be as safe as those in the United States, and accommodations should be carefully inspected for exposed wiring, pest poisons, paint chips, or inadequate stairway or balcony railings.

ALTITUDE

Children are as susceptible to altitude illness as adults (see Chapter 2, Altitude Illness). Young children who cannot talk can show nonspecific symptoms, such as loss of appetite and irritability. They may have unexplained fussiness and change in sleep and activity patterns. Older children may complain of headache or shortness of breath. If children demonstrate unexplained symptoms after an ascent, it may be necessary to

7

descend to see if they improve. Acetazolamide is not approved for pediatric use for altitude illness, but it is generally safe in children when used for other indications.

SUN EXPOSURE

Sun exposure, and particularly sunburn before age 15 years, is strongly associated with melanoma and other forms of skin cancer (see Chapter 2, Sun Exposure). Exposure to UV light is highest near the equator, at high altitudes, during midday (10 AM–4 PM), and where light is reflected off water or snow. Sunscreens are generally recommended for use in children aged >6 months. Sunscreens (or sun blocks), either physical (such as titanium or zinc oxides) or chemical (sun protection factor [SPF] ≥15 and providing protection from both UVA and UVB), should be applied as directed, and reapplied as needed after sweating and water exposure. Babies aged <6 months require extra protection from the sun because of their thinner and more sensitive skin; severe sunburn for this age group is considered a medical emergency. Babies should be kept in the shade and wear clothing that covers the entire body. A minimal amount of sunscreen can be applied to small exposed areas, including the infant's face and hands.

Sun-blocking shirts are available that are made for swimming and preclude having to rub sunscreen over the entire trunk. Hats and sunglasses also reduce sun injury to skin and eyes. If both sunscreen and a DEET-containing insect repellent are applied, the SPF of the sunscreen may be diminished by one-third, and covering clothing should be worn or time in the sun decreased accordingly.

OTHER CONSIDERATIONS

Travel Stress

Changes in schedule, activities, and environment can be stressful for children. Including children in planning for the trip and bringing along familiar toys or other objects can decrease these stresses. For children with chronic illnesses, decisions regarding timing and itinerary should be made in consultation with the child's health care providers.

Insurance

As for any traveler, insurance coverage for illnesses and injuries while abroad should be verified before departure. Consideration should be given to purchasing special medical evacuation insurance for airlifting or air ambulance to an area with adequate medical care (see Chapter 2, Travel Insurance, Travel Health Insurance, & Medical Evacuation Insurance).

Identification

In case family members become separated, each infant or child should carry identifying information and contact numbers in his or her own clothing or pockets. Because of concerns about illegal transport of children across international borders, if only 1 parent is traveling with the child, he or she may need to carry relevant custody papers or a notarized permission letter from the other parent.

BIBLIOGRAPHY

1. Ashkenazi S, Schwartz E, Ryan M. Travelers' diarrhea in children: what have we learnt? Pediatr Infect Dis J. 2016 Jun;35(6):698–700.

2. Bradley JS, Jackson MA, Committee on Infectious Diseases. The use of systemic and topical fluoroquinolones. Pediatrics. 2011 Oct;128(4):e1034–45.

3. Fedorowicz Z, Jagannath VA, Carter B. Antiemetics for reducing vomiting related to acute gastroenteritis in children and adolescents. Cochrane Database Syst Rev. 2011 Sep 7(9):1–71.

4. Goldman-Yassen AE, Mony VK, Arguin PM, Daily JP. Higher Rates of misdiagnosis in pediatric patients versus adults hospitalized with imported malaria. Pediatr Emerg Care. 2016 Apr;32(4):227–31.

5. Hagmann S, Neugebauer R, Schwartz E, Perret C, Castelli F, Barnett ED, et al. Illness in children after international travel: analysis from the GeoSentinel Surveillance Network. Pediatrics. 2010 May;125(5):e1072–80.

6. Herbinger KH, Drerup L, Alberer M, Nothdurft HD, Sonnenburg F, Loscher T. Spectrum of imported infectious diseases among children and adolescents returning from the tropics and subtropics. J Travel Med. 2012 May-Jun;19(3):150–7.

7. Hunziker T, Berger C, Staubli G, Tschopp A, Weber R, Nadal D, et al. Profile of travel-associated illness in children, Zurich, Switzerland. J Travel Med. 2012 May-Jun;19(3):158–62.

8. Kamimura-Nishimura K, Rudikoff D, Purswani M, Hagmann S. Dermatological conditions in international pediatric travelers: epidemiology, prevention and management. Travel Med Infect Dis. 2013 Nov-Dec;11(6):350–6.

9. Krishnan N, Purswani M, Hagmann S. Severe dengue virus infection in pediatric travelers visiting friends and relatives after travel to the Caribbean. Am J Trop Med Hyg. 2012 Mar;86(3):474–6.

10. van Rijn SF, Driessen G, Overbosch D, van Genderen PJ. Travel-related morbidity in children: a prospective observational study. J Travel Med. 2012 May-Jun;19(3):144–9.

VACCINE RECOMMENDATIONS FOR INFANTS & CHILDREN

Michelle S. Weinberg

Vaccinating children for travel requires careful evaluation. Whenever possible, children should complete the routine immunizations of childhood on a normal schedule. However, travel at an earlier age may require accelerated schedules. **Not all travel-related vaccines are effective in infants, and some are specifically contraindicated.**

The recommended childhood and adolescent immunization schedule is available at www.cdc.gov/vaccines/schedules/downloads/child/0-18yrs-schedule.pdf. The catch-up schedule for children and adolescents who start their vaccination schedule late or who are >1 month behind can also be accessed at www.cdc.gov/vaccines/schedules/downloads/child/catchup-schedule-pr.pdf. This table also describes the recommended minimum intervals between doses for children who need to be vaccinated on an accelerated schedule, which may be necessary before international travel.

Country-specific vaccination recommendations and requirements for departure and entry vary over time. For example, proof of yellow fever vaccination is required for entry into certain countries. Meningococcal vaccination is required for travelers entering Saudi Arabia for the annual Hajj. The World Health Organization issued temporary vaccination requirements for residents of and long-term visitors to countries with active wild poliovirus transmission. Clinicians should check the CDC website for up-to-date requirements and recommendations (www.cdc.gov/travel).

Additional information about diseases and routine vaccination is available in the disease-specific sections in Chapter 3. Interactive tools for determining routine and catch-up childhood vaccination are available at www.cdc.gov/vaccines/schedules/hcp/child-adolescent.html.

MODIFYING THE IMMUNIZATION SCHEDULE FOR INADEQUATELY IMMUNIZED INFANTS AND YOUNGER CHILDREN BEFORE INTERNATIONAL TRAVEL

Several factors influence recommendations for the age at which a vaccine is administered, including age-specific risks of the disease and its complications, the ability of people of a given age to develop an adequate immune response to the vaccine, and potential interference with the immune response by passively transferred maternal antibodies.

The routine immunization schedules for infants and children in the United States do not provide specific guidelines for those traveling internationally before the age when specific vaccines and toxoids are routinely recommended. Recommended age limitations are based on potential adverse events (yellow fever vaccine), lack of efficacy data or inadequate immune response (polysaccharide vaccines and influenza vaccine), maternal antibody interference (measles-mumps-rubella [MMR] vaccine), or lack of safety data. In deciding when to travel with a young infant or child, parents should be advised that the earliest opportunity to receive routinely recommended immunizations in the United States (except for the dose of hepatitis B vaccine at birth and age 1 month) is at age 6 weeks. In general, live-virus vaccines (MMR, varicella, yellow fever) should be administered on the same day or spaced ≥28 days apart.

Routine Infant and Childhood Vaccinations

Children should receive routine vaccination for hepatitis A virus; hepatitis B virus; diphtheria, tetanus, pertussis; *Haemophilus influenzae* type b (Hib); human papillomavirus; influenza; MMR; *Neisseria meningitidis*; polio; rotavirus; *Streptococcus pneumoniae*; and varicella. In order to complete vaccine series before travel, vaccine doses can be administered at the minimum intervals. Parents should be informed that infants and children who have not received all recommended doses might not be fully protected. Rotavirus vaccine is unique among the routine vaccines given to US infants because it has maximum ages for the first and last doses; specific consideration should be given to the timing of an infant's travel so that the infant will still be able to receive the vaccine series, if at all possible.

Travel-specific vaccine considerations include the following:

- **Hepatitis A vaccine:** Although hepatitis A is usually mild or asymptomatic in infants and children aged <5 years, infected children may transmit the infection to older children and adults, who are at risk for severe disease. Vaccination should be ensured for all children traveling to areas where there is an intermediate or high risk of hepatitis A. Because of the potential interference by maternal antibodies, the hepatitis A vaccine is not approved for children aged <1 year. The vaccine series consists of 2 doses ≥6 months apart. One dose of monovalent hepatitis A vaccine administered at any time before departure can provide adequate protection for most healthy children.

The second dose is necessary for long-term protection.

- **Immune globulin (IG) for hepatitis A protection:** Children aged <1 year or who are allergic to a vaccine component and who are traveling to high-risk areas can receive IG. One dose of 0.02 mL/kg intramuscularly provides protection for up to 3 months, and 1 dose of 0.06 mL/kg IM provides protection for 3–5 months. Children should receive a second dose after 5 months if travel continues. For optimal protection, children aged ≥1 year who are immunocompromised or have chronic medical conditions and who are planning to depart to a high-risk area in <2 weeks should receive the initial dose of vaccine along with IG at a separate anatomic injection site. IG does not interfere with the response to yellow fever vaccine but can interfere with the response to other live injected vaccines (such as MMR and varicella vaccines). Administration of MMR and varicella vaccines should be delayed for >3 months after administration of IG for hepatitis A prophylaxis. IG should not be administered <2 weeks after MMR or varicella vaccines unless the benefits exceed those of vaccination. If IG is given during this time, the child should be revaccinated with the live MMR or varicella vaccines but not sooner than 3 months after IG administration. When travel plans do not allow adequate time to administer live vaccines and IG before travel, the severity of the diseases and their epidemiology at the destination will help determine the course of preparation.

- **Hepatitis B vaccine:** Vaccine can be administered with an accelerated schedule of 4 doses of vaccine given at 0, 1, 2, and 12 months; the last dose may be given on return from travel.

- **Influenza vaccine:** Influenza viruses circulate predominantly in the winter months in temperate regions (typically November–April in the Northern Hemisphere and April–September in the Southern Hemisphere) but can occur year-round in tropical climates. Since influenza viruses may be circulating at any time of the year, travelers aged ≥6 months who were not vaccinated during the influenza season of their country of residence should be vaccinated ≥2 weeks before departure if vaccine is available. Children aged 6 months through 8 years who are receiving influenza vaccine for the first time require 2 doses administered ≥4 weeks apart. Check the CDC website annually for updated recommendations about seasonal influenza vaccination.

- **MMR or MMRV vaccine:** Children traveling abroad may need to be vaccinated at an earlier age than is routinely recommended. Infants aged 6–11 months should receive 1 dose of MMR vaccine before departure, then be vaccinated with MMR or MMRV (measles-mumps-rubella-varicella) vaccine at 12–15 months (≥28 days after the initial dose) and again at 4–6 years, according to the routinely recommended schedule. Children aged ≥12 months should have 2 doses of MMR vaccine before traveling overseas. Children who have received 1 dose should receive their second dose before departure, provided the 2 doses are separated by ≥28 days.

- **Meningococcal vaccine:** Epidemics of meningococcal disease, caused by the bacterium *Neisseria meningitidis*, occur in sub-Saharan Africa during the dry season, December through June (see Map 3-11). CDC recommends that travelers be vaccinated before traveling to this region. Meningococcal vaccination is a requirement to enter Saudi Arabia when traveling to Mecca during the annual Hajj. Health requirements and recommendations for US travelers to the Hajj are available each year on the CDC Travelers' Health website (www.cdc.gov/travel). Meningococcal vaccine is also recommended for children aged 2 months through 18 years who travel to or reside in areas where *N. meningitidis* is hyperendemic or epidemic; for these children, providers should take care to use a meningococcal vaccine that is licensed for the child's age group and contains all 4 serotypes (A, C, Y, W-135). The schedule for the primary series and booster doses varies depending on which meningococcal vaccine is administered (see CDC's

Immunization Schedules website at www.cdc.gov/vaccines/schedules for additional information).

Adolescents and young adults aged 16 through 23 years may also be vaccinated with a serogroup B meningococcal (MenB) vaccine to provide short-term protection against most strains of serogroup B meningococcal disease. The preferred age for MenB vaccination is 16–18 years. ACIP also recommends routine use of MenB vaccine for people aged ≥10 years who are at increased risk for meningococcal disease, including people who have persistent complement component deficiency and people who have functional or anatomic asplenia. MenB vaccine is not recommended for people who travel to or reside in meningitis belt countries, as serogroup B disease is rare in this region. MenB vaccine is not routinely recommended for travel to other regions of the world unless an outbreak of serogroup B disease has been reported. Although MenB vaccine is not licensed in the United States for children <10 years of age, some European countries have recently introduced MenB vaccine as a routine immunization for infants. Infants who will be residing in these countries may consider MenB vaccination according to the routine infant immunization recommendations of that country.

- **Polio vaccine:** Polio vaccine is recommended for travelers to countries with evidence of wild poliovirus (WPV) circulation (during the last 12 months) and for travelers with a high risk of exposure to someone with imported WPV infection when traveling to some countries that border areas with WPV circulation. Refer to the CDC Travelers' Health website destination pages for the most up-to-date polio vaccine recommendations (wwwnc.cdc.gov/travel/destinations/list). Clinicians should ensure that travelers have completed the recommended age-appropriate polio vaccine series and have received a single lifetime booster dose, if necessary. See Chapter 3, Poliomyelitis and CDC's Immunization Schedules website (www.cdc.gov/vaccines/schedules) for information about accelerated schedules for completing the routine series. Young adults (≥18 years of

7

age) who are traveling to areas where polio vaccine is recommended and who have received a routine series with either inactivated polio vaccine (IPV) or live oral polio vaccine in childhood should receive a single lifetime booster dose of IPV before departure. Available data do not indicate the need for more than a single lifetime booster dose with IPV. However, requirements for long-term travelers may apply when departing certain countries.

- In May 2014, the World Health Organization (WHO) declared the international spread of polio to be a Public Health Emergency of International Concern (PHEIC) under the authority of the International Health Regulations (2005). To prevent further spread of disease, WHO issued temporary polio vaccine recommendations for long-term travelers (staying >4 weeks) and residents departing from countries with WPV transmission ("exporting WPV" or "infected with WPV"). Clinicians should be aware that long-term travelers and residents may be required to show proof of polio vaccination when departing from these countries. All polio vaccination administration should be documented on an International Certificate of Vaccination or Prophylaxis (ICVP). The polio vaccine must be received between 4 weeks and 12 months before the date of departure from the polio-infected country. Country requirements may change, so clinicians should check for updates on the CDC Travelers' Health website. Refer to the Clinical Update: Interim CDC Guidance for Travel to and from Countries Affected by the New Polio Vaccine Requirements (wwwnc.cdc.gov/travel/news-announcements/polio-guidance-new-requirements) for a list of affected countries, guidance on meeting the vaccination requirements, and instructions on how to order and fill out the ICVP.

Other Vaccines

JAPANESE ENCEPHALITIS VACCINE

Japanese encephalitis (JE) virus is transmitted by mosquitoes and is endemic throughout most of Asia and parts of the western Pacific. The risk can be seasonal in temperate climates and year-round in more tropical climates. The risk to short-term travelers and those who confine their travel to urban centers is low. JE vaccine is recommended for travelers who plan to spend a month or longer in endemic areas during the JE virus transmission season. JE vaccine should be considered for short-term (<1 month) travelers whose itinerary or activities might increase their risk for exposure to JE virus. The decision to vaccinate a child should follow the more detailed recommendations in Chapter 3, Japanese Encephalitis.

An inactivated Vero cell culture–derived JE vaccine (Ixiaro [Valneva]) was licensed by the Food and Drug Administration in 2009 for use in the United States for travelers aged ≥17 years. In 2013, the recommendations were expanded and the vaccine was licensed for use in children starting at age 2 months.

The primary series is 2 intramuscular doses administered 28 days apart. Information on age-appropriate dosing is available at www.cdc.gov/japaneseencephalitis/vaccine/vaccineChildren.html. For people aged ≥17 years, ACIP recommends that if the primary series was administered >1 year previously, a booster dose may be given before potential JE virus exposures. Although studies are being conducted on the need for a booster dose following a primary series of Ixiaro in children, data are not yet available.

RABIES VACCINE

Rabies virus causes an acute viral encephalitis that is virtually 100% fatal. Traveling children may be at increased risk of rabies exposure, mainly from dogs that roam the streets in developing countries. Bat bites carry a potential risk of rabies throughout the world. There are 2 strategies to prevent rabies in humans:

- Avoiding animal bites or scratches.
- Use of preexposure and postexposure prophylaxis. A 3-dose preexposure immunization series may be given on days 0, 7, and 21 or 28. In the event of a subsequent possible rabies virus exposure, the child will require 2 more doses of rabies vaccine on days 0 and 3. The decision whether to obtain preexposure immunization for children should follow the recommendations in Chapter 3, Rabies.

7

Children who have not received preexposure immunization and may have been exposed to rabies require a weight-based dose of human rabies immune globulin and a series of 4 rabies vaccine doses on days 0, 3, 7, and 14.

TYPHOID VACCINE

Typhoid fever is caused by the bacterium *Salmonella enterica* serotype Typhi. Vaccination is recommended for travelers to areas where there is a recognized risk of exposure to *Salmonella* Typhi.

Two typhoid vaccines are available: Vi capsular polysaccharide vaccine (ViCPS) administered intramuscularly, and oral live attenuated vaccine (Ty21a). Both vaccines induce a protective response in 50%–80% of recipients. The ViCPS vaccine can be administered to children who are aged ≥2 years, with a booster dose 2 years later if continued protection is needed. The Ty21a vaccine, which consists of a series of 4 capsules (1 taken every other day) can be administered to children aged ≥6 years. A booster series for Ty21a should be taken every 5 years, if indicated. The capsule cannot be opened for administration but must be swallowed whole. All 4 doses should be taken ≥1 week before potential exposure.

YELLOW FEVER VACCINE

Yellow fever, a disease transmitted by mosquitoes, is endemic in certain areas of Africa and South America (see Maps 3-14 and 3-15). Proof of yellow fever vaccination is required for entry into some countries (see Chapter 3, Yellow Fever & Malaria Information, by Country). Infants and children aged ≥9 months can be vaccinated if they travel to countries within the yellow fever–endemic zone. In February 2015, the CDC Advisory Committee on Immunization Practices (ACIP) approved a new recommendation that a single dose of yellow fever vaccine provides long-lasting protection and is adequate for most travelers. The updated recommendations also identify specific groups of travelers who should receive additional doses and others for whom additional doses may be considered. More information, including how to access yellow fever vaccine in the United States, is available in Chapter 3, Yellow Fever.

Infants aged <9 months are at higher risk for developing encephalitis from yellow fever vaccine, which is a live virus vaccine. Studies conducted during the early 1950s identified 4 cases of encephalitis out of 1,000 children aged <6 months vaccinated with yellow fever vaccine. An additional 10 cases of encephalitis associated with yellow fever vaccine administered to infants aged <4 months were reported worldwide during the 1950s.

Travelers with infants aged <9 months should be advised against traveling to areas within the yellow fever–endemic zone. ACIP recommends that yellow fever vaccine *never* be given to infants aged <6 months. Infants aged 6–8 months should be vaccinated only if they must travel to areas of ongoing epidemic yellow fever and if a high level of protection against mosquito bites is not possible. Clinicians considering vaccinating infants aged 6–8 months may contact their respective state health departments or CDC toll-free at 800-CDC-INFO (800-232-4636) or wwwn.cdc.gov/dcs/ContactUs/Form.

7

BIBLIOGRAPHY

1. CDC. General recommendations on immunization—recommendations of the Advisory Committee on Immunization Practices (ACIP). MMWR Recomm Rep. 2011 Jan 28;60(2):1–64.

2. CDC. Use of Japanese encephalitis vaccine in children: recommendations of the Advisory Committee on Immunization Practices, 2013. MMWR Morb Mortal Wkly Rep. 2013 Nov 15;62(45):898–900.

3. CDC. Prevention and control of meningococcal disease: recommendations of the Advisory Committee on Immunization Practices (ACIP). MMWR Recomm Rep. 2013 Mar 22;62(RR-2):1–28.

4. CDC. Interim CDC guidance for polio vaccination for travel to and from countries affected by wild poliovirus. MMWR Morb Mortal Wkly Rep. 2014 Jul 11;63(27):591–4.

5. CDC. Yellow fever vaccine: recommendations of the Advisory Committee on Immunization Practices (ACIP). MMWR Recomm Rep. 2015 Jun 19;64(23):647–50.

6. Global Polio Eradication Initiative. Polio public health emergency: temporary recommendations to reduce international spread of poliovirus. Geneva: Global Polio Eradication Initiative; 2016 [cited 2016 Apr. 18]; Available from: http://www.polioeradication.org/Keycountries/PolioEmergency.aspx.

7. Jackson BR, Iqbal S, Mahon B, Centers for Disease Control and Prevention (CDC). Updated recommendations for the use of typhoid vaccine—Advisory Committee on Immunization Practices, United States, 2015. MMWR Morb Mortal Wkly Rep. 2015 Mar 27;64(11):305–8.

8. MacNeil JR, Rubin L, Folaranmi T, Ortega-Sanchez IR, Patel M, Martin SW, et al. Use of serogroup B meningococcal vaccines in adolescents and young adults: recommendations of the Advisory Committee on Immunization Practices, 2015. MMWR Morb Mortal Wkly Rep. 2015 Oct 23;64(41):1171–6.

9. Red Book. 2015 Report of the Committee on Infectious Diseases. 30th ed. Kimberlin DW, Brady MT, Jackson MA, editors. Elk Grove Village, IL: American Academy of Pediatrics; 2015.

TRAVEL & BREASTFEEDING

Katherine R. Shealy

The medical preparation of a traveler who is breastfeeding differs only slightly from that of other travelers and depends in part on whether the mother and child will be separated or together during travel. Most mothers should be advised to continue breastfeeding their infants throughout travel. Before departure, mothers may wish to compile a list of local breastfeeding resources at their destination to have on hand. Clinicians and travelers can use the Find a Lactation Consultant Tool (www.ilca.org/why-ibclc/falc) to find contact information for experts at their destination. Map 7-1 shows destinations with English-language breastfeeding support groups facilitated by accredited volunteer mothers. Clinicians and travelers can use La Leche League International's interactive map (www.llli.org/search/groups) to find specific location and contact information for breastfeeding support group leaders and groups worldwide.

Mothers who plan to use an electric breast pump while traveling may need an electrical current adapter and converter and should have a back-up option available, including information on hand expression techniques (detailed hand expression instructions are available at www.workandpump.com/handexpression.htm).

TRAVELING WITH A BREASTFEEDING CHILD

Breastfeeding provides unique benefits to mothers and children traveling together. Health care providers should explain clearly to breastfeeding mothers the value of continuing breastfeeding during travel. For the first 6 months of life, exclusive breastfeeding is recommended. This is especially important during travel because exclusive breastfeeding means feeding only breast milk, no other foods or drinks, which potentially protects infants from exposure to contamination and pathogens via foods or liquids. Additionally, feeding only at the breast protects infants from potential exposure to contamination from containers (bottles, cups, utensils).

Breastfeeding infants require no water supplementation, even in extreme heat environments. Breastfeeding protects children from eustachian tube pain and collapse during air travel, especially during ascent and descent, by allowing them to stabilize and gradually equalize internal and external air pressure.

Clinicians should offer information to breastfeeding mothers so that they are better able to continue breastfeeding during travel. Frequent, unrestricted breastfeeding opportunities ensure the mother's milk supply remains ample and the child's nutrition and hydration are ideal. Mothers who are concerned about breastfeeding away from home may feel more comfortable breastfeeding the child in a fabric carrier. In many countries around the world, breastfeeding in public places is more widely practiced than in the United States. US federal legislation protects mothers' and children's right to breastfeed anywhere they are otherwise authorized to be while on federal property, which includes US Customs areas, embassies, and consulates overseas.

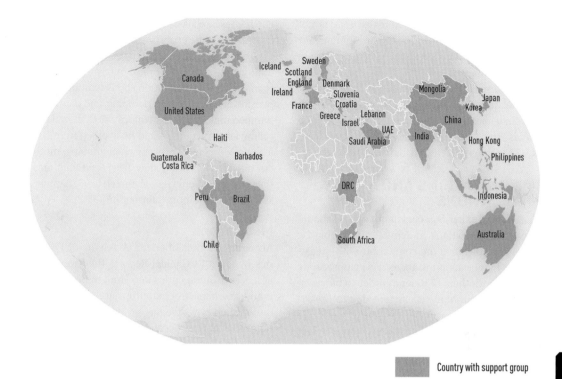

Country with support group

MAP 7-1. Breastfeeding support group locations[1]

[1] La Leche League Groups facilitated by accredited volunteer breastfeeding mothers. Country- and group-specific information available at www.llli.org/search/groups.

AIR TRAVEL

X-rays used in airport screenings have no effect on breastfeeding, breast milk, or the process of lactation. The Food and Drug Administration states that there are no known adverse effects from eating food, drinking beverages, or using medicine screened by x-ray. Airlines typically consider breast pumps as personal items to be carried onboard, similar to laptop computers, handbags, and diaper bags.

Before departure, mothers who will be traveling by air and expect to have expressed milk with them during travel need to carefully plan how they will transport their milk. Airport security regulations for passengers carrying expressed milk vary internationally and are subject to change. In the United States, expressed milk and related infant and child feeding items are exempt from Transportation Security Administration (TSA) regulations limiting quantities of other liquids and gels. The Infant and Child Nourishment Exemption permits passengers to carry with them all expressed milk, ice, gel packs (frozen or unfrozen), and other accessories required to transport expressed milk through airport security checkpoints and onboard flights, regardless of whether the breastfeeding child is also traveling. At the beginning of the screening process, travelers should inform the TSA officer and separate their expressed milk and related accessories from the liquids, gels, and aerosols that are limited to 3.4 oz (100 mL) each. Travelers may find that having on hand the related TSA regulations (available at www.tsa.gov/travel/special-procedures/traveling-children) facilitates the screening process.

Travelers carrying expressed milk in checked luggage should refer to cooler pack storage guidelines in "Proper Handling and Storage of Human Milk" on CDC's website (www.cdc.gov/breastfeeding/recommendations/handling_breastmilk.htm) to protect milk during travel. Expressed milk is not considered a biohazard. International Air Transport Authority regulations for shipping category B biological substances (UN 3373) do not apply to expressed milk; it is considered a food for individual use. Travelers shipping frozen milk should follow guidelines for shipping other frozen foods and liquids. Expressed milk does not need to be declared at US Customs upon return to the United States.

IMMUNIZATIONS AND MEDICATIONS

In almost all situations, clinicians can and should select immunizations and medications for the nursing mother that are compatible with breastfeeding. In most circumstances, it is inappropriate to counsel mothers to wean in order to be vaccinated or to withhold vaccination due to breastfeeding status.

Breastfeeding and lactation do not affect maternal or infant dosage guidelines for any immunization or medication; children always require their own immunization or medication, regardless of maternal dose. In the absence of documented risk to the breastfeeding child of a particular maternal medication, the known risks of stopping breastfeeding generally outweigh a theoretical risk of exposure via breastfeeding.

Immunizations

Breastfeeding mothers and children should be vaccinated according to routine, recommended schedules. Administration of most live and inactivated vaccines does not affect breastfeeding, breast milk, or the process of lactation. Only 2 vaccines, vaccinia (smallpox) and yellow fever, require special consideration. Preventive vaccinia (smallpox) vaccine is contraindicated for use in breastfeeding mothers.

SPECIAL CONSIDERATION: YELLOW FEVER VACCINATION

Breastfeeding is a precaution for yellow fever vaccine administration. Three cases of yellow fever vaccine–associated neurologic disease (YEL-AND) have been reported in exclusively breastfed infants whose mothers were vaccinated with yellow fever vaccine. All 3 infants were diagnosed with encephalitis and aged <1 month at the time of exposure.

Further research is needed to document the risk of potential vaccine exposure through breastfeeding. Data about possible excretion of vaccine virus and duration of excretion in breast milk are insufficient to make a recommendation about temporary suspension of breastfeeding, pumping, and discarding pumped milk. Until more information is available, yellow fever vaccine should be avoided in breastfeeding women. However, when nursing mothers must travel to a yellow fever–endemic area, these women should be vaccinated (see Chapter 3, Yellow Fever, for more information).

Medications

According to the American Academy of Pediatrics (AAP) 2013 Clinical Report: The Transfer of Drugs and Therapeutics into Human Breast Milk, many mothers are inappropriately advised to discontinue breastfeeding or avoid taking essential medications because of fears of adverse effects on their infants. The AAP's Tips for Giving Accurate Information to Mothers (www2.aap.org/breastfeeding/files/pdf/Lactmed.pdf) advises that this is usually unnecessary because only a small proportion of medications are contraindicated in breastfeeding mothers or associated with adverse effects on their infants. The National Institutes for Health's database of information on drugs and lactation (LactMed) is an online database of clinical information about drugs and breastfeeding (http://toxnet.nlm.nih.gov/newtoxnet/lactmed.htm). It provides information about maternal levels of drugs in breast milk, infant levels in blood, potential effects in breastfeeding infants and on lactation itself, the AAP category indicating the level of compatibility of the drug with breastfeeding, and alternate drugs to consider. The pharmaceutical reference guide, Medications and Mothers' Milk, is updated every 2 years and provides a comprehensive review of the compatibility or effects on breastfeeding of approximately 1,000 drugs, including concerns such as risk categories, pharmacologic properties, interactions with other drugs, and suitable alternatives.

SPECIAL CONSIDERATION: ANTIMALARIAL MEDICATIONS

Since chloroquine and mefloquine may be safely prescribed to infants, both are considered compatible with breastfeeding. Most experts consider short-term use of doxycycline compatible with breastfeeding. Primaquine may be used for breastfeeding mothers and children with normal G6PD levels. The mother and infant should be tested for G6PD deficiency before primaquine is given to the breastfeeding mother. Because data are not yet available on the safety of atovaquone-proguanil prophylaxis in infants weighing <11 lb (5 kg), CDC does not recommend it to prevent malaria in women who are breastfeeding infants weighing <11 lb (5 kg).

SPECIAL CONSIDERATION: TRAVELERS' DIARRHEA

Exclusive breastfeeding protects infants against travelers' diarrhea. Breastfeeding is ideal rehydration therapy. Children who are suspected of having travelers' diarrhea should breastfeed more frequently. Children in this situation should not be offered other fluids or foods that replace breastfeeding. Breastfeeding mothers with travelers' diarrhea should continue breastfeeding and increase their own fluid intake. The organisms that cause travelers' diarrhea do not pass through breast milk. Breastfeeding mothers should carefully check the labels of over-the-counter antidiarrheal medications to avoid using bismuth subsalicylate compounds, which can lead to the transfer of salicylate to the child via breast milk. Fluoroquinolones and macrolides, which are commonly used to treat travelers' diarrhea, are excreted in breast milk. The decision about the use of antibiotics such as fluoroquinolones and macrolides in nursing mothers should be made in consultation with the child's primary health care provider. Most experts consider the use of short-term azithromycin compatible with breastfeeding. Use of oral rehydration salts by breastfeeding mothers and their children is fully compatible with breastfeeding.

SPECIAL CONSIDERATION: ZIKA VIRUS

CDC encourages mothers with Zika virus infection and living in or traveling to areas with ongoing Zika virus transmission to breastfeed their infants. Current evidence suggests that the benefits of breastfeeding outweigh the theoretical risks of Zika virus transmission through breast milk. Updated information is available at www.cdc.gov/zika/hc-providers/infants-children.html.

TRAVELING WITHOUT A BREASTFEEDING CHILD

Before departure, a breastfeeding mother traveling without her breastfeeding infant or child may wish to express and store a supply of milk to be fed to the infant or child during her absence. Building a supply to be fed in her absence takes time and patience and is most successful when begun gradually, many weeks in advance of the mother's departure.

A mother's milk supply can diminish if she does not express milk while away from her nursing child, but this does not need to be a reason to stop breastfeeding. Clinicians should help mothers determine the best course for breastfeeding based on a variety of factors, including the amount of time she has to prepare for her trip, her flexibility of time while traveling, her options for expressing and storing milk while traveling, the duration of her travel, and her destination. A mother who returns to her nursing infant or child can continue breastfeeding and, if necessary, supplement as needed until her milk supply returns to its prior level. Often, after a mother returns from travel, her nursing infant or child will help bring her milk supply to its prior level. However, nursing infants or children who are separated from their mother for an extended time may have difficulty transitioning back to breastfeeding.

BIBLIOGRAPHY

1. Academy of Breastfeeding Medicine (ABM) Protocol Committee. ABM clinical protocol #8: human milk storage information for home use for full-term infants. Breastfeed Med. 2010 Jun;5(3):127–30.

2. Fleming-Dutra KE, Nelson JM, Fischer M, Staples JE, Karwowski MP, Mead P, et al. Update: interim guidelines for health care providers caring for infants and children with possible Zika virus infection—United States, February 2016. MMWR Morb Mortal Wkly Rep 2016 Feb 26;65(7):182–7.

3. Hale TW, Rowe HE. Medications and Mothers' Milk 2016: A Manual of Lactational Pharmacology. 17th ed. Plane, TX: Hale Pub; 2016.

4. Kuhn S, Twele-Montecinos L, MacDonald J, Webster P, Law B. Case report: probable transmission

of vaccine strain of yellow fever virus to an infant via breast milk. CMAJ. 2011 Mar 8;183(4):e243–5.

5. Sachdev HP, Krishna J, Puri RK, Satyanarayana L, Kumar S. Water supplementation in exclusively breastfed infants during summer in the tropics. Lancet. 1991 Apr 20;337(8747):929–33.

6. Section on Breastfeeding. Breastfeeding and the use of human milk. Pediatrics. 2012 Mar;129(3):e827–41.

7. Staples JE, Gershman M, Fischer M. Yellow fever vaccine: recommendations of the Advisory Committee on Immunization Practices (ACIP). MMWR Recomm Rep. 2010 Jul 30;59(RR-7):1–27.

INTERNATIONAL ADOPTION

Mary Allen Staat, Heather Burke

OVERVIEW

In the past 15 years, >250,000 children have come to the United States to join their families through international adoption. Families traveling to unite with their adopted child, siblings who wait at home for the child's arrival, extended family members, and childcare providers are all at risk for acquiring infectious diseases secondary to travel or resulting from contact with the newly arrived child. International adoptees may be underimmunized and are at increased risk for infections such as measles, hepatitis A, and hepatitis B because of crowded living conditions, malnutrition, lack of clean water, lack of immunizations, and exposure to endemic diseases that are not commonly seen in the United States. Challenges in providing care to internationally adopted children include the absence of a complete medical history, lack of availability of a biological family history, questionable reliability of immunization records, variation in preadoption living standards, varying disease epidemiology in the countries of origin, the presence of previously unidentified medical problems, and the increased risk for developmental delays and psychological issues in these children.

TRAVEL PREPARATION FOR ADOPTIVE PARENTS AND THEIR FAMILIES

A pretravel clinic visit is strongly recommended for prospective adoptive parents. In preparation, the travel health provider must know the disease risks in the adopted child's country of origin and the medical and social histories of the adoptee (if available), as well as which family members will be traveling, their immunization and medical histories, the season of travel, the length of stay in the country, and the itinerary while in country.

Family members who remain at home, including extended family, should be current on their routine immunizations. Protection against measles, varicella, tetanus, diphtheria, pertussis, hepatitis A, hepatitis B, and polio must be ensured for everyone who will be in the household or in close contact by providing care for the adopted child. Measles immunity or 2 doses of measles-mumps-rubella (MMR) vaccine separated by ≥28 days should be documented for all people born in or after 1957. Varicella vaccine should be given to those without a history of varicella disease or documentation of 2 doses of varicella vaccine ≥3 months apart. Adults who have not received the tetanus-diphtheria-acellular pertussis (Tdap) vaccine, including adults >65 years old, should receive a single dose of Tdap to protect against *Bordetella pertussis* in addition to tetanus and diphtheria. Unprotected family members and close contacts of the adopted child should be immunized against hepatitis A virus (HAV) before the child's arrival. Most adult family members and caretakers will need to be immunized with hepatitis B vaccine, since it has only been routinely given since 1990.

If the adopted child is from a polio-endemic area, family members and caretakers should ensure they have completed the recommended age-appropriate polio vaccine series. A one-time inactivated polio booster for adults who have completed the primary series in the past is recommended if they are traveling to these areas and can be considered for adults who remain at home but who will be in close contact caring for the child. Additional polio vaccination requirements for long-term travelers (staying >4 weeks) and residents departing from countries with polio transmission may affect travel (see Chapter 3, Poliomyelitis).

Prospective adoptive parents and any children traveling with them should receive advice on travel safety, food safety, immunization, malaria chemoprophylaxis, diarrhea prevention and treatment, and other travel-related health issues, as outlined elsewhere in this book. Instructions on car seats, injury prevention, food safety, and air travel apply equally to the adoptive child, so the travel health provider should also be familiar with and provide information on these child-specific issues.

OVERSEAS MEDICAL EXAMINATION OF THE ADOPTED CHILD

All immigrants, including children adopted internationally by US citizens, must undergo a medical examination in their country of origin, performed by a physician designated by the Department of State. The medical examination is used primarily to detect diseases or risk behaviors that may make the immigrant ineligible for a visa. Prospective adoptive parents should not rely on this medical examination to detect all possible disabilities and illnesses. Laboratory results from the country of origin may be unreliable. This examination should not replace the evaluation that is recommended once the child comes to the United States.

Additional information about the medical examination and the vaccination exemption form for internationally adopted children are available on the Department of State website at http://travel.state.gov/content/adoptionsabroad/en/us-visa-for-your-child/medical-examination.html and www.state.gov/documents/organization/80002.pdf, respectively.

FOLLOW-UP MEDICAL EXAMINATION AFTER ARRIVAL IN THE UNITED STATES

The adopted child should have a medical examination within 2 weeks of arrival in the United

States or earlier if the child has fever, anorexia, diarrhea, vomiting, or other medical concerns. Items to consider during medical examination of an adopted child include the following:

- Temperature (fever requires further investigation)

- General appearance: alert, interactive

- Anthropometric measurements: weight/age, height/age, weight/height, head circumference/age, body mass index

- Facial features: length of palpebral fissures, philtrum, upper lip (fetal alcohol syndrome: short palpebral fissures, thin upper lip, indistinct philtrum), other facial features suggestive of a genetic syndrome

- Hair: texture, color, areas of alopecia with dry patches (tinea capitis)

- Eyes: jaundice, pallor, strabismus, visual acuity screen

- Ears: hearing screen, otitis media

- Mouth: palate, thrush, presence of a uvula, teeth (number and condition)

- Neck: thyroid (enlargement secondary to hypothyroidism, iodine deficiency), lymph nodes

- Heart: murmurs

- Chest: symmetry, Tanner stage breasts

- Abdomen: liver or spleen enlargement

- Skin: Mongolian spots, scars, bacillus Calmette-Guérin (BCG) scar, birth marks, molluscum contagiosum, tinea capitis, tinea corporis

- Lymph nodes: enlargement suggestive of TB or other infections

- Back: scoliosis, sacral dimple

- Genitalia: Tanner stage, presence of both testicles, findings of sexual abuse

- Extremities: presence of bowing (rickets) or deformities

- Neurologic: presence and quality of reflexes

In addition, all children should receive a developmental screening by a clinician with experience in child development to determine if immediate referrals should be made for a more detailed neurodevelopmental examination and therapies. Further evaluation will depend on the country of origin, the age of the child, previous living conditions, nutritional status, developmental status, and the adoptive family's specific questions. Concerns raised during the preadoption medical review may dictate further investigation.

SCREENING FOR INFECTIOUS DISEASES

The current panel of tests for infectious diseases recommended by the American Academy of Pediatrics (AAP) for screening internationally adopted children is as follows:

- HAV serologic testing (IgG and IgM)

- Hepatitis B virus (HBV) serologic testing (repeat at 6 months if initial testing is negative)

- Hepatitis C antibody (repeat at 6 months if initial testing is negative)

- Syphilis serologic testing (treponemal and nontreponemal testing)

- HIV 1 and 2 serologic testing (antigen/ antibody)

- Complete blood cell count with differential and red blood cell indices

- Stool examination for ova and parasites (3 specimens)

- Stool examination for *Giardia intestinalis* and *Cryptosporidium* antigen (1 specimen)

- Tuberculin skin test (TST) (all ages) or interferon-γ release assay (IGRA) (for children >5 years of age) (repeat at 6 months if initial test is negative)

Additional screening tests may be useful, depending on the child's country of origin or specific risk factors. These screens may include Chagas disease serologic tests, malaria smears, or serologic testing for schistosomiasis, strongyloidiasis, and filariasis.

Gastrointestinal Parasites

Gastrointestinal parasites are commonly seen in international adoptees, but the prevalence varies by birth country and age. The highest rates of infection have been reported from Ukraine and Ethiopia and increase with older age. *Giardia intestinalis* is the most common parasite identified. Three stool samples collected in the early morning, 2–3 days apart and placed in a container with preservative are recommended for ova and parasite analysis. Only 1 of these samples needs to be analyzed for *Giardia* antigen and *Cryptosporidium* antigen. Although theoretically possible, transmission of intestinal parasites from internationally adopted children to family and school contacts has not been reported; however, good hand hygiene is recommended to prevent infection. Stool samples should be cultured for enteric bacterial pathogens for any child with fever and bloody diarrhea. Unlike refugees, internationally adopted children are not treated for parasites before departure.

Hepatitis A

HAV serology (IgG and IgM) should be considered for all internationally adopted children to identify children who may be acutely infected and shedding virus and to make decisions regarding HAV immunization. In 2007 and early 2008, multiple cases of hepatitis A secondary to exposure to newly arrived internationally adopted children were reported in the United States. Some of these cases involved extended family members who were not living in the household. Identification of acutely infected toddlers new to the United States is necessary to prevent further transmission. If a child is found to have acute infection, HAV vaccine or immunoglobulin can be given to close contacts to prevent infection. In addition, it is cost effective to identify children with past infection with serologic testing since they would not need to receive the HAV vaccine.

Hepatitis B

All internationally adopted children should be screened for HBV infection with serology for hepatitis B surface antigen (HBsAg) and hepatitis B surface antibody to determine past infection, current infection, or protection due to vaccination. HBV infection has been reported in 1%–5%

7

of newly arrived adoptees. Because of widespread use of the HBV vaccine, the prevalence of HBV infection has decreased over the years. Children found to be positive for HBsAg should be retested 6 months later to determine if the child has a chronic infection. Results of a positive HBsAg test should be reported to the state health department. HBV is highly transmissible within the household. All members of households adopting children with chronic HBV infection must be immunized and should have follow-up antibody titers to determine whether levels consistent with immunity have been achieved. Children with chronic HBV infection should receive additional tests for HBV e antigen, HBV e antibody, hepatitis D virus antibody, viral load, and liver function. They should be vaccinated for hepatitis A if they are not immune. They should also have a consultation with a pediatric gastroenterologist. Repeat screening at 6 months after arrival should be done on all children who initially test negative for HBV surface antibody.

Hepatitis C

Routine screening for hepatitis C virus (HCV) should be done, since most children with HCV infection are asymptomatic, screening for risk factors is not possible, effective treatments are available, and close follow-up of infected patients is needed to identify long-term complications. Antibody testing with an EIA should be done for screening. Since maternal antibody may be present in children <18 months of age, PCR testing should be done if the EIA is positive. Children with HCV infection should be referred to a gastroenterologist for further evaluation, management, and treatment.

Syphilis

Screening for *Treponema pallidum* is recommended for all internationally adopted children. Initial screening is done with both nontreponemal and treponemal tests. Treponemal tests remain positive for life in most cases even after successful treatment and are specific for treponemal diseases, which include syphilis and other diseases (such as yaws, pinta, and bejel) that can be seen in some countries. In children with a history of syphilis, the child's initial evaluation, treatment

(antibiotic type and treatment duration), and follow-up testing are rarely available; therefore, a full evaluation for disease must be undertaken and antitreponemal treatment given dependent upon the results.

HIV

HIV screening is recommended for all internationally adopted children. Positive HIV antibodies in children aged <18 months may reflect maternal antibody and not infection. Assaying for HIV DNA with PCR will confirm the diagnosis of HIV in the infant or child. Standard screening for HIV is with ELISA antibody testing, but some experts recommend PCR for any infant aged <6 months on arrival. If PCR testing is done, 2 negative results from assays administered 1 month apart, at least one of which is done after the age of 4 months, are necessary to exclude infection. Children with HIV infection should be referred to a specialist. Some experts recommend repeating the screen for HIV antibodies 6 months after arrival if the initial testing is negative.

Chagas Disease

Screening for Chagas disease should be considered for children arriving from a country endemic for Chagas disease. Chagas disease is endemic throughout much of Mexico, Central America, and South America (see Chapter 3, Trypanosomiasis, American [Chagas Disease]). The risk of Chagas disease varies by region within endemic countries. Although the risk of Chagas disease is likely low in adopted children from endemic countries, treatment of infected children is effective. Serologic testing when the child is aged 9–12 months will avoid possible false-positive results from maternal antibody. Testing by PCR can be done in children <9 months of age. If a child tests positive for Chagas disease, the child should be referred to a specialist for further evaluation and management.

Malaria

Routine screening for malaria is not recommended for internationally adopted children. However, thick and thin malaria smears should be obtained immediately for any febrile child newly arrived from a malaria-endemic area (see Chapter 3, Malaria).

Tuberculosis

All internationally adopted children should be screened for tuberculosis (TB) after arriving in the United States. Internationally adopted children are at 4–6 times the risk for TB than their US-born peers. The TST is indicated for all children, regardless of their BCG status. TST results must be interpreted carefully for internationally adopted children; guidelines may be found in the bibliography. For children aged ≥5 years, IGRA (such as QuantiFERON-TB Gold) is an acceptable screening alternative to the TST. IGRA has the advantage of not requiring a follow-up visit for testing or requiring individual interpretation of results (although results may be termed "indeterminate" by the laboratory). In addition, they appear to be more specific than the TST for *Mycobacterium tuberculosis* infection in children who have had BCG vaccination. The TST remains the most widely used screening test for TB in children. A chest radiograph and complete physical examination to assess for pulmonary and extrapulmonary TB are indicated for all children with positive TB screening results. Hilar lymphadenopathy is a more sensitive finding for TB in young children than are pulmonary infiltrates or cavitation. A repeat TST 3–6 months after arrival is recommended for children who initially test negative. Children who have a positive TST or IGRA result but have no evidence of active disease have latent tuberculosis infection (LTBI) and should generally be treated with isoniazid for 9 months. In consultation with TB experts, a shorter-course LTBI treatment regimen may be considered. Additional information is available at www.cdc.gov/tb/topic/treatment/ltbi.htm.

If active disease is found, every effort should be made to isolate the organism and determine sensitivities, particularly if the child is from a region of the world with a high rate of multidrug-resistant TB (see Chapter 3, Tuberculosis).

Eosinophilia

A complete blood count with a differential should be done on all internationally adopted children. An eosinophil count >450 cells/mm³ in an internationally adopted child may warrant further evaluation. Intestinal parasite screening will identify some helminths that may cause eosinophilia. Further investigation of the eosinophilia might include serologic evaluation for *Strongyloides stercoralis*, *Toxocara canis*, *Ancylostoma* spp., and *Trichinella spiralis*. For children arriving from countries endemic for *Schistosoma* spp. and filariasis, serologic testing should be done for these diseases as well.

SCREENING FOR NONINFECTIOUS DISEASES

Several screening tests for noninfectious diseases should be performed in all or in select internationally adopted children. All children should have a complete blood count with a differential, hemoglobin electrophoresis, and G6PD deficiency screening. Serum levels of thyroid-stimulating hormone and lead should be measured in all internationally adopted children. Testing for serum levels of iron, iron-binding capacity, transferrin, ferritin, and total vitamin D 25 hydroxy should be considered. All children should have vision and hearing screening and a dental evaluation. In certain circumstances, neurologic and psychological testing may also be considered.

IMMUNIZATIONS

The US Immigration and Nationality Act requires that any person seeking an immigrant visa for permanent residency must show proof of having received the Advisory Committee on Immunization Practices (ACIP)-recommended vaccines before immigration (www.cdc.gov/vaccines/schedules/downloads/child/0-18yrs-schedule.pdf). This requirement applies to all immigrant infants and children entering the United States, but internationally adopted children aged <10 years are exempt from the overseas immunization requirements. Adoptive parents are required to sign a waiver indicating their intention to comply with the immunization requirements within 30 days of the child's arrival in the United States. The vaccination exemption form can be found at www.state.gov/documents/organization/80002.pdf.

Most children throughout the developing world receive BCG, oral polio, measles, diphtheria, tetanus, and pertussis vaccines per the original immunization schedule of the United Nations Expanded Programme of Immunizations (begun in 1974). In many developing countries, HBV, *Haemophilus influenzae* type b (Hib), and rotavirus vaccines have become more widely available. Upon arrival in the United States, >90% of newly arrived internationally adopted children need catch-up immunizations to meet ACIP guidelines. Hepatitis A, Hib, human papillomavirus, mumps, pneumococcal conjugate, rotavirus, rubella, and varicella vaccines are often not available in developing countries. Reliability of vaccine records appears to differ by, and even within, country of origin. Some children may have an immunization record with documentation of the vaccines and dates they were given, and others may have incomplete documentation or no record at all. In addition, some children may be immune to vaccine-preventable diseases such as hepatitis A, measles, mumps, rubella, or varicella. A clinical diagnosis of any of these diseases should not be accepted as evidence of immunity.

Providers can choose 1 of 2 approaches for vaccination of internationally adopted children. The first is to reimmunize regardless of immunization record. The second, applicable to children aged ≥6 months, is to test antibody titers to the vaccines reportedly administered and reimmunize only for those diseases to which the child has no protective titers. Immunity to *B. pertussis* is an exception; antibody titers do not correlate with immune status to *B. pertussis*. However, protective antibody levels to diphtheria and tetanus imply protective antibody levels to *B. pertussis*. For children ≥6 months of age, testing can be done for diphtheria (IgG), tetanus (IgG), polio (neutralizing antibody to each serotype), hepatitis B (surface antibody), and Hib. Reimmunization for pneumococcus is recommended given that there are 13 serotypes in the vaccine. Most experts recommend serologic testing for infants and children aged ≥6 months. For children ≥12 months of age, testing can be done for measles, mumps, rubella, hepatitis A, and varicella. MMR is not given in most countries of origin; measles vaccine is often administered as a single antigen.

Immunizations should be given according to the current ACIP schedule for catch-up vaccination. If the infant is <6 months old and there is uncertainty regarding immunization status or validity of the immunization record, the child should be reimmunized according to the ACIP schedule.

BIBLIOGRAPHY

1. American Academy of Pediatrics. Medical evaluation of internationally adopted children for infectious diseases. In: Pickering LK, editor. Red Book: 2015 Report of the Committee on Infectious Diseases. 30th ed. Elk Grove Village, IL: American Academy of Pediatrics; 2015.

2. American Academy of Pediatrics Committee on Infectious Diseases. Recommendations for administering hepatitis A vaccine to contacts of international adoptees. Pediatrics. 2011 Oct;128(4):803–4.

3. CDC. Measles among adults associated with adoption of children in China—California, Missouri, and Washington, July–August 2006. MMWR Morb Mortal Wkly Rep. 2007 Feb 23;56(7):144–6.

4. CDC. CDC immigration requirements: technical instructions for tuberculosis screening and treatment: using cultures and directly observed therapy. 2009 [cited 2016 June 20]. Available from: http://www.cdc.gov/immigrantrefugeehealth/pdf/tuberculosis-ti-2009.pdf.

5. CDC. Recommended immunization schedules for persons aged 0 through 18 years—United States, 2014. MMWR Morb Mortal Wkly Rep. 2014 Feb. 7, 2014;63(5):108–9.

6. CDC, ACIP. Updated recommendations from the Advisory Committee on Immunization Practices (ACIP) for use of hepatitis A vaccine in close contacts of newly arriving international adoption. MMWR Morb Mortal Wkly Rep. 2009;58(36):1006–7.

7. Immigrant visas issued to orphans coming into the US. [database on the Internet]. US Department of State. 1999–2015 [cited 2016 Apr. 17]. Available from: http://adoption.state.gov/about_us/statistics.php.

8. Mandalakas AM, Kirchner HL, Iverson S, Chesney M, Spencer MJ, Sidler A, et al. Predictors of *Mycobacterium tuberculosis* infection in international adoptees. Pediatrics. 2007 Sep;120(3):e610–6.

9. Staat MA, Rice M, Donauer S, Mukkada S, Holloway M, Cassedy A, et al. Intestinal parasite screening in internationally adopted children: importance of multiple stool specimens. Pediatrics. 2011 Sep;128(3):e613–22.

10. Staat MA, Stadler LP, Donauer S, Trehan I, Rice M, Salisbury S. Serologic testing to verify the immune status of internationally adopted children against vaccine preventable diseases. Vaccine. 2010 Nov 23;28(50):7947–55.

11. Stadler LP, Donauer S, Rice M, Trehan I, Salisbury S, Staat MA. Factors associated with protective antibody levels to vaccine preventable diseases in internationally adopted children. Vaccine. 2010 Dec 10;29(1):95–103.

7

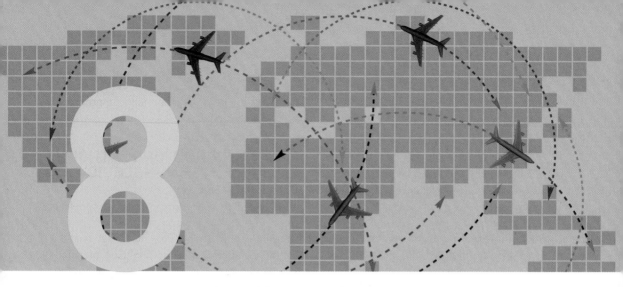

Advising Travelers with Specific Needs

IMMUNOCOMPROMISED TRAVELERS

Camille Nelson Kotton, Andrew T. Kroger, David O. Freedman

APPROACH TO THE IMMUNOCOMPROMISED TRAVELER

Immunocompromised travelers make up 1%–2% of travelers seen in US travel clinics. These travelers pursue itineraries largely similar to those of immunocompetent travelers. The pretravel preparation of travelers with immune suppression due to any medical condition, drug, or treatment must take into consideration several issues:

- What is the cause of the immune suppression? Different conditions and medications produce widely varying degrees of immune compromise, and there are many unknowns

in this field. Guidance regarding vaccination of immunocompromised travelers is less evidence-based than with other categories of travelers; this section provides recommendations based on the best available data and the practices of experienced clinicians.

- Is the traveler's underlying medical condition stable? The travel health care provider may need to contact the traveler's primary or specialty care providers (with the patient's permission) to discuss the traveler's fitness to travel, give specific medical advice for the proposed itinerary, verify the drugs and doses composing their usual maintenance regimen, and discuss whether any of the disease-prevention measures recommended for the proposed trip could destabilize the underlying medical condition, directly or through drug interactions.

- Do the conditions, medications, and treatments of the traveler constitute contraindications to, decrease the effectiveness of, or increase the risk for adverse events of any of the disease-prevention measures recommended for the proposed trip? Depending on the destination, such measures may include immunizations and drugs used for malaria chemoprophylaxis and management of travelers' diarrhea. Are there specific health hazards at the destination that would exacerbate the underlying condition or be more severe in an immunocompromised traveler? If so, can specific interventions be recommended to mitigate these risks?

- If an immunocompromised traveler were to become ill while traveling, what are the health care options (see Chapter 2, Obtaining Health Care Abroad)? What would the traveler do should medical evacuation be required? An immunocompromised traveler should have a plan for when and how to seek care overseas and how to pay for it.

The traveler's immune status is particularly relevant to immunizations. Overall considerations for vaccine recommendations, such as destination and the likely risk of exposure to disease, are the same for immunocompromised travelers as for other travelers. The risk of severe illness or death from a vaccine-preventable disease must be weighed against potential adverse events from administering a live vaccine to an immunocompromised patient. In some complex cases when travelers cannot tolerate recommended immunizations or prophylaxis, the traveler should consider changing the itinerary, altering the activities planned during travel, or deferring the trip.

For purposes of clinical assessment and approach to immunizations, immunocompromised travelers may be thought of as falling into 1 of 4 groups, based on mechanism and level of immune suppression. Vaccine recommendations for different categories of immunocompromised adults are shown in Table 8-1.

MEDICAL CONDITIONS WITHOUT SIGNIFICANT IMMUNOLOGIC COMPROMISE

With regard to travel immunizations, travelers whose health status places them in one of the following groups are not considered significantly immunocompromised and should be prepared as any other traveler, although the nature of the underlying disease needs to be kept in mind.

1. Travelers receiving corticosteroid therapy under any of the following circumstances:
   > Short- or long-term daily or alternate-day therapy with <20 mg of prednisone or equivalent.
   > Long-term, alternate-day treatment with short-acting preparations.
   > Maintenance steroids at physiologic doses (replacement therapy).
   > Steroid inhalers or topical steroids (skin, ears, or eyes).
   > Intraarticular, bursal, or tendon injection of steroids.
   > If >1 month has passed since high-dose steroids (≥20 mg per day of prednisone or equivalent for >2 weeks) have been used. After short-term (<2 weeks) therapy with daily or alternate-day dosing of ≥20 mg of prednisone or equivalent, some experts will still wait 2 weeks or more before administering live vaccines.
2. HIV patients without severe immunosuppression (for definitions of severe immunosuppression, see www.cdc.gov/mmwr/preview/mmwrhtml/rr6002a1.htm).
3. Travelers with a history of cancer who received their last chemotherapy treatment ≥3 months previously and whose malignancy is in remission.
4. Hematopoietic stem cell transplant recipients who are >2 years posttransplant, not on immunosuppressive drugs, with no evidence of ongoing malignancy, and without graft-versus-host disease.

Table 8-1. Immunization of immunocompromised adults

	HIV INFECTION, CD4 CELLS ≥200/mm³	SEVERE IMMUNOSUPPRESSION (HIV/AIDS), CD4 CELLS <200/mm³	SEVERE IMMUNOSUPPRESSION (NOT HIV-RELATED)	ASPLENIA	RENAL FAILURE	CHRONIC LIVER DISEASE, DIABETES
Live Vaccines						
Bacillus Calmette-Guérin (BCG)	X	X	X	U	U	U
Cholera	ND[1]	ND[1]	ND[1]	U	U	U
Influenza, live attenuated (LAIV)[2]	X	X	X	X	P	P
Measles-mumps-rubella (MMR)	R[3]	X[3]	X[3]	U	U	U
Typhoid, Ty21a	X	X	X	U	U	U
Varicella (adults)[4]	C[4]	X[4]	X[4]	U	U	U
Yellow fever[5]	P[5]	X[5]	X	U	OC[6]	OC[6]
Zoster	OC[7]	X[7]	X	U	U	U
Inactivated Vaccines						
Tdap, DTaP	U	U	U	U	U	U
Haemophilus influenzae type b (Hib)	U	U	OC[8]	R[9]	U	U
Hepatitis A[10]	U	U	U	U	U	U (diabetes), R (liver disease)
Hepatitis B[11]	R[12]	R[12]	U[12]	U[12]	R[12]	R[12,13]
Human Papillomavirus	U[14]	U[14]	U[14]	U	U	U

(continued)

8

Table 8-1. Immunization of immunocompromised adults (continued)

	HIV INFECTION, CD4 CELLS ≥200/mm³	SEVERE IMMUNOSUPPRESSION (HIV/AIDS), CD4 CELLS <200/mm³	SEVERE IMMUNOSUPPRESSION (NOT HIV-RELATED)	ASPLENIA	RENAL FAILURE	CHRONIC LIVER DISEASE, DIABETES
Influenza (inactivated)	R	R	R	R	R	R
Japanese encephalitis[15]	ND	ND	ND	ND	ND	ND
Meningococcal conjugate (ACWY)	R[16]	R[16]	U	R[16]	U	U
Meningococcal group B	C	C	C	R	C	C
PCV13 followed by PPSV23[17]	R	R	R	R	R	OC[18]
Polio (IPV)	U	U	U	U	U	U
Rabies	U	OC[19]	OC[19]	U	U	U
Td or Tdap	U	U	U	U	U	U
Typhoid, Vi	U	U	U	U	U	U

Abbreviations: X, Contraindicated (per the Advisory Committee on Immunization Practices [ACIP]); U, Use as indicated for normal hosts; R, Recommended for all in this patient category; P, Precaution (per ACIP); OC, Other considerations; C, Consider; ND, No data; PCV13, 13-valent pneumococcal conjugate vaccine; PPSV23, 23-valent pneumococcal polysaccharide vaccine.

[1] No safety or efficacy data exist regarding use of the current formulation of CVD 103-HgR vaccine in HIV-positive adults or people with severe immunosuppression. Limited data from an older formulation of the CVD 103-HgR suggest no association between the vaccine and serious or systemic adverse events, and slightly lower immunogenicity of the vaccine in HIV-positive versus HIV-negative adults.

[2] CDC did not recommend use of LAIV in the 2016–2017 season due to questions about LAIV effectiveness. Readers should consult the most recent guideline for recommendations in subsequent years.

[3] MMR vaccination is recommended for all HIV-infected patients aged ≥12 months with (for patients aged <6 years) CD4 percentage ≥15% or (for patients aged ≥6 years) CD4 percentage ≥15% and CD4 counts ≥200/mm³ for ≥6 months if they are without evidence of measles immunity. Immune globulin may be administered for short-term protection of those facing high risk of measles and for whom MMR vaccine is contraindicated. Additional guidance is available at www.cdc.gov/mmwr/preview/mmwrhtml/rr6204a1.htm.

[4] Varicella vaccine should not be administered to people who have cellular immunodeficiencies, but people with impaired humoral immunity (including congenital or acquired hypoglobulinemia or dysglobulinemia) may be vaccinated. HIV-positive adults with CD4 counts ≥200 cells/mm³ should be considered to receive 2 doses of vaccine spaced at 3-month intervals. VariZIG (varicella-zoster–specific immune globulin) is recommended for those exposed to varicella or herpes zoster if they do not have evidence of varicella immunity and have contraindications to vaccination.

[5] See details in Chapter 3, Yellow Fever. Yellow fever (YF) vaccination is a precaution for asymptomatic HIV-infected people with CD4 cell counts of 200–499/mm³. YF vaccination is not a precaution for people with asymptomatic HIV infection and CD4 cell counts ≥500/mm³. YF vaccine is also considered contraindicated by ACIP for symptomatic HIV patients without AIDS and with CD4 counts <200/mm³.

8

6 No data suggest increased risk of serious adverse events after use of YF vaccine in people with these conditions; however, varying degrees of immune deficit might be present, and providers should carefully weigh vaccine risks and benefits before deciding to vaccinate people with these conditions.

7 Also contraindicated by ACIP for symptomatic HIV patients without AIDS and with CD4 counts <200/mm3. No recommendation for asymptomatic HIV patients without AIDS and with CD4 counts ≥200/mm3.

8 Recipients of a hematopoietic stem cell transplant should be vaccinated with a 3-dose regimen 6–12 months after a successful transplant, regardless of vaccination history; at least 4 weeks should separate doses.

9 Only recommended for asplenic adults who have not previously received Hib vaccine.

10 Routinely indicated for all men who have sex with men, people with multiple sexual partners, hemophiliacs, patients with chronic hepatitis, injection drug users, and others.

11 Hepatitis B vaccination is indicated for people at risk for infection by sexual exposure, including sex partners of hepatitis B surface antigen (HBsAg)-positive people, sexually active people who are not in a long-term mutually monogamous relationship, people seeking evaluation or treatment for a sexually transmitted disease, men who have sex with men, people at risk for infection by percutaneous or mucosal exposure to blood, current or recent injection-drug users, household contacts of HBsAg-positive people, residents and staff of facilities for developmentally disabled people, health care and public safety workers with reasonably anticipated risk for exposure to blood or blood-contaminated body fluids, people with end-stage renal disease, international travelers to regions with high or intermediate levels (HBsAg prevalence >2%) of endemic HBV infection (see Map 3–4), people with chronic liver disease, and people with HIV infection.

12 Adult patients receiving hemodialysis or with other immunocompromising conditions should receive 1 dose of 40 µg/mL Recombivax HB administered on a 3-dose schedule at 0, 1, and 6 months or 2 doses of 20 µg/mL (Engerix-B) administered simultaneously on a 4-dose schedule at 0, 1, 2, and 6 months. Test for antibodies to hepatitis B virus surface antigen serum after vaccination and revaccinate if initial antibody response is absent or suboptimal (<10 mIU/mL). HIV-infected nonresponders may react to a subsequent vaccine course if CD4 cell counts rise to 500/mm3 after institution of highly active antiretroviral therapy. See text for discussion of other immunocompromised groups.

13 People with diabetes who are younger than 60 years as soon as feasible after diagnosis; people with diabetes who are age 60 years or older at the discretion of the treating clinician based on the likelihood of acquiring HBV infection, including the risk posed by an increased need for assisted blood glucose monitoring in long-term care facilities, the likelihood of experiencing chronic sequelae if infected with HBV, and the likelihood of immune response to vaccination; all people with chronic liver disease not caused by hepatitis B. At present, routine testing of antibody response after vaccination in people with diabetes or chronic liver disease is not recommended.

14 HPV vaccine should be administered as indicated for males and females but is additionally recommended for all in this patient category for men 22 through 26 years of age (otherwise male indication is through age 21 years). Female indication in each category is through 26 years of age.

15 No safety or efficacy data exist regarding the use of Ixiaro in immunocompromised people. In general, inactivated vaccines can be administered safely to people with altered immunocompetence, using the usual doses and schedules, but the effectiveness might be suboptimal. The inactivated, Vero cell–derived Japanese encephalitis vaccine, Ixiaro, is the only Japanese encephalitis vaccine available in the United States; other types of Japanese encephalitis vaccines, including live vaccines, are available internationally but are not included here.

16 Two doses ≥2 months apart recommended for patients with HIV infection if they are aged ≥2 years. If younger than 7 years old at previous dose, a patient should receive an additional dose of Menactra or Menveo 3 years after the primary series. Boosters should be repeated every 5 years thereafter. If aged ≥7 years at previous dose, a patient should receive an additional dose of Menactra or Menveo 5 years after the primary series. Boosters should be repeated every 5 years thereafter.

17 Previously unimmunized asplenic, HIV-infected, with chronic renal disease or nephrotic syndrome, or immunocompromised adults aged ≥5 years should receive 1 dose of 13-valent pneumococcal conjugate vaccine (PCV13) followed by 1 dose of pneumococcal polysaccharide vaccine (PPSV23) ≥8 weeks later. People with these conditions previously immunized with PPSV23 should follow catch-up guidelines per ACIP.

18 This is an indication for PPSV23 only (as opposed to both PCV13 and PPSV23).

19 For postexposure prophylaxis, both vaccine (5 doses at day 0, 3, 7, 14, 28) and immune globulin should be given to immunocompromised people, regardless of previous vaccination status.

8

5. Travelers with autoimmune disease (such as systemic lupus erythematosus, inflammatory bowel disease, or rheumatoid arthritis) who are not being treated with immunosuppressive or immunomodulatory drugs, although definitive data are lacking.

MEDICAL CONDITIONS AND TREATMENTS ASSOCIATED WITH LIMITED IMMUNE DEFICITS

Asymptomatic HIV Infection

Asymptomatic HIV-infected adults with CD4 cell counts of 200–499/mm^3 are considered to have limited immune deficits and should be vaccinated according to the guidelines in Table 8-1. Meningococcal (MenACWY), pneumococcal, and hepatitis B vaccines are recommended for HIV-positive patients regardless of travel plans. Many clinicians regard patients with CD4 cell counts ≥200/mm^3 who have undetectable viral loads as immunologically normal. More specific recommendations are available for MMR (measles-mumps-rubella) vaccine (www.cdc.gov/mmwr/preview/mmwrhtml/rr6204a1.htm). CD4 counts while on antiretroviral drugs, rather than nadir counts, should be used to categorize HIV-infected people. To achieve a maximal vaccine response with minimal risk, many clinicians advise a delay of 3 months after immune reconstitution (usually 6 months after initiation of antiretroviral therapy), if possible, before immunizations are administered; however, the optimal time to initiate vaccination after starting antiretroviral therapy has been identified as a gap in knowledge by the Infectious Diseases Society of America. For MMR vaccine, the recommendation is ≥6 months on antiretroviral therapy with the age- and CD4-based criteria. Although seroconversion rates and geometric mean titers of antibody in response to vaccines may be less than those measured in healthy controls, most vaccines can elicit protective levels of antibody in many HIV-infected patients in this category.

Transient increases in HIV viral load, which return quickly to baseline, have been observed after administration of several different vaccines to asymptomatic HIV-infected people. The clinical significance of these increases is not known, but they do not preclude the use of any vaccine.

Multiple Sclerosis (MS)

Inactivated vaccines, including influenza, hepatitis B, human papillomavirus, and tetanus vaccines, are generally considered safe for people with MS, although vaccination should be delayed during clinically significant relapses until patients have stabilized or begun to improve from the relapse, typically 4–6 weeks after it began. Published studies are lacking on the safety and efficacy of other vaccines, such as those against hepatitis A, meningococcal disease, pertussis, pneumococcal disease, polio, and typhoid. Inactivated vaccines are theoretically safe for people being treated with an interferon medication, glatiramer acetate, mitoxantrone, fingolimod, or natalizumab, although safety and efficacy data are lacking.

Modern MS therapy often includes aggressive and early immunomodulatory therapy for many MS patients, even those with stable disease. Live vaccines should not be given to people with MS during therapy with immunosuppressants such as mitoxantrone, azathioprine, methotrexate, or cyclophosphamide; during chronic corticosteroid therapy; or during therapy with immunosuppressive biologic agents. Patients on glatiramer acetate and interferon therapy have more limited immune deficits.

A few published studies suggest that mumps, measles, rubella, varicella, and zoster vaccines may be safe in people with stable MS if administered 1 month before starting or at the appropriate interval (see Duration of Iatrogenic Immune Compromise below) after discontinuing immunosuppressive therapy. One study suggests yellow fever vaccine can exacerbate symptoms in MS patients; this risk should be considered in consultation with the patient's neurologist before administering the vaccine.

Other Chronic Conditions

Chronic medical conditions that may be associated with varying degrees of immune deficit include asplenia, chronic renal disease, chronic liver disease (including hepatitis C), and diabetes mellitus. These patients should be vaccinated according to the guidelines in Table 8-1. Patients with complement deficiencies can receive any live or inactivated vaccine. Factors to consider in assessing the general level of immune competence of patients with chronic diseases include disease severity, duration, clinical stability, complications, comorbidities, and any potentially immune-suppressing treatment (see the next section in this chapter, Travelers with Chronic Illnesses).

Adults aged ≥19 years with most immunocompromising and some chronic conditions who have not previously received the 13-valent pneumococcal conjugate vaccine (PCV13) or the 23-valent pneumococcal polysaccharide vaccine (PPSV23) should receive a single dose of PCV13 followed by a dose of PPSV23 ≥8 weeks later; those who have previously received ≥1 dose of PPSV23 should receive a dose of PCV13 ≥1 year after the last PPSV23 dose was received. For adults who require additional doses of PPSV23, the first such dose should be given no sooner than 8 weeks after PCV13 and ≥5 years after the most recent dose of PPSV23.

A blunted response to hepatitis B vaccine has been reported in patients with immunosuppressive disease, which may include chronic hepatic or renal disease; a decreased response to hepatitis B vaccine has also been observed in patients with diabetes. Additional or higher doses of hepatitis B vaccine beyond the standard primary series may be necessary or indicated.

Asplenic patients are susceptible to overwhelming sepsis with encapsulated bacterial pathogens. Although response to vaccines may be diminished compared with people who have a functioning spleen, immunization against meningococcal (MenACWY and MenB), pneumococcal (see dosing above), and *Haemophilus influenzae* type b disease is recommended in these patients, regardless of travel plans.

- Dosing schedules for meningococcal ACWY conjugate vaccine in asplenic people differ for the 2 available vaccines. Menactra is indicated for both pediatric and adult populations aged ≥2 years, with 2 doses separated by ≥2 months. Menactra is licensed from 9 months through 55 years of age. For people with asplenia, the vaccine should be administered at 2 years through 55 years of age.

For children without asplenia aged 9 months through 2 years, Menactra should be administered at 0 months and 3 months, with an 8-week minimum interval between the doses. Booster recommendations vary by age. If younger than 7 years of age at the previous dose, a patient should receive a booster dose of Menactra or Menveo 3 years after the primary series; boosters should be repeated every 5 years thereafter. If 7 years old or older at the previous dose, a patient should receive an additional dose of Menactra or Menveo 5 years after the primary series; boosters should be repeated every 5 years thereafter.

- Menveo is recommended on a 2-dose schedule for asplenic adults and children aged ≥2 years and schedules of either 4 or 2 doses for children under the age of 2 depending on age at vaccine initiation; booster vaccinations should be repeated every 5 years if risk is ongoing.

- Serogroup B meningococcal (MenB) vaccine (Bexsero or Trumenba) is indicated for asplenic people ≥10 years of age. Travel itself is not an indication for vaccination with the serogroup B meningococcal vaccines. A booster interval has not been established.

- Asplenic people should receive a 1-time dose of *H. influenzae* type b (Hib) conjugate vaccine.

People with terminal complement deficiencies and those receiving eculizumab have increased susceptibility to meningococcal infections and should be immunized against meningococcal disease with both MenACWY and, if ≥10 years of age, MenB vaccine. The recommendations are the same as for patients with asplenia.

MEDICAL CONDITIONS AND TREATMENTS ASSOCIATED WITH SEVERE IMMUNE COMPROMISE

Severe Immune Compromise (Non-HIV)

Severely immunocompromised people include those who have active leukemia or lymphoma, generalized malignancy, aplastic anemia, graft-versus-host disease, or congenital immunodeficiency; others in this category include people who have received recent radiation therapy, those who have had solid-organ transplants and who are on active immunosuppression, and hematopoietic stem cell transplant recipients (within 2 years of transplantation or still taking immunosuppressive drugs). People who are severely immunocompromised should generally not be given live vaccines, and inactivated vaccines are less likely to be effective; these patients should consider postponing travel until their immune function improves. For people likely to travel in the future, usual travel-related vaccines may be considered before starting immunosuppressive therapies, if feasible.

People with chronic lymphocytic leukemia have poor humoral immunity, even early in the disease course, and rarely respond to vaccines. After hematopoietic stem cell transplant, complete revaccination with standard childhood vaccines should begin at 12 months, with the caveat that MMR and varicella vaccines should be administered 24 months after transplant and only if the recipient is assumed to be immunocompetent. Inactivated influenza vaccine should be administered beginning ≥6 months after hematopoietic stem cell transplant and annually thereafter; a dose of inactivated influenza vaccine can be given as early as 4 months after transplant if there is a community outbreak. A repeat dose of zoster vaccine may be administered after hematopoietic stem cell transplant if 24 months have passed since the transplant, the patient does not have graft-versus-host disease, and the patient is considered immunocompetent.

For solid-organ transplants, the risk of infection is highest in the first year after transplant, so travel to high-risk destinations should be postponed until after that time.

Doses of inactivated vaccines received while concurrently receiving potent immunosuppressive therapy (see below) or during the 2 weeks before starting therapy should not be counted toward completing the vaccination series or relied upon to induce adequate immune responses. At least 3 months after potent immunosuppressive therapy is discontinued, patients should be revaccinated with all indicated inactivated vaccines.

People taking any of the following categories of medications are considered severely immunocompromised:

- **High-dose corticosteroids**—Most clinicians consider a dose of either >2 mg/kg of body weight or ≥20 mg per day of prednisone or equivalent in people who weigh >10 kg, when administered for ≥2 weeks, as sufficiently immunosuppressive to raise concern about the safety of vaccination with live vaccines. Furthermore, the immune response to vaccines may be impaired. Clinicians should wait ≥1 month after discontinuation of high-dose systemic corticosteroid therapy before administering a live-virus vaccine.

- **Alkylating agents** (such as cyclophosphamide).

- **Antimetabolites** (such as azathioprine, 6-mercaptopurine, methotrexate). However, low-dose monotherapy (methotrexate ≤0.4 mg/kg/week, azathioprine ≤3 mg/kg/day, or 6-mercaptopurine ≤1.5 mg/kg/day) with these drugs does not preclude administration of zoster vaccine.

- **Transplant-related immunosuppressive drugs** (such as cyclosporine, tacrolimus, sirolimus, everolimus, azathioprine, and mycophenolate mofetil).

- **Cancer chemotherapeutic agents** are classified as severely immunosuppressive, as evidenced by increased rates of opportunistic infections and blunting of responses to certain vaccines among patient groups.[1]

- **Tumor necrosis factor (TNF) blockers** such as etanercept, adalimumab, certolizumab pegol, golimumab, and infliximab blunt the immune response to certain vaccines and certain chronic infections. When used alone or in combination regimens with other disease-modifying agents to treat rheumatoid

[1] Some of these agents are less immunosuppressive than others, such as tamoxifen or trastuzumab given to breast cancer patients, but clinical data to support safety with live vaccines are lacking.

8

disease, TNF blockers were associated with an impaired response to hepatitis A, influenza, and pneumococcal vaccines.

> Despite measurable impairment of the immune response, postvaccination antibody titers were often sufficient to provide protection for most people; therefore, treatment with TNF blockers does not preclude immunization against hepatitis A, influenza, and pneumococcal disease. When possible, all doses in the hepatitis A and pneumococcal series should be given before travel.

> The use of live vaccines is contraindicated according to the prescribing information for most of these therapies.

- **Other biologic agents** that are immunosuppressive or immunomodulatory may result in significant immunocompromise as outlined in Table 8-2. In particular, lymphocyte-depleting agents (thymoglobulin or alemtuzumab) and B cell–depleting agents (rituximab) are more significantly immunosuppressive. Consideration of the clinical context in which these were given is important, especially in hematologic malignancies.

DURATION OF IATROGENIC IMMUNE COMPROMISE

The period of time clinicians should wait after discontinuation of immunosuppressive therapies before administering a live vaccine is not consistent across all live vaccines. For cancer chemotherapy, radiation therapy, and highly immunosuppressive medications (exclusive of lymphocyte-depleting agents and organ transplant rejection prophylaxis), the waiting period is 3 months. For lymphocyte-depleting (alemtuzumab and rituximab) agents, the waiting period is ≥6 months, although many experts believe the waiting period should be ≥1 year. For steroid regimens considered immunosuppressive (see above), wait 1 month. Zoster vaccine is exceptional and may be given 1 month after any highly immunosuppressive agent, although many experts advocate waiting ≥1 year for anti–B cell antibodies and other lymphocyte-depleting agents. For agents not considered highly immunosuppressive (see Table 8-2), consultation with the prescribing clinician (and possibly a hospital pharmacist) is recommended to manage individual patients and estimate degree of immunosuppression. No basis exists for interpreting laboratory studies of immune parameters to evaluate vaccine safety or efficacy. Restarting immunosuppression after live vaccination has not been studied, but some experts would recommend waiting at least 1 month.

Severe Immune Compromise due to Symptomatic HIV/AIDS

Knowledge of the HIV-infected traveler's current CD4 T lymphocyte count is necessary for optimal pretravel consultation. HIV-infected people with CD4 cell counts <200/mm³, history of an AIDS-defining illness without immune reconstitution, or clinical manifestations of symptomatic HIV are considered to have severe immunosuppression (see Chapter 3, HIV Infection) and should not receive live viral or bacterial vaccines because of the risk that the vaccine could cause serious systemic disease.[2] The response to inactivated vaccines also will be suboptimal; thus, vaccine doses received by HIV-infected people while CD4 cell counts are <200/mm³ should be ignored, and the person should be revaccinated ≥3 months after immune reconstitution with antiretroviral therapy.

In newly diagnosed, treatment-naïve patients with CD4 cell counts <200/mm³, travel should be delayed pending reconstitution of CD4 cell counts with antiretroviral therapy and ideally complete suppression of detectable viral replication. Such postponement helps minimize risk of infection and avoid immune reconstitution illness during travel.

Household Contacts

The live vaccines MMR, varicella, and rotavirus vaccines should be administered to susceptible household contacts and other close contacts of immunocompromised patients when indicated. Zoster and yellow fever vaccine may

---

[2] For MMR vaccine, severe immunosuppression is defined as CD4 percentages <15% at any age in addition to CD4 count <200/mm³ for people aged >5 years. See www.cdc.gov/mmwr/preview/mmwrhtml/rr6204a1.htm.

Table 8-2. Immunosuppressive biologic agents that preclude use of live vaccines[1]

GENERIC NAME	TRADE NAME	MECHANISM/TARGET OF ACTION
Abatacept	Orencia	Anti-CD28/CTLA-4
Adalimumab	Humira	TNF blocker
Alemtuzumab	Campath	Anti-CD52
Anakinra	Kineret	IL-1 antagonist
Basiliximab	Simulect	IL-2R/CD25
Belatacept	Nulojix	CTLA-4
Bevacizumab	Avastin	VEGF
Certolizumab pegol	Cimzia	TNF blocker
Cetuximab	Erbitux	EGFR
Dasatinib	Sprycel	Bcr-Abl tyrosine kinase inhibitor
Dimethyl fumarate	Tecfidera	Activates the nuclear erythroid 2-related factor 2 transcriptional pathway
Etanercept	Enbrel	TNF blocker
Fingolimod	Gilenya	Aphingosine 1-phosphate receptor modulator
Glatiramer acetate	Copaxone	Immunomodulatory; target unknown
Golimumab	Simponi	TNF blocker
Ibritumomab tiuxetan	Zevalin	CD20 with radioisotope
Ibrutinib	Imbruvica	Tyrosine kinase inhibitor
Imatinib mesylate	Gleevec, STI 571	Signal transduction inhibitor/ protein-tyrosine kinase inhibitor
Infliximab	Remicade	TNF blocker
Interferon alfa	Pegasys, PegIntron	Block hepatitis C viral replication
Interferon beta-1a	Avonex, Rebif	Immunomodulatory; target unknown
Interferon beta-1b	Betaseron	Immunomodulatory; target unknown
Natalizumab	Tsabri	α4-integrin
Ofatumumab	Arzerra	CD20

(continued)

Table 8-2. Immunosuppressive biologic agents that preclude use of live vaccines[1] (continued)

GENERIC NAME	TRADE NAME	MECHANISM/TARGET OF ACTION
Panitumumab	Vectibix	EGFR
Lenalidomide	Revlimid	Immunomodulatory
Rilonacept	Arcalyst	IL-1
Rituximab	Rituxan	CD20
Secukinumab	Cosentyx	IL-17A
Sunitinib malate	Sutent	Multikinase inhibitor
Tocilizumab	Actemra	IL-6
Tofacitinib	Xeljanz	JAK kinase inhibitor
Trastuzumab	Herceptin	Human EGFR 2 (HER2)
Ustekinumab	Stelara	IL-12, IL-23
Vedolizumab	Entyvio	Binds integrin $\alpha_4\beta_7$

Abbreviations: CTLA, cytotoxic T-lymphocyte antigen; TNF, tumor necrosis factor; CD, cluster of differentiation; IL, interleukin; VEGF, vascular endothelial growth factor; EGFR, epidermal growth factor receptor.
[1] This table is based primarily on conservative expert opinion, given the lack of clinical data. Numerous agents are often given in combination with other agents (especially chemotherapy) and are immunosuppressive when given together. The list provides examples but is not inclusive of all biologic agents that suppress or modulate the immune system. Not all therapeutic monoclonal antibodies or other biologic agents result in immunosuppression; details of individual agents not listed here must be reviewed before determining whether live viral vaccines can be given. Some of these agents are less immunosuppressive than others; specifically, interferon used for hepatitis C and interferon and glatiramer acetate given to multiple sclerosis patients are immunomodulators, but clinical data to support safety with live vaccines are lacking.

8

be administered when indicated. Live attenuated influenza vaccine should not be administered. Smallpox vaccine (mostly for military personnel) is also transmissible to immunocompromised household and intimate contacts. Immunocompromised hosts should be cautious about contact with infants who have received the live rotavirus vaccine and children who may have received the oral polio vaccine; handwashing should be emphasized for prevention.

SPECIAL CONSIDERATIONS FOR IMMUNOCOMPROMISED TRAVELERS

Yellow Fever Vaccine

Unvaccinated travelers with severe immune compromise should be strongly discouraged from travel to destinations that present a true risk for yellow fever (YF). Significant immunosuppression is a contraindication to YF vaccination, as there is a risk of developing a serious adverse event, such as life-threatening yellow fever vaccine–associated viscerotropic disease.

If travel is unavoidable to an area where YF vaccine is recommended (see Maps 3-14 and 3-15) and the vaccine has not been given, these travelers should be informed of the risk of YF, carefully instructed in methods to avoid mosquito bites, and be provided with a vaccination medical waiver (see Chapter 3, Yellow Fever). Travelers should be warned that vaccination waiver documents might not be accepted by some countries and refusal of entry or quarantine is possible.

Patients with conditions that the Advisory Committee on Immunization Practices considers precautions (as opposed to contraindications) to administration of YF vaccine, such as asymptomatic HIV (see "Precautions" in Chapter 3, Yellow Fever), may be offered YF vaccine if travel to YF-endemic areas is unavoidable; recipients should be monitored closely for possible adverse effects. Studies show that higher CD4 cell counts and lower HIV viral loads seem to be the key determinants for development of protective neutralizing antibodies. Patients with undetectable viral loads respond well to YF vaccination regardless of CD4 count, although data are limited in those with CD4 counts <200 mm³. As vaccine response may be suboptimal, such vaccinees are candidates for serologic testing 1 month after vaccination. For information about serologic testing, contact your state health department or CDC's Division of Vector-Borne Diseases at 970-221-6400. Data from clinical and epidemiologic studies are insufficient at this time to evaluate the actual risk of severe adverse effects associated with YF vaccine among recipients with limited immune deficits. If international travel requirements, and not true exposure risk, are the only reasons to vaccinate a traveler with asymptomatic HIV infection or a limited immune deficit, the physician should provide a waiver letter.

Booster doses of YF vaccine are no longer recommended for most travelers, because a single dose of yellow fever vaccine provides long-lasting protection. However, additional doses of yellow fever vaccine are recommended for certain populations (such as hematopoietic stem cell transplant recipients and people with HIV) who might not have as robust or sustained immune response to yellow fever vaccine compared with other recipients. People who received a hematopoietic stem cell transplant after receiving a dose of yellow fever vaccine and who are sufficiently immunocompetent to be safely vaccinated should be revaccinated if travel puts them at risk of yellow fever. People who were infected with HIV when they received their last dose of yellow fever vaccine should receive a dose every 10 years if they continue to be at risk for yellow fever and if there are no precautions or contraindications based on their current CD4 cell counts. Recent data suggest that yellow fever vaccination before solid organ transplant, even long before transplant, generally provides protective antibody levels after transplant.

Response to Vaccination

Response to vaccination may be muted in severely immunocompromised hosts, and potential travelers should be informed about this. The decrease in response to vaccination is not particularly predictable based on the immunosuppressive regimen. Encouragingly, recent data in solid organ transplant recipients vaccinated before transplant suggests that a prolonged phase of protective antibody titers can exist after transplant. In general, serologic testing for response to most travel-related vaccines is not clinically recommended.

Malaria Chemoprophylaxis

Immunocompromised travelers to malaria-endemic areas should be prescribed drugs for malaria chemoprophylaxis and receive counseling about mosquito bite avoidance—the same as for immunocompetent travelers (see Chapter 3, Malaria). Special concerns for immunocompromised travelers include any of the following possibilities:

- Most current first-line regimens for HIV have few drug interactions, but some older maintenance regimens for HIV may interact with drugs used for malaria chemoprophylaxis. Notably, chloroquine, mefloquine, and primaquine may interact with older maintenance regimens for HIV. Potential interactions between a person's maintenance medication and antimalarial drugs should be considered and researched.

- The underlying medical condition or immunosuppressive regimen may predispose the immunocompromised traveler to more serious disease from malaria infection.

- A malaria infection and the drugs used to treat the malaria infection may exacerbate the underlying disease.

- The severity of malaria is increased in HIV-infected people; malaria infection increases HIV viral load and thus may exacerbate disease progression.

Commonly used integrase inhibitor (raltegravir, dolutegravir, elvitegravir)/NRTI combinations (brand names include Descovy-Tivicay, Truvada-Tivicay) have no known interactions with CDC-recommended chemoprophylactic drugs, although the cobicistat booster coformulated with elvitegravir (Stribild, Genvoya) may theoretically increase mefloquine levels. The rilpivirine, emtricitabine, TAF/TDF combinations (Odefsey and Complera) similarly have no interactions with antimalarials.

Of older drugs, efavirenz lowers serum levels of both atovaquone and proguanil, but there is no evidence for clinical failure of these agents when used concurrently. A number of older, now less commonly used drugs, especially protease inhibitors, have potential interactions. Extra care must be taken in researching potential interactions in people with HIV who are receiving highly active antiretroviral therapy.

For any patient on antiretroviral drugs, an interactive web-based resource for assessing possible drug interactions is found at the University of Liverpool website (www.hiv-druginteractions.org) and should always be consulted before adding a new drug to a patient on an anti-HIV regimen.

Antimalarial treatment regimens, including artemisinin derivatives, quinine/quinidine, lumefantrine (part of the artemether/lumefantrine combination, Coartem), and atovaquone and proguanil, may have potential interactions with many NNRTIs, PIs, and with the CCR5 receptor antagonist maraviroc. Expert advice should be sought when treating patients for malaria who are also on HAART.

In organ transplant recipients, malaria chemoprophylactic drugs may interact with calcineurin inhibitors and mTor inhibitors (tacrolimus, cyclosporine, sirolimus, everolimus). Mefloquine, chloroquine, primaquine, and doxycycline may cause elevated calcineurin inhibitor levels. Mefloquine, chloroquine, and calcineurin inhibitors may interact to prolong the QT interval. Some travel-related medications need to be dose-adjusted according to altered hepatic or renal function.

Some clinical case reports suggest that asplenic people may be at higher risk of acquisition and complications of malaria, so asplenic travelers to malarious areas should be counseled to adhere conscientiously to mosquito avoidance techniques and the malaria chemoprophylaxis regimen prescribed for them.

ENTERIC INFECTIONS

Many foodborne and waterborne infections, such as those caused by *Salmonella, Shigella, Campylobacter, Giardia, Listeria*, and *Cryptosporidium*, can be severe or become chronic in immunocompromised people. All travelers should follow safe food and beverage precautions; travelers' diarrhea can nonetheless occur despite strict adherence. Meticulous hand hygiene, including frequent and thorough handwashing with soap, is the best prevention against gastroenteritis. Hands should be washed after contact with public surfaces, after any contact with animals or their living areas, and before preparing food or eating. Because enteric pathogens, particularly *Shigella*, can also be acquired sexually, patients should be counseled about avoiding sex with people who have diarrhea; washing hands, genitals, and anus before and after sex; and using barriers during sex with partners who recently recovered from diarrhea. To reduce the risk of cryptosporidiosis, giardiasis, and other waterborne infections, patients should avoid swallowing water during swimming and other water-based recreational activities and should not swim in water that might be contaminated (with sewage or animal waste, for example). Travelers with liver disease should avoid direct exposure to salt water that may contain *Vibrio* spp., and all immunocompromised hosts should avoid raw seafood. Patients and clinicians should be aware of the augmented risk of infection or colonization with multidrug-resistant organisms during travel.

Antibiotic prophylaxis for a very limited duration may be considered for travelers with severe immune suppression. Selecting antimicrobials to be used for self-treatment of travelers' diarrhea, if indicated, may require special consideration of potential drug interactions among patients already taking medications for chronic medical conditions. Fluoroquinolones and rifaximin are active against several enteric bacterial pathogens and are not known to have significant interactions with HAART drugs. Macrolide antibiotics

8

> BOX 8-1.

BOX 8-1. Key patient education points for the immunocompromised traveler

- Develop plan in case of illness at destination (clinic or hospital that would be able to care for immunocompromised host; how to use embassy resources and medical evacuation insurance).
- Bring extra medications in case of travel delays; ensure medications are labeled.
- Avoid taking medications purchased at destination (drug interactions or substandard, spurious, falsely labeled, falsified, and counterfeit medical products).
- Augmented risk of infection with multidrug-resistant organisms during and after travel; highlight such travel to clinicians if ill afterwards.
- Vigilant use of sun protection given dramatically elevated rates of skin cancer in immunocompromised hosts, also high risk of photosensitivity from medications.
- Vigilant food and water precautions. Antibacterial hand wipes or an alcohol-based hand sanitizer containing at least 60% alcohol may be useful.
- Bring travel health kit.

may have significant interactions with HAART drugs and sometimes with organ transplant–related immunosuppression. Fluoroquinolones as well as azithromycin in combination with calcineurin inhibitors and mTor inhibitors may cause a prolonged QT interval.

Reducing Risk for Other Diseases

Geographically focal infections that pose an increased risk of severe outcome for immunocompromised people include visceral leishmaniasis and several fungal infections acquired by inhalation (such as *Talaromyces marneffei* [formerly *Penicillium marneffei*] infection in Southeast Asia and histoplasmosis and coccidioidomycosis in the Americas). Many developing areas have high rates of tuberculosis (TB), and

establishing the TB status of immunocompromised travelers going to such destinations may be helpful in the evaluation of any subsequent travel-associated illness. Depending on the traveler's degree of immune suppression, the baseline TB status may be assessed by obtaining a tuberculin skin test, *Mycobacterium tuberculosis* antigen-specific interferon-γ assay, or chest radiograph.

Patients with advanced HIV and transplant recipients frequently take either primary or secondary prophylaxis for one or more opportunistic infections (such as *Pneumocystis*, *Mycobacterium*, and *Toxoplasma* spp.). Adherence to all indicated prophylactic regimens should be confirmed before travel (see Chapter 3, HIV Infection).

Key points to stress with the immunocompromised traveler are summarized in Box 8-1.

BIBLIOGRAPHY

1. Agarwal N, Ollington K, Kaneshiro M, Frenck R, Melmed GY. Are immunosuppressive medications associated with decreased responses to routine immunizations? A systematic review. Vaccine. 2012 Feb 14;30(8):1413–24.

2. Barte H, Horvath TH, Rutherford GW. Yellow fever vaccine for patients with HIV infection. Cochrane Database Syst Rev. 2014 (1):Cd010929.

3. CDC. General recommendations on immunization—recommendations of the Advisory Committee on Immunization Practices (ACIP). MMWR Recomm Rep. 2011 Jan 28;60(2):1–64.

4. Dekkiche S, de Valliere S, D'Acremont V, Genton B. Travel-related health risks in moderately and severely immunocompromised patients: a case-control study. J Travel Med. 2016 Mar;23(3).

5. Farez MF, Correale J. Yellow fever vaccination and increased relapse rate in travelers with multiple sclerosis. Arch Neurol. 2011 Oct;68(10): 1267–71.

6. Garcia Garrido HM, Wieten RW, Grobusch MP, Goorhuis A. Response to hepatitis A vaccination in immunocompromised travelers. J Infect Dis. 2015 Aug 1;212(3):378–85.

7. Kotton CN, Hibberd PL. Travel medicine and transplant tourism in solid organ transplantation. Am J Transplant. 2013 Mar;13 Suppl 4:337–47.

8. Loebermann M, Winkelmann A, Hartung HP, Hengel H, Reisinger EC, Zettl UK. Vaccination against infection in patients with multiple sclerosis. Nat Rev Neurol. 2011;8(3):143–51.

9. Luks AM, Swenson ER. Evaluating the risks of high altitude travel in chronic liver disease patients. High Alt Med Biol. 2015 Jun;16(2):80–8.

10. Masur H, Brooks JT, Benson CA, Holmes KK, Pau AK, Kaplan JE. Prevention and treatment of opportunistic infections in HIV-infected adults and adolescents: updated guidelines from the Centers for Disease Control and Prevention, National Institutes of Health, and HIV Medicine Association of the Infectious Diseases Society of America. Clin Infect Dis. 2014 May;58(9):1308–11.

11. Pacanowski J, Lacombe K, Campa P, Dabrowska M, Poveda JD, Meynard JL, et al. Plasma HIV-RNA is the key determinant of long-term antibody persistence after yellow fever immunization in a cohort of 364 HIV-infected patients. J Acquir Immune Defic Syndr. 2012 Apr 1;59(4):360–7.

12. Perry RT, Plowe CV, Koumare B, Bougoudogo F, Kotloff KL, Losonsky GA, et al. A single dose of live oral cholera vaccine CVD 103-HgR is safe and immunogenic in HIV-infected and HIV-noninfected adults in Mali. Bull World Health Organ. 1998;76(1):63–71.

13. Rubin LG, Levin MJ, Ljungman P, Davies EG, Avery R, Tomblyn M, et al. 2013 IDSA clinical practice guideline for vaccination of the immunocompromised host. Clin Infect Dis. 2014 Feb;58(3):309–18.

14. Schwartz BS, Rosen J, Han PV, Hynes NA, Hagmann SH, Rao SR, et al. Immunocompromised travelers: demographic characteristics, travel destinations, and pretravel health care from the U.S. Global TravEpiNet Consortium. Am J Trop Med Hyg. 2015 Nov;93(5):1110–6.

15. Visser LG. TNF-α antagonists and immunization. Curr Infect Dis Rep. 2011 Jun;13(3):243–7.

16. Wieten RW, Goorhuis A, Jonker EF, de Bree GJ, de Visser AW, van Genderen PJ, et al. 17D yellow fever vaccine elicits comparable long-term immune responses in healthy individuals and immune-compromised patients. J Infect. 2016 Jun;72(6):713–22.

17. Wyplosz B, Burdet C, Francois H, Durrbach A, Duclos-Vallee JC, Mamzer-Bruneel MF, et al. Persistence of yellow fever vaccine-induced antibodies after solid organ transplantation. Am J Transplant. 2013 Sep;13(9):2458–61.

TRAVELERS WITH CHRONIC ILLNESSES

Deborah Nicolls Barbeau

GENERAL TRAVEL PREPARATION: PRACTICAL CONSIDERATIONS

Although traveling abroad can be relaxing and rewarding, the physical demands of travel can be stressful, particularly for travelers with underlying chronic illnesses. With adequate preparation, however, such travelers can have safe and enjoyable trips. General recommendations for advising patients with chronic illnesses include:

- Ensure that any chronic illnesses are well controlled. Patients with an underlying illness should see their health care providers to ensure that the management of their illness is optimized.

- Encourage patients to seek pretravel consultation ≥4–6 weeks before departure to ensure adequate time to respond to immunizations and, in some circumstances, to try medications before travel (see the Immunocompromised Travelers section earlier in this chapter).

- Advise patients to consider a destination where they have access to care for their condition.

- Ask about previous health-related issues encountered during travel, such as complications during air travel.

- Advise the traveler about packing a health kit (see Chapter 2, Travel Health Kits).

- Advise travelers to pack medications and medical supplies (such as pouching for ostomies) in their original containers in carry-on luggage and to carry a copy of their prescriptions. Ensure the traveler has sufficient quantities of medications for the entire trip, plus extra in case of unexpected delays. Since medications should be taken based on elapsed time and not time of day, travelers may need guidance on scheduling when to take medications during and after crossing time zones.

- Advise travelers to check with the US embassy or consulate to clarify medication restrictions in the destination country. Some countries do not allow visitors to bring certain medications into the country, especially narcotics and psychotropic medications.

- Educate travelers regarding drug interactions (see Chapter 2, Interactions among Travel Vaccines & Drugs). Medications (such as warfarin) used to treat chronic medical illnesses may interact with medications prescribed for self-treatment of travelers' diarrhea or malaria chemoprophylaxis. Discuss all medications used, either daily or on an as-needed basis.

- Provide a clinician's letter. The letter should be on office letterhead stationery and should outline existing medical conditions, medications prescribed (including generic names), and any equipment required to manage the condition.

- Suggest supplemental insurance. Three types of insurance policies can be considered: 1) trip cancellation in the event of illness; 2) supplemental insurance so that money paid for health care abroad may be reimbursed, since most medical insurance policies do not cover health care in other countries; and 3) medical evacuation insurance (see Chapter 2, Travel Insurance, Travel Health Insurance, & Medical Evacuation Insurance). Travelers may need extra help in finding supplemental insurance, as some plans will not cover costs for preexisting conditions.

- Encourage travelers with underlying medical conditions to consider choosing a medical assistance company that allows them to store their medical history so it can be accessed worldwide (see Chapter 2, Obtaining Health Care Abroad).

- Help travelers devise a health plan. This plan should give instructions for managing minor problems or exacerbations of underlying illnesses and should include information about medical facilities available in the destination country (see Chapter 2, Obtaining Health Care Abroad).

- Advise travelers to wear a medical alert bracelet or carry medical information on his or her person (various brands of jewelry or tags, even electronic, are available).

- Advise travelers to stay hydrated, wear loose-fitting clothing, and walk and stretch at regular intervals during long-distance travel (see Chapter 2, Deep Vein Thrombosis & Pulmonary Embolism).

- Consider advising the traveler to use a mobile application to track certain chronic illnesses, such as diabetes, while traveling.

SPECIFIC CHRONIC ILLNESSES

Issues related to specific chronic medical illnesses are addressed in Table 8-3. These recommendations should be used in conjunction with the other recommendations given throughout this book. Below is a noninclusive list of additional resources for information:

- American Association of Kidney Patients (www.aakp.org)

- American Diabetes Association (www.diabetes.org)

- American Heart Association (www.heart.org)

- American Lung Association (www.lung.org)

- American Society of Clinical Oncology, Cancer.Net (www.cancer.net)

- American Thoracic Society (www.thoracic.org)

- Anticoagulation Forum (www.acforum.org)

- British Thoracic Society (www.brit-thoracic.org.uk)

Table 8-3. Special considerations for travelers with chronic medical illnesses

CONDITION	ABSOLUTE AND RELATIVE CONTRAINDICATIONS TO AIRLINE TRAVEL	PRETRAVEL CONSIDERATIONS	IMMUNIZATION CONSIDERATIONS	MISCELLANEOUS
Cancer	Severe anemia Cerebral edema due to intracranial tumor ≤6 weeks since cranial surgery Cardiovascular, pulmonary, or gastrointestinal complications referred to below	Emphasize food and water precautions Plan for self-management of dehydration DVT precautions Supplemental oxygen Wear loose-fitting clothing to prevent worsening of lymphedema	Immunosuppressive medications may alter response to immunizations Live attenuated vaccines may be contraindicated Revaccination may be necessary following cancer treatment	Check for medication restrictions in the destination country, especially if controlled medications are required for pain management See the Immunocompromised Travelers section later in this chapter
Cardiovascular diseases	Following acute coronary syndrome: • those at very low risk and within 3 days after event • medium risk and within 10 days after event • high risk or awaiting further intervention or treatment—should defer air travel until disease is stable Unstable angina CHF, severe, decompensated Uncontrolled hypertension CABG within 14 days CVA within 2 weeks Elective percutaneous coronary intervention within 2 days Uncontrolled arrhythmia Eisenmenger syndrome Severe symptomatic valvular heart disease	Supplemental oxygen Plan for self-management of dehydration and volume overload; may include adjusting medications Bring copy of recent EKG Bring pacemaker or AICD card DVT precautions	Influenza Pneumococcal Hepatitis B	Have sublingual nitroglycerine available in carry-on bag Mefloquine not recommended for people with cardiac conduction abnormalities, particularly for those with ventricular arrhythmias Self-monitoring and management of INR should be tailored to the individual patient by the anticoagulant primary provider

8

(continued)

Table 8-3. Special considerations for travelers with chronic medical illnesses (continued)

CONDITION	ABSOLUTE AND RELATIVE CONTRAINDICATIONS TO AIRLINE TRAVEL	PRETRAVEL CONSIDERATIONS	IMMUNIZATION CONSIDERATIONS	MISCELLANEOUS
Pulmonary diseases	Severe, labile asthma Recent hospitalization for acute respiratory illness Bullous lung disease Active lower respiratory infection Pneumothorax within 2–3 weeks Pleural effusion within 14 days High supplemental oxygen requirements at baseline Major chest surgery within 10–14 days	Supplemental oxygen Discuss with airline need for other equipment on plane (such as nebulizer) Plan for self-management of exacerbations (including COPD, asthma) DVT precautions	Influenza Pneumococcal Hepatitis B	Consider carrying a short course of antibiotics and steroids for exacerbations Consider advising an inhaler be available in carry-on bag, even if not routinely used
Gastrointestinal diseases	Surgery, including laparoscopic, within 10–14 days Gastrointestinal bleed within 24 hours Colonoscopy within 24 hours Partial bowel obstruction Liver failure (especially cirrhosis or heavy alcohol use)	Emphasize food and water precautions Consider prescribing prophylactic antibiotic for TD Recommend avoiding undercooked seafood, if cirrhosis or heavy alcohol use (Vibrio vulnificus)	Influenza Pneumococcal Hepatitis A Hepatitis B	May experience increased colostomy output during air travel H₂ blockers and PPIs increase susceptibility to TD Use mefloquine with caution in any chronic liver disease For YF vaccine, see the Immunocompromised Travelers section later in this chapter
Renal failure and chronic renal insufficiency	None	Emphasize food and water precautions Plan for self-management of dehydration, which can worsen renal function Arrange dialysis abroad, if needed Adjust medications for CrCl	Influenza Pneumococcal Hepatitis B	Know HIV, hepatitis C, and hepatitis B status Atovaquone-proguanil contraindicated when CrCl <30 mL/min AAKP and Global Dialysis websites can help with finding dialysis centers; check for accreditation For YF vaccine, see the Immunocompromised Travelers section later in this chapter

8

Condition		Management	Vaccines/Immunizations	Travel considerations
Diabetes mellitus	None	Plan for self-management of dehydration, diabetic foot, and pressure sores Insulin adjustments Should check FSBG at 4- to 6-hour intervals during air travel Discuss changes in insulin regimen or oral agent with diabetes specialist Provide physician's letter stating need for all equipment, including syringes, glucose meter, and supplies	Influenza Pneumococcal Hepatitis B	Keep insulin and all glucose meter supplies in carry-on bag Bring food and supplies needed to manage hypoglycemia during travel Check feet daily for pressure sores For YF vaccine, see the Immunocompromised Travelers section later in this chapter
Severe allergic reactions	None	Plan for managing allergic reactions while traveling and consider bringing a short course of steroids for possible allergic reactions Should carry injectable epinephrine and antihistamines (H_1 and H_2 blockers)—always have on person		Many airlines already have policies in place for dealing with peanut allergies Make sure to carry injectable epinephrine in case of a severe reaction while in flight
Autoimmune and rheumatologic diseases	None	Should have a baseline TST or IGRA before starting TNF blockers	Immunosuppressive medications and TNF blockers may alter response to immunizations Live attenuated vaccines may be contraindicated	Particular emphasis should be placed on food and water precautions and hand hygiene

Abbreviations: DVT, deep vein thrombosis; CHF, congestive heart failure; CABG, coronary artery bypass graft; CVA, cerebrovascular accident; EKG, electrocardiogram; AICD, automatic implantable cardioverter defibrillators; INR, international normalized ratio; COPD, chronic obstructive pulmonary disease; TD, travelers' diarrhea; PPIs, proton-pump inhibitors; YF, yellow fever; CrCl, creatinine clearance; AAKP, American Association of Kidney Patients; FSBG, fingerstick blood glucose; TST, tuberculin skin test; IGRA, interferon-γ release assay; TNF, tumor necrosis factor.

8

- Crohn's and Colitis Foundation of America (www.ccfa.org)

- Global Dialysis (www.globaldialysis.com)

- International Narcotics Control Board (www.incb.org)

- International Self-Monitoring Association of Oral Anticoagulated Patients (www.ismaap.org)

- National Multiple Sclerosis Society (www.nationalmssociety.org)

- Transportation Security Administration (www.tsa.gov)

- Department of State (www.state.gov)

Travelers may also want to investigate international health care accreditation agencies for centers that have been awarded recognition for high standards and good patient safety records. If travelers or their health care providers have concerns about fitness for air travel or the need to obtain a medical certificate before travel, the medical unit affiliated with the specific airline is a valuable source for information. Remember to notify the airline in advance if oxygen or other equipment is needed on the plane. The TSA Cares Helpline (toll-free at 855-787-2227) can also provide information on how to prepare for the airport security screening process with respect to a particular disability or medical condition.

BIBLIOGRAPHY

1. Aerospace Medical Association. Medical Guidelines for Airline Travel. 2nd ed. Alexandria, VA: Aerospace Medical Association; 2003 [cited 2016 Sep. 27]. Available from: http://www.asma.org/asma/media/asma/Travel-Publications/medguid.pdf.

2. Exemption from import/export requirements for personal medical use. 21 CFR Part 1301; 2004 [cited 2016 Sep. 27]; Available from: http://www.deadiversion.usdoj.gov/fed_regs/rules/2004/fr0914.htm.

3. IATA. Medical Manual. 2015 [cited 2016 Sept 27]; 7th:[Available from: www.iata.org/publications/Pages/medical-manual.aspx.

4. Josephs LK, Coker RK, Thomas M, British Thoracic Society Air Travel Working Group. Managing patients with stable respiratory disease planning air travel: a primary care summary of the British Thoracic Society recommendations. Prim Care Respir J. 2013 Jun;22(2):234–8.

5. McCarthy AE, Burchard GD. The travelers with pre-existing disease. In: Keystone JS, Freedman DO, Kozarsky PE, Connor BA, Nothdurft HD, editors. Travel Medicine. 3rd ed. Philadelphia: Saunders Elsevier; 2013. pp. 257–63.

6. Perdue C, Noble S. Foreign travel for advanced cancer patients: a guide for healthcare professionals. Postgrad Med J. 2007 Jul;83(981):437–44.

7. Pinsker JE, Becker E, Mahnke CB, Ching M, Larson NS, Roy D. Extensive clinical experience: a simple guide to basal insulin adjustments for long-distance travel. J Diabetes Metab Disord. 2013;12(1):59.

8. Ringwald J, Strobel J, Eckstein R. Travel and oral anticoagulation. J Travel Med. 2009 Jul-Aug;16(4):276–83.

9. Smith D, Toff W, Joy M, Dowdall N, Johnston R, Clark L, et al. Fitness to fly for passengers with cardiovascular disease. Heart. 2010 Aug;96 Suppl 2:ii1–16.

PREGNANT TRAVELERS

Diane F. Morof, I. Dale Carroll

During pregnancy, women experience physiologic changes that require special consideration during travel. With careful preparation, however, most pregnant women are able to travel safely.

PRETRAVEL EVALUATION

The pretravel evaluation of a pregnant traveler (Box 8-2) should begin with a careful medical and obstetric history, with particular attention to gestational age and evaluation for high-risk conditions.

8

BOX 8-2. **Pretravel consultation checklist for pregnant travelers**

- Check for immunity to infectious diseases, for example, hepatitis A and B, rubella, varicella, measles, pertussis; update immunizations as needed
- Policies and necessary paperwork
  > Supplemental travel insurance, travel health insurance, and medical evacuation insurance (research specific coverage information and limitations for pregnancy-related health issues)

  > Check airline and cruise line policies for pregnant women
  > Letter confirming due date and fitness to travel
  > Copy of medical records
- Preparing for obstetric care at destination
  > Check medical insurance coverage
  > Arrange for obstetric care at destination, as needed
- Review signs and symptoms requiring immediate care
  > Pelvic or abdominal pain
  > Bleeding
  > Rupture of membranes

  > Contractions or preterm labor
  > Symptoms of preeclampsia (unusual swelling, severe headaches, nausea and vomiting, vision changes)
  > Vomiting, diarrhea, dehydration
  > Symptoms of potential deep vein thrombosis or pulmonary embolism (unusual swelling of leg with pain in calf or thigh, unusual shortness of breath)

A visit with an obstetrician should be a part of the pretravel assessment, to ensure routine prenatal care as well as identify any potential problems. The traveler should be provided with a copy of her prenatal records and physician's contact information. Checking for immunity to various infectious diseases may obviate the need for some vaccines.

A review of the pregnant woman's travel itinerary, including destinations, accommodations, and activities, should guide pretravel health advice. Preparation includes educating the pregnant woman regarding avoidance of travel-associated risks, the management of minor pregnancy discomforts, and recognition of more serious complications. Bleeding, severe pelvic or abdominal pain, contractions or premature labor, premature rupture of the membranes, symptoms of preeclampsia (unusual swelling, severe headaches, nausea and vomiting, vision changes), severe vomiting, diarrhea, dehydration, and symptoms of potential deep vein thrombosis (unusual swelling of leg with pain in calf or thigh) or pulmonary embolism (unusual shortness of breath) require urgent medical attention.

Pregnant travelers should pack a health kit that includes items such as prescription medications, hemorrhoid cream, antiemetic drugs, antacids, prenatal vitamins, medication for vaginitis or yeast infection, and support hose, in addition to the items recommended for all travelers (see Chapter 2, Travel Health Kits). Pregnant travelers should consider packing a blood pressure monitor if travel may limit access to a health center with blood pressure monitoring available.

CONTRAINDICATIONS FOR TRAVEL DURING PREGNANCY

Although travel is rarely contraindicated during a normal pregnancy, complicated pregnancies require extra consideration and may warrant a recommendation that travel be delayed (Box 8-3). Pregnant travelers should be advised that the risk of obstetric complications is highest in the first and third trimesters.

PLANNING FOR EMERGENCY CARE

Obstetric emergencies often are sudden and life-threatening. Travel to areas where obstetric care may be less than the standard at home is inadvisable. For a woman in the third trimester of pregnancy, it is advisable to identify a medical facility at her destination that could manage complications of pregnancy, delivery, a caesarean section,

BOX 8-3. Contraindications to travel during pregnancy

- **Absolute Contraindications**
  - > Abruptio placentae
  - > Active labor
  - > Incompetent cervix
  - > Premature labor
  - > Premature rupture of membranes
  - > Suspected ectopic pregnancy
  - > Threatened abortion, vaginal bleeding
  - > Toxemia, past or present

- **Relative Contraindications**
  - > Abnormal presentation
  - > Fetal growth restriction
  - > History of infertility
  - > History of miscarriage or ectopic pregnancy
  - > Maternal age <15 or >35 years
  - > Multiple gestation
  - > Placenta previa or other placental abnormality

and neonatal problems. Some complications may be managed so the mother could travel to a facility where she could receive advanced obstetric care, but some conditions are contraindications for any travel (Box 8-3). In such cases, it may be preferable to bring help to the patient rather than transport the patient.

Many health insurance policies do not cover complications of pregnancy or the newborn overseas. Supplemental travel health insurance should be strongly considered to cover pregnancy-related problems and care of the neonate, as needed. Evacuation insurance that includes coverage of pregnancy-related complications is also highly encouraged.

TRANSPORTATION CONSIDERATIONS

Pregnant women should be advised to wear seat belts, when available, on all forms of transport, including airplanes, cars, and buses. A diagonal shoulder strap with a lap belt provides the best protection. The shoulder belt should be worn between the breasts with the lap belt low across the upper thighs. When only a lap belt is available, it should be worn low, between the abdomen and the pelvis.

Air Travel

Most commercial airlines allow pregnant travelers to fly until 36 weeks' gestation. Some limit international travel earlier in pregnancy, and some require documentation of gestational age. Pregnant travelers should check with the airline for specific requirements or guidance. Cabins of most commercial jetliners are pressurized to 6,000–8,000 ft (1,829–2,438 m) above sea level; the lower oxygen tension should not cause fetal problems in a normal pregnancy, but women with preexisting cardiovascular problems, sickle cell disease, or severe anemia (hemoglobin <8.0 g/dL) may experience the effects of low arterial oxygen saturation. Risks of air travel include potential exposure to communicable diseases, immobility, and the common discomforts of flying. Abdominal distention and pedal edema frequently occur. The pregnant traveler may benefit from an upgrade in airline seating and should seek convenient and practical accommodations (such as close proximity to the toilet) and aisle seating so she can move about frequently. Loose clothing and comfortable shoes are recommended.

Some experts report that the risk of deep vein thrombosis in pregnancy is 5–10 times higher than for nonpregnant women. Preventive measures include frequent stretching, walking and isometric leg exercises, and wearing graduated compression stockings.

Cosmic radiation during air travel poses little threat, but may be a consideration for pregnant travelers who are frequent fliers (such as air crew). Older airport security machines are magnetometers and are not harmful to the fetus. Newer security machines use backscatter x-ray scanners, which emit low levels of radiation. Most experts agree that the risk of complications from radiation exposure from these scanners is extremely low.

Cruise Ship Travel

Most cruise lines restrict travel beyond 28 weeks of pregnancy, and some as early as 24 weeks.

Pregnant travelers may be required to carry a physician's note stating that they are fit to travel and including the estimated date of delivery. Pregnant women should check with the cruise line for specific requirements or guidance. The pregnant traveler planning a cruise should be advised regarding motion sickness, gastrointestinal and respiratory infections, and the risk of falls on a moving vessel.

ENVIRONMENTAL CONSIDERATIONS

Air pollution may cause more health problems during pregnancy, as ciliary clearance of the bronchial tree is slowed and mucus more abundant. Body temperature regulation is not as efficient during pregnancy, and temperature extremes can cause more stress on the gravid woman. In addition, an increase in core temperature, such as with heat prostration or heat stroke, may harm the fetus. The vasodilatory effect of a hot environment might also cause fainting. For these reasons, accommodation should be sought in air-conditioned quarters and activities restricted in hot environments.

Pregnant women should avoid activities at high altitude unless trained for and accustomed to such activities; women unaccustomed to high altitudes may experience exaggerated breathlessness and palpitations. The common symptoms of acute mountain sickness (insomnia, headache, and nausea) are frequently also associated with pregnancy, and it may be difficult to distinguish the cause of the symptoms. Most experts recommend a slower ascent with adequate time for acclimatization. No studies or case reports show harm to a fetus if the mother travels briefly to high altitudes during pregnancy. However, it may be prudent to recommend that pregnant women not stay at sleeping altitudes >12,000 ft (3,658 m), if possible. Probably the largest concern regarding high-altitude travel in pregnancy is that many such destinations are inaccessible and far from medical care (see Chapter 2, Altitude Illness).

ACTIVITIES

Pregnant travelers should be discouraged from undertaking unaccustomed vigorous activity. Swimming and snorkeling during pregnancy are generally safe, but waterskiing has resulted in falls that inject water into the birth canal. Most experts advise against scuba diving for pregnant women because of risk of fetal gas embolism during decompression. Riding bicycles, motorcycles, or animals presents risk of trauma to the abdomen.

INFECTIOUS DISEASES

Respiratory and urinary infections and vaginitis are more likely to occur and to be more severe in pregnancy. Pregnant women who develop travelers' diarrhea or other gastrointestinal infections may be more vulnerable to dehydration than are nonpregnant travelers. Strict hand hygiene and food and water precautions should be stressed (see Chapter 2, Food & Water Precautions). Bottled or boiled water is preferable to chemically treated or filtered water. Iodine-containing compounds should not be used to purify water for pregnant women because of potential effects on the fetal thyroid (see Chapter 2, Water Disinfection for Travelers). The treatment of choice for travelers' diarrhea is prompt and vigorous oral hydration; however, azithromycin may be given to pregnant women if clinically indicated. Use of bismuth subsalicylate is contraindicated.

Hepatitis A and E are both spread by the fecal-oral route. Hepatitis A has been reported to increase the risk of placental abruption and premature delivery. Hepatitis E is more likely to cause severe disease during pregnancy and may result in a case-fatality ratio of 15%–30%; when acquired during the third trimester, it is also associated with fetal complications and fetal death. Some foodborne illnesses of particular concern during pregnancy include toxoplasmosis and listeriosis; the risk during pregnancy is that the infection will cross the placenta and cause spontaneous abortion, stillbirth, or congenital or neonatal infection. The pregnant traveler should be warned, therefore, to avoid unpasteurized cheeses and undercooked meat products. Risk of fetal infection increases with gestational age, but severity of infection is decreased. Parasitic diseases are less common but may cause concern, particularly in women who are visiting friends and relatives in developing areas. In general, intestinal helminths rarely cause enough illness to warrant treatment during pregnancy. Most, in fact, can safely be addressed

8

with symptomatic treatment until the pregnancy is over. On the other hand, protozoan intestinal infections, such as *Giardia, Entamoeba histolytica*, and *Cryptosporidium*, often do require treatment. These parasites may cause acute gastroenteritis, severe dehydration, chronic malabsorption resulting in fetal growth restriction, and in the case of *E. histolytica*, invasive disease, including amebic liver abscess and colitis. Pregnant women should avoid swimming or wading in freshwater lakes, streams, and rivers that may harbor schistosomes.

Pregnant women should avoid mosquito bites when traveling in areas where vectorborne diseases are endemic. Preventive measures include use of bed nets, insect repellents, and protective clothing (see Chapter 2, Protection against Mosquitoes, Ticks, & Other Arthropods). A recent concern for pregnant women is Zika virus infection. Zika virus is spread primarily through the bite of an infected *Aedes* mosquito (*Ae. aegypti* and *Ae. albopictus*). The illness associated with Zika is usually mild, but in pregnant women, Zika virus infection can cause fetal microcephaly and other congenital abnormalities. Because of the risk of birth defects, CDC recommends pregnant women not travel to areas where Zika is present and take precautions to avoid sexual transmission of the virus. If travel cannot be avoided, pregnant women should strictly follow steps to prevent mosquito bites. Additional information, including the most current list of countries and territories where Zika virus is a risk, is available at www.cdc.gov/travel. Guidance for pregnant women can be found at the CDC Zika website (www.cdc.gov/zika/pregnancy/index.html).

MEDICATIONS

Various systems are used to classify drugs in regard to their safety in pregnancy. In most cases, it is preferable to refer to specific data regarding the effects of a given drug during pregnancy rather than simply to depend on a classification.

Analgesics that can be used during pregnancy include acetaminophen and some narcotics. Aspirin may increase the incidence of abruption, and other anti-inflammatory agents could cause premature closure of the ductus arteriosus. Constipation may require a mild bulk laxative. Several simple remedies are often effective in relieving the symptoms of morning sickness.

Nonprescription remedies include ginger, which is available as a powder that can be mixed with food or drinks such as tea. It is also available in candy, such as lollipops. Similarly, pyridoxine (vitamin B6) is effective in reducing symptoms of morning sickness and is available in tablet form, as well as lozenges and lollipops. Antihistamines, such as meclizine and dimenhydrinate, are often used in pregnancy for morning sickness and motion sickness and appear to have a good safety record.

VACCINES

In the best possible scenario, a woman should be up-to-date on routine vaccinations before she becomes pregnant. The most effective way of protecting the infant against many diseases is to immunize the mother. Tetanus, diphtheria, and pertussis (Tdap) vaccine should be given **during each pregnancy** irrespective of the woman's history of receiving Tdap. To maximize maternal antibody response and passive antibody transfer to the infant, **optimal timing for Tdap administration is between 27 and 36 weeks of gestation,** although it may be given at any time during pregnancy. Annual influenza vaccine (inactivated) is recommended during any trimester for all women who are or will be pregnant during influenza season. For travelers, vaccination is recommended ≥2 weeks before departure if vaccine is available. Certain vaccines, including meningococcal and hepatitis A and B vaccines that are considered safe during pregnancy, may be indicated based on risk. No adverse effects of inactivated polio vaccine (IPV) have been documented among pregnant women or their fetuses; however, vaccination of pregnant women should be avoided because of theoretical concerns. IPV can be administered in accordance with the recommended schedules for adults if a pregnant woman is at increased risk for infection and requires immediate protection against polio. Rabies postexposure prophylaxis with rabies immune globulin and vaccine should be administered after any moderate- or high-risk exposure to rabies; preexposure vaccine may be considered for travelers when the risk of exposure is substantial.

Most live-virus vaccines, including measles-mumps-rubella vaccine, varicella vaccine, and live attenuated influenza vaccine, are contraindicated during pregnancy; the exception is yellow fever vaccine, for which pregnancy is considered a precaution by the Advisory Committee on Immunization Practices (ACIP). If travel is unavoidable, and the risks for yellow fever virus exposure are felt to outweigh the risks of vaccination, a pregnant woman should be vaccinated. If the risks for vaccination are felt to outweigh the risks for yellow fever virus exposure, pregnant women should be issued a medical waiver to fulfill health regulations. Because pregnancy might affect immunologic function, serologic testing to document an immune response to yellow fever vaccine should be considered. Postexposure prophylaxis of a nonimmune pregnant woman exposed to measles or varicella may be provided by administering immune globulin (IG) within 6 days for measles or varicella-zoster IG within 10 days for varicella. Women planning to become pregnant should be advised to wait 4 weeks after receipt of a live-virus vaccine before conceiving. For certain travel-related vaccines, including Japanese encephalitis vaccine and typhoid vaccine, data are insufficient for a specific recommendation for use in pregnant women. A summary of current ACIP guidelines for vaccinating pregnant women is available at www.cdc.gov/vaccines/pregnancy/hcp/guidelines.html.

MALARIA CHEMOPROPHYLAXIS

Malaria may be much more serious in pregnant than in nonpregnant women and is associated with high risks of illness and death for both mother and child. Malaria in pregnancy may be characterized by heavy parasitemia, severe anemia, and sometimes profound hypoglycemia, and may be complicated by cerebral malaria and acute respiratory distress syndrome. Placental sequestration of parasites may result in fetal loss due to abruption, premature labor, or miscarriage. An infant born to an infected mother is apt to be of low birth weight, and, although rare, congenital malaria is a concern.

Because no prophylactic regimen provides complete protection, pregnant women should avoid or delay travel to malaria-endemic areas. However, if travel is unavoidable, pregnant women should take precautions to avoid mosquito bites, and use of an effective prophylactic regimen is essential.

Chloroquine and mefloquine are the drugs of choice for pregnant women for destinations with chloroquine-sensitive and chloroquine-resistant malaria, respectively. Doxycycline is contraindicated because of teratogenic effects on the fetus after the fourth month of pregnancy. Primaquine is contraindicated in pregnancy because the infant cannot be tested for G6PD deficiency, putting the infant at risk for hemolytic anemia. Atovaquone-proguanil is not recommended because of lack of available safety data. A list of the available antimalarial drugs and their uses and contraindications during pregnancy can be found in Table 3-10 and in Chapter 3, Malaria.

8

BIBLIOGRAPHY

1. ACOG Committee on Obstetric Practice. ACOG Committee Opinion No. 443: Air travel during pregnancy. Obstet Gynecol. 2009 Oct;114(4):954–5.

2. Carroll ID, Williams DC. Pre-travel vaccination and medical prophylaxis in the pregnant traveler. Travel Med Infect Dis. 2008 Sep;6(5):259–75.

3. CDC. Guidelines for vaccinating pregnant women. Atlanta: CDC; 2014 [cited 2016 Sep 27]; Available from: http://www.cdc.gov/vaccines/pubs/preg-guide.html.

4. Dotters-Katz S, Kuller J, Heine RP. Parasitic infections in pregnancy. Obstet Gynecol Surv. 2011 Aug;66(8):515–25.

5. Hezelgrave NL, Whitty CJ, Shennan AH, Chappell LC. Advising on travel during pregnancy. BMJ. 2011;342:d2506.

6. Irvine MH, Einarson A, Bozzo P. Prophylactic use of antimalarials during pregnancy. Can Fam Physician. 2011 Nov;57(11):1279–81.

7. Magann EF, Chauhan SP, Dahlke JD, McKelvey SS, Watson EM, Morrison JC. Air travel and pregnancy outcomes: a review of pregnancy regulations and outcomes for passengers, flight attendants, and aviators. Obstet Gynecol Surv. 2010 Jun;65(6):396–402.

8. Mehta P, Smith-Bindman R. Airport full-body screening: what is the risk? Arch Intern Med. 2011 Jun 27;171(12):1112–5.

9. Rasmussen SA, Jamieson DJ, Honein MA, Petersen LR. Zika virus and birth defects—reviewing the evidence for causality. N Engl J Med. 2016 May 19;374(20):1981–7.

10. Rasmussen SA, Watson AK, Kennedy ED, Broder KR, Jamieson DJ. Vaccines and pregnancy: past, present, and future. Semin Fetal Neonatal Med. 2014 Jun;19(3):161–9.

11. Roggelin L, Cramer JP. Malaria prevention in the pregnant traveller: a review. Travel Med Infect Dis. 2014 May-Jun;12(3):229–36.

TRAVELERS WITH DISABILITIES

Kira A. Barbre

OVERVIEW

According to the Americans with Disabilities Act, a person has a disability if he or she has a physical or mental impairment that substantially limits at least 1 major life activity. Nonetheless, with proper preparation many travelers with disabilities can travel internationally. Some travelers with disabilities, including those experiencing reduced mobility, may require special attention and adaptation of transportation services. The following recommendations may assist in ensuring safe, accessible travel for travelers with disabilities:

- Assess each international itinerary on an individual basis, in consultation with specialized travel agencies or tour operators.

- Consult travel health providers for additional recommendations.

- Plan ahead to ensure that necessary accommodations are available throughout the entire trip.

AIR TRAVEL

Regulations and Codes

In 1986, Congress passed the Air Carrier Access Act (ACAA) to ensure that people with disabilities are treated without discrimination in a way consistent with the safe carriage of all air passengers. The regulations established by the Department of Transportation (DOT) apply to all flights of US airlines and flights to or from the United States by foreign carriers.

Because of this act, carriers may not refuse transportation on the basis of a disability. However, there are a few exceptions; for example, the carrier may refuse transportation if the person with a disability would endanger the health or safety of other passengers or if transporting the person would be a violation of Federal Aviation Administration safety rules.

(Travelers and their clinicians can learn more about these exceptions and other aspects of the act at http://airconsumer.ost.dot.gov/publications/horizons.htm.) Air carriers are also obliged to accept a declaration by a passenger that he or she is self-reliant. A medical certificate, which is a written statement from the passenger's health care provider saying that the passenger is capable of completing the flight safely without requiring extraordinary medical care or endangering other passengers, can be required only in specific situations (for example, if a person intends to travel with a possible communicable disease, will require a stretcher or oxygen, or if the person's medical condition can be reasonably expected to affect the operation of the flight).

Many non-US airlines voluntarily adhere to codes of practice that are similar to US legislation based on guidelines from the International Civil Aviation Organization. However, these guidelines are not identical to those outlined in US legislation, and the degree of implementation may vary by airline and location. If a traveler's plans include flying between foreign countries while abroad, one must check with the overseas airlines to ensure that the carriers adhere to accessibility standards that are adequate for that traveler's needs.

The US Transportation Security Administration (TSA) has established a program for screening travelers with disabilities and their equipment, mobility aids, and devices. TSA permits prescriptions, liquid medications, and other liquids needed by people with disabilities and medical conditions. Travelers who have disabilities or medical conditions that may affect TSA screening may use notification cards to discreetly communicate with the officer. Notification cards are available at www.tsa.gov/sites/default/files/disability_notification_card_508.pdf. Travelers can learn more about the TSA guidelines for travelers with disabilities at www.tsa.gov/travel/special-procedures.

Assistance and Accommodations

Under the guidelines of the ACAA, when a traveler with disability requests assistance, the airline is obliged to meet certain accessibility requirements. For example, carriers must provide access to the aircraft door (preferably by a level entry bridge), an aisle seat, and a seat with removable armrests. However, aircraft with <30 seats are generally exempt from these requirements. Any aircraft with >60 seats must have an onboard wheelchair, and personnel must help move the wheelchair from a seat to the lavatory area. However, airline personnel are not required to transfer passengers from wheelchair to wheelchair, wheelchair to aircraft seat, or wheelchair to lavatory seat. In addition, airline personnel are not obliged to assist with feeding, visiting the lavatory, or dispensing medication to travelers. Only wide-body aircraft with ≥2 aisles are required to have fully accessible lavatories. Travelers with disabilities who require assistance should travel with a companion or attendant. However, carriers may not, without reason, require a person with a disability to travel with an attendant.

Airlines may not require advance notice of a passenger with a disability; however, they may require up to 48 hours' advance notice and 1-hour advance check-in for certain accommodations that require preparation time, such as the following services (if they are available on the flight):

- Medical oxygen for use on board the aircraft

- Carriage of an incubator

- Hook-up for a respirator to the aircraft electrical power supply

- Accommodation for a passenger who must travel in a stretcher

- Transportation of an electric wheelchair on a flight scheduled on an aircraft with <60 seats

- Provision by the airline of hazardous material packaging for a battery used in a wheelchair or other assistive devices

- Accommodation for a group of ≥10 people with disabilities who travel as a group

- Provision of an onboard wheelchair to be used on an aircraft that does not have an accessible lavatory

DOT maintains a toll-free hotline (800-778-4838 [voice] or 800-455-9880 [TTY], available 9 AM to 5 PM Eastern Time, Monday through Friday, except federal holidays) to provide general information to consumers about the rights of air travelers with disabilities and to assist air travelers with time-sensitive disability-related issues.

Patients with Respiratory Conditions

Travelers with certain respiratory conditions that cause low blood oxygen levels may need supplemental oxygen to make up for the reduced air pressure in the cabin during flight. More information about air travel for people who may need supplemental oxygen is available at www.uptodate.com/contents/supplemental-oxygen-on-commercial-airlines-beyond-the-basics.

Service Animals

Under the ACAA, carriers must permit guide dogs or other service animals with identification to accompany a person with a disability on a flight. Carriers must permit a service animal to accompany a traveler with a disability to any assigned seat, unless the animal obstructs an aisle or other area that must remain clear to facilitate an emergency evacuation, in which case the passenger will be assigned another seat. However, service animals are not exempt from compliance with quarantine regulations and may not be allowed to travel to all international destinations. They are also subject to US animal import regulations on return (see Chapter 6, Taking Animals & Animal Products across International Borders).

CRUISE SHIPS

US companies or entities conducting programs or tours on cruise ships have obligations regarding access for travelers with disabilities, even if the ship itself is of foreign registry. However, all travelers with disabilities should check with individual cruise lines regarding availability of requested or needed items before booking. Cruise operators and travel agents that cater to travelers with special needs also exist.

USEFUL LINKS

- Department of Transportation, Aviation Consumer Protection Division
  - > New Horizons Information for the Air Traveler with a Disability (http://airconsumer.ost.dot.gov/publications/horizons.htm)
  - > Aviation Consumer Protection and Enforcement Rules (see links under Part 382, Passengers with Disabilities) (http://airconsumer.ost.dot.gov/rules/rules.htm)
  - > Passengers with Disabilities (site provides a summary of the main points of the DOT rule, Title 14 CFR Part 382) (http://airconsumer.ost.dot.gov/publications/disabled.htm)
- Transportation Security Administration— Disabilities and medical conditions (www.tsa.gov/travel/special-procedures)
- MossRehab ResourceNet (www.mossrehab.com/patients-and-visitors/information-for-out-of-town-visitors/travel-resources)
- American Council of the Blind—Travel Resources(www.acb.org/node/1643)
- Society for Accessible Travel and Hospitality (www.sath.org)
- Aerospace Medical Association— Medical publications for airline travel (www.asma.org/publications/medical-publications-for-airline-travel)
- Mobility International USA (www.miusa.org)

BIBLIOGRAPHY

1. International Civil Aviation Organization. Manual on access to air transport by persons with disabilities. Montréal: International Civil Aviation Organization; 2013 [cited 2016 Sep 27]. Available from: http://www.passepartouttraining.com/uploads/2013/03/ICAO-Manual-Doc-9984-1st-Edition-alltext-en_published_March-2013.pdf

2. Josephs LK, Coker RK, Thomas M, British Thoracic Society Air Travel Working Group. Managing patients with stable respiratory disease planning air travel: a primary care summary of the British Thoracic Society recommendations. Prim Care Respir J. 2013 Jun;22(2):234–8.

3. Nondiscrimination on the basis of disability in air travel. 2003 [cited 2016 Sep. 27]; Available from: http://airconsumer.dot.gov/rules/382short.pdf.

IMMIGRANTS RETURNING HOME TO VISIT FRIENDS & RELATIVES (VFRs)

Jay S. Keystone

DEFINITION OF VFR

A traveler categorized as a VFR is an immigrant, ethnically and racially distinct from the majority population of the country of residence (a higher-income country), who returns to his or her home country (lower-income country) to visit friends or relatives. Included in the VFR category are family members, such as the spouse or children, who were born in the country of residence. Some experts have recommended that the term VFR refer to all those visiting friends and relatives regardless of the traveler's country of origin; however, this proposed definition may be too broad and not take into consideration cultural, economic, and attitudinal issues. Therefore, this review uses the more classic definition.

DISPROPORTIONATE INFECTIOUS DISEASE RISKS IN VFRS

Altered migration patterns to North America in the past 30 years have resulted in many immigrants originating from Asia, Southeast Asia, and Latin America instead of Europe. Although 13% of the US population is foreign born, in 2014, 37% of overseas international travelers from the United States listed VFR as a reason for travel. VFRs experience a higher incidence of travel-related infectious diseases, such as malaria, typhoid fever, tuberculosis, hepatitis A, and sexually transmitted diseases, than do other groups of international travelers, for a number of reasons:

- Lack of awareness of risk

- ≤30% have a pretravel health care encounter

- Financial barriers to pretravel health care

- Lack of access to clinics

- Cultural and language barriers with health care providers

- Lack of trust in the medical system

- Last-minute travel plans and longer trips

- Travel to higher-risk destinations

- High-risk trip characteristics, such as staying in homes and living the local lifestyle, which often includes lack of safe food and water and not using bed nets

Malaria

In 2012, 54% of imported malaria cases in US civilians occurred among VFRs. Data from the GeoSentinel Surveillance Network show that among ill travelers who present for medical care, VFRs are 8 times more likely to be diagnosed with malaria than are tourist travelers. Reports from the United Kingdom show similar results for VFR versus tourist travelers to West Africa. Many VFRs assume they are immune; however, in most VFRs, especially those who left their countries of origin years previously, immunity has waned and is no longer protective. In recent years, a number of VFRs have died of malaria on their return to North America; in the United States in 2012, 55% of those with severe malaria for whom the purpose of travel was known were VFRs, mostly returned from West Africa.

Other Infections

From 2008 through 2012 in the United States, 85% of typhoid and 88% of paratyphoid A cases occurred in VFRs, mostly from southern Asia. Most isolates were resistant or showed decreased susceptibility to fluoroquinolone antibiotics. Similar rates of resistant infections were noted in imported cases in Switzerland from the Indian subcontinent.

VFR children aged <15 years are at highest risk for hepatitis A, and many are asymptomatic. A Canadian study found that 65% of hepatitis A cases were in VFRs aged <20 years, and in a Swedish study of 636 cases of imported infection, 52% were in VFRs, of whom 90% were <14 years old. Other diseases, such as tuberculosis, hepatitis B, cholera, and measles, occur more commonly in VFRs after travel.

PRETRAVEL HEALTH COUNSELING FOR VFRS

Table 8-4 summarizes VFR health risks and prevention recommendations. It is important to increase awareness among VFR travelers regarding their unique risks for travel-related infections and the barriers to travel health services. If possible, clinics should incorporate culturally sensitive educational materials, provide language translators, and provide handouts in multiple languages. However, studies in the United Kingdom aimed at preventing malaria among VFRs showed that increased awareness and availability of medications do not necessarily increase use of malaria chemoprophylaxis, highlighting the complex socioecological context in which VFRs make travel health decisions.

Vaccinations

Travel immunization recommendations and requirements for VFRs are the same as those for

US-born travelers. It is crucial, however, to first try to establish whether the immigrant traveler has had routine immunizations (such as measles and tetanus) or has a history of specific diseases. Adult travelers, in the absence of documentation of immunizations, may be considered to be susceptible.

Table 8-4. Diseases for which VFR travelers are at increased risk, proposed reasons for risk variance, and recommendations to reduce risks[1]

DISEASES	REASON FOR RISK VARIANCE[2]	RECOMMENDATIONS TO STRESS WITH VFR TRAVELERS
Foodborne and waterborne illness	Social and cultural pressure (eat the meal served by hosts)	Frequent handwashing Avoid high-risk foods (dairy products, undercooked foods) Simplify treatment regimens (single dose, such as azithromycin, 1,000 mg, or ciprofloxacin, 500 mg) Discuss food preparation
Fish-related toxins and infections	Eating high-risk foods Less pretravel advice	Avoidance counseling about specific foods (such as raw freshwater fish)
Malaria	Longer stays Higher-risk destinations Less pretravel advice leading to less use of prophylaxis and fewer personal protection measures Belief that one is already immune	Education on malaria, mosquito avoidance, and the need for prophylaxis Consider cost of prophylaxis Use of insecticide-treated bed nets
Tuberculosis (particularly multidrug-resistant)	Increased close contact with local population Increased contact with HIV-coinfected people	Check PPD 2–3 months after return if history of negative tuberculin skin test and long stay (>3 months) Educate about tuberculosis signs, symptoms, and avoidance
Bloodborne and sexually transmitted diseases	More likely to seek substandard local care Cultural practices (tattoos, body modification practices) Longer stays and increased chance of blood transfusion Higher likelihood of sexual encounters with local population	Discuss high-risk behaviors, including tattoos, piercings, dental work, sexual encounters Encourage purchase of condoms before travel Consider providing syringes, needles, and intravenous catheters for long-term travel
Schistosomiasis and soil-transmitted helminths	Limited access to piped-in water in rural areas for bathing and washing clothes	Avoid freshwater exposure Use liposomal DEET preparation with freshwater exposures[3] Discourage children from playing in dirt Use ground cover Use protective footwear
Respiratory problems	Increased close exposure to fires, smoking, or pollution	Prepare for asthma exacerbations by considering stand-by bronchodilators and steroids

(continued)

Table 8-4. Diseases for which VFR travelers are at increased risk, proposed reasons for risk variance, and recommendations to reduce risks[1] (continued)

DISEASES	REASON FOR RISK VARIANCE[2]	RECOMMENDATIONS TO STRESS WITH VFR TRAVELERS
Zoonotic diseases (such as rickettsial infections, leptospirosis, viral fevers, leishmaniasis, anthrax, Chagas disease)	Rural destinations Staying with family where animals are kept Increased exposure to insects Increased exposure to mice and rats Sleeping on floors	Avoid animal contact Wash hands Wear protective clothing and use insect repellent Check for ticks daily Avoid thatched roofs and mud walled accommodation and fresh sugar cane juice in Latin America Avoid sleeping at floor level
Envenomations (snakes, spiders, scorpions)	Sleeping on floors	Avoid sleeping at floor level Wear shoes outdoors at night
Toxin ingestion (medication adverse events, heavy metal ingestion)	Purchase of local medications Use of traditional therapies Use of contaminated products (such as pottery with lead glaze) Eating contaminated freshwater fish	Anticipate need and purchase medications before travel Counsel avoidance of known traditional medications (such as Hmong bark tea with aspirin) and high-risk items (such as large reef fish)
Yellow fever and Japanese encephalitis (risk is decreased in adults)	Unclear, partial immunity from previous exposure or vaccination	Avoid mosquitoes by taking protective measures and receiving vaccination when appropriate
Dengue (especially risk of severe dengue)	Severe dengue occurs on repeat exposure to a different serotype of dengue; VFRs more likely to have had previous exposure	Avoid mosquitoes by taking protective measures

Abbreviations: VFR, visiting friends and relatives; PPD, tuberculin purified protein derivative; DEET, N,N-diethyl-m-toluamide.
[1] Adapted from: Bacaner N, Stauffer W, Boulware DR, Walker PF, Keystone JS. Travel medicine considerations for North American immigrants visiting friends and relatives. JAMA. 2004;291(23):2856–64.
[2] Hypothesis unless referenced to support assertions.
[3] In animal models, DEET (liposomal preparations) prevents *Schistosoma* cercariae from penetrating the skin.

Age-appropriate vaccinations (or serologic studies to check for antibody status) should be provided, with 2 caveats:

- Immunity to hepatitis A should not be assumed; many young adults and adolescents from developing countries are still susceptible.

- Consider varicella immunization for people born outside the United States. Such travelers may be more susceptible because infection occurs at an older age in tropical than in temperate regions. Also, rates of death

and complications from varicella disease are higher in adults than in children.

Malaria Prevention

VFR travelers to endemic areas should not only be encouraged to take prophylactic medications but also should be reminded of the benefits of barrier methods of prevention, such as bed nets and insect repellents, particularly for children (see Chapter 2, Protection against Mosquitoes, Ticks, & Other Arthropods). VFRs should be advised that drugs such as chloroquine and pyrimethamine, as well as proguanil monotherapy, are no longer effective in most areas, especially in sub-Saharan Africa. These medications are often readily available and inexpensive in their home countries but are not efficacious.

VFRs should also be encouraged to purchase their medications before traveling to ensure good drug quality. Studies in Africa and Southeast Asia show that one-third to half of antimalarial drugs purchased locally are counterfeit or substandard.

HEADING HOME HEALTHY

The CDC-supported Heading Home Healthy program (www.HeadingHomeHealthy.org) is focused on reducing travel-related illnesses in VFR travelers. The program contains videos, informational resources, and health tools in multiple languages and was developed to assist not only VFR travelers but also their primary care health providers.

BIBLIOGRAPHY

1. Behrens RH, Neave PE, Jones CO. Imported malaria among people who travel to visit friends and relatives: is current UK policy effective or does it need a strategic change? Malar J. 2015;14:149.

2. Chaccour C, Kaur H, Del Pozo JL. Falsified antimalarials: a minireview. Expert review of anti-infective therapy. 2015 Apr;13(4):505–9.

3. Date KA, Newton AE, Medalla F, Blackstock A, Richardson L, McCullough A, et al. Changing patterns in enteric fever incidence and increasing antibiotic resistance of enteric fever isolates in the United States, 2008–2012. Clin Infect Dis. 2016 Aug 1;63(3):322–9.

4. Hendel-Paterson B, Swanson SJ. Pediatric travelers visiting friends and relatives (VFR) abroad: illnesses, barriers and pre-travel recommendations. Travel Med Infect Dis. 2011 Jul;9(4):192–203.

5. LaRocque RC, Deshpande BR, Rao SR, Brunette GW, Sotir MJ, Jentes ES, et al. Pre-travel health care of immigrants returning home to visit friends and relatives. Am J Trop Med Hyg. 2013 Feb;88(2):376–80.

6. Leder K, Tong S, Weld L, Kain KC, Wilder-Smith A, von Sonnenburg F, et al. Illness in travelers visiting friends and relatives: a review of the GeoSentinel Surveillance Network. Clin Infect Dis. 2006 Nov 1;43(9):1185–93.

7. Monge-Maillo B, Norman FF, Perez-Molina JA, Navarro M, Diaz-Menendez M, Lopez-Velez R. Travelers visiting friends and relatives (VFR) and imported infectious disease: travelers, immigrants or both? A comparative analysis. Travel Med Infect Dis. 2014 Jan-Feb;12(1):88–94.

8

HEALTH CARE WORKERS

Henry M. Wu, V. Ramana Dhara, Alan G. Czarkowski, Eric J. Nilles

RISKS FOR HEALTH CARE WORKERS PRACTICING DURING TRAVEL OUTSIDE THE UNITED STATES

Health care workers practicing outside the United States may face unique health hazards. Numerous infectious risks are associated with patient contact or handling clinical specimens. Various types of health care workers may be at risk:

- Physicians, nurses, and other ancillary clinical staff providing care in international settings, including clinics, hospitals, and field locations

- Medical students and other health care trainees participating in clinical rotations overseas

- Other people working in clinics, hospitals, or laboratories, including researchers, laboratory technicians, ancillary staff, and public health workers

Health care workers in all settings are at risk for exposure to numerous infectious diseases, including infections spread through blood and bodily fluids (such as HIV or hepatitis B) or through airborne or respiratory droplet routes (such as tuberculosis [TB] or influenza). Risks vary depending on the duties of the worker, the geographic location, and the practice setting. Increased risks are due to multiple factors including the following:

- Less stringent safety regulations or infection control standards.

- Limited availability of personal protective equipment (PPE) or safety-engineered devices.

- Unfamiliar practice conditions or equipment.

- Challenging practice conditions that can prevent providers from adhering to standard precautions (such as extremely resource-limited settings, natural disasters, or conflict zones) (see Box 8-4, Health care workers in extreme circumstances).

- Unfamiliar medical procedures.

- High prevalence of transmissible infections (such as HIV, hepatitis B, hepatitis C, or TB).

- Potentially high infectious burden and increased transmission risk from source patients (such as high HIV viral loads in untreated patients).

- Limited resources for evaluation and treatment after exposure to bloodborne pathogens.

- Potential to encounter uncommon or emerging infectious diseases that are highly transmissible in health care settings (such as Middle East respiratory syndrome [MERS] or Ebola virus disease).

- Increased psychological stress resulting from practicing in resource-limited settings, isolated areas, and long-term assignments.

BOX 8-4. Health care workers in extreme circumstances

Health care workers regularly provide care in a range of extreme circumstances, which may be characterized by limited or absent medical and public health infrastructure, lack of fundamental hygiene supplies (such as soap and water for handwashing), increased infectious disease transmission, extreme environmental conditions, and high levels of violence. Violent attacks on humanitarian workers have increased substantially in the past 20 years, and kidnappings of aid workers increased 400% from 2002 through 2012.

Because of the increased risks and consequences of severe disease or injury, adequate prevention and preparation are essential. Health problems for the health care worker can have serious implications, both for the person and for those who depend on the health care worker for provision of health care. Detailed instructions on how to prepare for travel or work in developing countries or humanitarian environments is covered in detail in other sections, but additional key considerations

for the health care worker include the following:

1. Having reliable communication equipment: usually satellite phone, ensuring service provider contract for duration of the mission. Consider portable solar recharging capabilities unless power supply is guaranteed, which is rare in most extreme circumstances.

2. Acquiring evacuation insurance and having a plan if ill or injured: depending on the deploying organization, evacuation insurance (see Chapter 2, Travel Insurance, Travel Health Insurance, and Medical Evacuation Insurance) and a detailed evacuation contingency plan may or may not be provided. Both are critical, and the health care worker should be familiar with all details.

3. Considering underlying health conditions: provider's health should be monitored closely and treatment initiated early, if necessary. Any indication that a potentially serious

condition is not responding to treatment should warrant rapid planning for potential medical evacuation.

4. Being psychologically stable and knowing whom to contact if problems arise: providers in conflict and disaster zones typically work long hours in dangerous conditions and are exposed to profound suffering. These experiences can be intensely stressful, leading to increased rates of depression, posttraumatic stress disorder, and anxiety. Before deployment, providers should think about coping strategies and, as much as possible, stay in contact with a support network of family and friends.

5. Inquiring about availability of antidotes to chemical warfare: although rare, health care workers may be exposed to chemical warfare agents while caring for patients, as recently documented in Syria. If exposure to these agents is a possibility, antidotes (such as atropine) should be immediately available.

These challenges should be taken into account by all health care workers when they consider and prepare for international missions.

PRETRAVEL VACCINATION AND SCREENING

In addition to vaccinations specifically indicated for the country visited and routine age-appropriate vaccines, all health care workers should be up-to-date on all recommended vaccinations for employment in health care settings. These include vaccinations (or documented immunity) for the following:

- Measles, mumps, and rubella

- Influenza

- Varicella

- Tetanus, diphtheria, and pertussis

- Hepatitis B

For hepatitis B, postvaccination serologic testing is recommended for health care workers; of those who do not respond to a primary vaccine series, 25%–50% respond to an additional vaccine dose, and 44%–100% respond to a 3-dose revaccination series. Inactivated polio vaccine (given as an adult booster dose) or meningococcal vaccine may be indicated for specific locations experiencing high incidence or outbreaks of these infections. Providers should consult country-specific recommendations and travel alerts on the CDC Travelers' Health website (www.cdc.gov/travel) for updated vaccination recommendations.

Regular screening for latent TB infection with tuberculin skin test or interferon-γ release assay is recommended for health care workers, and testing before and after travel is particularly important when the provider is working in a country with a high prevalence of TB infection or in a setting of high TB exposure, such as in prisons (see Chapter 3, Tuberculosis). Routine vaccination of health care workers with bacillus Calmette-Guérin (BCG) is not recommended in the United States; however, BCG vaccination may be considered for some health care workers who will work in settings with high TB transmission risk and a high prevalence of strains resistant to isoniazid and rifampin. Baseline testing for HIV and hepatitis C before travel is not routinely recommended, although it should be considered if risk of exposure will be high and reliable testing will not be available locally in the event of an exposure.

PPE AND INFECTION CONTROL

Health care workers should consistently follow standard precautions whenever possible and apply other precautions (contact, droplet, or airborne) as needed. PPE, including gloves, gowns, aprons, surgical masks, fit-tested N95 respirator masks, and protective eyewear, may be necessary to achieve personal protection. Workers untrained in infection control practices should not participate in clinical activities, handle clinical specimens, or handle contaminated medical equipment. Needlestick injuries are a common mode of percutaneous exposure to bloodborne pathogens, and practices known to increase risk of needlestick injuries, such as recapping syringes or using needles to transfer a bodily fluid between containers, should be avoided whenever possible, even if they are commonly practiced locally. The traveling health care worker should be aware of the local practice environment in advance of travel, since limited use of PPE or even reuse of equipment that would not be acceptable in the United States is common.

For further details, guidelines, and training materials on standard precautions and PPE, see www.cdc.gov/HAI/prevent/ppe.html and www.cdc.gov/hicpac/2007IP/2007isolationPrecautions.html. Specific PPE advice may be recommended for certain infections that pose high risk to health care workers (such as MERS, avian influenza, and Ebola virus; see disease-specific websites at www.cdc.gov for further advice).

In preparation, traveling health care workers should:

- Ensure they are properly trained for all anticipated procedures, considering the locally available equipment.

- Maintain strict safety standards, even if local standards are less stringent.

- Bring their own supply of PPE or safety-engineered medical devices if they are unsure of local availability.

8

- Assess the local availability of postexposure prophylaxis (PEP) for HIV, and consider bringing a supply for personal use if unavailable (see Postexposure Prophylaxis, below).

INFECTIONS TRANSMITTED BY AIRBORNE OR DROPLET ROUTES

Health care workers are at risk of acquiring numerous airborne and droplet-transmitted infections from patients. Although some of these pathogens are vaccine preventable (such as measles, influenza, and varicella), airborne or droplet isolation precautions for patients suspected of having some respiratory infections are a mainstay of infection control in the United States. These precautions include PPE such as surgical masks for droplet precautions and fit-tested N95 respirator masks and negative-pressure isolation rooms for airborne precautions. Health care workers should inquire about the availability of isolation facilities when working internationally. Bringing a personal supply of PPE for use while working overseas might be prudent (see above, PPE and Infection Control).

TB is a particular concern for health care workers working overseas in high-incidence areas. Although fit-tested N95 respirators are protective for individual providers, identifying the situations where their use is indicated can be difficult when diagnosis and isolation of patients with active tuberculosis is suboptimal.

Traveling health care workers should be aware that they may encounter patients with unusual or emerging respiratory pathogens, such as MERS or avian influenza. Review of the disease-specific CDC websites at www.cdc.gov and the CDC Traveler's Health website (www.cdc.gov/travel) is important for the most up-to-date information on the epidemiology and infection control recommendations for emerging pathogens.

INFECTIONS TRANSMITTED THROUGH BLOOD OR BODILY FLUIDS

Health care workers are at risk for numerous infections transmitted through exposure to blood or bodily fluids via percutaneous, mucous membrane, or nonintact skin exposures. These include bloodborne pathogens such as HIV, hepatitis B virus (HBV), and hepatitis C virus (HCV). The risk of HIV transmission is approximately 0.3% after a percutaneous exposure to HIV-infected blood and approximately 0.09% after a mucous membrane exposure. Health care workers who have received hepatitis B vaccine and have developed immunity to the virus are at virtually no risk for infection; for an unvaccinated person the risk of HBV transmission from a single needlestick or a cut exposure to HBV-infected blood ranges from 6%–30% and depends on the hepatitis B e antigen status of the source individual. Based on limited studies, the estimated risk for HCV transmission after a needlestick or cut exposure to HCV-infected blood is approximately 1.8%. Other bodily fluids that may transmit HIV and viral hepatitis include cerebrospinal fluid, synovial fluid, pericardial fluid, pleural fluid, peritoneal fluid, amniotic fluid, semen, and vaginal secretions. Saliva, urine, sputum, nasal secretions, tears, feces, vomitus, and sweat are not considered infectious for HIV and HCV unless they are visibly bloody. Typically, exposures occur as a result of percutaneous exposure to contaminated sharps, including needles, lancets, scalpels, and broken glass (from capillary or test tubes). The risk of infection after percutaneous exposures is considered increased with exposure to larger blood volumes (visible blood on the injuring device, hollow-bore needles, deeper injuries, or procedures that involved direct cannulation of an artery or vein). Skin exposures to potentially infectious bodily fluids are only considered to be at risk for bloodborne pathogen infection if there is evidence of compromised skin integrity (for example, dermatitis, abrasion, or open wound). Higher circulating viral load in the source patient is also thought to increase the risk of transmission, and this can be of particular concern in resource-poor settings where treatment for HIV and viral hepatitis is limited.

Hepatitis B vaccination, standard precautions, PPE, and safety-engineered devices are important preventative measures (see above sections, Pretravel Vaccination and Screening and PPE and Infection Control). Numerous other infections have also been transmitted to health care workers via blood or bodily fluids, including many that are uncommon or not endemic in the United States,

8

such as viral infections (including Ebola virus, dengue), parasitic infections (including malaria), and brucellosis. Although standard infection control precautions and avoidance of needlestick injuries are effective in preventing most infections that are spread via blood or bodily fluids, enhanced levels of PPE are necessary for some infectious diseases (including Ebola virus disease) that pose high risk for health care workers (see above, PPE and Infection Control).

Health care workers who may have been occupationally exposed to blood or bodily fluids should immediately perform the following steps:

- Wash the exposed area with soap and water thoroughly. If mucous membrane exposure has occurred, flush the area with copious amounts of water or saline.

- If possible, assess the HIV and HCV status of the source patient. HBV testing of the source patient may be indicated if the health care worker is not a documented responder to hepatitis B vaccination.

- Rapid HIV testing of the source patient is preferred. Exposures originating from source patients who test HIV negative are considered not to have HIV transmission risk, unless they have clinical evidence of primary HIV infection or HIV-related disease.

- Baseline HIV (and potentially HCV and HBV) testing of the exposed health care worker should be performed at the time of the exposure. Seek qualified medical evaluation as soon as possible to guide decisions on HIV PEP (see below).

Postexposure Prophylaxis (PEP)

PEP after percutaneous and mucous membrane exposures to potentially infectious bodily fluids from patients with known or potential HIV infection is recommended to reduce the chance of transmission. A number of medication combinations are available for PEP (see the Updated US Public Health Service Guidelines for the Management of Occupational Exposures to HIV and Recommendations for Postexposure Prophylaxis at http://aidsinfo.nih.gov/guidelines).

The decision of whether or not to initiate PEP must weigh numerous factors. These include the timing, nature, and source of the exposure; regimen choice as affected by drug availability; the exposed person's medical history; potential drug interactions; and the possibility of exposure to a drug-resistant strain. Expert consultation is important when considering PEP. When expert advice is not immediately available, the National Clinicians' Postexposure Prophylaxis Hotline (PEPline) can be reached toll-free at 888-448-4911 (9 AM to 12 AM Eastern Time daily) for assistance in managing occupational exposures to HIV and hepatitis B and C (http://nccc.ucsf.edu/clinician-consultation/pep-post-exposure-prophylaxis). Other considerations when initiating HIV PEP include the following:

- Initiate HIV PEP as soon as possible after exposure.

- PEP can be stopped if new information changes the decision to treat.

- PEP recipients should be counseled regarding drug toxicities, drug interactions, and the importance of adherence.

Consider and manage other potentially infectious exposures in the source material. For example, if the health care worker is not a documented serologic responder to hepatitis B vaccination or is incompletely vaccinated, postexposure testing of the source patient and health care worker may be indicated, as well as PEP with hepatitis B immune globulin and vaccination (see www.cdc.gov/mmwr/preview/mmwrhtml/rr6210a1.htm).

Postexposure Testing and Counseling

Postexposure counseling and medical evaluation should be provided, whether or not the exposed person receives HIV or HBV PEP. This may include:

- Baseline and follow-up testing for HIV at 6 weeks, 3 months, and 6 months (follow-up to at 6 weeks and 4 months is acceptable if a fourth-generation combination HIV p24 antigen-HIV antibody test is used). Extended HIV follow-up testing for up to 12 months is recommended for those who

8

become infected with HCV after exposure to a source coinfected with HIV and HCV.

- Baseline and follow-up testing for HCV for those with known or potential exposure to HCV. Perform a baseline test for HCV antibody and if positive perform confirmatory RNA test. Follow-up testing should include either a test for HCV RNA at 3 or more weeks after exposure or a test for HCV antibody at 6 or more months after exposure with a confirmatory RNA test if positive.

- Baseline and follow-up testing for HBV for those with known or potential exposure to HBV if the health care worker is not a documented serologic responder to hepatitis B vaccination or is incompletely vaccinated. Baseline testing based on hepatitis B surface antigen and total core antibody tests should be performed as soon as possible after exposure with follow-up testing approximately 6 months after exposure.

- During the first 12 weeks after exposure, health care workers should take precautions to avoid secondary transmission (such as abstaining from sexual contact, using condoms or other barriers to prevent infection, avoiding blood or tissue donations, and breastfeeding, if possible).

- Monitoring for adverse reactions from HIV PEP (when initiated).

- Monitoring for other transmissible infections that were diagnosed or suspected in the source patient.

- Psychological counseling, which should be considered essential since the emotional effect of occupational exposures can be substantial and exacerbated by stressors inherent to the overseas work environment.

BIBLIOGRAPHY

1. CDC. Healthcare-associated infections (HAIs). Atlanta: CDC; 2014 [cited 2016 Sep. 27]; Available from: http://www.cdc.gov/HAI/prevent/ppe.html.

2. CDC. Hepatitis C and health care personnel. 2016 [cited 2016 Sep. 27]; Available from: http://www.cdc.gov/hepatitis/hcv/hcvfaq.htm#section6.

3. CDC. Information for healthcare personnel exposed to hepatitis C virus (HCV). Recommended testing and follow-up. Atlanta 2016; Available from: http://www.cdc.gov/hepatitis/hcv/management.htm.

4. Clinicians Consultation Center. Post-exposure prophylaxis (PEP): timely answers for urgent exposure management. San Francisco: UCSF; 2014 [cited 2016 Sep. 27]; Available from: http://nccc.ucsf.edu/clinician-consultation/post-exposure-prophylaxis-pep/.

5. Connorton E, Perry MJ, Hemenway D, Miller M. Humanitarian relief workers and trauma-related mental illness. Epidemiol Rev. 2012 Jan;34(1):145–55.

6. Grinnell M, Dixon MG, Patton M, Fitter D, Bilivogui P, Johnson C, et al. Ebola virus disease in health care workers—Guinea, 2014. MMWR Morb Mortal Wkly Rep. 2015 Oct 2;64(38):1083–7.

7. Human Rights Watch, Safeguarding Health in Conflict Coalition. Under attack: violence against health workers, patients, and facilities. 2014 [cited 2016 Sep. 27]; Available from: https://www.msh.org/sites/msh.org/files/hhr0514_brochure_lowres.pdf.

8. Kuhar DT, Henderson DK, Struble KA, Heneine W, Thomas V, Cheever LW, et al. Updated US Public Health Service guidelines for the management of occupational exposures to human immunodeficiency virus and recommendations for postexposure prophylaxis. Infect Control Hosp Epidemiol. 2013 Sep;34(9):875–92.

9. Lee R. Occupational transmission of bloodborne diseases to healthcare workers in developing countries: meeting the challenges. J Hosp Infect. 2009 Aug;72(4):285–91.

10. Lyon RM, Wiggins CM. Expedition medicine—the risk of illness and injury. Wilderness Environ Med. 2010 Dec;21(4):318–24.

11. Mohan S, Sarfaty S, Hamer DH. Human immunodeficiency virus postexposure prophylaxis for medical trainees on international rotations. J Travel Med. 2010 Jul-Aug;17(4):264–8.

12. Schillie S, Murphy TV, Sawyer M, Ly K, Hughes E, Jiles R, et al. CDC guidance for evaluating health-care personnel for hepatitis B virus protection and for administering postexposure management. MMWR Recomm Rep. 2013 Dec 20;62(RR-10):1–19.

13. Vaid N, Langan KM, Maude RJ. Post-exposure prophylaxis in resource-poor settings: review and recommendations for pre-departure risk assessment and planning for expatriate healthcare workers. Trop Med Int Health. 2013 May;18(5):588–95.

8

ADVICE FOR AIR CREWS

Phyllis E. Kozarsky

OVERVIEW

As airlines expand their reach and air crews are asked to travel to more exotic destinations, these travelers need to prepare ahead of time for the exposures they may encounter. To some degree, air crews are similar to all travelers to such destinations, but the differences require some modifications of travel health guidance for several reasons:

- Layovers are short, often 24–48 hours.

- Travel is frequent.

- Travel to new destinations may be on short notice.

- Despite short travel times, air crews may be more adventuresome and thus have more risk than typical tourists.

- Air crews may perceive themselves to be low risk because of their generally healthy status and because their in-country exposure time is short.

Given these factors, it is worth noting some guidelines for this special group. In general, air carriers traveling to destinations in the developing world try to inform their crews about health issues they may face. However, airlines do not necessarily have available on their staff occupational health or other providers who are experts in travel medicine, and may not be aware of special risks at the destinations they serve. Therefore, airlines may wish to avail themselves of professionals who are knowledgeable in the field and who can help determine recommendations for the various destinations served.

Pilots are often aware of some of the medications and classes of medications that may interfere with their flight capacity. Medications that affect the central nervous system should not be prescribed, and pilots should take a trial between trips of any new medications or those that could have side effects that may interfere with flying. Pilots and flight attendants should also be aware that certain foods and beverages contain trace amounts of products that could cause a drug screen to turn positive. If questions arise, an FAA-certified aeromedical examiner (AME) should be consulted (www.faa.gov/pilots/amelocator) who will know which medications can and cannot be taken. Sometimes medication decisions are made on a case-by-case basis. AMEs examine pilots regularly and are responsible for certifying that pilots are fit to fly.

Although any travel health provider can see and advise flight crews, it is important to ask the crew member what the airline may require, in addition to what is required or recommended to maintain the person's health while traveling. If in doubt, the travel health provider should contact the airline medical director or occupational health department for guidance. For example, some air crews primarily fly domestic routes or routes to Western Europe or Japan, so would not fly to a region of yellow fever risk in their normal daily work. However, an airline may require that crew members without contraindications be vaccinated against yellow fever, so that the airline has flexibility to shift crews and be able to address any urgent needs.

GENERAL HEALTH MEASURES

Although pilots are required to have periodic provider visits to ensure they are fit to fly, these may not address some issues that may affect them when they travel internationally, particularly to destinations in the developing world. Flight attendants and others should also consider asking their health care providers about these recommendations:

- Administering a periodic tuberculin skin test if traveling frequently to destinations where the prevalence of tuberculosis is much higher than in the United States, where the incidence of antimicrobial resistance is higher, or where the crew member will be in close contact with crowds (www.who.int/tb/areas-of-work/drug-resistant-tb/en).

8

- Checking at each visit to make sure that routine immunizations are up-to-date (see below).

- Immunizing against seasonal influenza every year when the vaccine becomes available.

In addition, all medications for chronic conditions should be carried in extra quantities, as they may not be available at some locations, and even if available and less costly, may be counterfeit or of poor quality (see Chapter 2, *Perspectives: Pharmaceutical Quality & Falsified Drugs*). The business of manufacturing counterfeit medications in developing countries is huge and growing; it is impossible to tell from the packaging or pills if they are counterfeit. Some counterfeit drugs contain little or no active ingredient, and others contain toxic contaminants.

Vaccinations

Because of the frequency of travel to international destinations, air crews may be exposed to various diseases that are not common in the United States. For example, measles can be a life-threatening illness for adults; it is more common in most of the world, including Europe, because of lack of mandatory childhood immunization against the disease in many countries. In addition, flight crews may not have had chickenpox as children and may not have been immunized. This illness often occurs at a later age in the tropics; thus, if there is interaction with local populations in these destinations, risk for infection will be higher. International flight crews should consider a travel health visit to ensure as complete protection as possible. Some may have short notice before traveling to new destinations; thus, air crew members should be asked about this possibility during their visit, so that vaccinations for an upcoming trip—that may not be imminent—may be given, or a series may be started early. Providers should educate travelers about health risks in the various destinations; whether certain vaccinations are administered will depend on the traveler's tolerance for risk.

All travelers should make sure they are up-to-date with routine vaccinations. These vaccines include measles-mumps-rubella (MMR) vaccine, diphtheria-tetanus-pertussis vaccine, varicella (chickenpox) vaccine, polio vaccine, and the seasonal influenza vaccine (see the separate sections on these diseases in Chapter 3).

Although there are no established guidelines or recommendations for the use of travel vaccinations in pilots and other air crew members, for some it may be reasonable to offer meningococcal, Japanese encephalitis, yellow fever, and typhoid vaccines because of their frequent, short-stay, and at times unpredictable travel and destinations. Hepatitis A is advisable for all travelers and may be stressed for air crews, since limited data suggest they have low rates of protection. Hepatitis B is advisable for frequent travelers because of the unpredictability of exposure. Air crews are generally a group who travel frequently beyond work, so they should always be asked during a consultation whether they plan other travel itineraries that can be addressed at the same time.

Malaria Prophylaxis

Crew members are typically informed by their airline as to which destinations harbor malaria. Some European and Asian air carriers have longer experience flying to destinations where malaria is endemic, and these airlines have various policies with respect to its prevention. Although there may be malaria transmission in some areas of destination countries, sometimes there is none in the capitals or the larger urban areas to which the major American carriers fly (such as in China or the Philippines). This is generally not the case in sub-Saharan Africa, where there can be substantial exposure during a short 24-hour layover (although in Ethiopia, there is no malaria risk in Addis Ababa). Although there may be little risk in the hotels at the destination, risk may be increased at the international airports, during unpredictable delays in transit, and during outings on layovers. Even during short single stops (for example, in West Africa on the way to South Africa), there is some risk when the aircraft doors are open. Little published data are available on the risk of malaria for flight crews with short layovers, but some information suggests that it is less than that for tourists.

Unfortunately, experience in American and European air crews to malaria-endemic destinations has shown that air crews continue to acquire malaria, as well as develop severe and complicated disease. Some illness may result from lack of awareness of airline recommendations, failure to take precautions against mosquito bites, lack of compliance with antimalarial prophylaxis, or inaccurate information regarding toxicity of medication. Transmission can be focal and intermittent, so prophylaxis for every trip to a highly endemic region should be stressed.

Flight crew members should have easy access to educational materials and prophylaxis and, if desired, should be able to have an individual risk assessment for preventive measures. For destinations where the prevalence of malaria is high (countries in West Africa, for example), crew members should take prophylaxis for layovers. For other destinations where crews are thought to be at low risk based on local intensity of transmission, accommodations, and personal behaviors, they may be advised to use insect repellents and take other precautions to avoid mosquito bites (see Chapter 2, Protection against Mosquitoes, Ticks, & Other Arthropods) but take no prophylaxis. Flight crews should always:

- Educate themselves as much as possible about malaria.

- Understand the importance of personal protective measures such as repellents, and use them properly.

- Take prophylaxis if recommended.

- Know that if fever or chills occur after exposure, it is a medical emergency.

- Know how they can get medical assistance at their destinations or at home in the event of symptoms or signs of malaria.

There are several options for malaria prophylaxis, depending on the destination city, although needed duration of prophylaxis and adverse effects profiles of some of the drugs make them less than desirable for air crews. Country-specific recommendations can be accessed either in this text (see Chapter 3, Yellow Fever & Malaria Information, by Country) or on the CDC Travelers' Health website (www.cdc.gov/travel).

International airlines generally prefer the combination drug atovaquone-proguanil; its adverse effect profile and its dosing make it the most suitable for air crews.

Additional information on malaria prevention may be found in Chapter 3, Malaria.

Other Vectorborne Diseases

In the last decade, several mosquitoborne viruses have emerged or reemerged, including dengue, chikungunya, and Zika (see the individual disease sections in Chapter 3). Preventing mosquito bites in tropical and subtropical destinations is critical to preventing disease. Because Zika virus infection during pregnancy can cause severe birth defects, airlines should develop flight destination policies for pilots and flight attendants who are pregnant, plan to become pregnant, or have a partner who is or may become pregnant.

Food and Water Precautions and Travelers' Diarrhea

Pilots and air crew members should follow the same safe food and water precautions and prevention and management of travelers' diarrhea as other travelers (see Chapter 2, Travelers' Diarrhea). They should also be well versed in the recognition and self-treatment of moderate to severe travelers' diarrhea to shorten the duration of illness that could affect their job performance.

Bloodborne and Sexually Transmitted Infections

Although these risks and preventions are addressed in more detail in other sections, it is worth reiterating that frequent travelers have an increased likelihood of engaging in casual and unprotected sex. It is common to think that people from all Western countries would have the same risk of HIV and other sexually transmitted infections; however, travelers have far higher rates of such infections. The risk of acquisition may be higher not only for diseases such as gonorrhea and chlamydia but also for chronic illnesses such as hepatitis B and C. Dental procedures and activities such as acupuncture, tattooing, and piercing also are ill-advised during travel to developing countries.

8

BIBLIOGRAPHY

1. Bagshaw M, Barbeau DN. The aircraft cabin environment. In: Keystone JS, Freedman DO, Kozarsky PE, Connor BA, Nothdurft HD, editors. Travel Medicine. 3rd ed: Saunders Elsevier; 2013. pp. 405–12.

2. Byrne N. Urban malaria risk in sub-Saharan Africa: where is the evidence? Travel Med Infect Dis. 2007 Mar;5(2):135–7.

3. Byrne NJ, Behrens RH. Airline crews' risk for malaria on layovers in urban sub-Saharan Africa: risk assessment and appropriate prevention policy. J Travel Med. 2004 Nov-Dec;11(6):359–63.

4. CDC. Notes from the field: malaria imported from West Africa by flight crews—Florida and Pennsylvania, 2010. MMWR Morb Mortal Wkly Rep. 2010 Nov 5;59(43):1412.

5. Schwartz MD, Macias-Moriarity LZ, Schelling J. Professional aircrews' attitudes toward infectious diseases and aviation medical issues. Aviat Space Environ Med. 2012 Dec;83(12):1167–70.

6. Selent M, de Rochars VMB, Stanek D, Bensyl D, Martin B, Cohen NJ, et al. Malaria prevention knowledge, attitudes, and practices (KAP) among international flying pilots and flight attendants of a US commercial airline. J Travel Med. 2012 Dec;19(6):366–72.

HUMANITARIAN AID WORKERS

Brian D. Gushulak

OVERVIEW

Through organizations and agencies or individual activities, many thousands of people are involved in the delivery of humanitarian and disaster relief aid in diverse locations every year. After large-scale events such as earthquakes or tsunamis, the number of those traveling to provide humanitarian aid and assistance can increase. Additionally, many others already engaged in international missionary or faith-based activities often become involved in humanitarian and disaster relief efforts. Maintaining the health of humanitarian aid workers is important to ensure that they are able to deliver care to those in need and avoid additional strain on local health services.

In common with other travelers, people who travel to provide humanitarian aid or disaster relief must first address their personal health and welfare before, during, and after travel. This includes knowledge of and preparation for all the usual elements associated with travel to the area. Additionally, aid workers can experience specific risks and situations related to the provision of humanitarian care, such as:

- Exposure to the environment that precipitated or sustains a crisis or event, such as a natural disaster or conflict

- Working long hours under adverse or extreme conditions, often in close contact with the affected population

- Damaged or absent infrastructure, including limits in the availability of food, water, lodging, transportation, and health services

- Reduced levels of security and protection

- Stress, ethical, and moral challenges related to the event and the resource capacities of the situation

Humanitarian service can damage personal health. Studies involving long-term humanitarian workers have noted that >35% report that their personal health status deteriorated during the mission. Accidents and violence are documented risks for humanitarian aid workers and cause more deaths than disease and natural causes. Recent estimates place the risk of violence-related deaths, medical evacuations, and hospitalizations at approximately 6 per 10,000 person-years among aid workers. Conditions and outcomes vary by location, nature of the humanitarian event, and time spent in the field.

A study of American Red Cross workers noted a 10% ratio of injury or accident and an exposure to violence of 16%. The same study also showed that >40% found the experience more stressful than expected. An earlier study of deaths among Peace Corps volunteers noted that unintentional injuries were the cause of nearly 70% of deaths, followed by homicide at 17%. Illness was responsible for 14% of the Peace Corps fatalities.

However, risks to humanitarian aid workers are not uniformly distributed across the spectrum of humanitarian aid. Ongoing surveillance of violence directed against humanitarian and disaster relief aid workers continues to demonstrate that a small number of insecure locations (Afghanistan, Pakistan, South Sudan, Syria, and the Central African Republic) account for most of these events.

PRETRAVEL CONSIDERATIONS

Evaluation and Pretravel Medical Care

Giving careful attention to pretravel evaluation, both medical and psychological, in addition to educating travelers, can reduce the likelihood of illness and the need for emergency repatriation. Comprehensive medical examinations can prepare travelers by helping identify previously unrecognized conditions and allowing for treatment before travel. Careful evaluation of risk factors (family history, history of alcohol or substance abuse, sexually transmitted diseases, and psychiatric illness) may direct additional evaluation and identify previously unrecognized psychological problems or chronic conditions. Identifying alcohol or substance dependence, depression, or other psychiatric illness is important, as these conditions may be exacerbated by the stress of the mission and are often the reason for emergency repatriation. People planning long-term assignments should have their dental condition assessed and any problems dealt with before departure.

Missionaries and faith-based workers may have additional issues that need to be considered by health care providers. Their service may involve extended periods of time abroad, possibly their entire professional lives, so the provider must consider the implications of long-term residence in areas of health risk. Additionally, they may be accompanied by family members, including young children. Both of these factors engender additional travel health considerations that may be different than those encountered by short-term humanitarian and disaster relief workers. For more information, see the next section in this chapter, Long-Term Travelers & Expatriates.

Those who will be providing medical care or participating in clinical research as part of their humanitarian activities should be evaluated in terms of occupational risk and the need for preventive preexposure or postexposure interventions. They should also be reminded that providing aid during outbreak situations may involve contact with infected people who are asymptomatic or have nonspecific symptoms, requiring more attention to infection control protocols. Disaster relief and humanitarian aid workers destined for areas of active conflict or limited police presence may benefit from specialized security briefings, either provided by the employing agency or private sources. Medical facilities may be compromised by the disaster or overwhelmed in responding to it. Therefore, volunteers with underlying conditions likely to require care and pregnant women should be counseled against travel and encouraged to support the response in other ways. Travelers planning to participate in animal rescue should review information available in Chapter 6, Taking Animals and Animal Products across International Borders, and discuss rabies preexposure prophylaxis with a health care provider (see Chapter 3, Rabies).

Travelers who will be caring for people ill with potentially life-threatening infections such as Ebola virus disease or other diseases spread by contact with blood or other body fluids should be familiar with infection control measures specific for the disease. They should also ensure that their organization provides personal protective equipment (PPE), such as masks, gloves, gowns, and eye protection.

Regardless of the area of the world in which the aid worker will be deployed, certain basics should be addressed in the pretravel encounter, including routine vaccinations, malaria chemoprophylaxis (if appropriate), food and water precautions, self-treatment for travelers' diarrhea, risks from insect bites, behavioral risk avoidance, and injury prevention.

8

Counseling and Advice

Predeployment education and training are essential, as personal illness or injury burdens the community the worker has come to support. Injuries and motor vehicle accidents are common risks for travelers anywhere in the world; thus, travelers should be sensitive to their surroundings and carefully select the type of transportation and hour of travel, if possible. In disaster and emergency situations, the traveler should also be aware of physical hazards such as debris, unstable structures, downed power lines, environmental hazards, and extremes of temperature. Although rare, emergency situations in developed nations may involve unusual exposures, such as radiation exposures observed after damage to nuclear facilities after the earthquake in Japan in 2011.

Travelers to conflict areas should be aware of landmines and other potential hazards associated with unexploded ordnance. In situations associated with damage or destruction to local services and facilities, humanitarian aid workers should expect, anticipate, and plan for limited accommodations, logistics, and personal support. Disaster relief and humanitarian aid workers destined for low-resource areas or situations may benefit from pretravel training and counseling regarding the moral complexities of providing service in these environments.

Preparation

HEALTH ITEMS

The traveler should be advised to prepare a travel health kit that is more extensive than the typical kit and should also be familiar with basic first aid to self-treat any injury until medical attention can be obtained. Aid workers may need to disinfect their own water and may want to carry high-energy, nonperishable food items for emergency use. Humanitarian and disaster relief workers should research the available resources in the destination to tailor how extensive their packed supplies should be.

Those with underlying medical conditions requiring treatment should ensure that, if possible, they travel with prescriptions and medications sufficient for the duration of their service.

As not all pharmaceuticals are globally available, travelers who will be on extended deployment should review alternative preparations or compounds should their normal formulations not be available. It is a good practice to separate and store medications in 2 separate allotments in case of loss or theft. People with dental crowns or bridgework may wish to carry temporary dental adhesive for short-term management of a dislodged dental appliance. In addition to a basic travel health kit (see Chapter 2, Travel Health Kits), humanitarian aid workers should consider bringing the following items:

TOILETRIES

- Toothbrush and toothpaste
- Skin moisturizer
- Soap, shampoo
- Lip balm
- If corrective lenses are used:
  - > Extra pair of prescription glasses in a protective case and a copy of the prescription
  - > Eyeglasses cleaning supplies and repair kit
  - > Extra contact lenses and lens cleaner
- Disposable razor, extra cartridges
- Nail clippers
- Toilet paper
- Menstrual supplies

PROTECTIVE CLOTHING

- Comfortable, lightweight clothing
- Long pants
- Long-sleeved shirts
- Hat
- Boots
- Shower shoes
- Rain gear
- Bandana or handkerchief
- Towel (highly absorbent travel towel if possible)

- Gloves (leather gloves if physical labor will be performed; rubber gloves if handling blood or body fluids)
- Safety goggles

ITEMS FOR DAILY LIVING

- Sunglasses
- Sunscreen
- Insect repellent
- Waterproof watch
- Flashlight
- Spare batteries
- Sewing kit
- Laundry detergent
- Small clothesline and clothespins
- Travel plug or voltage adapters for electronics
- Knife, such as a Swiss Army knife or Leatherman[1]
- If traveling to an area where food and water may be contaminated:
  > Bottled water or water filters/purification system/water purification tablets
  > Nonperishable food items
- If traveling to malaria-endemic areas:
  > Personal bed net (insecticide-impregnated)

SAFETY AND SECURITY

- Money belt
- Cash
- Cellular telephone, equipped to work internationally, or satellite telephone (with charger)
- Candles, matches, and lighter in a zip-top bag[2]
- Extra zip-top bags

PERSONAL ITEMS

Because of the loss of life, serious injuries, missing and separated families, and destruction often associated with disasters, humanitarian aid workers should recognize that situations they encounter may be extremely stressful. Keeping a personal item nearby, such as a family photo, favorite music, or religious material, can offer comfort in such situations. Checking in with family members and close friends from time to time is another means of support. Satellite telephones are small, can work almost anywhere in the world, and can be rented for <$10 per day.

IMPORTANT DOCUMENTS

It is often useful to have extra passport-style photos, which may be required for certain types of visas or for additional work permits or extensions. Travelers should bring photocopies of important documents, such as passports and credit cards, as well as copies of their medical, nursing, or other professional license, if applicable. Medical information, such as immunization records and blood type, is also helpful to have at hand. The traveler should carry copies and also leave copies with someone back home. In addition, they should carry contact information for the person who should be notified in an emergency.

REGISTRATION WITH EMBASSIES

Travelers should enroll in the Department of State's Smart Traveler Enrollment Program (STEP, https://step.state.gov/step) to register with the US embassy in the destination country before departure. This will ensure that the local consulate is aware of their presence, they can receive notifications, and they may be accounted for and included in evacuation plans. Travelers providing humanitarian assistance should review and understand medical, evacuation, and life insurance provided by their employing agency. They should also consider supplemental travel, travel health, and medical evacuation insurance to cover medical care and evacuation should they become ill or injured.

---

[1] Pack these items in checked baggage, since they are considered sharp objects and will be confiscated by airport or airline security if packed in carry-on bags.
[2] See www.tsa.gov for restrictions on traveling with lighters and matches.

POST-TRAVEL CONSIDERATIONS

Returning disaster relief and humanitarian aid workers should be advised to seek medical care if they sustained injuries during their travel or become ill after returning. To ensure proper evaluation, they should advise their providers of the nature of their recent travel.

Depending upon the length of time away or their activities (such as working in health care), returning aid workers may benefit from a complete medical review. Those involved in situations of infectious disease outbreaks should be made aware of post-travel illness monitoring recommendations or requirements. Homecoming has also been identified as a risk period for difficulties in psychological adjustment, and treatment or counseling should be sought. Workers who witnessed or were involved in situations of mass casualties, deaths, or serious injuries or who have been victims of violence (assault, kidnapping, or serious road traffic crash) should be considered for referral for critical incident counseling. They should also be advised that the psychological effects of traumatic experiences may present long after return.

Studies have indicated that >30% of aid workers report depression shortly after returning home. The adjustment process can be assisted by a skilled debriefing. Generally, humanitarian aid and disaster relief workers are able to adapt to the acute and chronic stressors of their work and demonstrate considerable resilience, but they will also benefit from proper rest and support to help them fully adjust back into the home environment.

BIBLIOGRAPHY

1. Aid Worker Security Database (AWSD): figures at a glance [database on the Internet]. Humanitarian Outcomes; 2015 [cited 2016 Sep. 27]; Available from: http://reliefweb.int/sites/reliefweb.int/files/resources/ho_aidworkersecuritypreview2015_0.pdf.

2. Brooks SK, Dunn R, Sage CA, Amlot R, Greenberg N, Rubin GJ. Risk and resilience factors affecting the psychological wellbeing of individuals deployed in humanitarian relief roles after a disaster. J Ment Health. 2015 Dec;24(6):385–413.

3. Callahan MV, Hamer DH. On the medical edge: preparation of expatriates, refugee and disaster relief workers, and Peace Corps volunteers. Infect Dis Clin North Am. 2005 Mar;19(1):85–101.

4. CDC. Coping with a traumatic event: information for the public. Atlanta: CDC; 2009 [cited 2016 Sep. 27]; Available from: http://www.cdc.gov/masstrauma/factsheets/public/coping.pdf.

5. Connorton E, Perry MJ, Hemenway D, Miller M. Humanitarian relief workers and trauma-related mental illness. Epidemiol Rev. 2012 Jan;34(1):145–55.

6. Kortepeter MG, Seaworth BJ, Tasker SA, Burgess TH, Coldren RL, Aronson NE. Health care workers and researchers traveling to developing-world clinical settings: disease transmission risk and mitigation. Clin Infect Dis. 2010 Dec 1;51(11):1298–305.

7. McFarlane CA. Risk associated with the psychological adjustment of humanitarian aid workers. Australas J Disaster Trauma Stud [Internet]. 2004;[cited Sep. 27 2016]. Available from: http://www.massey.ac.nz/~trauma/issues/2004-1/mcfarlane.htm.

8. Mitchell AM, Sakraida TJ, Kameg K. Critical incident stress debriefing: implications for best practice. Disaster Manag Response. 2003 Apr-Jun;1(2):46–51.

9. Nurthen NM, Jung P. Fatalities in the Peace Corps: a retrospective study, 1984 to 2003. J Travel Med. 2008 Mar-Apr;15(2):95–101.

10. Peytremann I, Baduraux M, O'Donovan S, Loutan L. Medical evacuations and fatalities of United Nations High Commissioner for Refugees field employees. J Travel Med. 2001 May-Jun;8(3):117–21.

8

LONG-TERM TRAVELERS & EXPATRIATES

Lin H. Chen, Davidson H. Hamer

The risk of illness or injury increases with duration of travel, so special consideration should be given to travelers who are planning long-term visits (≥6 months is a common definition) to low- or middle-income countries, whether they are expatriates with definite plans or adventurers with open itineraries. Points to discuss in the pretravel consultation include accessing care at the destination, vaccines, infectious diseases not prevented by vaccines, injury prevention, and psychological and cultural issues that long-term travelers may encounter.

ACCESSING CARE ABROAD

Before departure, all long-term travelers should undergo complete medical and dental examinations. It also may be beneficial to have a psychological evaluation, as early repatriation is often due to psychological issues that could be addressed prior to travel. Travelers should anticipate that they will need care at some point during their stay, and they should plan where they will get it and how they will pay for it. Those traveling for work or with an organization (such as a university or the Peace Corps) may have a predetermined source of care and some may access advice from the international expatriate community. In contrast, other travelers should identify a source in advance (see Chapter 2, Obtaining Health Care Abroad). Long-term travelers should also determine if they will need supplemental travel health insurance and evacuation insurance (see Chapter 2, Travel Insurance, Travel Health Insurance, & Medical Evacuation Insurance), since health insurance can be a challenge to procure locally.

In some countries, travelers are likely to encounter poor-quality (substandard, falsified, counterfeit, or expired) medications. Because the pills and packaging may be nearly indistinguishable from their legitimate counterparts, travelers should bring a sufficient supply of their routine medications (antihypertensive or antihyperlipidemic drugs, for example) from the United States (see Chapter 2, *Perspectives:* Pharmaceutical Quality & Falsified Drugs). There are different options to obtain sufficient medications: (1) request an override from the insurance company to dispense the entire quantity of medication, (2) pay out of pocket for the full amount of medication needed and then submit to insurance company for reimbursement, or (3) rely on friends or family members who visit to bring refilled medication supplies.

VACCINES

Routine vaccines, including influenza vaccine, should be updated. In addition, long-term travelers should be aware of any vaccine requirements at their destination for employment, schooling, or entry. A number of travel-related vaccines warrant consideration:

- Hepatitis A and typhoid vaccines are appropriate given the cumulative risk, although the traveler should be aware that the latter does not provide full protection.

- Travel-associated hepatitis B infections are rare, but the risk for travelers may be higher than for nontravelers, and the vaccine should be considered for all long-term travelers and expatriates.

- Meningococcal disease is more likely in travelers with prolonged exposure to local populations in endemic or epidemic areas; quadrivalent vaccine should be considered for those at risk.

- Japanese encephalitis is associated with longer stays in endemic areas, and the vaccine is recommended for travelers who plan to reside in endemic areas or travel for ≥1 month to endemic areas, or travelers anticipating

8

outdoor activities in endemic areas after dusk (see Chapter 3, Japanese Encephalitis).

- Rabies preexposure prophylaxis is an important consideration for people spending a prolonged time in endemic countries, especially in areas where rabies immune globulin is not available (which is true of many resource-limited countries). Vaccinating children who will be living in high-risk areas is a priority.

- Numerous unvaccinated Chinese expatriates have recently fallen ill from yellow fever while working in Angola, illustrating the importance of yellow fever vaccination for travelers who will be staying in an endemic area or a country with a vaccine requirement.

In addition to the intended destination, consider disease risk in surrounding areas, since long-term travelers may be likely to travel locally. For example, a short-term traveler to Seoul would not be considered at risk for Japanese encephalitis, but an expatriate living in Seoul may have opportunities to visit the Korean countryside or other areas in Asia where he or she could be exposed.

INFECTIOUS DISEASES NOT PREVENTED BY VACCINES

Malaria

Data suggest that the incidence of malaria increases and the use of preventive measures decreases with increasing length of stay. For instance, malaria incidence in British travelers returning from West Africa after a stay of 6–12 months was 80 times that of the incidence in travelers who had stayed only 1 week. Among expatriate corporate employees in Ghana, adherence to malaria prophylaxis deteriorated with increasing duration of stay, and all those who had been on the site for >1 year had abandoned prophylaxis. About half of the cohort used insect repellent only intermittently, and more than one-third never used repellent. Even though most British expatriates from the UK Foreign and Commonwealth Office had good knowledge about malaria and its prevention strategies, they adhered to malaria prophylaxis <25% of the time; only 25% reported rigorous compliance, and 13% reported having contracted malaria. Given the

high relative risk of malaria for travelers in Africa, these data on long-term travelers and expatriates highlight worrisome risks and practices.

A traveler who will be residing in an area of continuous malaria transmission should continue to use malaria prophylaxis for the entire stay. It is important to reassure the traveler that the drugs are safe and effective. Doxycycline has been well-tolerated for long-term malaria prophylaxis in the military, and CDC has no recommended limits on its duration of use for malaria prophylaxis. Mefloquine has been used frequently during prolonged stays by Peace Corps volunteers, with a discontinuation rate of 0.9%. Mefloquine may be appropriate for long-term prophylaxis in chloroquine-resistant areas because of its convenient weekly dosing, but concern has increased regarding its neuropsychiatric side-effect profile, especially the recent Food and Drug Administration label indicating that neurologic side effects may persist. Atovaquone-proguanil has shown good long-term tolerability in post-marketing surveillance, with a discontinuation rate of only 1% because of diarrhea. Peace Corps Volunteers prescribed atovaquone-proguanil adhered to prophylaxis best when compared with those given doxycycline and mefloquine. If long-term use (>5 years) of chloroquine is planned, a baseline ophthalmic examination with biannual follow-up is recommended to screen for potential retinal toxicity.

The possibility of pregnancy requires careful consideration for long-term female travelers to malarious areas (see the Pregnant Travelers section earlier in this chapter). Malaria infection during pregnancy can result in severe complications to both mother and fetus. When pregnancy is anticipated, prophylaxis options may need to be adjusted. Ideally, this possibility should be explored before travel with all female long-term travelers of childbearing age. For women who are pregnant or plan to become pregnant during long-term travel, mefloquine is considered safe in all trimesters. Data from published studies in pregnant women have shown no increase in the risk of teratogenic effects or adverse pregnancy outcomes after mefloquine prophylaxis during pregnancy. Chloroquine has also been used long-term without ill effect on pregnancy. If a woman traveling long-term is taking atovaquone-proguanil, doxycycline, or primaquine, she should discontinue her medication and begin weekly mefloquine (or chloroquine in those areas where it remains efficacious) and wait at least 3–4 weeks to conceive so that a therapeutic blood level of mefloquine can build up.

Women who become pregnant while taking antimalarial drugs do not need a therapeutic abortion but should be advised during the pretravel consultation of potential risks. The effect of atovaquone-proguanil on the fetus is unknown, but doxycycline is associated with fetal toxicity in animals and is contraindicated in pregnant women. Primaquine may harm a G6PD-deficient fetus, so it should not be used in pregnancy.

French service members deployed to Central African Republic for 4 months in 2013 experienced malaria at a rate of 150 cases/1,000 person-years; a survey found that prophylaxis compliance correlated with other prophylactic measures against malaria (bed net use, insecticide on clothing, taking prophylaxis at the same time every day), correct perception of malaria risk, positive perception of prophylaxis effectiveness, and peer-to-peer reinforcement. For long-term travelers, the need for adjuncts to prophylaxis should also be stressed, such as personal protection measures to avoid mosquito bites (sleeping under a bed net, using screens, and applying repellents). Travelers should bring a sufficient supply of antimalarial drugs from the United States, since drugs purchased at the destination may be of poor quality. Even with urging to adhere to personal protective measures and reassurance that long-term prophylaxis is safe and effective, adherence is likely to decline over time. Consequently, the pretravel consultation for a long-term traveler to a malarious area should stress the severity of malaria, its signs and symptoms, and the need to seek care immediately if they develop. Travelers could consider bringing a reliable supply of drugs to treat malaria if they are diagnosed with malaria. For additional discussion, see the next section in this chapter, *Perspectives:* Malaria in Long-Term Travelers & Expatriates.

Other Diseases

Because diarrhea and gastrointestinal diseases are common in long-term travelers, they should be educated about the management of acute diarrhea including rehydration, the use of antimotility agents, empiric antimicrobial therapy, and when to seek care.

Tuberculosis risk may rise to the level of the local population if the traveler or expatriate has a longer stay and intimate contact with the local population. A baseline tuberculin test or interferon-γ release assay, followed by the same test after travel, should be considered, especially for health care workers or those who may be working in hospitals, refugee camps, or in prisons.

Likewise, dengue seroconversion occurred at a rate of 3.4/1,000 people per month of stay in endemic areas among development aid workers. Other mosquitoborne viral illnesses are also a risk, so long-term travelers and expatriates should be advised to protect themselves from the mosquito vectors.

Risk for HIV and sexually transmitted infections are increased in travelers and expatriates, and the consistent use of condoms in expatriates is low (approximately 20%). Long-term travelers should be educated about the risk of HIV and sexually transmitted diseases in their destination, as well as preventive measures. The potential for occupational exposure to HIV is important to consider in health care workers; postexposure prophylaxis with antiretroviral therapy and risk avoidance should be included in the pretravel consultation (see the Health Care Worker section earlier in this chapter).

Transfusion is a potential source of hepatitis C infection in expatriates. The risk of hepatitis E, spread by the fecal-oral route, is highest in Asia, although it has been transmitted in many different tropical locations. Pregnant women are at highest risk of fulminant disease.

Other infections vary with location and include giardiasis, amebiasis, strongyloidiasis, schistosomiasis, cutaneous leishmaniasis, and filariasis. *Strongyloides stercoralis* infections can be prevented by not walking barefoot through soil, and schistosomiasis may be prevented by not swimming or wading in fresh water. This latter risk is difficult to communicate to long-term travelers who, for example, may be living in sub-Saharan Africa and who look forward to river rafting or vacationing at a lake. The risks of strongyloidiasis and

8

schistosomiasis increase with long-term travel, so screening on return (and also during long-term expatriate assignments for those with access to health care) should also be discussed. Cutaneous leishmaniasis and filariasis should be reviewed if a traveler has the potential geographic exposure risk. Compared with short-term travelers, long-term travelers experience more chronic diarrhea and postinfectious irritable bowel syndrome (possibly because some become less adherent to food and water precautions over time) and should be advised to continue food and water precautions in order to reduce the risk for these conditions.

INJURY

Since injuries are the leading cause of preventable death in travelers, long-term travelers should be educated about safety. Road and vehicle safety should be stressed, and travelers should choose the safest vehicle options available. Roads are often poorly constructed and maintained, traffic laws may not be enforced, vehicles may not have seatbelts or be properly maintained, and drivers may be reckless and poorly trained. See Chapter 2, Injury Prevention for strategies to reduce the risk of traffic and other injuries.

PSYCHOLOGICAL ISSUES

The stress of long-term travel can trigger or exacerbate psychiatric reactions. A long-term traveler should be assessed for preexisting psychiatric diagnosis, depressed mood, recent major life stressors, and use of medications that may have psychiatric effects. These conditions may suggest a need for further screening. All long-term travelers should be urged to take care of their physical and mental health by exercising regularly and eating healthfully. They should be able to recognize signs of anxiety and depression and have a plan for coping with them. Having photographs or other mementoes of friends and family at hand and staying in close contact with loved ones at home can alleviate the stress of long-term travel. For more information, see Chapter 2, Mental Health.

LONG-TERM TRAVELERS WITH OPEN ITINERARIES

Offering pretravel care to travelers with no itinerary (or those who present with only vague travel plans) presents unique challenges. These travelers benefit from broad immunization coverage for all potential exposures to vaccine-preventable diseases, although some prioritization may be necessary. Because their plans are unclear, these travelers must understand that they may need to diagnose and treat themselves for common ailments, including travelers' diarrhea, upper respiratory tract infections, urinary tract infections, vaginitis, skin disorders, and musculoskeletal problems (see Chapter 2 for details on a variety of self-treatable conditions). For travelers such as backpackers who may go in and out of malarious areas, a sensible approach is to provide a supply of atovaquone-proguanil with instructions on how to administer it when they do visit risk areas. In addition to strategies to prevent health problems and injuries during their long sojourns, traveler education is imperative regarding health resources, signs and symptoms that require urgent medical evaluation, and medical evacuation.

SCREENING LONG-TERM TRAVELERS AND EXPATRIATES AFTER RETURN

Long-term travelers, whether they are expatriate workers, Peace Corps volunteers, or highly adventurous travelers, need a thorough medical interview to assess potential infectious exposures after return to their country of origin. A careful itinerary-specific history with detailed questioning about potential high-risk exposures including food, water, animal, and human contact is the foundation of the post-travel evaluation. A physical examination focused on specific signs and symptoms and a selected array of tests, including tuberculin skin test or interferon-γ release assay for tuberculosis screening, a complete blood count with differential, hepatic transaminases, and serologic markers depending on types of exposure (but most importantly for strongyloidiasis and schistosomiasis), are helpful to detect subclinical infections and determine whether seroconversion to the more common pathogens (where treatment would be advised) has occurred (see Chapter 5, Screening Asymptomatic Returned Travelers). A benefit of the post-travel evaluation is preventive counseling for potential future travel.

8

BIBLIOGRAPHY

1. Brown ML, Henderson SJ, Ferguson RW, Jung P. Revisiting tuberculosis risk in Peace Corps Volunteers, 2006–13. J Travel Med. 2015 Dec 18;23(1).

2. Chen LH, Wilson ME, Davis X, Loutan L, Schwartz E, Keystone J, et al. Illness in long-term travelers visiting GeoSentinel clinics. Emerg Infect Dis. 2009 Nov;15(11):1773–82.

3. Chen LH, Wilson ME, Schlagenhauf P. Prevention of malaria in long-term travelers. JAMA. 2006 Nov 8;296(18): 2234–44.

4. Créach M-A, Velut G, de Laval F, Briolant S, Aigle L, Marimoutou C, et al. Factors associated with malaria chemoprophylaxis compliance among French service members deployed in Central African Republic. Malaria J. 2016;15:174.

5. Cunningham J, Horsley J, Patel D, Tunbridge A, Lalloo DG. Compliance with long-term malaria prophylaxis in British expatriates. Travel Med Infect Dis. 2014 Jul–Aug;12(4):341–8.

6. Hamer DH, Ruffing R, Callahan MV, Lyons SH, Abdullah AS. Knowledge and use of measures to reduce health risks by corporate expatriate employees in western Ghana. J Travel Med. 2008 Jul–Aug;15(4):237–42.

7. Landman KZ, Tan KR, Arguin PM; Centers for Disease Control and Prevention (CDC). Knowledge, attitudes, and practices regarding antimalarial chemoprophylaxis in U.S. Peace Corps Volunteers—Africa, 2013. MMWR Morb Mortal Wkly Rep. 2014 Jun 13;63(23):516–7.

8. Lim PL, Han P, Chen LH, MacDonald S, Pandey P, Hale D, et al. Expatriates ill after travel: results from the Geosentinel Surveillance Network. BMC Infect Dis. 2012;12:386.

9. Pierre CM, Lim PL, Hamer DH. Expatriates: special considerations in pretravel preparation. Curr Infect Dis Rep. 2013 Aug;15(4):299–306.

10. Visser JT, Edwards CA. Dengue fever, tuberculosis, human immunodeficiency virus, and hepatitis C virus conversion in a group of long-term development aid workers. J Travel Med. 2013 Nov-Dec;20(6):361–7.

8

MALARIA IN LONG-TERM TRAVELERS & EXPATRIATES

Lin H. Chen

Long-term travelers and expatriates in malarious areas are at risk for severe malaria throughout their stay, but sometimes they do not recognize the continued need for reducing risk through prophylaxis and personal protective measures. Even those with knowledge of the need for preventive practices may be unable to adhere to them or may opt to discontinue them. Guidelines for malaria prevention might be interpreted as focusing on preventing *Plasmodium falciparum* malaria in short-term travelers. Optimal malaria prevention in long-term travelers poses dilemmas because of diverse traveler characteristics and itineraries (including traveling in and out of malarious areas), the heterogeneous quality of and access to medical care, and the limited reports on long-term safety and efficacy of antimalarial drugs. Moreover, parasite resistance, seasonality, and the intensity of transmission evolve with environmental and population alterations.

For this discussion, long-term travelers are defined as nonimmune travelers staying in malaria-endemic countries for ≥6 months. A review summarized published data on the risk of malaria in long-term travelers, evidence for personal protective measures, and safety and tolerability of malaria prophylaxis during long-term use (Box 8-5).

INDIVIDUALIZED RISK CONSIDERATIONS

Some travelers have preconceived notions about malaria prevention for their long-term journey or stay in an endemic region that may shape their acceptance of standard recommendations. Even when educational efforts appear successful in convincing such travelers to take prophylaxis, they often meet other travelers or locals who convince them that the medication is either not necessary or is in some way detrimental to their health. Additionally, adherence to malaria prophylaxis

among Peace Corps volunteers was associated with forgetting the medication, fear of long-term adverse effects, and experiencing adverse events attributed to the drug. Nonetheless, taking a detailed assessment of the traveler's risk and attitude may help the clinician determine the traveler's likelihood of adherence to preventive actions during long-term travel. Consider asking about the following:

- Traveler's beliefs regarding personal protective measures

- Traveler's knowledge and preferences toward continuous prophylaxis

- Travel characteristics, including the quality of accommodations, activities, and social support and network

- Economic considerations

- Destination-specific infrastructure, including medical service, access to high-quality care, medication supply, and availability of repellents, insecticides, and nets

(continued)

PRACTICAL RECOMMENDATIONS
Personal Protective Measures

Preventing malaria in all travelers is a complex issue and particularly so for long-term travelers and expatriates, who require personalized expert advice. For long-term travelers and expatriates, malaria prevention must stress the role of personal protective measures as an adjunct to prophylaxis, including adapting behaviors to minimize mosquito exposure, staying in housing with screened windows and doors, using air conditioning, sleeping under an insecticide-treated bed net, applying insecticide sprays in the residence, managing the environment to reduce vector breeding, using effective repellent, and wearing long sleeves and pants when practical (Box 8-6).

Malaria Prophylaxis

Prophylaxis decreases the risk of illness, hospitalization, and death. However, some travelers may disregard prophylaxis recommendations. Working with the traveler to overcome his or her concerns, providing insight into the severity of malaria, and deriving a feasible and sensible prophylaxis plan are recommended (Box 8-7). For example, a long-term traveler or expatriate based in a malaria-endemic country with highly seasonal or geographically focal malaria transmission may rely primarily on personal protective measures at some times and target periods of prophylaxis during

8

BOX 8-5. **Key findings from a review of studies relevant to long-term travelers and expatriates[1]**

- Long-term travelers are at higher risk for malaria than short-term travelers.
- Long-term travelers underuse personal protective measures and often abandon continuous prophylaxis.
- Travelers use a variety of unproven strategies during long stays: discontinuing prophylaxis after the initial period of stay, using different medications for prophylaxis in succession, relying on standby emergency self-treatment, or taking prophylaxis intermittently during high-transmission periods or locations.
- All the prophylaxis strategies have advantages and disadvantages, but prophylaxis is recommended for at least high-transmission destinations and seasons. People who elect to take prophylaxis only for high-transmission destinations and seasons should ensure they have access to a reliable supply of a full course of an approved malaria treatment regimen (Box 3-3 and Table 3-8).
- Poor-quality drugs (including antimalarial drugs) threaten the health of long-term travelers who obtain their medications in developing countries.
- Primaquine (in people with adequate levels of G6PD) can be used as presumptive antirelapse therapy after long exposures in areas with high *Plasmodium vivax* prevalence.

[1] Adapted from: Chen LH, Wilson ME, Schlagenhauf P. Prevention of malaria in long-term travelers. JAMA. 2006;296(18):2234–44.

BOX 8-6. Practical advice on personal protective measures for clinicians counseling long-term travelers and expatriates

- Instruct on treating clothing and bed nets with a pyrethroid insecticide.
- Discuss the effectiveness of applying repellent.
- Review experience regarding efficacy and safety of repellents: in >60 years since

DEET came into wide use, no adverse effects attributed to long-term use have been published.
- Discuss mosquito-proofing methods for use in accommodations, including maintenance

of drains, elimination of mosquito breeding sites, installation of screens, and applying insecticide indoors.
- Advise on the biting habits of the local *Anopheles* mosquito populations.

---

the transmission season or when venturing into endemic areas. However, a traveler who will be staying in an area of high continuous malaria transmission should continue to use malaria prophylaxis for the entire stay.

Another scenario that may arise and merits discussion with long-term travelers is whether they should continue malaria prophylaxis if they develop fever during travel. Rapid diagnostic tests are unreliable for self-diagnosis in travelers because most travelers are not able to use and read the test correctly. (In the United States, rapid diagnostic tests are only approved for laboratory use.) Because fever has numerous possible causes besides malaria, travelers should continue their recommended prophylaxis

provided that they are tolerating it well. In addition, they should be tested for malaria even if taking prophylaxis. Clearly the possibility of other treatable causes of fever should be explored. Travelers who will be >24 hours from adequate medical care should consider carrying a full course of malaria medication for emergency self-treatment when malaria is suspected, regardless of whether they take continuous prophylaxis. Travelers who might self-administer treatment should be told that they still require follow-up care as soon as they are able to access it.

Unfortunately, in many countries malaria is a frequent diagnosis in people who do not have malaria. In addition to receiving

unnecessary treatment, long-term travelers and expatriates who are misdiagnosed with malaria may stop taking their prophylaxis because they erroneously believe that it did not work. It is difficult to relay such a concept during the pretravel consult, but the attempt should be made.

SUMMARY

Recommendations for malaria prevention in all travelers must be personalized. Tailoring advice by assessing the traveler's preferences and concerns and determining the traveler's possible adherence, along with education regarding malaria, will likely result in better adherence than simply prescribing a course of

(continued)

BOX 8-7. Practical advice on malaria prophylaxis for long-term travelers and expatriates

- Reassure travelers that long-term use of prophylaxis is safe and effective.
- Chloroquine used long-term (5–6 years of weekly dosing) raises concern for retinal toxicity. A baseline ophthalmologic examination is recommended, with follow-up every 6–12 months after 5 years of use.
- Encourage travelers to take their prophylaxis for as long as they are living in areas with malaria transmission.
  > For people living in countries with only seasonal or focal areas of malaria transmission, use prophylaxis during high-transmission seasons or for travel to endemic areas.
  > Assess whether traveler should carry a reliable supply of malaria treatment medication. If malaria is diagnosed, the traveler will have an effective medicine that will not interact with other medicines (see Chapter 3, Malaria).
  > Beware of the wide availability of poor-quality (substandard, falsified, or counterfeit) antimalarial drugs, especially in Asia and sub-Saharan Africa. All medications should be obtained from the home country or a reliable and reputable local source.
- Discuss *Plasmodium vivax* malaria with travelers who may have prolonged exposure in high-prevalence areas (for example, a traveler who has been in Papua New Guinea for 6 months).
  > Check G6PD to determine whether an expatriate can take presumptive antirelapse therapy after leaving an endemic area.

prophylaxis. The following messages should be conveyed to the long-term traveler regarding malaria prevention:

- Adherence to prophylaxis in high-risk areas is essential.

- Use of personal protective measures, such as bed nets and screens, is critical (as many will not use repellents long term).

- Reliable medical facilities at the destination should be located as soon as feasible.

- Data support the safety of long-term use of prophylaxis.

- Supplies of antimalarial drugs should be brought from home, because poor-quality drugs (substandard, falsified, or counterfeit) are prevalent in malaria-endemic countries.

- Fever is a worrisome sign, and malaria must be considered and ruled out (see Chapter 5, Fever in Returned Travelers).

- A medical evacuation insurance policy should be purchased if the traveler will be in an area with inadequate medical facilities.

- Although individual use of rapid diagnostic tests is not advised, carrying standby treatment with

8

follow-up medical care may be appropriate for some.

- Presumptive antirelapse therapy may be appropriate for exposure in areas with intense *P. vivax* transmission (after a normal level of G6PD is documented).

- Misconceptions regarding malaria are pervasive in malaria-endemic countries among expatriates and local residents, and long-term travelers should trust health advice only from reputable and respected sources.

BIBLIOGRAPHY

1. Berg J, Visser LG. Expatriate chemoprophylaxis use and compliance: past, present and future from an occupational health perspective. J Travel Med. 2007 Sep–Oct;14(5):357–8.

2. Chen LH, Wilson ME, Davis X, Loutan L, Schwartz E, Keystone J, et al. Illness in long-term travelers visiting GeoSentinel clinics. Emerg Infect Dis. 2009 Nov;15(11):1773–82.

3. Chen LH, Wilson ME, Schlagenhauf P. Prevention of malaria in long-term travelers. JAMA. 2006 Nov 8;296(18):2234–44.

4. Chen LH, Wilson ME, Schlagenhauf P. Controversies and misconceptions in malaria prophylaxis for travelers. JAMA. 2007 May 23;297(20):2251–63.

5. Cunningham J, Horsley J, Patel D, Tunbridge A, Lalloo DG. Compliance with long-term malaria prophylaxis in British expatriates. Travel Med Infect Dis. 2014 Jul–Aug;12(4):341–8.

6. Landman KZ, Tan KR, Arguin PM. Adherence to malaria prophylaxis among Peace Corps Volunteers in the Africa region, 2013. Travel Med Infect Dis. 2015 Jan–Feb;13(1):61–8.

7. Lengeler C. Insecticide-treated bed nets and curtains for preventing malaria. Cochrane Database Syst Rev. 2004(2):CD000363.

8. Renschler JP, Walters KM, Newton PN, Laxminarayan R. Estimated under-five deaths associated with poor-quality antimalarials in sub-Saharan Africa. Am J Trop Med Hyg. 2015 Jun;92(6 Suppl):119–26.

9. Tusting LS, Thwing J, Sinclair D, Fillinger U, Gimnig J, Bonner KE, Bottomley C, Lindsay SW. Mosquito larval source management for controlling malaria. Cochrane Database Syst Rev. 2013 Aug 29;8:CD008923.

10. Tusting LS, Ippolito MM, Willey BA, Kleinschmidt I, Dorsey G, Gosling RD, Lindsay SW. The evidence for improving housing to reduce malaria: a systematic review and meta-analysis. Malar J. 2015 Jun 9;14:209.

8

Perspectives sections are written as editorial discussions aiming to add depth and clinical perspective to the official recommendations contained in the book. The views and opinions expressed in this section are those of the author and do not necessarily represent the official position of CDC.

LAST-MINUTE TRAVELERS

Gail A. Rosselot

Ideally, travelers should seek medical advice at least 4–6 weeks before departure, but clinicians are frequently asked to provide pretravel care to travelers leaving on short notice, sometimes within days or even hours. "Last-minute travelers" can refer to people who are leaving on short notice (such as some business travelers or immigrants returning to their home country for a family emergency), or it may refer to people who have planned a trip for some time but delayed seeking pretravel care. Regardless of the reason, clinicians can offer travelers support for their upcoming trip even on short notice. This support could include vaccination with standard or accelerated immunization schedules, health counseling, prescriptions, and referrals to services at the destination.

VACCINATIONS

Consider the traveler's itinerary and activities at the destination when assessing which vaccines might be indicated. Note that immunity generally takes approximately 2 weeks to develop after vaccination (although this duration is shorter after booster vaccinations), so travelers might not be adequately protected if they are vaccinated immediately before travel. Counsel travelers to adhere to preventive behaviors regarding food, water, and insects (see the Food & Water Precautions and Protection against Mosquitoes, Ticks, & Other Arthropods sections in Chapter 2) in case they are incompletely protected, as well as to prevent diseases for which no vaccine is available.

Routine Vaccinations

Most travelers who attended school in the United States have received standard routine vaccinations. If the traveler is not completely up-to-date on age-appropriate routine vaccines, administer first or additional doses of these. Throughout the season and while supplies remain, provide the seasonal influenza vaccination, if needed. Depending on the age and medical conditions of the traveler, pneumococcal, meningococcal, and *Haemophilus influenzae* type b vaccines may also be indicated. Note that if the traveler needs >1 live-virus vaccine (yellow fever, measles-mumps-rubella, varicella, intranasal influenza, zoster), they must be given on the same day or separated by ≥28 days.

Recommended Vaccinations: Single-Dose Protection

Even when a traveler has limited time before departure, research supports the use of certain single-dose vaccines, if indicated, to initiate protection. These include hepatitis A (monovalent), typhoid (injectable), polio (inactivated), cholera, and quadrivalent (ACWY) meningococcal meningitis vaccines. The booster dose of the hepatitis A vaccine should be given ≥6 months after the first dose is administered.

Recommended Vaccinations: Multiple Doses Needed

Last-minute travelers often cannot complete the full course of vaccines that require multiple doses to induce full protection. If a traveler needs protection against hepatitis B, Japanese encephalitis, or rabies, the clinician can consider alternative approaches.

HEPATITIS B

As time allows, complete the accelerated monovalent hepatitis B (Engerix-B) schedule (0, 1, and 2 months, plus a 12-month booster) or the super-accelerated combination hepatitis A/B (Twinrix) schedule (0, 7, 21–30 days, plus a 12-month booster). If an accelerated schedule cannot be completed before travel, start the vaccination series and schedule a follow-up visit to complete it, or, for extended-stay travelers or expatriates, help them identify resources at the destination to complete the series.

JAPANESE ENCEPHALITIS

At present, no accelerated schedule for Japanese encephalitis vaccine (Ixiaro) has been approved in the United States. A study of adults given 2 doses of Ixiaro 7 days apart found that 99% were protected, and the vaccine has been licensed in Europe for use on this schedule (days 0 and 7). However, people who receive only 1 dose may have a suboptimal response and may not be protected. Travelers who cannot complete the primary vaccine series ≥1 week before travel should be counseled to adhere rigidly to mosquito precautions if they will be at risk for Japanese encephalitis. Alternatively, the clinician can help them identify resources for vaccination with Ixiaro or alternative vaccines at their destination.

RABIES

Because of the multiple immunizations required to complete a primary rabies vaccine series (0, 7, and 21 or 28 days), it may be difficult for last-minute travelers to complete the series before departure. A person who starts but does not complete a primary series and is potentially exposed should receive the same postexposure prophylaxis as a completely unimmunized person. Counsel travelers about the importance of avoiding animals,

8

washing any bite thoroughly with soap and water, and seeking immediate medical care. Travelers to developing or remote destinations should consider medical evacuation insurance in case evacuation is needed to receive timely postexposure prophylaxis.

Required Vaccinations

Documentation of a yellow fever vaccine becomes valid 10 days after administration. If a yellow fever vaccine is required by a country in the traveler's itinerary and the traveler lacks sufficient time, it may be necessary to rearrange the order of travel or reschedule the trip. Otherwise, the traveler risks entry problems at the country's border or risks yellow fever vaccination at the border. Additionally, the traveler who receives the yellow fever vaccine <10 days before entering a yellow fever risk area risks yellow fever infection. Travelers for whom the yellow fever vaccination is contraindicated can be issued a medical waiver letter.

Quadrivalent (ACWY) meningococcal vaccine is required of all adults and children aged >2 years traveling to Saudi Arabia for religious pilgrimage, including Hajj. Hajj visas cannot be issued without proof that applicants received meningococcal vaccine ≥10 days and ≤3 years (≤8 years for conjugate vaccine) before arriving in Saudi Arabia.

The World Health Organization has asked certain countries to require travelers leaving those countries to show proof of polio vaccination before they leave, if they have been in the country >4 weeks. The proof of vaccination should be documented on an International Certificate of Vaccination or Prophylaxis and is valid from 4 weeks to 1 year after the vaccine is administered. This requirement should not present a problem to travelers receiving the vaccine at the last minute, since if they stay for >4 weeks, the vaccination will be valid, even if administered on the day of travel. However, if travelers stay in the country for >1 year, they should be advised to get revaccinated >4 weeks before they plan to leave. Countries with this requirement can change. Consult the CDC website (wwwnc.cdc.gov/travel/news-announcements/polio-guidance-new-requirements) for a current list. For more information, see Chapter 3, Poliomyelitis.

MALARIA

Effective malaria chemoprophylaxis is possible for the last-minute traveler. The choice of antimalarial agent depends on a number of factors, including itinerary, drug resistance at the destination, medication contraindications and precautions, cost, and patient preference. Chloroquine and mefloquine should be initiated 1–2 weeks before departure, so most clinicians recommend doxycycline or atovaquone-proguanil for travelers who are departing in <1–2 weeks. Both doxycycline and atovaquone-proguanil can be started 1–2 days before arriving in an endemic area. Instruct the traveler to purchase malaria medication before departure, and reinforce the importance of minimizing insect bites and of seeking medical care if a febrile illness occurs during or after the trip.

HEALTH COUNSELING

Pretravel counseling is critical for last-minute travelers. Determine prior knowledge and experience with travel health risks, and direct your advice accordingly. Focus on major risks of the trip, and deliver simple, customized messages about prevention and self-care. Provide travelers with education and prescriptions for travelers' diarrhea, such as a fluoroquinolone or macrolide, as well as education and prescriptions for altitude illness, if indicated. Last-minute travelers may be tempted to buy medications at their destination. Encourage them to purchase all medications in the United States before departure to avoid buying medications that may be counterfeit.

Counsel the traveler on these topics (see related in-depth discussions on the following topics in Chapters 2 and 3):

- Destination- and activity-specific risks

- Unintentional injuries, including motor vehicle accidents (the leading cause of preventable death in healthy travelers), and personal safety

- Accessing health care abroad and the need to consider travel health and evacuation insurance

- Packing a carry-on travel health kit that includes an extra supply of usual prescriptions and over-the-counter medications

- Insect precautions

- Rabies avoidance and what to do in the event of an animal bite

- Food and water safety

- Sexually transmitted diseases

- Issues related to long flights, including venous thromboembolism (for at-risk travelers) and jet lag

- The State Department's Smart Traveler Enrollment Program (STEP, https://step.state.gov/step)

- Resources for further travel health information, including those from CDC (www.cdc.gov/travel)

Clinicians should also encourage last-minute travelers to schedule an appointment after the trip to complete any needed vaccinations and to initiate preparation for the next potential "spur of the moment" trip. For travelers likely to have future last-minute trips, preemptive vaccinations or "pre-loading" for certain itineraries might also be considered.

SPECIAL CHALLENGES AND ADDITIONAL CONSIDERATIONS

The Traveler Leaving in a Few Hours: If time does not permit an appointment, the clinician can still provide general prevention messages by telephone or secure digital messaging. Refer the traveler to useful websites such as CDC (www.cdc.gov/travel), the Department of State (www.travel.state.gov), the Heading Home Healthy Program (www.headinghomehealthy.org), and the International Society of Travel Medicine clinic directory (www.istm.org). Emphasize and reassure the traveler that many travel health risks can be prevented by adhering to healthy behaviors. Recommend travel health kit items that can be purchased at the airport, if necessary. Some international airports now have travel health or vaccination clinics; suggest the traveler try to visit one before departure.

The Traveler with Preexisting Medical Conditions: These patients may be at increased risk for travel-related illness if they have inadequate time for preparation. They should consider purchasing travel health insurance, trip insurance, and possibly medical evacuation insurance, and should carry a sufficient supply of all medications and a portable medical record. Emphasize the importance of a pretravel appointment or conversation with their treating clinician. Some conditions, such as pregnancy and immunosuppression, often require additional discussion and advance planning and may warrant delaying departure.

The Last-Minute, Extended-Stay Traveler: Advise these travelers to arrange an early visit with a qualified clinician at their destination for additional evaluation and education. A last-minute consultation does not provide an expatriate with adequate time for a full medical and psychological evaluation.

Requests for Off-Label Vaccine Dosing: Because of time constraints, some travelers may ask for a vaccine to be administered off-label (different schedule, double dosing, partial series). Using a vaccine in a nonstandard manner can have consequences that include medical-legal issues and inducing a false sense of protection in the traveler.

Recurring Last-Minute Travelers: Any clinic that frequently sees last-minute travelers may want to address this as a management issue. One option is to build some flexibility into the appointment schedule. Another option, which may be particularly relevant for clinics that are part of a corporation or university, is to attempt early identification of people who are likely to travel internationally and to intervene proactively.

BIBLIOGRAPHY

1. Centers for Disease Control and Prevention. Epidemiology and Prevention of Vaccine-Preventable Diseases. Hamborsky J, Kroger A, Wolfe S, eds. 13th ed. Washington D.C. Public Health Foundation; 2015 [cited 2016 Mar. 23]; Available from: http://www.cdc.gov/vaccines/pubs/pinkbook/index.html.

2. Chen LH, Leder K, Wilson ME. Business travelers: vaccination considerations for this population. Expert Rev Vaccines. 2013 Apr; 12(4):453–66.

3. Cramer JP, Jelninek T, Paulke-Korinek M, Reisinger EC, Dieckmann S, Alberer M, et al. One-year immunogenicity kinetics and safety of a purified chick embryo

cell rabies vaccine and inactivated Vero cell-derived Japanese encephalitis vaccine administered concomitantly according to a new, 1-week, accelerated primary series. J Travel Med. 2016 Mar;23 (3).

4. Sanford CA and EC Jong. Immunizations. Med Clin N Am. 2016;100: 247–259.

5. Zuckerman JN, Van Damme P, Van Herck K, Loscher T. Vaccination options for last-minute travellers in need of travel-related prophylaxis against hepatitis A and B and typhoid fever: a practical guide. Travel Med Infect Dis. 2003 Nov;1(4):219–26.

SPECIAL CONSIDERATIONS FOR US MILITARY DEPLOYMENTS

Mark Fukuda, Gregory A. Raczniak, Mark S. Riddle, Michael Forgione, Alan J. Magill

The US military, as a matter of policy, follows most of the recommendations in the CDC Yellow Book. However, certain situations apply only to the US military, and some policies or recommendations differ from what is recommended in the Yellow Book for civilian travel. Active-duty military physicians generally manage predeployment medicine, but civilian physicians may interact with people who are on reserve status, home on leave, recently discharged from active duty, or veterans. Predeployment and postdeployment information, policies, and guidelines for clinicians, service members and their families, and veterans can be found on the Deployment Health Clinical Center website (www.pdhealth.mil). The purpose of this section is to inform US military medical corps officers, who routinely consult the Yellow Book, about these differences. An additional purpose is to provide civilian clinicians who frequently see military personnel with background and available information sources regarding these differences and to emphasize their role in informing relevant findings to military care providers.

In many countries, one of the largest traveling populations is their military personnel. The military should be considered a special population with demographics, destinations, and needs that may differ from those of civilian travelers. This section focuses on the unique aspects of using pretravel vaccines and malaria chemoprophylaxis in the military population and on special considerations relevant to returning service members with health concerns. The specific examples will be from the US military, but the concepts may be applicable to other militaries. In 2016, approximately 1.3 million US military members were on active duty, and approximately 800,000 were in the reserve forces.

Several characteristics of the military force differ from those of the civilian population (Table 8-5). In general, the active duty military population is younger, in better health than the population at large, and predominately male.

FORCE HEALTH PROTECTION

Force health protection (FHP) is an important concept in military medicine. FHP is defined as all measures taken by commanders, supervisors, individual service members, and the military health system to promote, protect, improve, conserve, and restore the mental and physical well-being of service members across the range of military activities and operations. Delivery of vaccines and the use of malaria chemoprophylaxis agents are 2 aspects of FHP.

Medical interventions for FHP are the responsibility of the unit commander, with advice from the unit medical officer. When predeployment vaccines or malaria chemoprophylaxis are indicated, the commander includes such requirements in the mission plan. Service members are then required to receive these interventions under proper medical supervision. If a particular vaccine or drug is medically contraindicated, alternative

8

Table 8-5. Differences between military populations and civilian traveling populations

CHARACTERISTIC	TRAVEL MEDICINE	MILITARY MEDICINE
Primary focus	Individual	Unit
Goal	Optimizing advice and interventions for individual travelers	Ensuring mission success; optimizing advice and interventions for each person is difficult
Adherence	Strongly encouraged but travelers are free to choose	Required; vaccines and malaria chemoprophylaxis are part of force health protection (FHP)
Education	One-on-one encounters	Unit education
Population	Not prescreened; travel health providers see all ages and people with preexisting medical conditions	Prescreened; people with serious medical problems are not allowed to join the military or be deployed
Special populations	Infants, children, pregnant women, elderly people, people with renal or hepatic impairment and often taking other medications	Less frequent in military population or deployments
Disease comorbidity	Similar to civilian population	Limited, generally healthy
Sex	50% male, 50% female	85% male
Unusual activities	Adventure activities, such as trekking, climbing, scuba diving, spelunking	Housed in barracks or other group settings, aviators, Special Forces, operating complex weapons systems, hostile and extreme environments, stress of combat operations, night operations, and use of night-vision goggles
Duration of malaria chemoprophylaxis use	Mostly short term, 2–3 weeks	The US military often uses chemoprophylaxis for longer periods of time than do short-term travelers. Many deployments are for 1 year or longer.

agents may be employed if they are available. The unit medical officer documents which military personnel have not received standard preventive measures, so these people may receive additional monitoring or treatment if they become ill.

FHP policy positions in the Department of Defense (DoD) are issued as directives and instructions. All directives and instructions can be found online at www.dtic.mil/whs/directives. The Policy and Program for Immunizations to Protect the Health of Service Members and Military Beneficiaries is found in directive 6205. O2E (September 19, 2006) at www.dtic.mil/whs/ directives/corres/pdf/620502p.pdf. Although policy may be made at higher levels in Washington, DC, the final decision to use vaccines or malaria chemoprophylaxis under FHP is made by commanders in the field, guided by their medical staff. In certain circumstances, individual service members may be exempt from vaccination. There are 2 types of exemptions from immunization: medical and administrative. Granting medical exemptions is a medical function that can only be validated by a health care professional. Granting administrative exemptions is a nonmedical function, usually controlled by the person's unit commander.

ROUTINE AND TRAVEL-RELATED IMMUNIZATION

DoD policy states that the recommendations for immunization from CDC and the Advisory Committee for Immunization Practices shall generally be followed, consistent with requirements and guidance of the Food and Drug Administration (FDA) and with consideration for the unique needs of military settings and exposure risks. The Defense Health Agency (DHA) Immunization Healthcare Branch (IHB) [formerly the Military Vaccine Agency (MILVAX)] supports 5 branches of the US Armed Services to enhance military medical readiness by coordinating DoD immunization (vaccination) programs worldwide. A valuable source of service-specific information on immunizations for all branches of the US military is found at the DHA IHB website (www.health.mil/vaccines).

GEOGRAPHIC AREAS OF RESPONSIBILITY

The US military issues FHP recommendations based on geographic areas of responsibility (AOR) (www.vaccines.mil/QuickReference). Command and control over US military personnel in each AOR are under a unified combatant command, which is a joint (all branches of the US military) command that provides recommendations for all service members being deployed to that AOR. For example, Afghanistan is in the Central Command (CENTCOM) AOR. All personnel on orders to deploy or travel to Afghanistan should receive the vaccines listed in the "Vaccine Recommendations" tab of the above quick reference web page unless there is a medical contraindication.

MALARIA CHEMOPROPHYLAXIS

Preventing malaria in military units deployed to endemic areas is an essential objective of FHP. Malaria can be prevented through 1) education and training; 2) use of personal protection measures, which include individual bed nets, permethrin-impregnated uniforms, and insect repellents; and 3) use of chemoprophylaxis where indicated. The joint instruction on immunization and chemoprophylaxis stipulates that medical commanders designate trained staff to provide comprehensive malaria prevention counseling to military and civilian personnel considered to be at risk of contracting malaria and that such counseling "include instruction on how to take prescribed antimalarial medications, the importance of compliance with the prescribed medication schedule, information about potential adverse effects, and the need to seek medical care if these adverse effects occur."

Malaria cases seen in returning US military personnel reflect the current deployments around the world. In 2015, the number of malaria cases was the lowest in >20 years (30 cases). The number of cases declined with the continued drawdown of deployed personnel to Afghanistan from 2012 through 2015. The risk of *Plasmodium falciparum* malaria, which accounted for 43% of cases in 2015, is substantial for people with frequent training and development missions to sub-Saharan Africa (www.afhsc.mil/documents/pubs/msmrs/2016/v23_n01.pdf).

Several features of malaria chemoprophylaxis under FHP that are unique to the US military are derived from the activities and stressors of military deployments. When antimalarial drugs are used for chemoprophylaxis as part of FHP, the military can only use FDA-approved chemoprophylaxis agents in accordance with the specific FDA-approved indications. Off-label use of drugs is not allowed when given under FHP. If off-label use is felt to be in the best interest of the person or unit, trained and knowledgeable clinicians must provide one-on-one medical evaluations, document in the medical record the rationale for such use, and provide a by-name prescription for the drug or vaccine to each person.

In September 2011, United States Africa Command (AFRICOM) issued a policy change recommending atovaquone-proguanil (Malarone) as the recommended malaria chemoprophylaxis option for all personnel for both short- and long-term deployments in high-transmission areas of Africa. High-transmission areas for the purpose of this policy are defined by the National Center for Medical Intelligence. For practical purposes, this includes most of sub-Saharan Africa. For people who are unable to receive atovaquone-proguanil because of intolerance or contraindication, doxycycline is the preferred second-line therapy. Use of mefloquine as prophylaxis is a third-line recommendation for those unable to receive either atovaquone-proguanil or doxycycline. Before prescribing mefloquine for prophylaxis, absolute and relative contraindications as described in the approved product label must be considered.

In April 2013, the Assistant Secretary of Defense (Health Affairs) issued new guidance on medications to prevent malaria. Atovaquone-proguanil and doxycycline are both first-line choices in areas other than sub-Saharan Africa. Mefloquine should be reserved for people with intolerance or contraindications to both first-line medications. Before using mefloquine for prophylaxis, care should be taken to identify any contraindications on an individual basis and ensure required FDA mefloquine medication guide (www.accessdata.fda.gov/drugsatfda_docs/label/2013/076523s007lbl.pdf) is given to people prescribed mefloquine.

As a matter of policy, the US military routinely uses primaquine for presumptive antirelapse treatment (PART) in returning military populations to prevent the late relapse of *P. vivax* malaria or *P. ovale* malaria. PART is also referred to as "terminal prophylaxis." In PART, primaquine is given to otherwise healthy people on their departure from an endemic area. Primaquine is used for this indication much more frequently in the military than in most civilian travelers.

The FDA-approved regimen for PART is 15 mg (base) given daily for 14 days. This regimen was approved in 1952 and has not been revisited since. In the intervening decades, an overwhelming amount of data has accumulated to show that the total dose of primaquine to eliminate the dormant hypnozoite stages responsible for late relapses is dependent on the infecting *P. vivax* strain and the weight of the patient; therefore, the optimal human dose should be based on weight and adjusted for the infecting *P. vivax* strain.

In 2003, CDC recommended 30 mg (base) of primaquine daily for 14 days for PART based on available evidence, but the FDA-approved regimen remains the lower dose. Adherence to the daily 14-day regimen is poor unless primaquine is given under directly observed therapy, which is rarely done. As a result of noncompliance and subtherapeutic dosing with the 15 mg (base) for 14 days regimen, periodic outbreaks of relapsed

P. vivax malaria continue to occur in returning military personnel. Use of the higher-dose primaquine regimen for PART is now recommended for military personnel. This recommendation is consistent with the spirit of DoD issuance 6200.02 (February 17, 2008), in that the higher-dose recommendation for primaquine when used as PART is "standard medical practice in the United States."

Although primaquine is included as an acceptable alternative by CDC for primary prophylaxis in some countries where the risk of malaria is exclusively or mostly *P. vivax* malaria, primaquine is not FDA-approved for primary prophylaxis. Because use of primaquine for primary prophylaxis constitutes off-label use, it cannot be prescribed for a deploying group under FHP, but it can be prescribed by a licensed medical provider on an individual basis as part of medical practice.

The most important risk of using primaquine is hemolytic anemia in those who are deficient in G6PD. Current policy is for all US military personnel to be screened for G6PD deficiency on entry into military service. However, some people, such as reservists, may have deployed without testing, or clinicians may not be able to confirm results for all people in a unit requiring PART. Clinicians should be aware that hemolytic reactions to primaquine may occur in those with unrecognized G6PD deficiency.

A recurrent issue for military medicine is the correct timing of primaquine when given as PART in conjunction with the standard chemoprophylaxis drug being taken. Primaquine can be given at any time after personnel leave an endemic area. For convenience and for enhancing adherence to the 14-day regimen of primaquine, it is often best for military units to prescribe primaquine in the immediate 2 weeks after return. During this time, the units are often still at their home base completing their in-processing before block leave. Once personnel depart on leave, adherence and monitoring for side effects are more difficult.

Under FHP, military personnel are required to take their chemoprophylaxis agents as prescribed to maintain mission readiness. Individual soldiers do not have the right to refuse an order given under FHP. There is great variability in practice as to how seriously individual commanders enforce

8

these policies, however, and continued outbreaks of malaria occur in military populations because of poor compliance.

Differences between civilian and US military use of chemoprophylaxis drugs are summarized in Table 8-6.

Table 8-6. Differences between CDC recommendations and US military's use of malaria chemoprophylaxis

	CDC RECOMMENDATION	US MILITARY POLICY
Choice of malaria chemoprophylaxis agent	Chemoprophylaxis guidelines do not recommend one drug versus another, but rather emphasize the goal of tailoring the recommendation for the individual traveler on the basis of past experience, itinerary, possible drug interaction, potential side effects, costs, and medical contraindications such as drug allergies.	Individualizing advice and recommendations for large military deployments is rarely logistically possible or feasible. Recognizing this reality, in April 2013, the US military adopted a new policy on the use of malaria chemoprophylaxis in the US military. Atovaquone-proguanil and doxycycline are now the first-line drugs of choice to prevent malaria in deployed US military forces in all areas other than sub-Saharan Africa. Atovaquone-proguanil is the drug of choice for short-term travel (up to 2 or 3 weeks) and for people who travel frequently, to minimize long postexposure prophylaxis treatment courses. In September 2011, AFRICOM policy changed to recommending atovaquone-proguanil for most destinations in sub-Saharan Africa.
Doxycycline	An option for chemoprophylaxis in all areas.	Recommended first-line chemoprophylaxis choice in all areas other than sub-Saharan Africa.
Mefloquine	An option for chemoprophylaxis in all areas except Southeast Asia.	Mefloquine is not recommended as a primary option. It should be reserved for people with intolerance or contraindications to atovaquone-proguanil and doxycycline. Before using mefloquine for prophylaxis, care should be taken to identify any contraindications on an individual basis and ensure the required FDA mefloquine medication guide (www.accessdata.fda.gov/drugsatfda_docs/label/2013/076523s007lbl.pdf) is given to people prescribed mefloquine.
Atovaquone-proguanil	An option for chemoprophylaxis in all areas.	Atovaquone-proguanil is the drug of choice for sub-Saharan Africa and a first-line option in all other areas.
Primaquine chemoprophylaxis	CDC recommends the use of primaquine as primary chemoprophylaxis in geographic areas with mainly *Plasmodium vivax* malaria.	There is no FDA-approved indication for the use of primaquine to prevent malaria. Therefore, the US military cannot use primaquine as a chemoprophylaxis agent under current FHP guidelines.
PART	Primaquine at 30 mg (base) for 14 days.	There is no FDA-approved indication for the use of primaquine at the higher dose of 30 mg (base) for 14 days. However, primaquine is an FDA-approved drug with an indication for PART. The CDC-recommended (higher) dose is recommended, as it is the standard of medical practice in the United States.

Abbreviations: AFRICOM, African Command; FDA, Food and Drug Administration; FHP, Force Health Protection; PART, presumptive antirelapse treatment.

UNIQUE NEEDS FOR THE MILITARY

US military personnel may encounter threats, such as biological warfare agents, that are not usually considered for civilian travelers. Vaccines, immunoglobulins, drug prophylaxis, and drug treatment regimens can be given under FHP, but only in accordance with FDA-licensed products and regimens and for FDA-approved indications.

Products not approved by the FDA are given to soldiers only with voluntary informed consent under an institutional review board-approved protocol and in accordance with a current and FDA-approved investigational new drug application.

Only under exceptional circumstances would products not approved by the FDA be given to soldiers without informed consent. This circumstance is governed by emergency use authorization procedures. Section 564 of the Federal Food, Drug, and Cosmetic Act (21 USC 360bbb-3), as amended by the Project BioShield Act of 2004 (Public Law 108–276), permits the FDA commissioner to authorize the use of an unapproved medical product or an unapproved use of an approved medical product during a declared emergency involving a heightened risk of attack on the public or US military forces, or when there is a potential to affect national security.

THE RETURNING SERVICE MEMBER WITH HEALTH CONCERNS

Symptoms and health concerns after a deployment may be similar to health issues reported from nonmilitary returning travelers. However, deployment presents a different set of circumstances from the civilian traveler such as differential vaccination recommendations, physical and psychological stress and trauma of combat, environmental exposures, and infections that may cause unique health concerns. In 2002, the US Department of Defense developed and mandated the use of the Post-Deployment Health Clinical Practice Guideline (PDH-CPG) under Health Affairs Policy 02-007. The PDH-CPG is designed to help clinicians implement specific approaches to address these distinctive experiences and exposures and includes clinical tools and resources to evaluate and manage patients with the full spectrum of deployment-related concerns. The goal of the PDH-CPG is to promote evidence-based management of people with postdeployment health concerns, identify the critical decision points in managing patients with postdeployment health concerns, allow flexibility so that local policies or procedures such as those regarding referrals to or consultation with specialists, and improve local management of patients with postdeployment health concerns and thereby improve patient outcomes.

DISCLOSURE

Drs. Forgione, Fukuda, and Riddle are employees of the Department of Defense and as such, the views expressed in this section are those of the authors and do not necessarily reflect the official policy or position of the Departments of the Air Force, Army, or Navy, nor the Department of Defense.

BIBLIOGRAPHY

1. Armed Forces Health Surveillance Center. Update: Malaria, U.S. Armed Forces, 2015. MSMR. 2016 Jan;23(1):2–6.

2. Brisson M, Brisson P. Compliance with antimalaria chemoprophylaxis in a combat zone. Am J Trop Med Hyg. 2012 Apr;86(4):587–90.

3. Carr ME, Jr., Fandre MN, Oduwa FO. Glucose-6-phosphate dehydrogenase deficiency in two returning Operation Iraqi Freedom soldiers who developed hemolytic anemia while receiving primaquine prophylaxis for malaria. Mil Med. 2005 Apr;170(4):273–6.

4. Food and Drug Administration. Emergency use authorization of medical products. Rockville, MD: Food and Drug Administration; 2007 [cited 2016 Sep. 27]; Available from: http://www.fda.gov/RegulatoryInformation/Guidances/ucm125127.htm.

5. Office of the Assistant Secretary of Defense (Health Affairs). HA-Policy 13-002. Guidance on medications for prophylaxis of malaria. Washington, DC 2013 Apr 15; [cited 2016 Sep. 27]; Available from: http://www.health.mil/~/media/MHS/Policy%20Files/Import/13-002.ashx.

6. Townell N, Looke D, McDougall D, McCarthy JS. Relapse of imported *Plasmodium vivax* malaria is related to

primaquine dose: a retrospective study. Malar J. 2012 Jun 22;11(1):214.

7. US Africa Command. Force Health Protection procedures for deployment and travel 2011; [cited 2016 Sep. 27]; Available from: http://www.med.navy.mil/sites/nepmu2/Documents/threat_assessment/AFRICOM-FHP-Guidance-22SEP11.pdf.

8. US Department of Defense. Department of Defense directive: Force Health Protection (FHP), no. 6200.04. Washington, DC: US Department of Defense; 2004 [updated 2007 Apr 23; cited 2016 Sep. 27]; Available from: http://www.dtic.mil/whs/directives/corres/pdf/620004p.pdf

9. US Department of Defense. Department of Defense instruction: application of Food and Drug Administration (FDA) rules to Department of Defense Force Health Protection programs, no 6200.02. Washington, DC: US Department of Defense; 2008 [cited 2016 Sep. 27]; Available from: http://www.dtic.mil/whs/directives/corres/pdf/620002p.pdf.

10. Whitman TJ, Coyne PE, Magill AJ, Blazes DL, Green MD, Milhous WK, et al. An outbreak of *Plasmodium falciparum* malaria in US Marines deployed to Liberia. Am J Trop Med Hyg. 2010 Aug;83(2):258–65.

STUDY ABROAD & OTHER INTERNATIONAL STUDENT TRAVEL

Gary Rhodes, Inés DeRomaña, Bettina N. Pedone

Study abroad can be a life-changing and positive experience. However, with increasing numbers of students choosing to study in regions where health and safety concerns differ from those in the United States, students and their families must plan for and understand the risks of such travel. This planning should include researching the policies of the study-abroad program administrator, learning about health and safety risks at the destination, making plans to mitigate those risks, and obtaining advice from a health care professional before departure.

Study-abroad programs vary in structure and staffing, the support provided by the program, and obligations placed on students. Some institutions have several employees dedicated to supporting study-abroad programs while others have no full-time staff members. Some hire specialized professionals to focus on health and safety issues; others have no staff dedicated to such support. Some institutions require students to carry insurance that includes accident and illness coverage, 24-hour emergency assistance, emergency medical evacuation, and repatriation. Other institutions may recommend obtaining travel insurance for study abroad but may provide limited or no information about available options.

Whether or not a university offers pretravel health clinic support, students should consult with a medical professional as a part of the planning process. This consultation should include information on endemic health issues in the host country, travel vaccinations, availability and legality of medications commonly prescribed in the United States, and information on how to obtain medical care abroad.

PREDEPARTURE PLANNING

Program professionals should collaborate with institutional health practitioners to provide students with comprehensive pretravel consultations that include an assessment of the student's health and immunization history, length of program, destination country, activities, and other travel the student will undertake while abroad. The consultation should also cover the following:

- Country- and region-specific health and environmental information

- A plan for continued treatment while abroad

- Gender-specific health information

- Required, recommended, and routine vaccinations

- Recommended prophylactic and self-treatment medications and first aid kit (see Chapter 2, Travel Health Kits)

- Advice and resources for students with special needs, including specific plans for students with preexisting conditions that include provisions for medications, ongoing care, and emergency treatment

- Information about physiologic and psychological consequences students may encounter as a result of culture shock or changes in routine

- General advice on nutrition and dietary deficiencies

- Cautions about alcohol and drug use and a specific plan for those with preexisting dependency issues

- Rabies education (avoid feeding or petting animals, and postexposure measures)

- Bloodborne pathogens precautions (needles, blood products, tattoos, piercing, surgeries, acupuncture) and safe sex (including emergency contraception)

- General instructions for emergency medical situations, including locating a physician abroad (see Chapter 2, Obtaining Health Care Abroad)

- Illness and accident insurance policies and emergency assistance coverage information, including medical and evacuation insurance

- Pretravel medical and dental exams and treatment as indicated

Before departure, program professionals and health practitioners should encourage students to learn about the countries they will visit to better understand the health and safety issues there, as well as the cultural and political climate. The information in the Humanitarian Aid Workers section earlier in this chapter can be useful for students participating in study abroad, internships, field studies, community service projects, or research in the developing world.

The Department of State's online resource for students (http://studentsabroad.state.gov) includes information to help students plan healthy and safe experiences abroad. Their travel website (http://travel.state.gov) provides country-specific information, including guidance on crime and transportation safety. Advise students to be aware of possible travel warnings or travel alerts and to consider this information when making travel decisions. Students also should know how to get help from a US embassy or consulate in an emergency. Encourage students who are not US citizens to contact their country's embassy or consulate in the United States and in the countries where they will be traveling to find out what support their country may provide.

Before departure, students should register with the Department of State's Smart Traveler Enrollment Program (STEP, https://step.state.gov/step). Program professionals may be able to register their students as a group with STEP.

The CDC Travelers' Health website (www.cdc.gov/travel) contains advice for travelers on the most current health recommendations for international destinations. Other resources for study abroad are provided in Table 8-7.

HEALTH AND SAFETY WHILE ABROAD

Food and Water Safety

Food and water contamination is one of the leading causes of illness for travelers. Basic precautions can minimize the risk of diarrhea and other illnesses. Specific food and water recommendations depend on the destination country. In most developing countries, the only safe sources of water are factory-sealed bottles or water that has been purified (see Chapter 2, Water Disinfection for Travelers). Advise students to avoid ice in drinks, as the ice may have been made with unsafe water.

Cooked foods should be eaten hot; raw fruits and vegetables should be eaten only if they have been washed in clean water or peeled by the traveler. Poor refrigeration, undercooked meat, and food purchased from street vendors could pose problems related to food contamination. See Chapter 2, Food and Water Precautions for more information. Travelers may also wish to download CDC's Can I Eat This? app (wwwnc.cdc.gov/travel/page/apps-about) for on-the-go safe food and water guidance.

Table 8-7. Study-abroad resources

ORGANIZATION	DESCRIPTION
NAFSA: Association of International Educators www.nafsa.org	Useful information for institutions implementing study-abroad programs, as well as information for students to support their health and safety
Responsible Study Abroad: Good Practices for Health & Safety, by the Interorganizational Task Force for Safety and Responsibility in Study Abroad www.nafsa.org/Professional_Resources/Browse_ by_Interest/Education_Abroad/Network_Resources/ Education_Abroad/Responsible_Study_Abroad__ Good_Practices_for_Health___Safety/	Advice for developing plans and procedures to implement good practices for program sponsors, students, and parents/guardians/families, especially those pertaining to health and safety issues
Council on Standards for International Educational Travel (CSIET) http://csiet.org	Standards for exchange programs for US high school and middle school students going abroad Health and safety good practices
Center for Global Education, SAFETI (Safety Abroad First–Educational Travel Information) Clearinghouse http://globaled.us/safeti	Resources to support study-abroad program development and implementation, emphasizing health and safety issues and resources for US colleges and universities offering study abroad
SAFETI Program Audit Checklist http://globaled.us/SAFETI/program_audit_checklist.asp http://studentsabroad.com	List of health and safety and study-abroad issues to guide institutions' policies and procedures Resource website for students that includes a country-specific handbook
GlobalScholar.us and GlobalStudent.us: Online Learning for Study Abroad http://globalscholar.us http://globalstudent.us	University and high school–level online courses that provide students with helpful information, including health and safety information before, during, and after study abroad
Forum on Education Abroad www.forumea.org	Standards of good practice, a code of ethics, and health and safety and other resources for institutions and organizations that sponsor and support study-abroad programs
Federal Bureau of Investigation https://www.fbi.gov/file-repository/student-travel-brochure-pdf.pdf/view	A brochure that introduces students to threats they may face and provides tips on avoiding unsafe situations

Adherence to Host Country Laws and Codes of Conduct

The rules and regulations of the host country, city, region, and institution may differ from those at home. Students should be counseled that they must abide by the legal system of their host country. Additional information on host country laws may be found on the Department of State website (http://travel.state.gov).

Mental and Physical Health

International travel can be stressful for many reasons. Dealing with stressful situations abroad may be difficult for students away from their familiar support systems and could trigger mental and physical issues. Existing health conditions can be made worse when adjusting to unfamiliar food, a different climate, and different time zones. To minimize potential problems, students must consider their own mental and physical well-being when deciding on an experience abroad and discuss their destination, local resources, and any existing medical or mental health issues with their families and health professionals.

The NAFSA: Association of International Educators' publication, "Best Practices in Addressing Mental Health Issues Affecting Education Abroad Participants" (www.nafsa.org/mentalhealth) encourages study-abroad programs "to sensitively offer support that connects the student to professional help before a problem reaches a crisis state or seriously derails the student's academic and career plans."

Students should be encouraged to disclose any chronic physical or mental health conditions or accommodation needs before departure. Program professionals can encourage students' disclosure by assuring confidentiality and explaining that the information is needed to facilitate a safe experience while abroad—not to prevent them from going.

Once a student has disclosed a chronic or mental health condition, health care professionals can assist with planning for care while abroad. Engaging students in a discussion about potential scenarios they may encounter can help determine their acumen for problem solving and can reveal areas that need further attention before departure. Mobility International USA (www.miusa.org) provides information and resources to support study abroad by students with special needs and can be contacted directly for assistance.

Prescription Medication

Medications commonly prescribed in the United States may not be legal or available in the host country. Well before departure, students should check with the US embassy or consulate in the host country or the International Narcotics Control Board (https://www.incb.org) regarding the legality of their prescription medications—particularly if they take narcotic or psychotropic drugs. They also should discuss with their health care providers whether some medications should be changed, and allow sufficient time to make adjustments before departure. Students should avoid switching medications immediately before departure and should not discontinue prescribed

medications while abroad unless instructed by a health care professional.

Students must travel with a signed prescription for all medications. The prescription must indicate the name of the student, the name of the medication (both brand name and generic), and the dosage and quantity prescribed. The student should also have a letter from the US treating physician explaining the recommended dosage, the student's diagnosis, and the treatment. This is especially important for controlled substances and injectable medications. Translations of these documents to the host country language may be helpful. It is a good idea to leave copies of prescriptions with a family member or friend at home. In most countries, arriving with quantities exceeding those prescribed for personal use is prohibited. Students should pack all medications in the original, labeled containers in their carry-on baggage.

Many countries consider marijuana to be illegal. A student possessing marijuana, even with a valid US prescription, may be arrested, prosecuted, and jailed or deported.

If the anticipated term of study exceeds 90 days, students should ask if their doctor can write prescriptions for more than 90 days of medication and should fill all prescriptions before departure, if possible. This reduces the need to purchase medication overseas and lowers the risk of exposure to counterfeit or poor-quality medications abroad (see Chapter 2, *Perspectives: Pharmaceutical Quality & Falsified Drugs*).

US prescriptions are not accepted by pharmacies overseas. Shipping or mailing medications may not be viable options because many countries' laws prohibit the mailing of drugs, including prescription medicines. Students who anticipate the need to refill a prescription while abroad must plan to be assessed by a local doctor to obtain a local prescription. Students need to determine whether these appointments will be covered by their insurance policy, as they may be considered preventive care and thus not covered by the policy.

How to Access Medical Care Abroad

Adequate medical care may not be available at all destinations. Providing information to students about quality-of-care issues abroad is important. Serious medical problems may require emergency medical evacuation, which is why students should have accident and illness travel insurance that includes medical evacuation coverage. Many foreign doctors and hospitals may require full cash payment in advance of treatment, as they do not accept US insurance policies. Insurance requirements and limitations may reduce reimbursements. Many students who will need ongoing care while abroad may have to make special arrangements with their insurance travel assistance provider before departure, particularly if the continued care will be expensive. Frank discussions about these issues should take place well in advance of departure.

If the student is covered by travel insurance while abroad, the plan provider may be able to issue a referral for a local doctor. US embassies and consulates maintain a list of doctors and medical facilities in the regions they serve. To locate a US embassy or consulate, visit www.usembassy.gov. Once on the website, look for the lists under the US Citizens Services section of the embassy or consulate website.

For more detailed information, consult Chapter 2: Obtaining Health Care Abroad and Travel Insurance, Travel Health Insurance, & Medical Evacuation Insurance.

Emergency Contacts and Emergency Preparedness

Instruct students to print and fill out an emergency information card with contact numbers and personal information and carry a copy with them at all times. If one is not provided by the program, a sample can be found at http://studentsabroad.com/emergencycard.asp. Students should provide friends and family members at home with emergency contact information for their destination, and should provide study-abroad program officials and the host school with their emergency contacts at home. Students may want to consider programming emergency contact information into their smartphones, if available.

Students should keep program staff and home emergency contacts informed of their whereabouts and activities and provide them with copies of their travel documents (passport, visa, plane tickets, prescriptions) and itinerary. Developing an emergency plan and testing it soon after arrival abroad can help students respond more effectively if a health or safety incident occurs. Resources to help develop and implement an emergency action plan can be found at http://studentsabroad.com/handbook/crisis-management.php.

Sexual Harassment and Sexual Violence

Student travelers will need predeparture information about sexual harassment and assault abroad. Sexual assault can happen to anyone and at any time and any place. Encourage students to watch out for one another and to get advice and information from program administrators.

Transportation and Pedestrian Safety

Traffic crashes are a major cause of injury to students while traveling abroad. Vehicular traffic is not always regulated to the extent it is in the United States, and traffic laws may differ. For instance, students should be made aware of countries where traffic travels on the left side of the road instead of the right as in the United States. If not aware, students may look in the wrong direction for oncoming traffic and risk being hit by a car.

Students should also be counseled to choose safe and legitimate modes of travel in their destination countries. Each US Department of State country information sheet includes "Traffic Safety and Road Conditions" content to help assess conditions in a specific country. A good source of information on transportation safety is the Association for Safe International Road Travel at www.asirt.org.

Water and Swimming Safety

Students must be careful and informed about water safety before approaching unfamiliar bodies of water. Warn students not to swim alone or on beaches where there are no lifeguards or warning signs.

Swimming in contaminated water can put students at risk for contracting certain infectious diseases. Inform students about common waterborne pathogens, especially those in freshwater.

Building and Fire Safety

Students should think about building safety at their destination, including the potential impact of earthquakes, wind damage or flooding, and substandard building standards or maintenance practices. Fire safety is of particular concern. Students should evaluate buildings for the presence of functioning smoke alarms, fire extinguishers, emergency ladders, and fire exits.

Air Pollution

Air pollution is a problem in many cities around the world and can exacerbate symptoms for students with chronic health conditions. Even if students are healthy, they may experience temporary symptoms such as irritation of the eyes, nose, and throat; coughing; phlegm; chest tightness; and shortness of breath.

Alcohol and Drugs

The misuse of alcohol and drugs can increase the risk of accidents, injury, unwanted attention, and theft. Being in a foreign environment requires the ability to respond to new and changing circumstances, which can be impaired under the influence of drugs or alcohol. Many students are not of legal drinking age in the United States but are in the host country. Many do not receive adequate alcohol- and drug-prevention education explaining the consequences of risky drinking and drug abuse before departure. Violating drug laws abroad may result in serious consequences. In some countries, being found guilty of violating drug laws can lead to life in prison or the death penalty. Study-abroad professionals, in collaboration with institutional experts, should conduct a proper orientation about the risks associated with drinking and using drugs abroad.

Bloodborne Pathogens and Safe-Sex Precautions

Advise students on risk factors associated with the use of needles, blood products, tattoos, piercing, surgeries, and acupuncture. Most people are aware of the risk of contaminated needles, but students also need to know that the water used to create tattoo ink is often shared and can be contaminated with bloodborne pathogens.

Students should be encouraged to be prepared. Have frank conversations about safe sex (bring adequate condoms, birth control, and emergency contraception) and encourage students to educate themselves on social customs of their host city and country with regard to dating, public displays of affection, and sexual intimacy.

BIBLIOGRAPHY

1. Forum on Education Abroad. Code of ethics for education abroad. Carlisle, PA: Forum on Education Abroad; 2008 [cited 2016 Sep. 27]; Available from: https://forumea.org/resources/standards-of-good-practice/code-of-ethics/.

2. Gore J, Green J. Issues and advising responsibilities. NAFSA's Guide to Education Abroad for Advisors and Administrators. 3rd ed. Washington, DC: NAFSA Association of International Educators; 2005. p. 261.

3. Institute of International Education. Americans study abroad in increasing numbers. New York: Institute of International Education; 2009 [cited 2016 Sep. 27]; Available from: http://www.iie.org/en/Who-We-Are/News-and-Events/Press-Center/Press-Releases/2009/2009-11-16-Americans-Study-Abroad-Increasing.

4. Institute of International Education. Host regions of US study abroad students, 2012/13-2013/14. New York: Institute of International Education; 2013 [cited 2016 Sep. 27]; Available from: http://www.iie.org/Research-and-Publications/Open-Doors/Data/US-Study-Abroad/Leading-Destinations/2012-14.

5. Interorganizational Task Force on Safety and Responsibility in Study Abroad. Responsible study abroad: good practices for health and safety. Washington, DC: NAFSA: Association of International Educators; 2002 [cited 2016 Sep. 27]; Available from: http://www.nafsa.org/Find_Resources/Supporting_Study_Abroad/Network_Resources/Education_Abroad/Responsible_Study_Abroad__Good_Practices_for_Health___Safety/.

6. NAFSA: Association of International Educators. Best practices in addressing mental health issues affecting education abroad participants. Washington, DC: NAFSA: Association of International Educators; 2006 [cited 2016 Sep. 27]; Available from: http://www.nafsa.org/mentalhealth.

7. Pedersen ER, LaBrie JW, Hummer JF. Perceived behavioral alcohol norms predict drinking for college students while studying abroad. J Stud Alcohol Drugs. 2009;70(6):924–8.

TRAVEL TO MASS GATHERINGS

Joanna Gaines, Gary W. Brunette

OVERVIEW

Mass gatherings are typically defined as a large number of people (1,000 to >25,000) at a specific location, for a specific purpose. More practically speaking, a mass gathering can be thought of as any assembly of people that is large enough to strain local resources. Travelers to mass gatherings face unique risks because these events are associated with environmental hazards, increased infectious disease transmission due to the influx of attendees, crowding, poor hygiene from temporary food and sanitation facilities, and challenging security situations.

CHARACTERISTICS OF MASS GATHERINGS

Medical providers preparing travelers and travelers themselves should understand the characteristics of any mass gathering a patient will attend. These events can be spontaneous, such as a political protest; others are planned events. Some mass gatherings regularly occur at different locations, such as the Olympic Games or the FIFA World Cup, while others recur in the same location, such as the Hajj or Wimbledon. Mass gatherings can be effectively described in terms of their location, venue, purpose, size, participants, duration, timing, activities, and capacity.

- **Location:** Factors to consider include the host country, available infrastructure, the local environment, and the adequacy of security arrangements.

- **Venue:** Facilities vary widely, and events may be held indoors or outdoors. Facilities, including food, water, and sanitation, may be of varying quality.

- **Purpose:** Mass gatherings can be political, religious, social, or athletic; the purpose of an event can affect the activities and mood of participants.

- **Size:** Densely packed crowds may facilitate disease spread or induce riots or crowd crush disasters.

- **Participants:** Attendees may represent a unique demographic or may vary by features such as sex or age.

- **Duration:** The longer an event lasts, the more likely local resources will become strained.

- **Timing:** Mass gatherings and local capacity are affected by the timing of an event. Weather, heavy tourism, and other factors can affect the ability of a host to organize a safe mass gathering.

- **Activities:** Understand the activities that the traveler may participate in: some may be risky or strenuous or may involve alcohol or drug use.

- **Capacity:** Hosts differ in terms of their ability to detect, respond to, and prevent public health emergencies. Understanding what health outcomes have been previously associated with recurring mass gatherings can help travelers prepare for future events.

HEALTH CONCERNS RELATED TO MASS GATHERINGS

Existing medical conditions may be exacerbated during a mass gathering. Emergency medical services are often involved in preparations and are usually equipped to address acute medical conditions such as myocardial infarction and asthma. Conditions such as heat exhaustion, dehydration, hypothermia, or sunburn are usually handled on site as well.

Catastrophic incidents are of particular concern with mass gatherings. Numerous casualties at mass gatherings have occurred as the result of poor crowd management, structural collapses, fires, and violence.

Mass gathering attendees also are at risk for infectious disease. Previous mass gatherings have been associated with outbreaks of influenza, meningococcal disease, and norovirus. Mass gatherings also have implications for global health security. Travelers to mass gatherings may import diseases to a host site as well as spread disease when they return home.

GUIDANCE FOR CLINICIANS
Assessing Risk

- **Ask travelers about their itineraries and activities.** Verify a traveler's itinerary to identify risks beyond those associated with the event. Patients may add side trips or extend travel beyond the mass gathering.

- **Consider your patient's unique characteristics.** Chronic health conditions may be exacerbated by activities at a mass gathering. Patients should ensure they have adequate supplies of medication for the duration of their trip as well as documentation for any prescriptions.

Mitigating Risk

- **Identify requirements** for mass gathering attendees beyond those required for entry to a country. For example, all participants in the Hajj, the Islamic pilgrimage to Mecca, are required to have meningococcal vaccinations, whereas other travelers to Saudi Arabia are not required to have these.

- **Identify recommendations** for attendees, as host sites may make additional recommendations on the basis of public health concerns. After the emergence of the Middle East respiratory syndrome (MERS) coronavirus, Saudi Arabia recommended that elderly or immunocompromised people delay their pilgrimage.

- **Educate travelers on preventive measures.** These may include the use of insect repellent or advice on how to choose safe food and water from vendors. All travelers to mass gatherings should be educated on the importance of regular handwashing and the use of alcohol-based sanitizer when sanitation facilities are not available.

- **Visit the CDC Travelers' Health website at** www.cdc.gov/travel. This website is regularly updated with travel health notices; information may also be provided on mass gatherings such as the Hajj or Olympic Games.

GUIDANCE FOR TRAVELERS

- **Consult a travel medicine provider at least 4–6 weeks before the departure date.** This should allow adequate time to receive most vaccinations. Discuss your itinerary and any planned activities with your provider so that he or she can make more accurate recommendations to ensure your health and safety. If a travel medicine provider is not locally available, a primary care provider should be able to assist you with ensuring you have the adequate vaccinations and health information necessary.

- **Register with the Department of State's Smart Traveler Enrollment Program (STEP, https://step.state.gov/step).** Travelers can subscribe for notifications on travel warnings, travel alerts, and other information for their specific destination(s), as well as ensure that the Department of State is aware of a traveler's presence in the event of serious legal, medical, or financial difficulties while traveling. In the event of an emergency at home, STEP can also help friends and family reach travelers abroad.

- **Ensure any existing medical conditions are well controlled before departure.** Travelers should discuss their medical history with their medical provider during the pretravel consultation.

- **Visit the CDC Travelers' Health website at** www.cdc.gov/travel. Learn more about specific destinations and view any travel notices for your destination.

BIBLIOGRAPHY

1. Abubakar I, Gautret P, Brunette GW, Blumberg L, Johnson D, Poumerol G, et al. Global perspectives for prevention of infectious diseases associated with mass gatherings. Lancet Infect Dis. 2012 Jan;12(1):66–74.

2. Arbon P. Mass-gathering medicine: a review of the evidence and future directions for research. Prehosp Disaster Med. 2007 Mar-Apr;22(2):131–5.

3. Emergency Management Australia. Safe and healthy mass gatherings: a health, medical and safety planning manual for public events. Fyshwick (Australia): Commonwealth of Australia; 1999 [cited 2016 Sep. 28]; Available from: http://www.health.sa.gov.au/pehs/publications/ema-mass-gatherings-manual.pdf.

4. Lombardo JS, Sniegoski CA, Loschen WA, Westercamp M, Wade M, Dearth S, et al. Public health surveillance for mass gatherings. Johns Hopkins APL Technical Digest. 2008;27(4):1–9.

5. McCloskey B, Endericks T. Learning from London 2012: a practical guide to public health and mass gatherings. London: 2013 2016 Sep 28. Report No.

6. Milsten AM, Maguire BJ, Bissell RA, Seaman KG. Mass-gathering medical care: a review of the literature. Prehosp Disaster Med. 2002 Jul-Sep;17(3):151–62.

7. Steffen R, Bouchama A, Johansson A, Dvorak J, Isla N, Smallwood C, et al. Non-communicable health risks during mass gatherings. Lancet Infect Dis. 2012 Feb;12(2):142–9.

8. World Health Organization. Communicable disease alert and response for mass gatherings: key considerations. Geneva: World Health Organization; 2008 [cited 2016 Sep 28]; Available from: http://www.who.int/csr/Mass_gatherings2.pdf.

NEWLY ARRIVED IMMIGRANTS & REFUGEES

Michelle Russell, Hope Pogemiller, Elizabeth D. Barnett

8

More than 1 million immigrants obtained legal permanent resident status in the United States during fiscal year (FY) 2014. The Department of Homeland Security reported that 535,126 of these immigrants were already living in the United States, and 481,392 arrived directly from their country of origin. In addition, 69,987 refugees were admitted into the US during FY 2014. Table 8-8 lists the top 10 countries of origin for refugee and new immigrant arrivals in FY 2014.

The Immigration and Nationality Act (INA) mandates that all immigrants and refugees undergo a medical screening examination to identify inadmissible health conditions. This examination is performed by authorized physicians in the applicants' countries of origin or in the United States for applicants adjusting their status after arrival. A panel physician is a medical doctor practicing outside the United States who has an agreement with a US embassy or consulate general to conduct preimmigration medical screening; >600 panel physicians perform these examinations internationally. A civil surgeon is a US physician authorized by US Citizenship and Immigration Services (USCIS) to perform official immigration medical examinations required for the adjustment of status after arrival in the United States (the process of becoming a permanent US resident).

CDC's Division of Global Migration and Quarantine (DGMQ) issues *Technical Instructions* to panel physicians and civil surgeons who conduct the required medical examinations for immigrants and refugees. CDC also issues recommendations for premigration health interventions for special populations, such as refugees, before travel to the United States; these recommended health interventions are not required under the INA (such as treatment for parasitic diseases). CDC's predeparture recommendations for refugees are implemented based on risk in the origin country and when funding and logistical support are available. CDC's premigration guidelines for refugee populations are available at www.

Table 8-8. Top 10 countries of birth for newly arriving refugees and immigrants (from overseas locations), fiscal year 2014

REFUGEE ARRIVALS		IMMIGRANT ARRIVALS	
COUNTRY OF BIRTH	NUMBER OF ARRIVING REFUGEES	COUNTRY OF BIRTH	NUMBER OF ARRIVING IMMIGRANTS
Iraq	19,651	Mexico	61,862
Burma	14,578	Dominican Republic	36,839
Somalia	9,011	China, People's Republic	36,562
Bhutan	8,316	Philippines	31,275
Dem. Rep. Congo	4,502	India	27,046
Cuba	4,063	Vietnam	25,260
Iran	2,833	Pakistan	14,117
Eritrea	1,445	Bangladesh	13,313
Sudan	1,307	El Salvador	11,661
Afghanistan	758	Jamaica	11,174

cdc.gov/immigrantrefugeehealth/guidelines/overseas/overseas-guidelines.html. Refugees are not required by federal regulations to repeat health screening upon arrival in the United States; however, systems are in place in all states for refugees to receive a health assessment shortly after arrival. These may be carried out by any qualified health professional and are usually done in coordination with resettlement volunteer agencies and local health departments. CDC's postarrival guidelines for refugee screening are available at www.cdc.gov/immigrantrefugeehealth/guidelines/domestic/domestic-guidelines.html. Specific protocols may vary by state and are usually available on the websites of the departments of health in the state or region.

The prearrival medical exam is only performed by panel physicians for those applicants who apply for immigrant or refugee status prior to arrival in the United States. US health care providers may encounter a larger number of immigrants in their clinical practice who have not entered the United States on an immigrant or refugee visa (some categories of temporary visitors and undocumented migrants) and, therefore, have not received this immigrant medical exam.

BEFORE ARRIVAL IN THE UNITED STATES

Overseas Medical Examination and Treatment

CDC provides *Technical Instructions* to panel physicians and monitors the quality of the premigration medical examination process. The purpose of the mandated medical examination is to detect inadmissible conditions, including communicable diseases of public health significance, mental disorders associated with harmful behavior, and substance-use or substance-induced disorders (www.cdc.gov/immigrantrefugeehealth/exams/ti/panel/technical-instructions-panel-physicians.

html). For certain refugee populations, a visit to the panel physician also provides an opportunity for health interventions such as presumptive therapy for parasitic diseases, including nematode infections and malaria (www.cdc.gov/immigrantrefugeehealth/guidelines/refugee-guidelines.html).

The medical examination includes a physical examination, mental health evaluation, syphilis serologic testing, review of vaccination records, and chest radiography followed by acid-fast bacillus smears and sputum cultures if the chest radiograph is consistent with tuberculosis (TB). Chest radiographs are required for all applicants ≥15 years of age. Applicants 2–14 years of age from high-TB-burden countries (incidence rate ≥20 cases per 100,000 population as estimated by the World Health Organization) must be tested for TB infection using either a tuberculin skin test (TST) or interferon-γ release assay (IGRA); chest radiographs are required for those who have a positive TST or IGRA. For people diagnosed with active TB, CDC's *Technical Instructions* require *Mycobacterium tuberculosis* culture, drug susceptibility testing, and directly observed therapy through the end of treatment before immigration. Treatment is also required before immigration for certain other inadmissible conditions, such as specific sexually transmitted diseases (such as syphilis) and Hansen disease.

Proof of Vaccination

IMMIGRANTS

Applicants who apply for a US immigrant visa outside the United States are required to receive all age-appropriate immunizations before immigrating to the United States. Vaccines are administered by panel physicians according to CDC's *Vaccine Technical Instructions*. These requirements are based on the Advisory Committee on Immunization Practices (ACIP) recommendations, with some modifications for immigrant populations. For example, immigrants are not required to complete all doses of a multidose vaccine series as long as they have received the next dose in the series before arrival in the United States. New immigrant arrivals should be encouraged to complete vaccination schedules according to ACIP recommendations after arrival in the United States.

CDC's *Vaccine Technical Instructions* are available at www.cdc.gov/immigrantrefugeehealth/exams/ti/panel/vaccination-panel-technical-instructions.html.

CHILDREN ADOPTED INTERNATIONALLY

Parents adopting children internationally may request to delay immunization of children <10 years of age by agreeing to begin immunizations within 30 days of arrival in the United States. Adopting families should be aware that vaccinating children before arrival in the United States reduces the risk of importing diseases of public health concern, such as measles, which was reported in unvaccinated children adopted from China in 2004, 2006, and 2013.

REFUGEES

Refugees are not required to meet the INA immunization requirements before entry into the United States; however, CDC is working with domestic and international migration partners to implement a vaccination program for US refugees. Program updates and population-specific schedules can be found at www.cdc.gov/immigrantrefugeehealth/guidelines/overseas/interventions/immunizations-schedules.html. Refugees are required to show proof of vaccination when they apply for permanent US residence (adjustment of status exam performed by a US civil surgeon), typically 1 year after arrival.

Classification of Medical Conditions

Medical conditions of public health significance are categorized into those that preclude an immigrant or refugee from entering the United States (class A) or those that indicate a departure from normal well-being and for which follow-up after arrival is recommended (class B). An immigrant or refugee who has an inadmissible class A condition may still be issued a visa after the illness has been treated or after a waiver of the visa ineligibility has been approved by USCIS.

Notifications and Follow-Up on Arrival

The results of the immigrant medical exam are collected at US ports of entry when immigrants and refugees arrive. CDC then notifies state or

8

local health departments of all arriving refugees, as well as immigrants with notifiable class A (with waiver) and class B conditions who may need follow-up evaluation after arrival. State and local health departments are asked to report follow-up evaluation results back to CDC, as well as any serious conditions of public health concern identified among recently arrived immigrants and refugees. Such reporting enables CDC to track epidemiologic patterns of disease in recently arrived immigrants and refugees and allows for monitoring of the quality of the overseas medical examinations.

AFTER ARRIVAL IN THE UNITED STATES: SCREENING & HEALTH ASSESSMENT

A comprehensive postarrival health assessment is an opportunity to screen for communicable and noncommunicable diseases, provide preventive services (such as immunizations and treatment for latent tuberculosis) and individual counseling (such as nutritional and mental health), establish ongoing primary care and a medical home, and orient new arrivals to the US health care system.

Challenges for health professionals in providing comprehensive health assessments for new arrivals include lack of familiarity with CDC screening recommendations and diseases endemic to a migrant's country of origin, inability to find trained interpreters, and lack of knowledge of social and cultural beliefs of new migrant groups. Immigrants and refugees often have other priorities related to their new environment, such as English classes, school, housing, and work, which may take precedence over accessing health care services. Several organizations can facilitate health screenings for refugees (such as the Association of Refugee Health Coordinators [ARHC]), and networks of clinicians who serve refugees and immigrants are growing. Additional resources are provided in the online Yellow Book (see Box 8-8).

Medical Screening

Newly arrived immigrants and refugees may have undiagnosed infectious diseases or untreated chronic health conditions, such as hypertension, diabetes, or hypercholesterolemia. Ideally, each new migrant should receive a complete health assessment that includes screening for migration-associated illness plus the age-appropriate screening and health care recommended for anyone residing in the United States. Clinicians caring for migrants who are not recent arrivals should still ensure that migrant screening has been completed, especially for diseases of long latency such as TB, hepatitis B, and HIV, and complete any missing tests. It would also be ideal to be able to screen each individual for diseases specific to his or her country of origin, migration route, and individual epidemiologic risk. Described below are guidelines available for the 2 populations for which there are the most data to guide screening efforts (refugees and children adopted internationally), followed by an approach to performing health assessments for other categories of immigrants.

HEALTH ASSESSMENT OF REFUGEES

Evidence-based guidelines for refugees have been developed by CDC in collaboration with the Department of Health and Human Services Administration for Children and Families' Office of Refugee Resettlement (ORR), clinical and subject matter experts outside of CDC, and representatives of ARHC. The full guidelines and a summary checklist of the postarrival exam components and recommended testing are available at www.cdc.gov/immigrantrefugeehealth/guidelines/domestic/domestic-guidelines.html. CDC has also developed population-specific health profiles for certain populations (such as Bhutanese or Congolese refugees), available at www.cdc.gov/immigrantrefugeehealth/profiles/index.html.

Another function of the postarrival medical screening is to arrange and coordinate ongoing primary care. Many refugees have not had age-appropriate screening for chronic diseases such as heart disease, diabetes, cancer, or hearing, vision, or dental problems; these needs should be addressed at early follow-up visits. Several cancers are more prevalent in migrant populations, such as cervical, liver, stomach, and nasopharyngeal cancers. Refugees should be educated regarding age-appropriate cancer screening tests, such as mammography, colonoscopy and Papanicolaou tests during the postarrival exam.

8

BOX 8-8.
Additional migrant health resources for clinicians

Visit this section in the online edition of the Yellow Book at www.cdc.gov/travel for a comprehensive list of resources for clinicians and organizations that serve immigrants, refugees, asylum seekers, and international adoptees, including up-to-date patient care guidelines, online education materials, and print resources.

HIV testing was removed from the requirements for US admission in January 2010, but HIV screening is highly encouraged in all newly arriving refugees and routinely recommended in the guidelines from the United States Public Health Service (USPHS) and the American Academy of Pediatrics (AAP). Culturally sensitive counseling regarding HIV testing is critical.

Nutritional deficiencies occur commonly in refugee populations. For example, one study found that the prevalence of vitamin B12 deficiency in newly arrived Bhutanese refugees from Nepal was 64% in those tested premigration and 27%–32% in those tested after arrival in the United States. Clinicians should be aware of the possibility of malnutrition and micronutrient deficiencies and screen and treat accordingly.

CDC recommends checking blood lead levels of all refugee children aged 6 months to 16 years of age at the time of arrival, with follow-up blood lead testing for children 6 months to 6 years of age 3–6 months after settling into a permanent residence. Potential lead exposures include using lead-containing gasoline, burning fossil fuels and waste, and using lead-containing traditional remedies, cosmetics, foods, ceramics, or utensils. Ongoing lead exposure among refugee children after arrival in the United States also has been documented.

Mental health screening for refugees is another component of the postarrival exam and, when clinically indicated, a more detailed social history including any history of trauma, torture, or rape. Risk factors that may predispose refugees to psychiatric symptoms and disorders include exposure to war, state-sponsored violence and oppression, loss of family members, and the stress of adapting to a new culture.

Refugees may qualify for state Medicaid programs to cover medical screening and any ongoing medical care that may be needed. Refugees determined ineligible for Medicaid are eligible for Refugee Medical Assistance in many states, which provides for their medical care needs for up to 8 months from their date of arrival. For more information, clinicians and refugees can contact their state health departments and can access more information through the ORR, which administers this program (www.acf.hhs.gov/programs/orr/programs/cma).

Other published resources available to clinicians include consensus documents on evidence-based screening for newly arriving refugees to Canada, provided by the Canadian Collaboration for Immigrant and Refugee Health. A list of resources can be found in the online edition of the Yellow Book (see Box 8-8).

HEALTH ASSESSMENT OF CHILDREN ADOPTED INTERNATIONALLY

There are many similarities in health conditions between international adoptees and refugees. One difference is that refugees generally remain in their own cultural group for some time after arrival and may have limited interactions with the wider community, whereas international adoptees frequently enter households and communities that are clinically naïve to infections common in resource-poor settings. This distinction is particularly pertinent for conditions that may continue to be infectious for weeks to months after arrival (such as hepatitis A or B and giardiasis). Clinicians should encourage updating immunizations prior to the adoption for those who travel internationally to meet their adopted children and travel home with them, as well as close family members and caregivers (even if they do not travel). The AAP offers guidance in the *Red Book: Report of the Committee on Infectious Diseases* for clinicians who will serve this population after their arrival in the United States (the *Red Book* may be accessed for free by AAP members at http://aapredbook.aappublications.org). More information is available in Chapter 7, International Adoption. Most families who adopt children internationally are required to have health insurance for the child effective upon arrival, so funding for the postarrival health assessment poses fewer problems than for other immigrant groups.

HEALTH ASSESSMENT FOR OTHER IMMIGRANTS

All newly arrived immigrants would benefit from a comprehensive postarrival health assessment and introduction to the US health system. Because immigrants enter the country in so many different ways, they access health care at multiple different points and with providers who have differing levels of expertise in immigrant medicine. Since there is no formal mechanism or funding source available for a standard comprehensive health assessment, immigrants may never receive any health assessment that targets conditions they may have acquired in their country of birth or during their migration process unless every health professional assumes the responsibility and has the knowledge to assess these issues when caring for patients born outside the United States. A list of screening tests that should be considered for immigrant health assessments is included in Table 8-9.

Most experts agree that testing for TB, hepatitis B, and HIV should be performed for most new arrivals to the United States. Clinicians should also make a habit of ensuring that this screening has been done for every new–US-born patient they see, regardless of time since the person's arrival.

Vaccine records, laboratory evidence of immunity, and history of vaccine-preventable diseases should be obtained and age-appropriate vaccines be given as indicated. Vaccine series do not need to be restarted if documentation of prior doses is available.

Basic mental health screening, including coping strategies and support systems, can be included in the assessment so that referrals to resources can be made within the medical home.

A complete blood count with differential and urinalysis is appropriate for most new arrivals for diagnosis of anemia or eosinophilia or to identify evidence of hemoglobinopathy. A basic metabolic panel may be indicated, especially for those of appropriate age or with evidence of conditions such as renal disease or diabetes. Immigrant health care providers should continue to follow the age- and risk-based guidelines provided by the United States Preventive Services Task Force (USPSTF) for the general US population when continuing to care for immigrant patients over time. (See the Guide to Clinical Preventative Services 2014 at www.uspreventiveservicestaskforce.org, click on "Information for Health Professionals" and then on the "Guide to Clinical Preventive Services, 2014"). Per CDC lead screening guidelines for the US population, a blood lead level should be obtained for children 12 months old and 24 months old if resources allow. If a child has additional risks, screening should be started at 6 months. If an immigrant has never had a blood lead level and has lived in a highly industrialized city with potential for exposure to industrial waste, has a developmental delay, or has a medical condition consistent with lead exposure, he or she should be screened for blood lead level as well. Diagnostic testing should be considered if an immigrant presents with symptoms consistent with a particular parasite if endemic in the country of origin (malaria, intestinal parasites). STD screening (syphilis, gonorrhea, chlamydia, HIV), above that of the recommendations for the US general population, should be considered for immigrants if their migration history places them at significant risk. Known medical and family history should be recorded, and medications and treatments received prior to migration should be discussed.

Immigrants who travel back to their country of origin may be at higher risk of travel-related infectious diseases. Thus, travel vaccines can be considered in addition to age-appropriate vaccinations for these immigrants.

Table 8-9. Recommended postarrival laboratory screening tests for immigrants and refugees receiving medical care in the United States

TEST	AGE RANGE	GEOGRAPHIC AREA	COMMENTS
Tuberculosis: IGRA or TST	All	All	Test based on standard guidelines
HIV	>13 years[1]	All	Test based on standard guidelines
Hepatitis B: surface antigen	All	Where prevalence of hepatitis B infection in home country is >2%	Consider surface antibody if unimmunized. May consider core antibody. Current recommendations for refugees can apply to both immigrants and refugees.
STDs (syphilis, gonorrhea, chlamydia, others as indicated)	15–65 years or <15 if sexually active	All	Test choice based on standard guidelines. Consider for all immigrants, taking into account the migration history and if it adds increased risk.
CBC with differential and MCV	All	All	Screen for chronic anemias; look for absolute eosinophilia, as it can be evidence of parasitic infection.
Serology for parasites: schistosomiasis, strongyloidiasis, other soil-transmitted helminths	All	Where endemic if high risk of exposure	Consider screening with exposure history, unexplained eosinophilia. Some experts choose to treat empirically. Empiric treatment is recommended when at-risk immigrant is about to receive steroids or become immunocompromised, if testing is unavailable or when there is insufficient time to obtain results.
Malaria	All	Where malaria is endemic	Consider malaria if from highly endemic area within 3–6 months of arrival.
Blood lead level	<16 years or if clinical indication	All	Consider if never had a lead test and have additional risks: lived in a highly industrialized city with potential exposure to industrial waste, has a developmental delay, or has medical conditions consistent with lead exposure
Varicella antibody	>5 years	All, but especially those with history of varicella and older children and adults	
Urinalysis, basic metabolic panel	All adults or if clinical indication	All	Screening for renal failure and schistosomiasis (if from an endemic area)

Abbreviations: IGRA, interferon-γ release assay; TST, tuberculin skin test; STD, sexually transmitted disease; CBC, complete blood count; MCV, mean corpuscular volume
[1] Consider in younger children who have signs or symptoms of disease, risk factors for transmission, or mother is missing or deceased or has illness compatible with HIV.

8

BIBLIOGRAPHY

1. Barnett ED. Immunizations and infectious disease screening for internationally adopted children. Pediatr Clin North Am. 2005 Oct;52(5):1287–309, vi.

2. CDC. Vitamin B12 deficiency in resettled Bhutanese refugees—United States, 2008–2011. MMWR Morb Mortal Wkly Rep. 2011 Mar 25;60(11):343–6.

3. CDC. Technical instructions for panel physicians. Atlanta: CDC; 2014 [cited 2016 Sep. 28]; Available from: http://www.cdc.gov/immigrantrefugeehealth/exams/ti/panel/technical-instructions-panel-physicians.html.

4. Lowenthal P, Westenhouse J, Moore M, Posey DL, Watt JP, Flood J. Reduced importation of tuberculosis after the implementation of an enhanced pre-immigration screening protocol. Int J Tuberc Lung Dis. 2011 Jun;15(6):761–6.

5. Maloney SA, Fielding KL, Laserson KF, Jones W, Nguyen TN, Dang QA, et al. Assessing the performance of overseas tuberculosis screening programs: a study among US-bound immigrants in Vietnam. Arch Intern Med. 2006 Jan 23;166(2):234–40.

6. Miller LC. International adoption: infectious diseases issues. Clin Infect Dis. 2005 Jan 15;40(2):286–93.

7. Minnesota Department of Health. Lead poisoning in Minnesota refugee children, 2000–2002. Disease Control Newsletter [Internet]; 2004 [cited 2016 Sep. 28]; 32(2):13–5. Available from: http://www.health.state.mn.us/divs/idepc/newsletters/dcn/2004/0402dcn.pdf.

8. Nyangoma EN, Olson CK, Benoit SR, Bos J, Debolt C, Kay M, et al. Measles outbreak associated with adopted children from China—Missouri, Minnesota, and Washington, July 2013. MMWR Morb Mortal Wkly Rep. 2014 Apr 11;63(14):301–4.

9. Office of Immigration Statistics. Yearbook of Immigration Statistics: 2012. Washington, DC: US Department of Homeland Security; 2014 [cited 2016 Sep. 28]; Available from: https://www.dhs.gov/yearbook-immigration-statistics.

10. Posey DL, Blackburn BG, Weinberg M, Flagg EW, Ortega L, Wilson M, et al. High prevalence and presumptive treatment of schistosomiasis and strongyloidiasis among African refugees. Clin Infect Dis. 2007 Nov 15;45(10):1310–5.

11. Posey DL, Naughton MP, Willacy EA, Russell M, Olson CK, Godwin CM, et al. Implementation of new TB screening requirements for U.S.-bound immigrants and refugees—2007–2014. MMWR Morb Mortal Wkly Rep. 2014 Mar 21;63(11):234–6.

12. Pottie K, Greenaway C, Feightner J, Welch V, Swinkels H, Rashid M, et al. Evidence-based clinical guidelines for immigrants and refugees. CMAJ. 2011 Sep 6;183(12):E824–925.

13. Walker PF, Barnett ED, editors. Immigrant Medicine. Philadelphia: Saunders Elsevier; 2007.

8

WILDERNESS & EXPEDITION MEDICINE

Christopher Van Tilburg

Wilderness and expedition trips are a unique aspect of travel because of challenging terrain, extreme weather, remote locales, and long durations. Popular destinations include trekking to Everest Base Camp, climbing Mount Kilimanjaro, hiking the Inca Trail, sailing the South Pacific, and exploring the poles. Adventure travel often includes mountaineering, backpacking, cycling, diving, surfing, or river rafting. Travelers may be working, providing humanitarian relief, or completing scientific research.

The risks and consequences of injury and illness are often significantly increased in wilderness and expedition travel compared with other types of travel for several reasons:

- Destinations may be remote and lack access to care.

- Communication is often limited.

- Weather, climate, and terrain can be extreme.

- Travelers exert themselves physically, increasing caloric, fluid, and sleep requirements.

- Trips are often long: several weeks, months, or years.

- Expeditions are often goal oriented, which can cause travelers to exceed safety limits.

PRETRAVEL CONSIDERATIONS

In addition to routine travel medicine advice, providers should gather extra information and discuss precautions for wilderness and expedition travel.

Trip Type

Obtain details about the type, length, and remoteness of the trip. Guided trips may eliminate some of the need for complex logistics planning on the part of the traveler. However, participants in guided trips should ask key questions of the trip organizers including:

- Guide experience
- Type of medical kit carried by guides
- Contingency plan for emergencies
- Recommended medications and medical supplies to be carried by participants
- Type of insurance recommended
- Medical training of guides

In a few cases, such as polar cruises and Mount Everest expeditions, a formal medical officer with a comprehensive medical kit may be available.

Confirm if the skill level of the participant matches the trip type: beginners in an activity such as diving, mountaineering, skiing, or sailing should participate in instructional trips. Those with less experience or visiting a location for the first time should be encouraged to go on a guided trip. Most people will consult a travel medicine professional only after they have selected and paid for their adventure, but it may be possible to work with the organizer to change it to a trip more in line with the traveler's skill and experience.

For self-planned trips, the travel medicine practitioner may need to augment a comprehensive medical kit with prescription medication and offer more support with logistics, evacuation planning, and insurance.

Personal Health Requirements

Adequate nutrition, hydration, and sleep may be difficult to obtain, especially with increased demand because of weather, terrain, and exertion. Travelers should pay attention during the planning stages to how food and water will be obtained on the journey.

Pretravel screening should be completed for conditions that can be exacerbated by high altitude, extreme heat, extreme cold, exertion, and other environmental hazards. These include diabetes (particularly insulin-dependent diabetes), asthma, any cardiac disease (such as hypertension, arrhythmias, and coronary artery disease), chronic pain treated with opiates, recent surgery, anaphylaxis-level allergy, oxygen-dependent emphysema, and sleep apnea. Travelers who have battery-operated devices, such as a continuous positive airway pressure machine or an insulin pump, should be cautioned about device failure and have a backup plan. A past history of environmental illness—altitude illness, hypothermia, frostbite, heat exhaustion, or anaphylaxis—likely puts one at increased risk for recurrence.

Medical clearance for participation may be required for a guided trip. The treating physician should complete medical clearance for travelers with chronic disease. Travel health practitioners can complete pretravel medical clearance if it is a usual function of their practice and the patient has no chronic disease or medications. If possible, travelers should get medications for chronic illness from the treating physician. For example, travelers with preexisting asthma should obtain their routine, rescue, and emergency self-treatment medications from the treating physician.

Money and Insurance

Rescue, evacuation, and repatriation may require upfront payment, especially with aeromedical transport from remote locations. Travelers should bring sufficient emergency cash and a credit card with high credit and cash advance limits.

Insurance is widely variable and comes in many forms, but insurance does not guarantee rescue. Insurance may be contingent on limits including preexisting conditions, deductibles, maximum expenditures, and medical control approval.

8

Insurers may also not authorize helicopter or air-planes for in-country transport or repatriation. Insurance companies may deny claims involving chronic illness, drugs, alcohol, pregnancy, mental health, and acts of war or civil unrest.

Types of insurance include:

- Domestic health insurance, which may or may not be effective outside a home country.

- Travel insurance, which often includes medical, trip cancellation, evacuation, and repatriation benefits, but may exclude coverage for wilderness rescue and adventure sports like mountaineering, skiing, and diving. An adventure sports rider is available with some travel insurance policies, so travelers should confirm coverage for adventure sports.

- Wilderness rescue insurance (usually separate from travel insurance), such as policies through North American mountaineering clubs, outdoor and professional associations, and scuba dive organizations. Short-term rescue insurance is available in some countries, for example, through local helicopter rescue companies, ski resorts, and guides.

- Comprehensive expedition policies, including travel, medical, rescue, security, and repatriation services.

Training

If travelers have time before disembarking, they should consider completing a first aid and basic life support course. Such courses can be found through local community colleges and fire departments.

Emergency Resources

Before they go, travelers should know emergency escape routes, local rescue resources, embassy contacts, and local medical facilities.

If travel medicine practitioners are willing to accept phone calls, emails, and text messages from travelers who are abroad, give out contact information and approximate time of response. Make sure travelers understand this is not a substitute for local emergency care.

In a travel medicine encounter, physicians may only have a brief moment to educate travelers. Depending on the type, duration, and location of trip, a few key pearls may be worth discussing:

- Travelers should understand basic wound care, seek help with signs of infection—redness, swelling, pus, and warmth—and be educated on self-treatment with antibiotics.

- For hypothermia, cessation of shivering and mental status changes are dangerous signs. Frostbite can be treated with thrombolytics to aid reperfusion, but treatment needs to be initiated within 72 hours in a hospital (see Chapter 2, Problems with Heat & Cold).

- Heat stroke marked by a temperature of 40°C and mental status changes is a medical emergency.

- Snakes, spiders, scorpions, ticks, and jellyfish can deliver toxic venom, inoculate microbes, and cause anaphylaxis. For anaphylaxis (also caused by food), treatment with epinephrine can be life-saving if administered immediately. Regional antivenoms exist around the world for certain venomous snakes, spiders, scorpions, and jellyfish.

- Travel to high altitude may require prevention and treatment with acetazolamide, dexamethasone, and other medications. Mental status changes and ataxia are ominous signs of high-altitude cerebral edema. Breathlessness at rest is the sign of life-threatening high-altitude pulmonary edema.

WILDERNESS SUPPLIES

Communication and Route Finding

Travelers should carry a cell phone enabled with global positioning system (GPS), such as a smartphone. Importantly, not all North American cell phones are compatible with international networks. Travelers should check with their cell carrier before departing.

In many countries, a global-compatible phone can be used with an international plan purchased beforehand through the traveler's North American

8

cell carrier. Global-compatible phones use the Global System for Mobiles system commonly found with AT&T and T-Mobile services. Phones that use the Code Division Multiple Access system, such as Sprint, Verizon, and US Cellular services, often do not work internationally.

Alternatively, an unlocked (not restricted to any carrier) global-compatible cell phone can be used with a local SIM card in the country of travel. If one does not have a global-compatible phone and SIM card capability, travelers can buy an inexpensive local phone, which is best for travelers who expect frequent use of their phone, especially for data and local calls. Phones and SIM cards are usually available at kiosks and stores in major cities and in some airports. In some countries, registration to obtain a local SIM card requires fingerprinting and a passport picture.

Where cell phone service is not available, travelers may consider an unlocked (no frequency restrictions) VHF/UHF radio or a satellite phone. Advise travelers that restrictions exist and permits are required in many countries regarding use of handheld radios and satellite phones; they should check local restrictions prior to departing.

Remind travelers that electronics are not foolproof; often they are limited by battery power, dense cloud cover, deep canyons, government restrictions, and physical damage caused by impact, water, or extreme temperatures. A backup power source, such as a solar or dynamo charger, is useful.

For extreme terrain and remote locations, adventurers should carry and know how to use a GPS unit (or have GPS app installed on their phone), compass, altimeter, or local topographic map (the latter may need to be acquired in-country).

Clothing

Remind travelers that clothing helps prevent heat and cold illness as well as bites and stings from insects and arthropods.

Cold weather clothing should be polyester, nylon, Merino wool, or, in some circumstances, goose down. Layering typically consists of a base layer, insulating layers of heavy-pile polyester or nylon-encased polyester (goose down suffices if traveling to a location that is dry and cold), and a windproof, waterproof outer layer of tightly woven nylon with a durable water-repellent coating. Gloves, hat, neck warmer, warm socks, and goggles are vital to cover all exposed skin.

For hot weather, sun- and insect-protective clothing is important including loose-fitting, lightweight clothing made from nylon, polyester, or a cotton blend. Long-sleeve shirts and long pants offer the most protection. A wide brim sun hat and a bandana protect the head and neck. Sunglasses protect eyes. Clothing should be sprayed with permethrin to ward off insects and arthropods. Footwear should be activity-specific boots or shoes, equally important in a marine or mountain environment.

Emergency Kits

Expedition and wilderness adventures often require a comprehensive, yet compact, personal emergency kit for survival, medical care, and equipment repair. In addition to a basic travel health kit (see Chapter 2, Travel Health Kits), travelers should consider packing additional items due to the remote nature of their travel. Items may include additional first aid supplies (such as a pocket-size CPR mask), safety supplies, and a more robust variety of medications (see below). Standard kits may also need to be augmented for specific activities like undersea, ocean, jungle, polar, and high-altitude travel.

If travelers are on guided trips, they may only need a small personal medical kit. A list of recommended supplies and drugs, including antibiotic, analgesic, and anaphylaxis medications, should be available from the guide company and will likely need to be prescribed at the travel medicine encounter. Before they go, travelers should identify any available group emergency equipment such as an automatic external defibrillator, a portable stretcher, portable hyperbaric chamber, oxygen, and comprehensive medical kit.

Be cautious if asked to prescribe medications for guides to be stocked in the expedition medical kit intended for use on clients. Third-party use of prescription medication is unlawful in most jurisdictions and best left for the guide company medical director. If prescribing to a guide as a patient, clarify that the medication is for the guide's personal use.

8

MEDICATIONS

Travelers should be advised on self-treatment of disease such as gastroenteritis, febrile illness, wound infections, and respiratory illness. This may require prophylactic and self-treatment with antibiotics. In addition to medications recommended in a basic travel health kit (see Chapter 2, Travel Health Kits), travelers should consider a more comprehensive medication supply including opiate pain medication, ophthalmologic antibiotic ointment and anesthetic, and nondrowsy antihistamines.

SAFETY SUPPLIES

Wilderness and expedition travelers should consider packing additional safety equipment to supplement a travel health kit. These items can help in an emergency situation. Useful items include the following:

- Headlight with extra batteries
- Perlon cord
- Emergency sleeping sack or tarp
- Duct tape
- Multi-tool
- Safety pins
- Polyurethane straps
- Chemical heat packs
- Map, compass, altimeter
- Whistle
- Water purification tablets
- Oral hydration packs

BIBLIOGRAPHY

1. Iserson KV. Medical planning for extended remote expeditions. Wilderness Environ Med. 2013 Dec;24(4):366–77.

2. Lewin M, Jensen S, Platts-Mills T. Wilderness preparation, equipment, and medical supplies. In: Auerbach PS, editor. Wilderness Medicine. 6th ed. Philadelphia: Elsevier; 2012. pp. 1820–44.

3. Lipman GS, Eifling KP, Ellis MA, Gaudio FG, Otten EM, Grissom CK. Wilderness Medical Society practice guidelines for the prevention and treatment of heat-related illness: 2014 update. Wilderness Environ Med. 2014 Dec;25(4 Suppl):S55–65.

4. McIntosh SE, Opacic M, Freer L, Grissom CK, Auerbach PS, Rodway GW, et al. Wilderness Medical Society practice guidelines for the prevention and treatment of frostbite: 2014 update. Wilderness Environ Med. 2014 Dec;25(4 Suppl):S43–54.

5. Mellor A, Dodds N, Joshi R, Hall J, Dhillon S, Hollis S, et al. Faculty of Prehospital Care, Royal College of Surgeons Edinburgh guidance for medical provision for wilderness medicine. Extrem Physiol Med. 2015;4:22.

6. Quinn RH, Wedmore I, Johnson EL, Islas AA, Anglim A, Zafren K, et al. Wilderness Medical Society practice guidelines for basic wound management in the austere environment: 2014 update. Wilderness Environ Med. 2014 Dec;25(4 Suppl):S118–33.

7. Zafren K, Giesbrecht GG, Danzl DF, Brugger H, Sagalyn EB, Walpoth B, et al. Wilderness Medical Society practice guidelines for the out-of-hospital evaluation and treatment of accidental hypothermia: 2014 update. Wilderness Environ Med. 2014 Dec;25(4 Suppl):S66–85.

WORK-RELATED TRAVEL

Margaret Kitt, Kristin Yeoman, Casey Chosewood, John Gibbins, Leslie Nickels, Donna Van Bogaert, John Piacentino

Business travel is projected to grow an average 6.9% through 2016. Small- to midsized businesses are a growing part of the global business market. Through 2014, nearly 98% of all US identified exporters were small or midsized companies, a trend that has held steady since 2006. Building and maintaining that export business has created an increasing need to travel business staff overseas. Many large corporations have corporate medical offices or contract for services that provide travel assistance and preparation for business travelers. However, small and medium enterprises as well as self-employed travelers may not possess the resources to make comprehensive decisions regarding travel abroad.

PREPARING FOR TRAVEL

Employers and workers traveling internationally for job duties should take steps pretravel, during travel, and post-travel to prevent injury or illness. Risks associated with the type of work or the travel destination, as well as ways to protect and achieve optimal personal health and safety, should be identified during each of these three phases of travel.

Using checklists, planning tools, and various information sources, employers and workers can help maximize the likelihood that work-related travel is completed safely. This section cannot give specific information on the workplace hazards in every industry or travel location. Instead, the information in this chapter guides employers and workers in recognizing and mitigating common hazards, and it generally applies to all who travel for work.

PRETRAVEL

The pretravel period is the best time to identify risks and make plans to prevent occupational injury and illness. Planning needs vary depending on the type of work; for example, business meetings in a metropolitan office setting differ from site visits at a mine or work on a construction site in a remote location. The first step in pretravel planning is for employers and workers to confirm the need for international travel. Make a list of assessment topics tailored to a given travel assignment to guide this determination. These topics may include the following:

- Type of Work
  - ➤ Assess the trip's objectives and whether they could be met by using videoconferences, phone meetings, or other methods.
  - ➤ Assess duration of travel. Risks may increase as more time is spent on a trip. Requirements (such as work visas) or recommendations (such as immunizations)

also vary based on the expected length of stay.
  - ➤ Determine whether site visits to factories, industrial facilities, or other worksites will be needed. If so, evaluate the potential hazards at those sites and how those hazards can be minimized.

- Travel Destination
  - ➤ Assess the potential hazards of the travel destination, including hazards related to security concerns, natural disasters, infectious diseases, and climate extremes.
  - ➤ Assess the timing of the trip. Can the trip be postponed to a time when there may be less risk (such as after contentious elections, rainy seasons, or infectious disease outbreaks)?

- Personal Health
  - ➤ Assess whether the most appropriate personnel are selected for the trip. Think about technical and job expertise as well as current workload, responsibilities, and potential health concerns.
  - ➤ Ensure that travelers have opportunities to maintain optimal health during the trip and access to care and resources they may need while traveling.

If travel is judged as necessary, the next step is to give workers the information they need to stay healthy and safe. Employers and workers together can assess risks related to the type of work and make a plan that adequately addresses risks. Useful steps include the following:

1. Identify points of contact.
   - > At the home worksite, in case problems arise.
   - > At the international worksite, to assist with questions and problems; discuss the upcoming trip to ensure that workers bring adequate work clothes, equipment, and personal protective equipment (PPE).
   - > US embassy and consulate personnel.

2. Assess job tasks.
   - > Determine whether tasks will differ from the usual work at home.

> Determine where the job tasks will be performed (indoor/outdoor, rural/urban, office or other setting).

> Determine what PPE is needed, if the traveler needs to bring PPE, and if any additional training to use this PPE is required before departure.

> Evaluate whether differences in language, customs, or culture are likely to affect job tasks.

3. Review existing local health and safety rules and regulations.

> Determine if specific rules exist for possible work-related hazards such as exposure to chemicals.

In addition to assessing specific risks related to the type of work, employers and workers should remember to plan for common risks associated with the travel destination (such as risks associated with driving, personal safety, or infectious diseases) or opportunities to maintain optimal personal health. Workers may want to discuss their travel plans with their personal physician before departure. This is especially true for those with chronic health conditions. A health care provider can evaluate workers and guide them on issues such as food and water safety, vaccinations, prevention of exposure to infectious diseases and environmental hazards, and the potential impact of travel demands on personal health. Other sections of the Yellow Book give extensive guidance on these issues.

DURING TRAVEL

Once an employee arrives in a country, reassess whether conditions have changed since plans were put into place during the pretravel phase. Pretravel plans should be reassessed periodically throughout travel and whenever conditions change substantially. Common issues arising before and during travel include the following:

- Type of Work

  > Changes in working conditions that may have different potential hazards
  > Changes in requirements for personal protection
  > Changes or additions to work locations

- Travel Destination

  > Disease outbreaks
  > Severe weather and natural disasters that may affect travel
  > Changes in availability or nature of local transportation
  > Changes in local security situations due to protests, strikes, or armed conflicts
  > Changes in accommodations or in food/water availability

- Personal Health

  > Changes in personal health status, including worsening of existing conditions or onset of new illness

Each of the 3 factors to consider in work-related travel—type of work, travel destination, and personal health—need to be reassessed. Issues related to the travel destination and personal health may apply to either leisure or work-related travel, but some specifics related to the job need to be considered that may present challenges not encountered by typical leisure travelers.

POST-TRAVEL

Travel-related safety and health concerns do not necessarily end after returning home. The following issues should be considered in the post-travel setting: transitioning back to work and life at home, reporting of incidents and exposures, getting necessary medical care, and capturing lessons learned to ensure future travel is safe for other workers. In addition, certain elements of the pretravel and travel periods, such as completing vaccination series or resuming care of a personal health condition, may also need to be addressed after travel.

Transitioning Back to Work and Life at Home

Depending on the length and nature of travel, returning workers may need a transition period before resuming pretravel work activities. It is important that employers and workers discuss a plan for returning to regular duty that addresses the following employee needs:

- Time for rest, adjusting to the new time zone, and resuming a normal sleep cycle

- Time for adjusting to work or pace of activity that is different from travel

- Refresher training (or new training) on returning work tasks and any changes in safety procedures or PPE

- Time to reconnect with family or significant others or to catch up on home responsibilities

- Time to wrap up unfinished business with employers and workers at the international location

Returning workers can contact their employer's employee assistance program, if available, or they can consult with their health care provider, especially if the transition to home becomes difficult or adjustment challenges are prolonged.

Reporting Incidents and Exposures
Returning workers need to notify their employer of any work-related incidents that may have occurred during travel and take appropriate actions. Commonly occurring incidents that require reporting include the following:

- Work-related injuries or illnesses

- Health and safety-related exposures related to the work performed or the location visited, including physical hazards, chemical hazards, or infectious disease risks

- Incidents and close call mishaps related to the travel that could affect other workers at the site or future travelers

- Traffic crashes

- Property damage or loss

- Security incidents, thefts, personal violence or other crimes

- Legal issues that may have occurred during travel

Medical Care
Returning workers should immediately seek treatment for any lingering, worrisome, or new medical complaints, symptoms, or concerns that have arisen during travel or after. In addition to information related to travel history and destination that would normally be reported to health providers, workers should give information about specific job duties and hazards encountered in their work during international travel. Health providers should consider potential associations between new symptoms and both the work duties and the travel destination itself. Until proven otherwise, it is safest to assume new symptoms—especially fever or other signs of infection—are related to the travel.

Workers need to resume routine personal medical care upon return. This includes actively managing ongoing chronic conditions, illness or injury that may have occurred during travel, as well as check-ups, screenings, and medical or dental visits that may have been missed while on travel status.

Depending upon the nature of the work performed during travel, employers and returning workers should assess whether work-specific medical monitoring related to hazardous exposures is necessary. This may include medical examinations, surveillance questionnaires, laboratory work, or other medical monitoring. If needed, specific guidance on this issue can be obtained from a qualified occupational health specialist.

Lessons Learned: Revisit Travel Health and Safety Plan
It is important that workers returning from work-related travel share what they learned on travel with employers and coworkers to help assure the health and safety of future travelers. Revisions of pretravel safety and health plans can be guided by considering these issues:

- Unexpected events related to the type or location of job duties.

- Availability of all equipment and PPE.

- Unexpected weather, local conditions, safety, travel arrangements, and accommodations.

- Challenges related to culture, customs, and language.

- Unexpected sources of conflict or stress.

SUMMARY

During work-related travel, personal health factors and leisure activities not related to work are important to consider, along with job hazards at worksites abroad. Pretravel planning should assess risks related to the type of work, as well as the travel destination and opportunities to achieve optimal personal health. Other chapters in the Yellow Book give important information related to travel destinations (such as food and water precautions, sun exposure, environmental hazards, and infectious diseases) and personal health factors (such as chronic illnesses). Job duties, work locations and conditions, equipment needs, and conditions unrelated to work may change while traveling. While on the travel assignment, be sure to periodically reassess changes and develop strategies to reduce risks. Returning workers should address issues of transitioning back to work life, reporting incidents and exposures, determining whether medical monitoring is necessary based on travel-related work exposures, and documenting lessons learned for the benefit of future travelers. Carefully consider the special circumstances associated with work-related travel during the pretravel, travel, and post-travel phases. This gives employers and workers the information needed to help travelers both complete their work and stay safe and healthy.

BIBLIOGRAPHY

1. CDC. Qualitative risk characterization and management of occupational hazards: control banding (CB). [cited 2016 Sep. 28]; Available from: http://www.cdc.gov/niosh/docs/2009-152/pdfs/2009-152.pdf.

2. Global Business Travel Association. U.S. business travel volume projected to rise over next two years. 2015 [cited 2016 Sep. 28]; Available from: www.gbta.org/PressReleases/Pages/RLS_041515_USA.aspx.

3. International Labour Organization. International Chemical Safety Cards database. [cited 2016 Sep. 28]; Available from: www.ilo.org/safework/info/publications/WCMS_113134/lang--en/index.htm.

4. International Labour Organization. International hazard datasheets on occupation. [cited 2016 Sep. 28]; Available from: http://www.ilo.org/safework/info/publications/WCMS_113135/lang--en/index.htm.

5. Khan NM, Jentes ES, Brown C, Han P, Rao SR, Kozarsky P, et al. Pre-travel medical preparation of business and occupational travelers: an analysis of the Global TravEpiNet Consortium, 2009 to 2012. J Occup Environ Med. 2016 Jan;58(1):76–82.

6. Small Business & Entrepreneurship Council. Going global: resources for entrepreneurs and small businesses. [cited 2016 Sep. 28]; Available from: http://sbecouncil.org/resources/going-global/.

8

Appendices

APPENDIX A: PROMOTING QUALITY IN THE PRACTICE OF TRAVEL MEDICINE

Calvin Patimeteeporn, Stephen M. Ostroff

Travel medicine remains a young area of medical practice, but even as the field continues to mature based on a growing body of scientific and medical information, there remains no recognized specialty or subspecialty of travel medicine anywhere in the world, including the United States. Clinicians offering travel medicine services are not "board certified" in travel medicine. Instead, travel medicine providers generally have credentials in other disciplines, including infectious diseases, internal medicine, pediatrics, nursing, pharmacy, or family practice. Clinics in the United States that offer travel medicine services are also not specifically credentialed for this purpose.

Given these circumstances, how can travelers maximize the likelihood their provider will deliver quality travel-related medical care and that the advice, preventive measures, and treatment services they are given fall within accepted standards? Similarly, how can providers assure patients they have sufficient knowledge of the subject matter relevant to travel medicine?

Research into the quality of travel health care is limited, but several studies suggest that travelers who visit a clinician with training in travel medicine are more likely to receive pretravel and post-travel advice and care than if they see other clinicians for such services. Similarly, 2006 guidelines on travel medicine published by the Infectious Diseases Society of America recommend that pretravel and post-travel care be obtained from a clinician with expertise in travel medicine. This is especially relevant for travelers going to exotic destinations, engaging in adventure travel, or who have special needs or medical problems.

Providers can pursue training in travel medicine through a number of professional organizations. Providers may also look to the many open and excellent courses hosted by members of the International Society of Travel Medicine (ISTM), notably those in the United States, Canada, Ireland, Scotland, and Switzerland. They vary in length from days to a year, depending upon the depth of the course and credential offered. Many individuals looking for training beyond the textbook do so informally by spending time in a travel clinic learning the basics of the pretravel consultation. Post-travel care typically involves infectious disease and tropical medicine training.

Below is a partial list of resources for clinicians who wish to enhance their knowledge of travel medicine. People seeking travel-related medical services may want to inquire whether their provider or clinic participates in these organizations or activities.

TRAVEL MEDICINE–RELATED PROFESSIONAL ORGANIZATIONS

International Society of Travel Medicine (ISTM)

Founded in 1991, ISTM (www.istm.org) is the preeminent multinational organization dealing exclusively with travel medicine. ISTM has >3,500 members worldwide.

ISTM activities include the following:

- *Journal of Travel Medicine*

- An active listserv (TravelMed) where members share information and can ask questions

- Special-interest groups that include travel medicine nurses and travel medicine pharmacists

- A biennial travel medicine meeting and annual regional submeetings

- A directory of domestic and international travel clinics affiliated with ISTM members in 65 countries

- An online learning curriculum of >60 programs that cover a wide range of topics and webinars on selected topics

- ISTM Travel Medicine Continuing Professional Development Program

- An examination leading to a Certificate of Knowledge in Travel Medicine, available to physicians, nurses, pharmacists, and other professionals offering travel advice

The ISTM Body of Knowledge, which covers the scope of the specialty of travel medicine, forms the basis for Certificate of Knowledge in Travel Medicine examination questions. It is regularly updated by the ISTM Exam Committee. Content areas in the Body of Knowledge include the following:

- Epidemiology related to travel medicine

- Immunology and vaccinology (including travel-related vaccines)
  - Pretravel consultation and management
  - Patient evaluation
  - Travelers with special needs
  - Special itineraries
  - Prevention and self-treatment
  - Precautions

- Diseases contracted during travel
  - Vectorborne diseases
  - Diseases transmitted from person to person
  - Foodborne and waterborne diseases
  - Diseases related to bites and stings
  - Diseases due to environmental hazards

- Other conditions associated with travel
  - Conditions occurring during or after travel
  - Conditions due to environmental factors
  - Threats to personal safety and security
  - Psychocultural issues

- Post-travel management

- General travel medicine issues
  - Medical care abroad
  - Travel clinic management
  - Travel medicine information resources

The Certificate of Knowledge in Travel Medicine examination has been administered since 2003, and as of 2016 more than 3,500 exams have been administered. The society hosts periodic 2-day intensive exam preparation courses open to all qualified professionals (such as physicians, nurses, pharmacists, and physician assistants) who provide travel health–related services. Those who are successful in the examination are awarded a Certificate in Travel Health (CTH). Beginning with CTHs awarded in 2011, the certificate is good for 10 years and the awardee must be recertified either through professional development activities or by retaking the examination. Practitioners offering travel medicine services or interested in the subject should strongly consider membership in ISTM. ISTM practitioners are listed on the organization's website, and those who have the CTH are designated as such.

ISTM also offers research programs. These include research grants, travel awards, and support for such efforts as the GeoSentinel Surveillance Network.

American Society of Tropical Medicine and Hygiene (ASTMH)

Formed in 1951 through the merger of predecessor organizations dating back to 1903, ASTMH (www.astmh.org) has a subsection that deals exclusively with tropical and travel medicine, known as the American Committee on Clinical Tropical Medicine and Travelers' Health.

ASTMH activities include the following:

- *The American Journal of Tropical Medicine and Hygiene*

A

- An annual meeting

- An electronic distribution list

- A tropical and travel medicine consultant directory

- A biennial examination leading to a Certificate of Knowledge in Clinical Tropical Medicine and Travelers' Health, available to those with a current professional health care license and who have passed an ASTMH-approved tropical medicine diploma course or have sufficient tropical medicine experience

The content areas of the ASTMH Certificate of Knowledge in Clinical Tropic Medicine and Travelers' Health are as follows:

- Basic science and fundamentals

- Infectious and tropical diseases (including parasites, bacteria, fungi, and viruses)

- Other diseases and conditions

- Diagnostic and therapeutic approach to clinical syndromes

- Travelers' health

- Public health in the tropics

- Epidemiology and control of disease

- Laboratory diagnosis

More than 750 people who have passed the ASTMH examination are listed on the ASTMH website. The society offers an annual intensive update course in clinical tropical medicine and travelers' health, which is in part designed to prepare those planning to take the Certificate of Knowledge examination.

Wilderness Medical Society

Organized in 1983, this society (www.wms.org) focuses on adventure travel, including wilderness travel and diving medicine. Its activities include the following:

- The journal *Wilderness and Environmental Medicine*

- Practice guidelines for emergency care in wilderness settings

- Annual meetings, a world congress, and sub-specialty meetings

- Courses leading to certification in advanced wilderness life support

- Participation in courses that lead to a diploma in mountain medicine

- A wilderness medical curriculum that, when successfully completed, qualifies members for fellowship in the Academy of Wilderness Medicine

Infectious Diseases Society of America (IDSA)

IDSA (www.idsociety.org) is the largest organization representing infectious disease clinicians in the United States. Although IDSA deals with all infectious diseases, it has many active members with expertise in tropical and travel medicine or strong interests in these disciplines. In 2006, IDSA published extensive evidence-based guidelines on the practice of travel medicine in the United States. IDSA also publishes travel-related research in its journals: *The Journal of Infectious Diseases, Clinical Infectious Diseases*, and *Open Forum Infectious Diseases.*

International Society for Infectious Diseases (ISID)

ISID (www.isid.org) was formed in 1986 and has approximately 60,000 members in 155 countries around the world. Like IDSA, ISID does not specifically focus on travel medicine. However, its international reach, particularly in low-resource countries, makes travel medicine an important topic in ISID and a valuable source of information for infectious diseases clinicians in many overseas travel destinations. Activities relevant to travel medicine that are supported by ISID include the following:

- *International Journal of Infectious Diseases*

- The biennial meeting International Congress on Infectious Diseases

- The Program for Monitoring Emerging Diseases (Pro-MED), an open-source electronic reporting system for reports of emerging infectious diseases and toxins, including outbreaks (www.promedmail.org)

Aerospace Medical Association This organization (www.asma.org) represents professionals in the fields of aviation, space, and environmental medicine who deal with air and space travelers. Its activities include the following:

- The journal *Aviation, Space, and Environmental Medicine*

- An annual meeting

- Continuing medical education in topics related to aerospace medicine

BIBLIOGRAPHY

1. Boddington NL, Simons H, Launders N, Hill DR. Quality improvement in travel medicine: a programme for yellow fever vaccination centres in England, Wales and Northern Ireland. Qual Prim Care 2011 Jan;19(6):391–8.

2. Chiodini JH, Anderson E, Driver C, Field VK, Flaherty GT, Grieve AM, et al. Recommendations for the practice of travel medicine. Travel Med Infect Dis. 2012 May;10(3):109–28.

3. Hill DR, Ericsson CD, Pearson RD, Keystone JS, Freedman DO, Kozarsky PE, et al. The practice of travel medicine: guidelines by the Infectious Diseases Society of America. Clin Infect Dis. 2006 Dec 15;42(12):1499–539.

4. Kozarsky P. The Body of Knowledge for the practice of travel medicine--2006. J Travel Med 2006 Sep-Oct;13(5):251–4.

5. Kozarsky PE, Steffen R. Travel medicine education-what are the needs? J Travel Med. 2016 Jul 4;23(5).

6. LaRocque RC, Jentes ES. Health recommendations for international travel: a review of the evidence base of travel medicine. Curr Opin Infect Dis. 2011 Oct;24(5):403–9.

7. Ruis JR, van Rijckevorsel GG, van den Hoek A, Koeman SC, Sonder GJ. Does registration of professionals improve the quality of travelers' health advice? J Travel Med. 2009 Jun-Aug;16(4):263–6.

8. Schlagenhauf P, Santos-O'Connor F, Parola P. The practice of travel medicine in Europe. Clin Microbiol Infect. 2010 Mar;16(3):203–8.

9. Sistenich V. International emergency medicine: how to train for it. Emerg Med Australas. 2012 Aug;24(4):435–41.

A

APPENDIX B: TRAVEL VACCINE SUMMARY TABLE

David R. Shlim

Table B-1 is a quick reference for administering or prescribing travel-related vaccines. Before administering any vaccine, please pay particular attention to the dose and whether it is to be administered intramuscularly or subcutaneously. Also review detailed instructions, contraindications, precautions, and side effects under the specific vaccines discussed in this book or in the manufacturer's prescribing information. For other immunizations, refer to the corresponding disease section in Chapter 3.

Table B-1. Travel vaccine summary

VACCINE	TRADE NAME (MANUFACTURER)	AGE	DOSE	ROUTE	SCHEDULE	BOOSTER
Cholera CVD 103-HgR vaccine	Vaxchora (PaxVax)	18–64 y	100 mL (reconstituted)	Oral	1 dose	Undetermined[1]
Hepatitis A vaccine, inactivated	Havrix (GlaxoSmithKline)	1–18 y ≥19 y	0.5 mL (720 ELU) 1 mL (1,440 ELU)	IM IM	0, 6–12 mo 0, 6–12 mo	None None
Hepatitis A vaccine, inactivated	Vaqta (Merck & Co., Inc.)	1–18 y ≥19 y	0.5 mL (25 U) 1 mL (50 U)	IM IM	0, 6–18 mo 0, 6–18 mo	None None
Hepatitis B vaccine, recombinant[2]	Engerix-B (GlaxoSmithKline)	0–19 y (primary) 0–10 y (accelerated) 11–19 y (accelerated) ≥20 y (primary) ≥20 y (accelerated)	0.5 mL (10 µg HBsAg) 0.5 mL (10 µg HBsAg) 1 mL (20 µg HBsAg) 1 mL (20 µg HBsAg) 1 mL (20 µg HBsAg)	IM IM IM IM IM	0, 1, 6 mo 0, 1, 2 mo 0, 1, 2 mo 0, 1, 6 mo 0, 1, 2 mo	None 12 mo 12 mo None 12 mo
Hepatitis B vaccine, recombinant[2]	Recombivax HB (Merck & Co., Inc.)	0–19 y (primary) 11–15 y (adolescent accelerated) ≥20 y (primary)	0.5 mL (5 µg HBsAg) 1 mL (10 µg HBsAg) 1 mL (10 µg HBsAg)	IM IM IM	0, 1, 6 mo 0, 4–6 mo 0, 1, 6 mo	None None None
Combined hepatitis A and B vaccine	Twinrix (GlaxoSmithKline)	≥18 y (primary) ≥18 y (accelerated)	1 mL (720 ELU HAV + 20 µg HBsAg) Same as above	IM IM	0, 1, 6 mo 0, 7, 21–30 d	None 12 mo
Japanese encephalitis vaccine, inactivated	Ixiaro (Valneva)	≥17 y 3–16 y 2 mo–2 y	0.5 mL 0.5 mL 0.25 mL	IM IM IM	0, 28 d 0, 28 d 0, 28 d	>1 y after primary series[3] Awaiting FDA assessment Awaiting FDA assessment

A

Vaccine	Product	Age	Dose	Route	Schedule	Booster
Meningococcal polysaccharide diphtheria toxoid conjugate vaccine (MenACWY-D)[4]	Menactra (Sanofi Pasteur)	9–23 mo 2–55 y	0.5 mL 0.5 mL	IM IM	0, 3 mo 1 dose	If at continued risk[5]
Meningococcal oligosaccharide diphtheria CRM[197] conjugate vaccine (MenACWY-CRM)[4]	Menveo (GSK)	2–12 mo 7–23 mo 2–55 y	0.5 mL 0.5 mL 0.5 mL	IM IM IM	0, 2, 4, 10–13 mo 0, 3 mo (2nd dose administered in 2nd year of life) 1 dose	If at continued risk[5]
Meningococcal polysaccharide vaccine (MPSV4)	Menomune (Sanofi Pasteur)	≥2 y	0.5 mL	SC	1 dose	If at continued risk[6]
Polio vaccine, inactivated	Ipol (Sanofi Pasteur)	≥18 y	0.5 mL	SC or IM	1 dose if the patient has completed a pediatric series	Repeat boosters may be needed for long-term travelers to polio-affected countries; see Chapter 3, Poliomyelitis
Rabies vaccine (human diploid cell)	Imovax (Sanofi Pasteur)	Any	1 mL	IM	Preexposure series: 0, 7, and 21 or 28 d	None; see Chapter 3, Rabies for postexposure immunization
Rabies vaccine (purified chick embryo cell)	RabAvert (Novartis)	Any	1 mL	IM	Preexposure series: 0, 7, and 21 or 28 d	None; see Chapter 3, Rabies for postexposure immunization
Typhoid vaccine (oral, live, attenuated)	Vivotif (PaxVax)	≥6 y	1 capsule[7]	Oral	0, 2, 4, 6 d	Repeat primary series after 5 y

(continued)

A

Table B-1. Travel vaccine summary (continued)

VACCINE	TRADE NAME (MANUFACTURER)	AGE	DOSE	ROUTE	SCHEDULE	BOOSTER
Typhoid vaccine (Vi capsular polysaccharide)	Typhim Vi (Sanofi Pasteur)	≥2 y	0.5 mL	IM	1 dose	2 y
Yellow fever	YF-Vax (Sanofi Pasteur)	≥9 mo[8]	0.5 mL	SC	1 dose	Not recommended for most[9]

Abbreviations: ELU, ELISA units of inactivated HAV; HAV, hepatitis A virus; HBsAg, hepatitis B surface antigen; IM, intramuscular; U, units HAV antigen; SC, subcutaneous.

[1] In a clinical trial, vaccine efficacy was 90% at 10 days postvaccination and declined to 80% at 3 months postvaccination in prevention of severe diarrhea after oral cholera challenge. Long-term immunogenicity is unknown. Clinicians advising travelers who are at continued or repeated risk over an extended period may consider revaccination, although the appropriate interval and efficacy are unknown.

[2] Consult the prescribing information for differences in dosing for hemodialysis and other immunocompromised patients.

[3] If potential for Japanese encephalitis virus exposure continues. Data on the response to a booster dose administered ≥2 years after the primary series are not available.

[4] If an infant is receiving the vaccine before travel, 2 doses may be administered as early as 8 weeks apart.

[5] Revaccination with meningococcal conjugate vaccine (MenACWY-D or MenACWY-CRM) is recommended after 3 years for children who were previously vaccinated at ages 2 months through 6 years. Revaccination with meningococcal conjugate vaccine is recommended after 5 years for people who were previously vaccinated at ages 7–55 years and every 5 years thereafter for people who are at continued risk.

[6] Revaccination with meningococcal polysaccharide vaccine is recommended for adults aged >55 years who remain at increased risk 5 years after the last dose. For adults aged >55 years who have received meningococcal conjugate vaccine previously or for whom multiple doses are anticipated (such as people with asplenia), meningococcal conjugate vaccine is preferred.

[7] Must be kept refrigerated at 35.6°F–46.4°F (2°C–8°C); administer with cool liquid no warmer than 98.6°F (37°C).

[8] Special considerations apply in deciding whether to administer yellow fever vaccine to people aged <9 months or ≥60 years. Please review Chapter 3, Yellow Fever before administration.

[9] In 2014, the World Health Assembly (of the World Health Organization) adopted the recommendation to remove the 10-year booster dose requirement from the International Health Regulations as of July 2016. As of that time, a completed International Certificate of Vaccination or Prophylaxis is considered valid for the lifetime of the vaccinee. However, it is uncertain when and if all countries with yellow fever vaccination entry requirements will adopt this change. In February 2015, the Advisory Committee on Immunization Practices (ACIP) approved a new recommendation that a single dose of yellow fever vaccine provides long-lasting protection and is adequate for most travelers. The ACIP also identified specific groups of travelers who should receive additional doses and others for whom additional doses may be considered. For full details see Chapter 3, Yellow Fever.

Index

H

HAART (highly active antiretroviral therapy), 569, 570
HACE. *See* high-altitude cerebral edema (HACE)
Haemophilus influenzae, 67, 263
Haemophilus influenzae type b (Hib)
  immunization of children, 542, 555
  immunization of immunocompromised adults, 559*t*, 563
  meningitis and, 263, 264*t*
  vaccine, 19*t*, 32, 38*t*, 612
Haiti
  cholera outbreak in, 20*t*, 154, 450, 457
  destination map, 456*m*
  destination overview, 455–6
  earthquake of 2010, 457, 458
  health issues in, 456–8
  malaria information for, 234*m*, 396, 500*t*
  safety concerns, 458
  schistosomiasis in, 310*m*
  yellow fever information for, 396
  Zika in, 457
Hajj pilgrimage
  destination map, 431*m*
  destination overview, 430, 432
  disease spread during, 27, 262, 627–8
  health issues in, 432–5
  meningococcal vaccine, 19*t*, 27, 262, 265, 543, 613
halogens, water disinfection with, 73*t*, 75–6
hand, foot, and mouth disease, 180–1
hantaviruses, 104, 349–51
HAPE. *See* high-altitude pulmonary edema (HAPE)
HAV. *See* hepatitis A and hepatitis A virus (HAV)
HBV. *See* hepatitis B and hepatitis B virus (HBV)
HCV. *See* hepatitis C and hepatitis C virus (HCV)
HDCV (human diploid cell rabies vaccine). *See* rabies vaccine
health care abroad, 133–5
health care workers traveling outside the United States, 28, 588–93
health certificates, animals, 529
health insurance. *See* insurance
health kits, travel, 126–30, 577–9, 599–600
health screening
  asymptomatic returned travelers, 512
  immigrants and international adoptees, 633–4
  newly arrived refugees, 632–3
heat, water disinfection with, 72–4, 73*t*, 77*t*
heat disorders, 90–2, 454, 471. *See also* hot climate problems
Helicobacter pylori, 181–2
helminths, soil-transmitted, 182–3, 586*t*
hepatitis A and hepatitis A virus (HAV), 183–7
  adoptions, screening for, 550, 552

immigrants visiting friends and relatives, 585
pregnant travelers, 186, 579
hepatitis A vaccine, 12, 20*t*, 28, 31, 32, 35*t*, 38*t*, 185*t*, 184–6, 317, 612, 650*t*
  immunization of children, 542, 550, 552, 555
  immunization of immunocompromised adults, 559*t*
  long-term travelers/expatriates, 602
  vaccinations for air crews, 595
hepatitis B and hepatitis B virus (HBV), 187, 190–3
  adoptions, screening for, 552–3
  health care workers, 591–3
  immigrants visiting friends and relatives, 585
  interpretation of serologic test results for, infection, 190*t*
  last-minute travelers, 612
  prevalence of chronic, infection, 188–9*m*
hepatitis B vaccine, 19*t*, 21*t*, 32, 35*t*, 38*t*, 191, 192*t*, 316, 317, 650*t*
  immunization of children, 542, 550, 552–3, 555
  immunization of immunocompromised adults, 559*t*
  vaccinations for air crews, 595
hepatitis C and hepatitis C virus (HCV), 193, 196–7
  adoptions, screening for, 553
  health care workers, 591–3
  prevalence of chronic, infection, 194–5*m*
hepatitis E and hepatitis E virus (HEV), 198–9
  pregnant travelers, 579, 604
herpes B. *See* B virus
herpes zoster, recommended and minimum ages and intervals between doses, 38*t*
high-altitude cerebral edema (HACE), 57–8, 58*t*, 59–60, 60*t*, 61
high-altitude pulmonary edema (HAPE), 57, 58, 58*t*, 60, 60*t*, 61
highly active antiretroviral therapy (HAART), 569, 570
histoplasmosis, 199, 202
HIV. *See* human immunodeficiency virus (HIV) infection
Hiva Oa. *See* French Polynesia
Holy See. *See* Italy
homeopathy, 63, 118, 119
homicide, 94, 95*f*, 598
Honduras
  dengue distribution in, 163*m*
  malaria information for, 234*m*, 396
  yellow fever information for, 396
Hong Kong SAR (China), 207, 260, 385, 396, 474
hookworms, 159, 182–3, 462, 498, 509, 513, 538
hot climate problems, 89–92. *See also* cold climate problems
HPV. *See* human papillomavirus (HPV)

human diploid cell rabies vaccine (HDCV). *See* rabies vaccine
human immunodeficiency virus (HIV) infection, 7, 31, 202–5
  adoptions, screening for, 553
  asymptomatic infection in immunocompromised travelers, 562
  immunocompromised travelers and, 47, 558, 559*t*, 560*t*
  long-term travelers, 592
  occupational exposure to, 23, 588, 591–3
  postexposure prophylaxis, 205
  screening newly arrived refugees, 632–3
  testing requirements for US travelers entering foreign countries, 205
  yellow fever vaccine, 356
humanitarian aid workers, 597–601
human papillomavirus (HPV), 314
  catch-up immunization schedule, 555
  immunization of children, 541, 555
  vaccine, 19*t*, 32, 38*t*, 315
human rabies immune globulin (HRIG), 35*t*, 291, 294, 438, 447, 476, 480, 485, 487, 539, 545, 580
human trafficking, 318–19*b*
Hungary
  malaria and yellow fever information for, 396
  tickborne encephalitis in, 327
hydroxychloroquine, malaria chemoprophylaxis, 241*t*, 243, 244*t*, 248, 248*t*, 286. *See also* chloroquine
hyponatremia, 90–1
hypothermia, 92–3

I

ibuprofen, 61, 87, 128, 168, 172
Iceland, 397
immigrant and refugee health considerations, 629–35
  arrival in United States, health assessments and screening, 632–5
  before arrival in United States, examination and follow-up, 630–2
  returning home to visit friends and relatives, 584–8
immune globulin (IG), administration intervals, 35*t*
immunobiologics, spacing of, 34, 36
immunocompromised travelers, 37, 557–70
  asymptomatic HIV infection, 562
  enteric infections in, 569–70
  household contacts of, 565, 567
  immunization of, 559–60*t*
  immunosuppressive biologic agents, 566–7*t*
  malaria chemoprophylaxis, 568–9
  measles vaccine, 258–9
  medical conditions with limited immune deficits, 562–3
  medical conditions without immunologic compromise, 558, 562

Photography Credits

BANNER IMAGES FOR SELECT DESTINATIONS

East Africa (Safaris): Ashley K. Barnes/Personal Collection

Saudi Arabia (Hajj/Umrah Pilgrimage): Salim Parker/Personal Collection

South Africa: Gary W. Brunette/Personal Collection

Tanzania (Kilimanjaro): Shutterstock

Brazil: David Adam Roth/Personal Collection

Cuba: Jonatan Brandt/Personal Collection

Dominican Republic: Ashley K. Barnes/Personal Collection

Haiti: Gary W. Brunette/Personal Collection

Mexico: Shutterstock

Peru: Cusco, Machu Picchu, & Other Regions: Mark J. Sotir/Personal Collection

Burma (Myanmar): Logan Scholfield/Personal Collection

China: Zlatko Unger/Personal Collection

India: Apophia Funa/Personal Collection

Nepal: Gregg Taliaferro/Personal Collection

Thailand: Logan Scholfield/Personal Collection

Vietnam: Carolina Uribe/Personal Collection